Surgical Hip Dislocation

Michael Leunig • Hannes A. Rüdiger
Ira Zaltz • Reinhold Ganz
Editors

Surgical Hip Dislocation

A Comprehensive Approach to Modern Hip Surgery

Springer

Editors
Michael Leunig
Hip Service, Department of Orthopedics
Schulthess Clinic
Zürich, Switzerland

Hannes A. Rüdiger
Hip Service, Department of Orthopedics
Schulthess Clinic
Zürich, Switzerland

Ira Zaltz
Department of Orthopaedic Surgery
C.S. Mott Children's Hospital
University of Michigan
Ann Arbor, MI, USA

Reinhold Ganz
Emeritus, Faculty of Medicine
University of Berne
Berne, Switzerland

ISBN 978-3-031-70621-9 ISBN 978-3-031-70622-6 (eBook)
https://doi.org/10.1007/978-3-031-70622-6

This Springer imprint is published by the registered company Springer Nature Switzerland AG
The registered company address is: Gewerbestrasse 11, 6330 Cham, Switzerland

Foreword

In the dynamic field of orthopedic surgery, the pursuit of excellence is a constant journey. It is our distinct honor to present "The Surgical Hip Dislocation – A Comprehensive Approach to Modern Hip Surgery", a seminal work authored by Michael Leunig, Hannes A. Rüdiger, Ira Zaltz and Reinhold Ganz. This book is a testament to the ingenuity and pioneering spirit of Professor Ganz, who, by defining the anatomy of the primary blood supply from the medial femoral Circumflex artery, revolutionized the approach to surgical hip dislocation.

Divided into seven comprehensive sections, this volume guides the reader through Presurgical Interventions, Basic Surgical Techniques, Intraarticular Reconstruction/Repair, Specific Applications of Surgical Hip Dislocation, Trauma, Tumors, and Total Hip Replacement. Each chapter is meticulously crafted to provide the reader with a foundation in the anatomic, pathomechanical, and technical nuances that underpin the successful application of this transformative technique.

Surgical Hip Dislocation has dramatically expanded the horizons of hip joint reconstruction, offering orthopedic surgeons opportunities that were previously thought unattainable. It has not only enhanced the treatment modalities for the hip joint itself but also served as a catalyst for innovation, enhancing the efficacy of other surgical techniques, improving success rates, and reducing the incidence of failure.

This book is unique in its approach to combining rigorous scientific exploration with practical application. It includes detailed background information, clear surgical indications, and precise technical guidance, complemented by exceptional technical drawings and illustrative case examples. Such a resource is invaluable to practitioners across all levels of expertise, from the novice to the seasoned expert.

The editors have curated contributions from a cadre of world-renowned authors and leading surgeons, ensuring that the contents of this book are of extraordinary quality and practical value. "The Surgical Hip Dislocation" does more than just inform; it equips its readership to make informed decisions about joint preservation and to approach hip arthroplasty with a comprehensive understanding of the alternatives available.

In a field where joint replacement, despite its advancements, faces the limitation of prosthesis longevity, preserving a natural, well-functioning hip joint is of paramount importance. This book is an essential read for anyone involved in hip arthroplasty, providing the necessary insights to evaluate joint preservation possibilities thoroughly.

On a personal note, the editors of this book as well as many of the authors, have not only become close personal friends, but have been mentors, colleagues and thought partners, who have been transformational in our own careers and lives. We extend our heartfelt congratulations to the editors and authors for their exceptional work and dedication. Their contributions command the utmost respect and are sure to leave a lasting impact on the field of hip surgery. This book is not merely a resource but a cornerstone for any surgeon dedicated to the art and science of hip preservation and replacement.

New York, NY, USA/Berlin, Germany

Bryan T. Kelly
Carsten Perka

Preface

The correction of deformities of the human skeleton was first described by Hippocrates nearly 2500 years ago [1]. In 1741, Nicolas Andry [2] pointed out the importance of treating skeletal deformities to prevent secondary damage. However, he was primarily addressing parents and teachers of affected children rather than the medical profession [3]. Treatment at the time was nonsurgical and Andry's comparison to a crooked tree attempting to correct spinal deformities still serves as a symbol for many orthopedic societies around the world. More than a century later, a better understanding of antisepsis during surgery [4], improvements in general anesthesia, and the invention of radiography made deformity analysis and surgical correction possible.

The first joint-preserving skeletal procedures were directional corrections that treated major limb deformities resulting from improperly healed fractures or ankyloses with the goal of restoring the anatomic axis [5]. Initially, the corrected position was rarely stabilized/fixed and, if near a stiff joint, often resulted in the formation of pseudarthrosis [5, 6]. One of the first successful implants for stabilization/fixation at the hip joint was Smith-Petersen's nail described in 1925 [7]. Decades later, other fixation devices and techniques became available for proximal femoral osteotomy [8] that allowed more accurate correction and fixation of the osteotomy. In 1939, McMurray [9] was the first to describe the use of an osteotomy for the treatment of hip osteoarthritis. This procedure, with various inter- and subtrochanteric modifications, was routinely used until the 1970s [10], and publications reported good results in patients with advanced hip osteoarthritis [11]. With the introduction of total hip arthroplasty in the late 1960s, osteotomies became less commonly utilized. Even in young adults, there was an early belief in the durability of the prosthesis. Consequently, young orthopedic surgeons during the 1970s and 1980s rarely were exposed to hip osteotomies during their training.

Due to limitations of prosthetic replacement not initially foreseen in the early 1980s there has been a renaissance of hip osteotomies proving the continued importance of joint-preserving hip surgery. Furthermore, the relevance of osteotomies became more apparent because the general increase in sports activity, especially in young athletes, led to complaints about the hip related with morphologic variations and consequent anatomic limitations. At about the same time, there was a proliferation of publications describing worse outcomes of hip replacements in patients under 50 years of age [12]. In contrast to the classic indications for arthroplasty in patients with radiologically proven osteoarthritis, the main focus of hip joint preservation surgery shifted to the symptomatic young adult hip prior to radiologically apparent joint degeneration. With increased clinical experience and understanding of hip deformities, it quickly became clear that understanding the blood supply to the femoral was essential. Subsequent detailed anatomic and vascular studies of the blood supply to the femoral head enabled the development of new surgical approaches and techniques that have furthered both our clinical understanding of hip mechanics and our therapeutic capabilities.

Although the blood supply to the proximal femur, particularly the extent of medial femoral circumflex artery for perfusion of the femoral head, had been described [13, 14, 15, 16, 17], the topographic relationships and anastomostic branches were underappreciated and not well described. Consequently, there was long held a general objection to dislocation of the femoral head because of the perceived high risk of avascular necrosis [18]. Our studies initially led to the development of surgical hip dislocation (SHD), a procedure with low morbidity and few complications, that is now considered the basic approach for a number of intracapsular procedures because it protects the vascular supply and prevents head necrosis. In addition, SHD led to the conceptualization of femoroacetabular impingement and a greater understanding of hip pathomechanics. According to the recent review from Khalifa et al. [19] on 160 publications in 66 journals from 28 countries there is an increasing trend over the past two decades from countries worldwide on the use of SHD in traumatic and non-traumatic hip conditions. The number of publications increased by 10-fold comparing the period from 2001 to 2005 with 2018 to 2022. Switzerland and the United States of America contributed to more than 50% of the publications reflected by the contributing authors to this book.

Based on work involving many of the authors of this book between 1980 and 2022, we present a summary of developments in hip preservation surgery based on the technique of SHD. The book is intended to provide orthopedic surgeons interested in both joint-preserving but also hip replacement surgery with a detailed description of the breadth of complex intracapsular and juxtaarticular surgical techniques so that they can be performed correctly with a low risk of complications. The book; however, should not be viewed as a substitute for a detailed anatomical and surgical skill training provided by experts in these techniques.

Surgical indication is a sensitive issue that warrants experience, and, in case of doubt, expert consultation. Success can be immediate but should best be stated with long-term results. Return to sporting activities may be a financial success, but is not always a good decision in view of hip joint longevity.

Zürich, Switzerland — Michael Leunig
Zürich, Switzerland — Hannes A. Rüdiger
Ann Arbor, MI, USA — Ira Zaltz
Berne, Switzerland — Reinhold Ganz

Suggested Readings

1. Valentin B. Geschichte de Orthopadie. Stuttgart: Thieme, 1961.
2. Andry N. L'orthopedie ou l'arte de prevenir et de corriger dans les enfants, les difformities du corps. Paris: La Veuve Alix/Lambert & Durand, 1741 (in French).
3. Michel L. A propos du prochain bicentenaire de l'orthopédie. Rev Chir Orthop Reparatrice Mot 1938;25:282–286 (in French).
4. Lister J. On the antiseptic principle in the practice of surgery. Br Med J 1867;2:246– 248.
5. Milch H. Osteotomy of the upper end of the femur. Baltimore: Lippincott Williams & Wilkins, 1965.
6. Hoffa A. Die Nachbehandlung der nach abgelaufener Coxitis zurückgebliebenen Deformitäten. Leipzig: Breitkopf und Härtel, 1896 (in German).
7. Smith Petersen MN, Cave EF, van Gorder GW. Intracapsular fracture of the femoral neck of the femur: treatment by internal fixation. Arch Surg 1931;23:715–759.
8. Muller ME. Manual of internal fixation. Berlin, Heidelberg and New York: Springer; 1977.
9. McMurray TP. Osteoarthritis of the hip joint. J Bone Joint Surg 1939;21:1–11.
10. Morscher E. The intertrochanteric osteotomy for osteoarthritis if the hip: analysis of 2251 cases. Bern-Stuttgart-Wien: Huber; 1971.
11. D'Souza SR, Sadiq S, New AM, Northmore-Ball MD. Proximal femoral osteotomy as the primary operation for young adults who have osteoarthrosis of the hip. J Bone Joint Surg [Am] 1998;80-A:1428–1438.

12. Kärrholm J, Garellick G, Rogmark C, Herberts P. Swedish Hip Arthroplasty Register: Annual Report 2007. http://www.shpr.se (date last accessed 2 October 2013).
13. Chung SM. The arterial supply of the developing proximal end of the human femur. J Bone Joint Surg [Am] 1976;58-A:961–970.
14. Crock HV. The blood supply of the lower limb bones in man (descriptive and applied). Edinburgh: E&S Livingstone; 1967.
15. Judet J, Judet R, Lagrange J, Dunoyer J. A study of the arterial vascularization of the femoral neck in the adult. J Bone Joint Surg [Am] 1955;37-A:663–680.
16. Sevitt S, Thompson RG. The distribution and anastomoses of arteries supplying the head and neck of the femur. J Bone Joint Surg [Br] 1965;47-B:560–573.
17. Trueta J, Harrison MH. The normal vascular anatomy of the femoral head in adult man. J Bone Joint Surg [Br] 1953;35-B:442–461.
18. Gautier E, Ganz K, Krugel N, Gill T, Ganz R. Anatomy of the medial femoral circumflex artery and its surgical implications. J Bone Joint Surg [Br] 2000;82-B:679–683.
19. Khalifa, A.A., T.G. Hassan, and M.A. Haridy, The evolution of surgical hip dislocation utilization and indications over the past two decades: a scoping review. Int Orthop, 2023;47:3053–3062. doi: 10.1007/s00264-023-05814-w

Acknowledgement

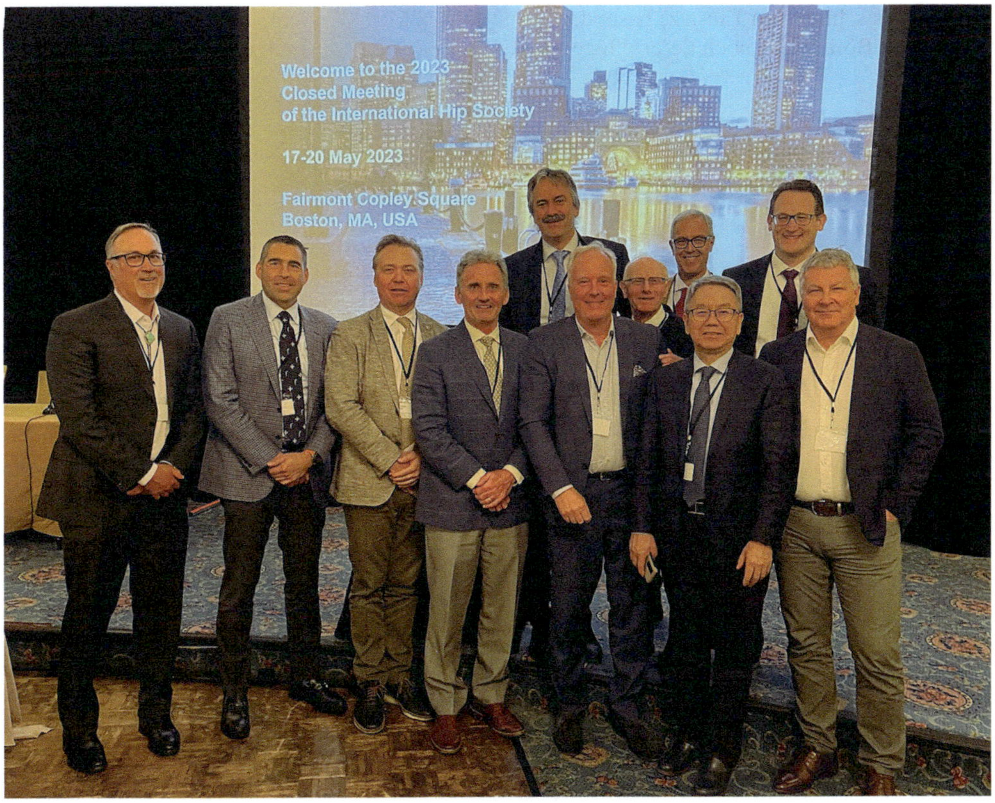

Photograph taken at the International Hip Society Meeting held 2023 in Boston with several chapter authors being members of this society. From left to right Chris L. Peters, Rafael J. Sierra, Paul Beaule, John C. Clohisy, Carsten Perka, Michael Leunig, Michael B. Millis, Alessandro Masse, Xiadong Chen, Moritz Tannast and Martin Beck.

Contents

Part 4 Specific Applications of SHD

Part 5 Trauma

Part 6 Tumors

Part 7 Total Hip Replacement

Part 1

Presurgical Interventions

Clinical Assessment of Hip Dysfunction

1

Hubert P. Nötzli and Ernest L. Sink

1.1 Introduction

The medical history, which includes pain location, quality, and triggers, is of eminent importance. A detailed clinical examination including provocative tests will help confirm or refute the differential diagnosis. The addition of the appropriate imaging is done based on the clinical findings. Various diagnoses treatable with joint preservation surgery are based not only on imaging but also on a clinical exam. As there are few radiological or clinical findings that are uniquely pathognomonic of impingement, all relevant clinical data must be interpreted collectively in order to differentiate clinical disorders. For example, an increased alpha angle is only an indication of possible impingement, but not yet proof, as it only describes the head/femoral neck and does not include femoral torsion, acetabular version, or extent of femoral head coverage.

1.2 Medical History

When a patient presents for the first time for the evaluation of "hip complaints," it is important to understand where the patient experiences pain and any potential patterns of pain radiation. Many patients do not know where the hip joint is located and think the trochanter, the pelvis, or the lower back is the hip. If the patient grasps laterally around the hip region and localizes the pain there in-depth, described as a C-sign, then an intra-articular hip problem is more likely than if their pain is located in the lower back, buttock, or over the trochanter.

The patient's historical recollection plays a crucial role in the diagnosis and should be sought in a structured and detailed manner. The first point of interest is when the pain first occurred and whether a traumatic event was associated with it. The mechanism of trauma must be asked in detail in order to be able to determine which structures might have been affected.

In the case of hip impingement without a traumatic event, the pain often begins insidiously and disappears quickly after a pain-provoking load. Over time, the pain episodes can become more frequent, intense, and prolonged. In some cases, stabbing groin pain occurs during uncontrolled movements of the hip. However, patients also report feelings of locking and sticking or the feeling that the leg is no longer supporting them for a moment (dead leg, giving way episodes). To be differentiated from this is pain in the trochanteric region, which typically occurs at rest and when lying on the side and radiates laterally to the knee.

On the occasion of the initial consultation, the following clinical complaints are important to query:

- Pain characteristic and location: e.g., groin pain of a sharp, stabbing, and shooting character
- Groin pain while sitting
- Groin pain during or after sports activities
- Painful adductor muscles with or without trauma
- Locking when arising from a sitting position
- Limited hip mobility or hypermobility of the hip and/or other joints
- Pain over the trochanter

Complaints are often triggered by

- Activities that involve rotational movements
- Prolonged hip flexion (prolonged sitting)
- Getting up from a seated position (pinching, locking)
- Symptoms from getting in and out of a car
- Sexual intercourse

H. P. Nötzli
Hip Service, Orthopedics Sonnenhof, Berne, Switzerland
e-mail: hubertnoetzli@sonnenhof.ch

E. L. Sink (✉)
HSS Hip Preservation and Pediatric Service, Hospital for Special Surgery, New York, NY, USA
e-mail: sinke@hss.edu

M. Leunig et al. (eds.), *Surgical Hip Dislocation*, https://doi.org/10.1007/978-3-031-70622-6_1

- Foot care including putting on shoes, socks, stockings, and so on (deep bending)
- Lying on the side
- Walking especially up or down inclines
- Sporting activities

There are many other historical factors that are important to assess. These include limitations in day-to-day activity and/or sports activities, dependence on pain medication, and/or the need for a walking aid. What type, frequency, and duration of physiotherapy has been attempted, and whether the therapy has influenced the complaints in any way? Have diagnostic or therapeutic joint injections been performed and have they had any effect on the patient's symptoms? What was done in the process and how did it affect the complaints? What operative and nonoperative treatments have been performed prior to evaluation and how have these interventions changed the patient's complaints? Are the complaints different now than before the surgery? If patients have had prior surgery, all operative notes and arthroscopic photographs or videos should be reviewed. In addition, evaluation of hip pain and dysfunction on mental health may also be important to consider, especially when considering certain surgical treatments.

The personal medical and developmental history is an important part of the initial evaluation. A history of infant DDH treatment such as double diapers, brace, or harness use can be important. In younger patients, it is of interest to know if walking commenced at an age-appropriate time or if special treatments were needed during infancy or childhood. In addition, a history of any childhood disorder, not necessarily just limited to the hip is of value. Not only should patients be questioned about disorders such as Legg-Calve-Perthes, slipped upper femoral epiphysis, sepsis, and osteomyelitis, but any history of neurologic, systemic inflammatory, or family history of premature arthrosis or genetic disorders of growth or stature can become important in establishing an accurate diagnosis and influential in any treatment plan.

1.3 Physical Exam

The initial physical exam should be comprehensive and detailed beginning with obtaining the height and weight, observing the overall body habitus, examining for signs of ligamentous laxity, and performing a general neurological evaluation. For adolescents of growing age, you want to know what stage of growth the patient is currently in, whether the patient is currently growing rapidly or growth is largely complete. Subsequently, the hip-specific portion of the examination commences with an evaluation of gait and progresses measuring supine and prone hip range motion, hip-specific muscular examination, and performance of hip-specific provocative tests. It may be recommended in many countries and cultures to have a second clinician or provider in the exam room to record and witness the exam when examining the hip region.

1.3.1 Inspection

Much can be gleaned by carefully inspecting the hip. Initially, the posture, pelvic position, and axial relationships between the spine and lower extremities should be evaluated. Next, the condition of the skin includes any previous surgical incisions, symmetry of soft tissues, especially muscle mass, and overall health and nutritional status. Abnormalities of connective tissue suggested by inspection include cutaneous translucency, hyperextension of the knees, ocular abnormalities, pectus deformity, scoliosis, and pes planus. Finally, the physician should carefully evaluate the patient in the standing position for evidence of a leg length inequality, scoliosis, or spinal imbalance that can affect hip function.

Gait is assessed from the side, front, and back. Limping (antalgic, leg length discrepancy, and abductor weakness (Duchenne/Trendelenburg)) is documented. Different phases of the gait are evaluated (stance and swing phases (Fig. 1.1). Observing the foot progression angle and knee rotation may give information on the version of the femur. An inward foot progression angle can occur because of femoral or rarely tibial torsion. An inward progression can also occur to stabilize a hip with anterior overload, especially toward the end of the stance phase.

A distinction is made between Trendelenburg limp, which is caused by a weakness of the abductors with a drop of the pelvis to the contralateral side, and Duchenne limp, in which the upper body is shifted over the affected hip to reduce the load on the hip by shortening the load arm. The shifting of the upper body takes time and the stance is prolonged, unlike the relief of a painful foot, where the relief happens with a shortened stance phase. A mixed picture of Trendelenburg and Duchenne limp is observed but only in patients with advanced hip disease. A subtle limp is often easier to hear than to see.

Single leg stance is used to assess for abductor weakness. The patient flexes the hip and knee to 45° of the not-affected leg for at least 6 seconds. The test is positive if the pelvis is lowered by more than 2 cm to the contralateral side (Fig. 1.2). A positive Trendelenburg sign is characterized by the lowering of the pelvis to the non-affected side with the upper body in a neutral position (Fig. 1.3). Note, however, that a negative Trendelenburg sign does not rule out abductor weakness, especially in young patients. A patient with a positive Duchenne sign is compensating for an abductor deficiency by moving the upper body over the affected hip to move the plumb line closer to the center of rotation of the affected hip

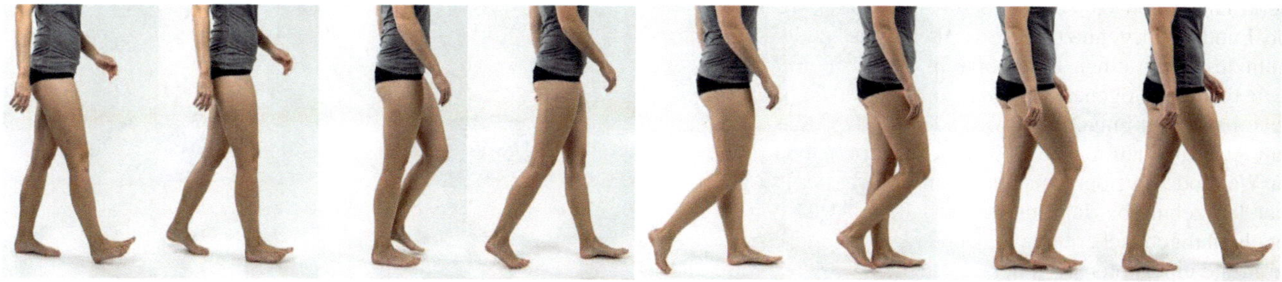

Fig. 1.1 Normal gait phases

Fig. 1.2 Normal abductor function. The pelvis remains horizontal during a single-leg stance

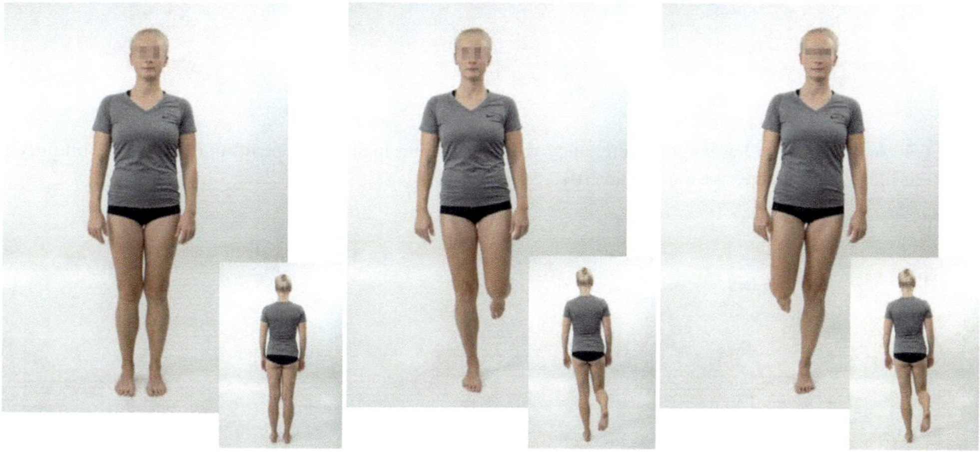

Fig. 1.3 Patients with abductor deficiencies may have a positive Trendelenburg sign with the pelvis tilting toward the contralateral side with the upper body in a neutral position. Some patients exert a Duchenne compensation by moving the plumb line over the affected hip to unload the affected abductor apparatus

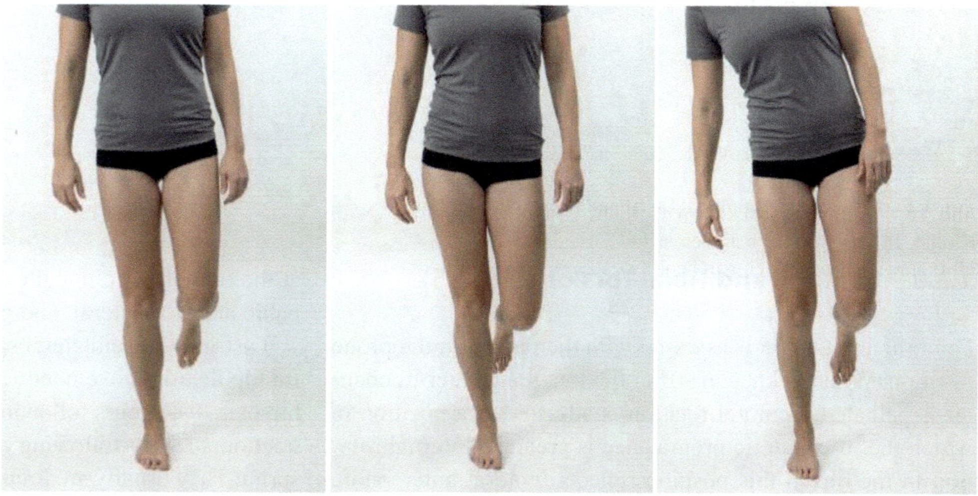

joint, thereby shortening the load arm. These tests are not suitable to detect subtle abductor weaknesses.

1.3.2 Assessment of Leg Length

Leg length may be assessed with the patient standing. The iliac crests are palpated (Fig. 1.4). With the patient in the supine position, the apparent limb lengths should also be evaluated as this may be a subtle sign of a hip abduction or flexion contracture. If a contracture is suspected, then specific tests including the Thomas test and Ober test are needed to elicit the type of contracture. Limited hip mobility for abduction, adduction, or extension may suggest a significant (functional) leg length discrepancy.

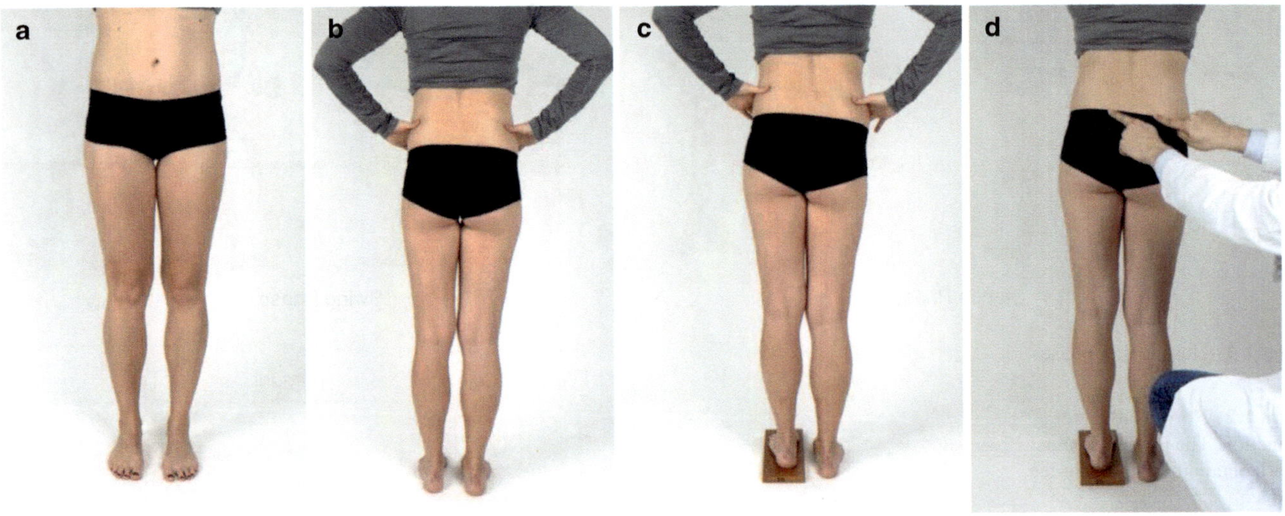

Fig. 1.4 Assessment of leg length discrepancy with the patient in standing position (**a**). Pelvic obliquity is assessed by palpating the iliac crests (**b**, **c**) or the posterior superior iliac spines (**d**)

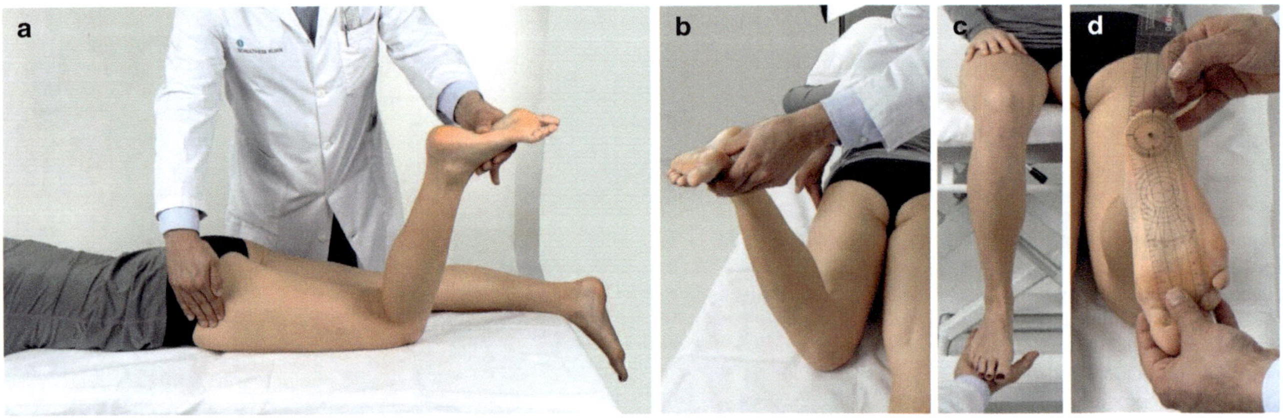

Fig. 1.5 Assessment of femoral (**a**, **b**) and tibial (**c**, **d**) torsion

1.3.3 Femoral and Tibial Torsion (Fig. 1.5)

Femoral antetorsion is assessed with the patient in the prone position. With the knee in 90° of flexion, the greater trochanter is palpated. Femoral rotation is adjusted to a position in which the trochanteric prominence is greatest. Internal rotation in the hip in this position reflects femoral antetorsion. Tibial torsion is best assessed by measuring the foot progression angle with the patient sitting and the knee in flexion (hanging leg).

1.3.4 Palpation (Figs. 1.6 and 1.7)

Palpation is part of every clinical exam of the hip and is performed in a bimanual technique. Bony and musculotendinous landmarks are first palpated anteriorly and then medial, lateral, and posterior. It is advised to palpate the tender region at the end of the clinical exam. Multiple landmarks are palpable anterior, lateral, and posterior.

Fast-growing athletes, especially those who perform forceful hip flexion movements, are referred to because of anterior hip pain that occurs following powerful eccentric muscle contraction such as following a soccer kick or after a powerful sprint. They usually are found to have tight muscles on clinical examination. When pressure is applied to the attachment area of the rectus femoris and/or adductors, pain is triggered, aggravated by active lifting/adducting of the leg against resistance. Passive stretching in the prone position can also provoke pain when pressure is applied to the attachment.

1.3.5 Range of Motion

Range-of-motion values reported in most textbooks including those recently published often significantly exceed the

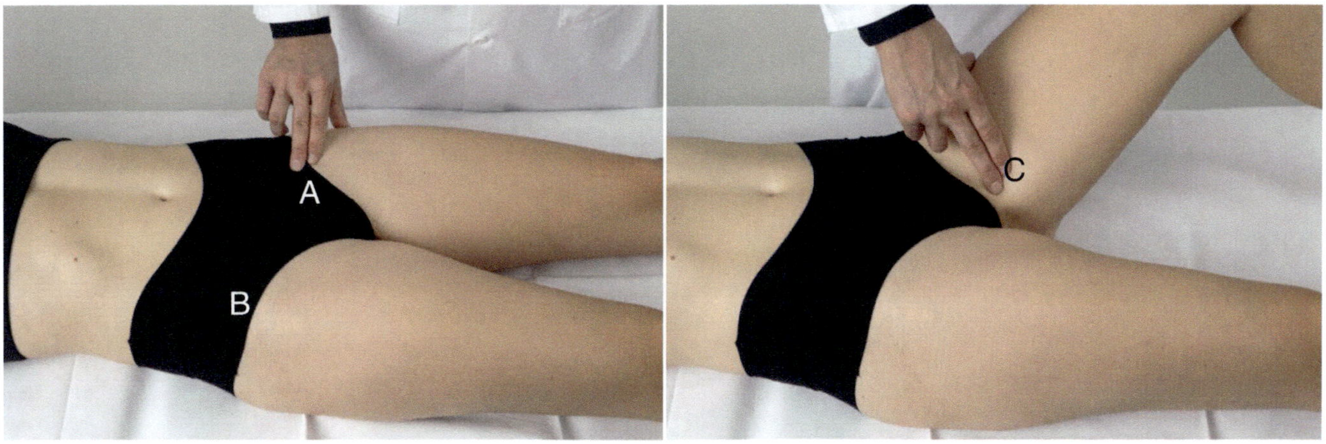

Fig. 1.6 (**a**) Pubic tubercle. (**b**) Anterior inferior iliac spine (rectus tendon). (**c**) Adductor tendons

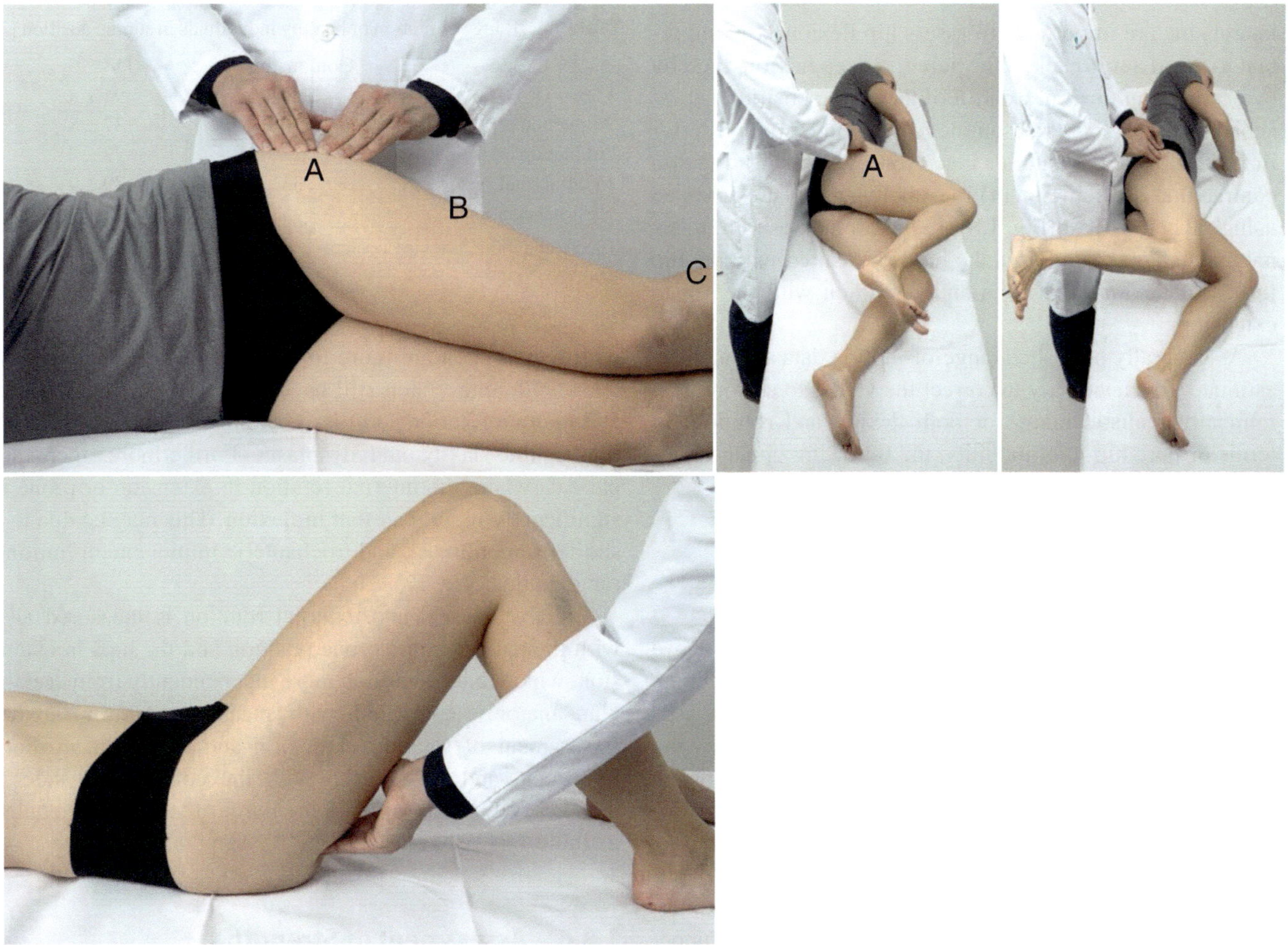

Fig. 1.7 (**a**) Greater trochanter. (**b**) Iliotibial band. (**c**) Gerdy's tubercle. With the patient in a lateral position, coxa saltans may be palpable over the greater trochanter during cycling motions of the upper leg. Insertion of the hamstrings at the tuber ischiadicum

actual anatomic hip movement because the clinically measured hip range of motion was not differentiated from the coupled movement of the lumbar spine.

Range-of-motion tests are performed passively, first in a supine then in a prone position. As the range of motion varies considerably among patients, comparisons with the contra-

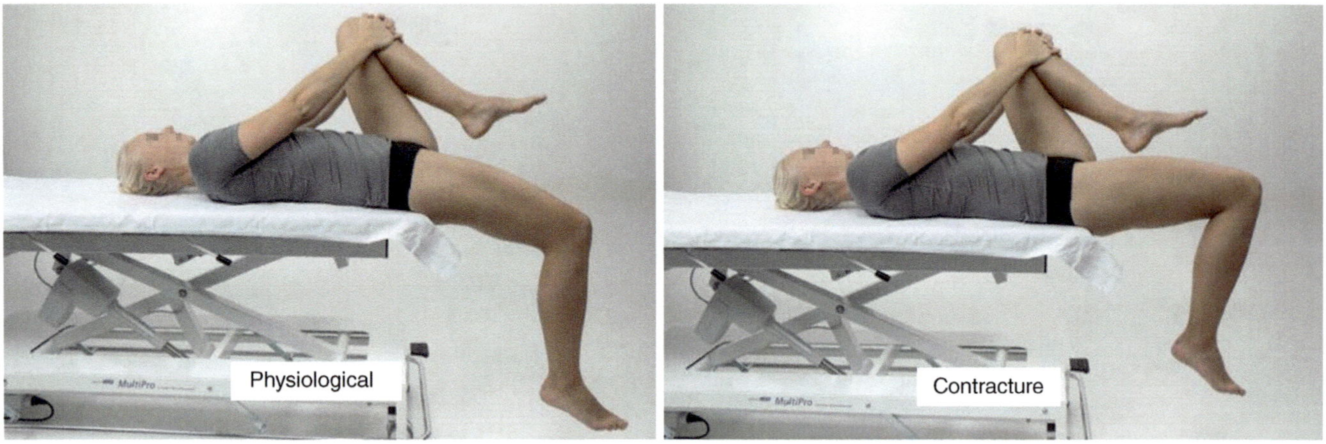

Fig. 1.8 Thomas test to evaluate flexion contractures of the hip. The patient is holding the pelvis in a neutral position by flexing the non-affected hip

lateral side are important. To assess hip flexion, it is important to avoid a roll-back of the pelvis in deep flexion, thereby overestimating flexion. Control of the pelvic position is best achieved by placing the examiner's hand under the posterior iliac crest or on the anterior iliac crest (not shown). Flexion contractures are common in hip pathologies and are assessed using a Thomas Test (Fig. 1.8). In the supine position, internal and external rotation of the hip is measured with the hip in 90° of flexion, abduction and adduction with the hip in extension.

As generally published range-of-motion data are an overestimate, it is necessary to correct the values to a more anatomically realistic range for both flexion and rotation. In terms of pure hip joint mobility, the following upper values can be expected on average in healthy individuals:

Flexion/extension	95°—0°—20°
External rotation/internal rotation	35°—0°—25°
Abduction/adduction	30°—0—15° [1]

If the values on clinical examination are significantly above this, dysplasia must be suspected. If there is less mobility, especially for internal rotation and/or flexion, a hip "at risk" for impingement must be assumed; however, many hips can have anatomic features consistent with both impingement and instability such that the physical examination alone is insufficient for the formulation of a definitive diagnosis.

The primary determination of internal and external rotation in the non-arthritic hip is complex and related to combinations of pelvic and acetabular morphology and upper femoral morphology and torsion. Patients with anteversion may have more hip flexion but specifically will have increased internal motion and decreased external rotation. The lack of external rotation may be a functional issue and also result in impingement in the posterior acetabulum or the posterior trochanter against the pelvis. Conversely, patients

Table 1.1 Range of motion of healthy individuals in supine position [2]

	Goniometer	ETS[a]
Flexion (°)	112 ± 11	94 ± 8
Abduction (°)	39 ± 7	37 ± 8
Adduction (°)	27 ± 6	22 ± 3
Internal rotation (°)	34 ± 10	29 ± 9
External rotation (°)	45 ± 5	35 ± 4

[a]Electromagnetic tracking system

with retroversion are more likely to impinge. Occasionally, those with anteversion still have excessive external rotation and internal rotation and those parameters are possible with ligamentous laxity and dysplasia. Furthermore, there are patients where the internal rotation in extension or prone is significantly more than that in flexion. This may be due to a shorter femoral neck and trochanteric impingement limiting range in flexion.

Finally, internal and external rotation is measured also with the patient in the prone position and the hips in extension, which reflects motion more independently from acetabular anatomy compared with measurements in flexion. Assessment of rotation in flexion and extension are both important, and comparison with the contralateral side is mandatory. Normal values or hip range of motion are detailed in Table 1.1.

1.3.6 Assessment of Strength

Strength of hip flexors (in the supine position) and abductors (in the lateral decubitus position) are part of every physical hip exam. Strength of hip flexion is assessed by asking the patient to lift the strength is tested with tal resistance (Fig. 1.9).

Many patients who are referred for hip complaints actually have a muscular problem, primarily related to weakness, with abductor strength deficit as the primary problem. Abductor weakness may be primary or secondary, and an initial examination may not be able to differentiate a primary problem from a secondary effect.

Abductor strength deficit is frequently accompanied by adductor hypertonicity presenting as medial groin pain accompanied by insertional tendinosis of the dorsal portions of the gluteus medius tendon and myelogelosis in the gluteus medius itself. This may be accompanied by insertional pain at the origin of the gluteus medius and trochanteric bursitis that may be associated with radiating pain along the outer side of the thigh to the tibial lateral tuberosity.

Accordingly, the first step is to palpate the various structures. It is best to start in the supine position with the adductors, which are typically indurated and tender to palpation. In certain cases, only the direct attachments to the bone are painful.

After turning to the lateral decubitus position, the trochanter region should be palpated. Bursitis makes the tissue over the trochanter appear more dense. Bursitis pain can be reproduced by a cycling movement in the lateral position. With the load on the foot while performing the movement, distal radiation can occasionally be provoked.

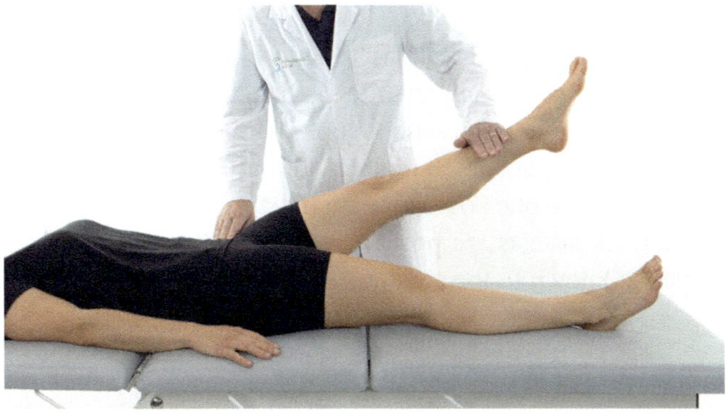

Fig. 1.9 Straight leg raise against resistance to test the strength of hip flexors

Abductor weakness may be associated with painful insertion of the dorsal tendon of the gluteus medius, which is often misinterpreted as "piriformis syndrome." Myelogeleosis in the gluteus medius is easy to palpate, as is tendinosis of the origin of the gluteus medius. As gluteus medius weakness often induces functional compensatory changes in the gluteus maximus and tensor fascia, these muscles may also demonstrate irritation.

However, testing abductor strength with the Trendelenburg sign is very inaccurate, especially in young patients with preserved strength but with muscular imbalance. As such, the Trendelenburg sign is unreliable for strength assessment even with long periods of testing in the single-leg stance.

Abductor strength is best tested with the patient in the lateral position (Fig. 1.10a). The goal is to test the hip abductor strength by isolating the gluteus medius as much as possible. This is best done with the hip in neutral extension but with the leg held horizontally in maximum internal rotation with simultaneous knee flexion of 30–45 degrees. By testing the gluteus medius with the leg positioned properly, the tensor and quadriceps cannot be activated to compensate for a weak gluteus medius. While testing, it is important to palpate the quadriceps and gluteus maximus to ensure that they are soft when testing resistance to vertical pressure on the distal upper thigh. We grade the force with the M-scale and divide it into M3 (hold against gravity), M4– (minimal resistance), M4 (weak resistance), M4+ near normal force but still surmountable or weaker than the opposite side), and M5 (normal force); however, M4 and M5 have poor interrater reliability. If the hip is brought in maximal internal rotation, a patient with an intact anterior gluteus medius is able to actively hold the leg in exactly this position (Fig. 1.10b). If the leg drops into external rotation, it is suggestive of a lesion

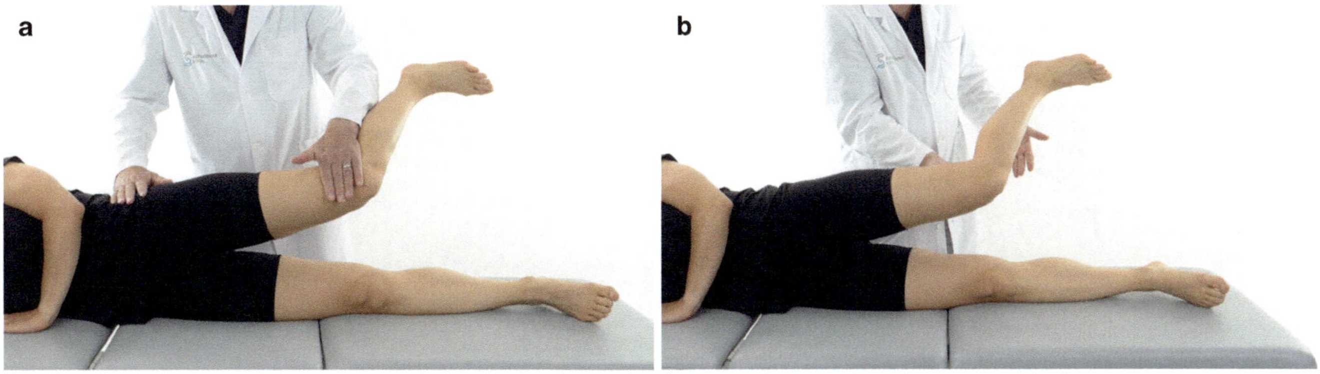

Fig. 1.10 Abductor strength assessment. (**a**) Straight leg raise against resistance with the hip internally rotated and the knee flexed to about 45° tests abductor strength. (**b**) The leg can be held in maximal internal rotation against gravity if the anterior portion of the gluteus medius muscle is intact. If the thigh drops in external rotation, it is suggestive of a deficiency of the anterior abductor apparatus (positive internal rotation lag sign)

of the anterior gluteus medius tendon (internal rotation lag sign).

In abductor weakness, patients have difficulty holding the leg in the position set by the examiner. They shake or deviate forward, thus activating the quadriceps (M4–). On the contrary, with normal force (M5), the patient can hold the leg in position without the examiner being able to push it down.

It is important to compare the abductor force of both sides, especially if one hip is symptomatic and the other is not.

This examination is usually not painful. If pain is stated in the groin, internal rotation is insufficient, so the adductors, which are already overstimulated, are activated. The same applies to the tensor. Therefore, the examiner must adjust the leg position in a way that no pain is triggered when holding the position.

1.3.7 Provocative Tests

Several tests aim to stress anatomical structures and provoke a "typical" pain known to the patient. Such tests include impingement, apprehension, and psoas tests.

1.3.7.1 Impingement Test (Fig. 1.11)

Historically, the impingement test was performed statically by holding the hip at 90° flexion, while adducting and internally rotating the proximal femur (Fig. 1.11a). By forceful sliding of the femoral neck over the anterior acetabular rim, this maneuver induces pain in many patients regardless of the status of the hip joint (Flexion/Adduction/Internal Rotation FADIR).

As we know that the impingement zone for each hip is different and based upon a complex combination of acetabular and femoral morphology, a contemporary impingement test should be performed as a dynamic test in which, starting at approximately 30° less than the 90° position up to maximum flexion, the femoral neck is brought into contact with the anterior acetabular rim by a flexion-adduction motion with the leg's own weight and not with force. Performing this movement in different flexion positions provides information concerning where the acetabular rim might be irritated, as it usually causes pain in higher degrees of flexion, which disappears at a certain point in lower flexion angles [3].

Only if the following three conditions are met, the test can be considered positive:

- The test must trigger pain.
- Pain should be similar to the pain the patient experiences (if he does not know it, the test is likely to have been performed too forcefully or incorrectly).
- Localization of the pain is described by the patient with the C-sign.

Posterior impingement is tested with the patient in the supine position, the affected leg is hanging over the edge of the table, and the contralateral hip is held in flexion with both hands by the patient. External rotation in full extensions is applied to provoke posterior pain (posterior impingement) or impingement tests are positive if they are triggering a pain, which is known to the patient (Fig. 1.11b).

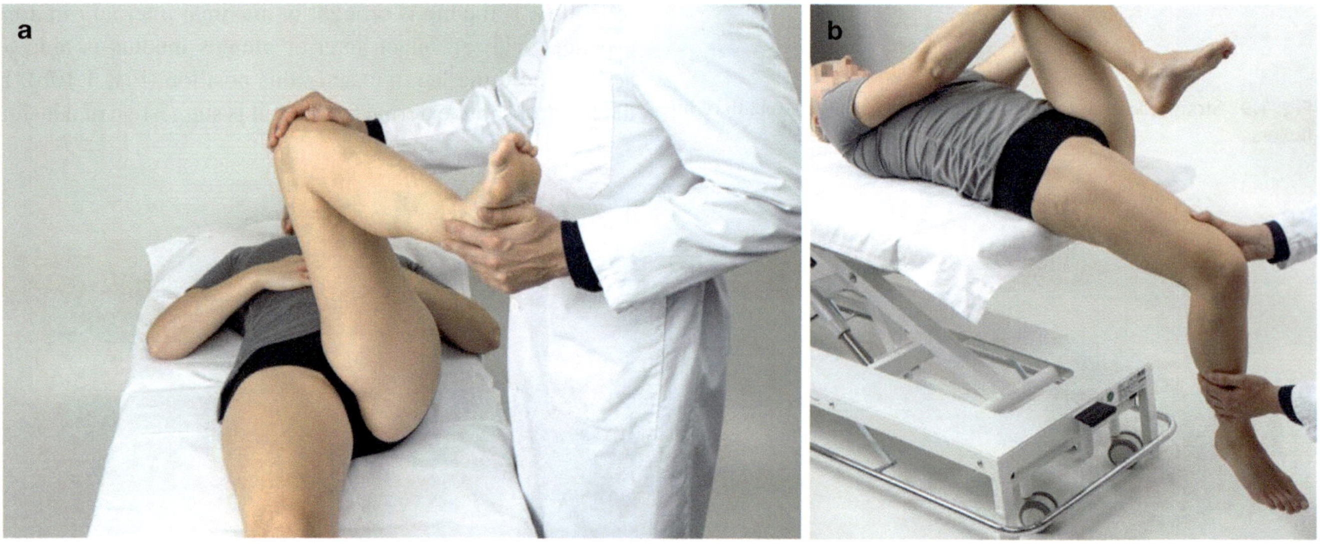

Fig. 1.11 Tests for anterior (**a**) and posterior impingement or apprehension (**b**). Anterior impingement is tested at various degrees of flexion and adduction

1.3.7.2 Anterior Apprehension (Fig. 1.11b)

This test is performed with the patient supine and the hip in extension. With external rotation of the leg, the patient will have discomfort in the anterior hip. Anecdotally, this test is positive 20% of the time with anterior overload and may be likely positive in patients with excessive femoral/acetabular anteversion or following hip arthroscopy with persistent anterior instability. The author commonly performs this test with hip ultrasound where it is assessed whether the femoral head becomes more prominent relative to the acetabulum in this position.

1.3.7.3 PART Test (Fig. 1.12)

The PART test (prone apprehension relocation test) has been shown to be associated with anterior acetabular undercoverage when comparing a positive test with CT scans. It is also beneficial when patients have continued hip pain after hip arthroscopy and there are concerns for anterior instability. In the prone position, the patient's leg is extended in neutral with the knee flexed and held by the examiner. An anterior force is applied by the examiner on the upper femur and a positive test is described when the patient has discomfort with the force, and it gets better when the force is released. The test has been shown to have significant intra-observer reliability [4].

1.3.7.4 Simple Test to Exclude an Inguinal Hernia (Fig. 1.13)

In the supine position, raise both legs at a shallow angle and cross the legs alternately. This leads to a high pressure in the abdomen and provocation of inguinal pain in the presence of a hernia. If there is no pain, an inguinal hernia can be excluded with a high degree of certainty.

1.3.7.5 Psoas Test (Fig. 1.14)

Psoas tendon dysfunction can produce groin and hip pain, especially in young hyperlax patients and in patients with tight musculature. These patients frequently complain of locking when arising from a sitting position or from a cross-legged position. The locking can be described as very painful and combined with the sensation of "giving-way" or that there is inadequate support in the affected leg. The blockage is often released by rotating the leg from side to side or shaking it and can frequently be associated with an audible clunk caused by the subluxated psoas tendon springing back over the iliopectineal eminence or over the femoral head. Intra-articular causes for blockages are rarely present except in advanced arthrosis or cases of loose bodies or displaced bucket handle-type labral displacement.

During the psoas test, the patient lies on his back and lifts the leg from the table, stretches it, and brings it back to its original position in a circular external rotation movement. It makes sense to have the patient perform this movement actively with one hand of the examiner positioned over the psoas tendon or the os pubis. With the second hand, the movement of the leg can and should also be performed passively. If the psoas sign is positive, the examiner feels a bounce with an often audible clunk or a barely audible rub. The clunk is more common in hyperlax patients, and the (painful) tendon rub is more common in muscle shortening. Psoas shortening can be easily detected by passively bending the knee when the patient is lying prone and observing the pelvis lifting off of the exam table.

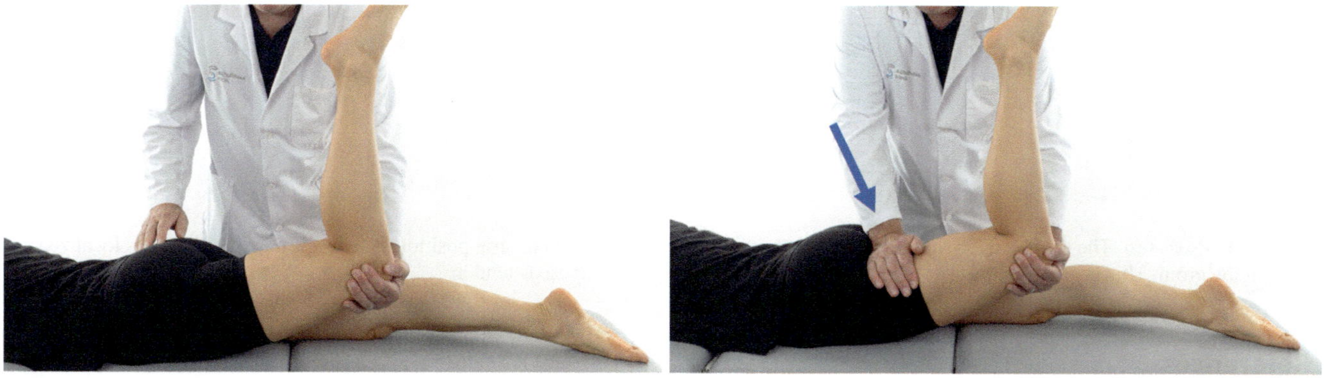

Fig. 1.12 The PART test performed with the patient in the prone position. The examiner holds the knee flexed and applies an anterior force on the upper femur

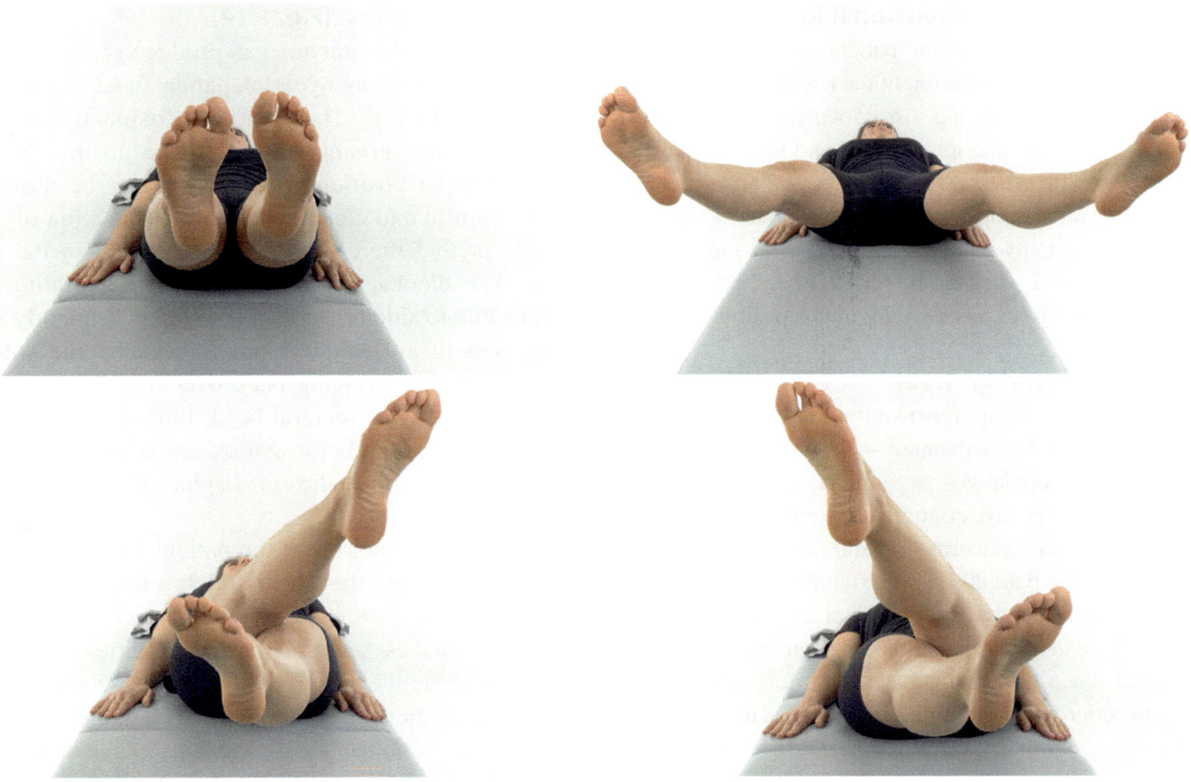

Fig. 1.13 In the supine position, raise both legs at a shallow angle and cross the legs alternately

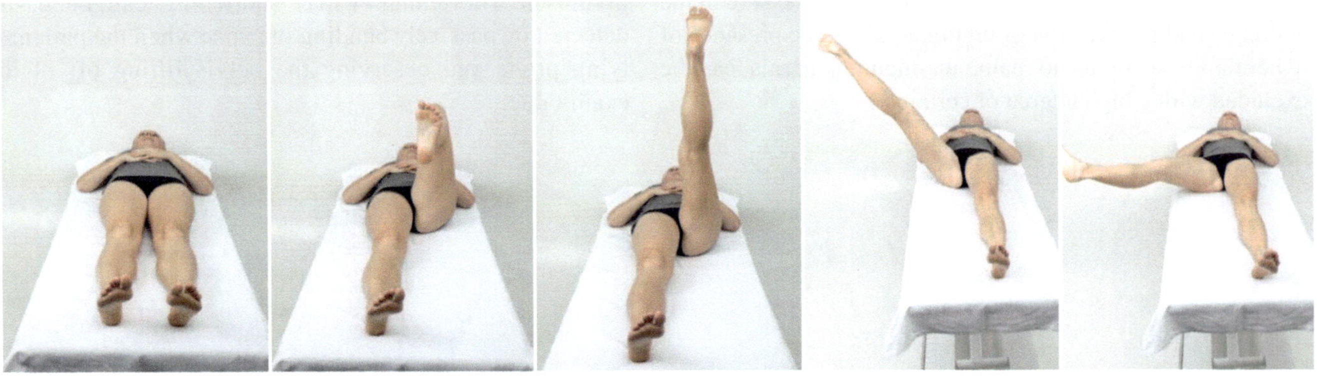

Fig. 1.14 Psoas test. The leg is actively moved in flexion then abduction and back to neutral position. The test is positive if there is localized pain deep in the groin. This is occasionally associated with an internal snapping of the psoas tendon

References

1. Tannast M, Kubiak-Langer M, Langlotz F, Puls M, Murphy SB, Siebenrock KA. Noninvasive three-dimensional assessment of femoroacetabular impingement. J Orthop Res. 2007;25(1):122–31. https://doi.org/10.1002/jor.20309.
2. Nussbaumer S, et al. Validity and test-retest reliability of manual goniometers for measuring passive hip range of motion in femoroacetabular impingement patients. BMC Musculoskelet Disord. 2010;11:194.
3. Lerch TD, Antioco T, Boschung A, et al. Hip impingement location in maximal hip flexion in patients with femoroacetabular impingement with and without femoral retroversion. Am J Sports Med. 2022;50(11):2989–97. https://doi.org/10.1177/03635465221110887.
4. Spiker AM, Fabricant PD, Wong AC, Suryavanshi JR, Sink EL. Radiographic and clinical characteristics associated with a positive PART (prone apprehension relocation test): a new provocative exam to elicit hip instability. J Hip Preserv Surg. 2020;7(2):288–297. Published 2020 Jun 29. https://doi.org/10.1093/jhps/hnaa021.

Further Reading

Macdonald SJ, Garbuz D, Ganz R. Clinical evaluation of the symptomatic young adult hip. Semin Arthroplast. 1997;8:3–9.

2 Radiographic Assessment

Moritz Tannast and Jeffrey J. Nepple

2.1 Introduction

Standardized plain radiographs of the hip remain the initial imaging modality in all patients with hip pain. This radiographic tool gives a reliable and simple overview of the osseous morphologies of the pelvis and the proximal femur. Radiographs are used in all phases of care for these patients: preoperatively, postoperatively, at long-term follow-up, and in many cases intraoperatively. In addition, they are versatile in that they allow functional views and are not subject to metal artifacts.

In comparison to computer tomography (CT) and magnetic resonance imaging (MRI), radiographs are widely available, need only a few minutes for acquisition, and are cost-effective when used to decide if further imaging is needed. It is essential to understand basic technical principles and standardized acquisition techniques to correctly interpret pathomorphologies and reproducibility of measurements.

This chapter describes the technical principles, different radiographic views, and techniques for assessment of osteoarthritis, proximal femoral and acetabular morphology, as well as the influence of pelvic tilt and rotation.

2.2 Technical Principles of Radiographic Imaging

For the correct interpretation of a radiograph, it is important to understand the acquisition techniques. Plain radiographs reduce a three-dimensional object to a two-dimensional image. In comparison to computer tomography (CT) and magnetic resonance imaging (MRI), radiographs are based on a single-point X-ray source which produces a conical projection.

- *Relevance of Film-Focus Distance*

  As the conical portion of the beam strikes an object, the closer a structure is positioned to the X-ray source the more lateral it appears on the radiograph (Fig. 2.1). To illustrate this point, with increasing film-focus distance, the acetabular anteversion increases, whereas with decreasing film-focus distance, the acetabulum appears increasingly retroverted (Fig. 2.2). The patient-film distance, on the contrary, exhibits only a minor influence on the projection of the hip joint onto the film, even in overweight patients.
- *Relevance of the Center of the X-Ray Beam*

  Well established, standardized anterior–posterior (AP) pelvis radiograph for hip preserving surgery is centered on the midpoint between the upper border of the symphysis and the line connecting the two anterior superior iliac spines (ASIS) (Fig. 2.3). By lowering the center of the X-ray beam (low-centered AP pelvis radiograph, e.g., used in total hip arthroplasty (THA) templating), the apparent acetabular anteversion increases and may mask the diagnosis of acetabular retroversion. The acetabular anteversion also increases

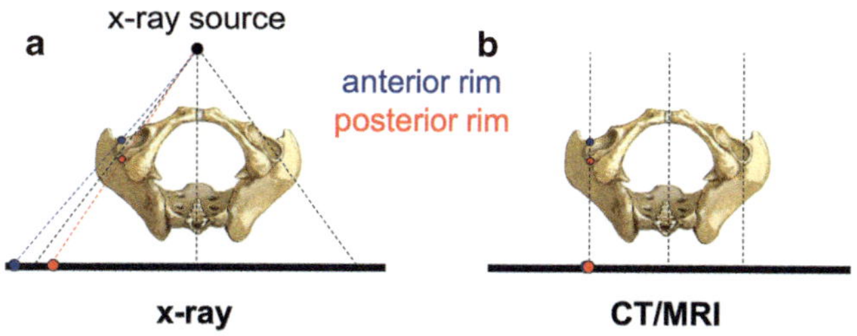

Fig. 2.1 (**a**) shows a conical X-ray source, as seen during the acquisition of pelvic radiographs. The anterior rim, which is closer to the source, appears more lateral on the X-ray film. In comparison, the more posterior rim appears more medial. (**b**) shows the typical acquisition technique of CT or MRI that uses parallel rays, reducing distortion

M. Tannast (✉)
Department of Orthopaedic Surgery and Traumatology, Inselspital, University of Berne, Berne, Switzerland
e-mail: moritz.tannast@insel.ch

J. J. Nepple
Department of Orthopaedic Surgery, Washington University School of Medicine, St. Louis, MO, USA
e-mail: nepplej@wustl.edu

M. Leunig et al. (eds.), *Surgical Hip Dislocation*, https://doi.org/10.1007/978-3-031-70622-6_2

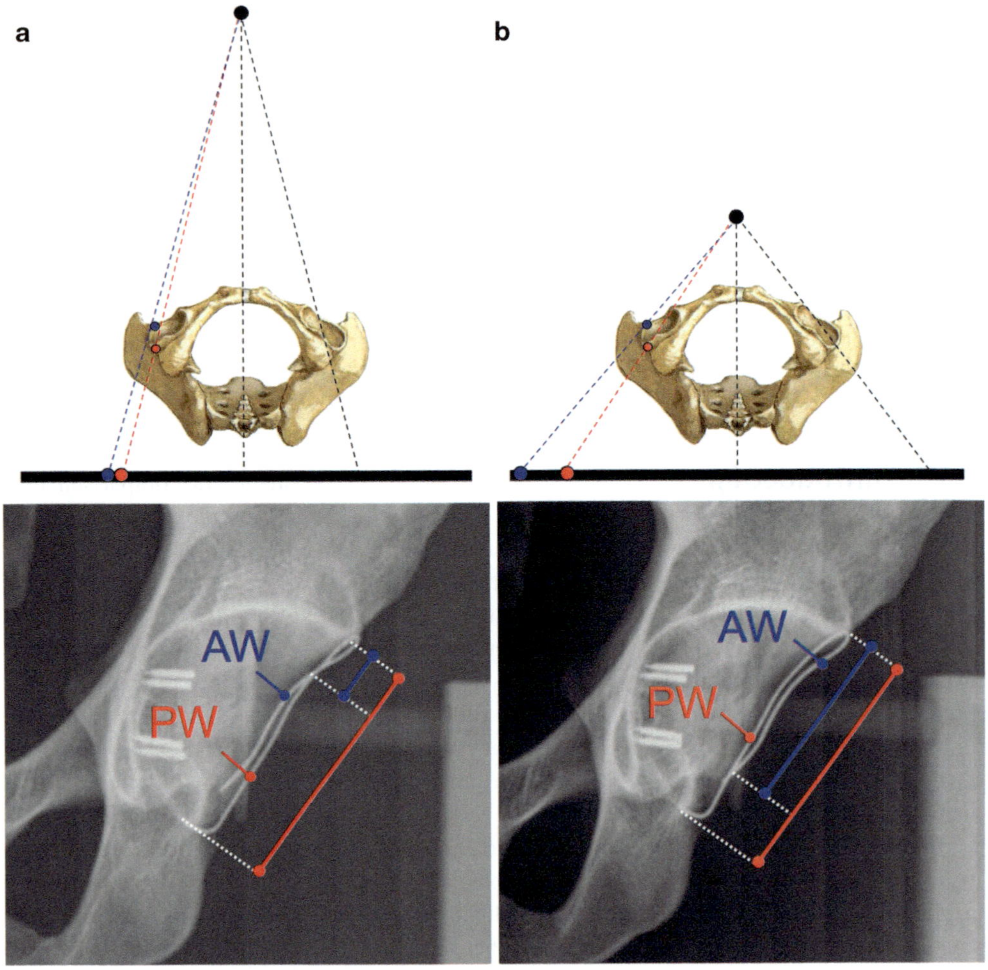

Fig. 2.2 (**a**) With the standard film-focus distance the anterior wall (AW) crosses the posterior wall (PW) in this example. (**b**) With decreasing film–focus distance, the retroversion becomes more notable with the anterior wall crossing the posterior wall more distally

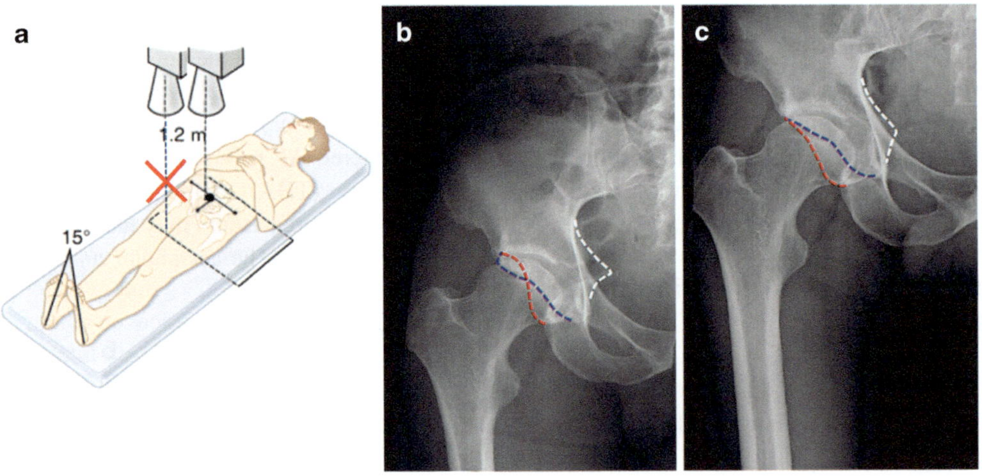

Fig. 2.3 (**a**) Standardized acquisition technique of a pelvis-centered radiograph with the legs 15° internally rotated and a film-focus distance of 120 cm. (**b**) Appropriately centered AP pelvis radiograph shows an acetabular retroversion with a crossover sign of the anterior (blue) and posterior wall (red). With a low-centered AP pelvis radiograph (**c**), the crossover sign is no longer apparent due to increasing anteversion with distalization of the X-ray beam

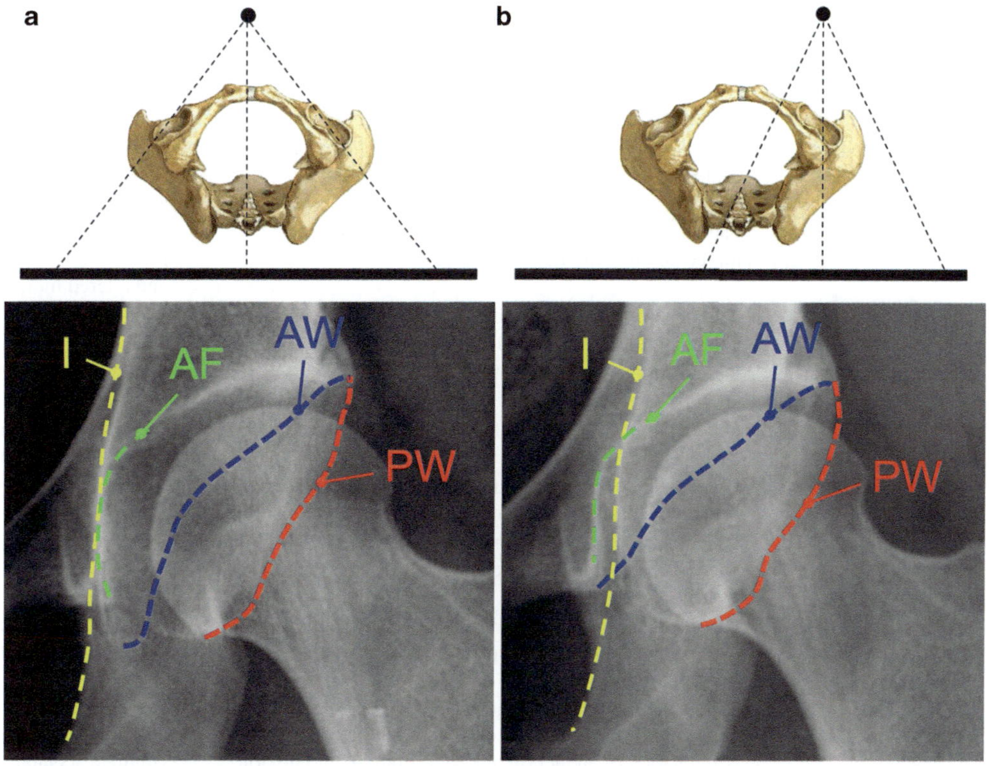

Fig. 2.4 Moving the beam center from the pelvis (**a**) to the hip (**b**) leads to an apparent increased acetabular anteversion. The posterior wall (PW) appears more lateral with increasing distance between the anterior (AW) and posterior wall (PW). Additionally, the acetabulum appears deeper with signs of a coxa profunda with the ilioischial line (I) appearing lateral to the acetabular fossa (AF)

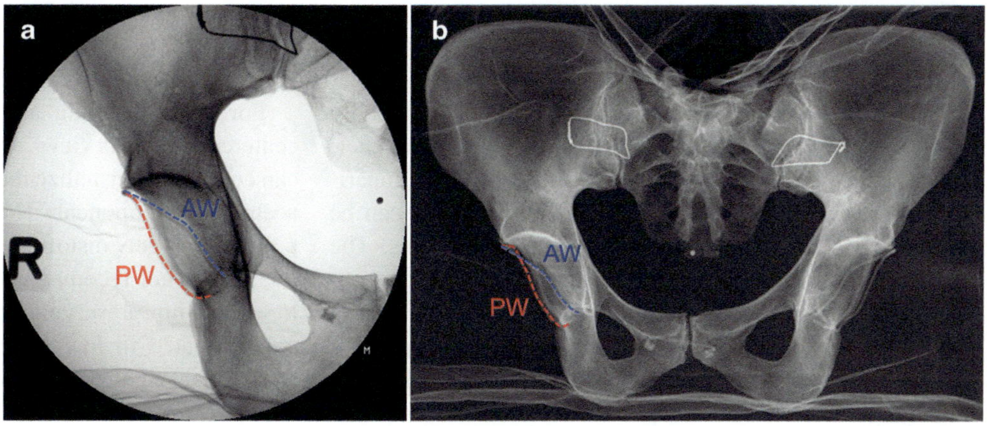

Fig. 2.5 (**a**) Shows a hip-centered fluoroscopic image. The distance between the anterior (AW) and posterior wall (PW) is large and no crossover sign is visible. (**b**) In comparison, the AP pelvis radiograph of the same specimen shows the anterior (AW) and posterior wall (PW) crosses cranially

by moving the beam from being centered on the pelvis to being centered on the hip joint (Fig. 2.4).

- *Fluoroscopy*

It is important to note how fluoroscopy differs in acquisition when compared with standardized AP pelvis radiographs. The differences must be understood to correctly interpret fluoroscopic images. The X-ray beam is posterior → anterior (PA) rather than anterior → posterior (AP). The fluoroscopic field of view is usually smaller than plain radiography which is why the fluoro beam is often hip-centered rather than pelvis-centered. Additionally, the tube-intensifier distance is decreased. The combination of these factors results in the appearance of a more anteverted acetabulum when comparing fluoroscopy to a standardized AP pelvis radiograph (Fig. 2.5).

2.3 Radiographic Projections of the Pelvis and the Hip

Standardized radiographs in two planes are the foundation of hip joint radiography. Well-established projections are the AP pelvis radiograph and the axial, cross-table view of the proximal femur. Additional radiographic projections can be added to address specific morphologic questions (Table 2.1 and Fig. 2.6).

Table 2.1 Overview of different radiographic projections of the hip

Projection	Technique	Features
Anteroposterior (AP) pelvis	Patient supine or standing, legs 15° internally rotated, centering of X-ray beam to the midpoint between the upper border of symphysis and a line connecting both ASIS	Basic radiographic evaluation of the hip for hip-preserving surgery, THA, or trauma surgery
Low-centered AP pelvis	Patient supine or standing, legs 15° internally rotated, centering of the X-ray beam below the symphysis	Performed in THA; not recommended for hip-preserving surgery due to different X-ray centering and altered morphology of the hip
Anteroposterior (AP) hip	Patient supine or standing, legs 15° internally rotated, hip-centered X-ray beam	Performed in THA; not recommended for hip-preserving surgery due to different X-ray centering and altered morphology of the hip
Axial cross-table	Patient supine, ipsilateral leg 15° internally rotated, contralateral hip flexed and elevated	Anterior and posterior femoral head–neck contour
Dunn–Rippstein	Patient supine, hips in 90° flexion and 20° abduction, knees in 90° of flexion, legs in holding device	Femoral antetorsion, anterior and posterior femoral head–neck contour
Modified Dunn	Patient supine, hips in 45° flexion and maximal abduction	Increased sensitivity to detect cam deformities in the anterosuperior head–neck area
Lauenstein	Patient supine, hip centered X-ray beam, hip and knee flexed, and hip in abduction	Anterior and posterior femoral head–neck contour
Frog-leg lateral	Patient supine, pelvis-centered X-ray beam, both hips and knee flexed, and the leg abducted so the soles of the feet contact	Anterior and posterior femoral head–neck contour
False profile	Patient standing, hip-centered X-ray beam, contralateral hip is tilted backward by 25°, ipsilateral foot remains parallel to the radiographic table	Anterior acetabular coverage, anterosuperior subluxation, quantification of posteroinferior joint space
Functional (abduction/adduction)	Patient positioning and centering of X-ray for AP pelvis view; additional abduction or adduction of the hip, possible combination of abduction, internal rotation, and flexion	Abduction view to differentiate between subluxation and true joint space narrowing in dysplastic hips, to simulate acetabular coverage following acetabular reorientation or femoral osteotomy

- *AP Pelvic Radiograph*

  The AP pelvis view is the standard radiographic modality in the frontal plane. It gives a good overview of hip and pelvis morphology and allows a direct, single-image comparison between both hip joints. AP pelvis radiographs can be performed in either the standing or supine positions. The authors prefer the supine position because it is more reproducible in the intraoperative setting and is not compromised during times of partial weight bearing such as in the postoperative setting. In addition, most of the reference values for radiographic predictors for periacetabular osteotomies or surgical hip dislocation as well as predictors for long-term follow-up in hip joint preservation surgery are based on supine radiographs. This contrasts with the Lisbon agreement, which recommends a standing film notwithstanding that the hip joint space does not depend on weight bearing. It has to be considered that pelvic tilt in general decreases with the patient standing, which directly influences the projected appearance of the hip joint morphology (Fig. 2.7). In selected cases, however, a standing radiograph has the advantage of detecting functional dysplasia in the presence of a leg length discrepancy (Fig. 2.8).

  For correct acquisition, the legs are rotated 15° internally to compensate for femoral torsion, and a film-focus distance of 120 cm is used. The beam is centered on the mid-point of the upper border of the symphysis and a line connecting the two ASIS (Fig. 2.9).

- *Low-Centered AP Pelvis View*

  For THA planning and postoperative evaluation, low-centered AP pelvis views are optimal because this projection can completely visualize the entirety of the femoral stem and acetabular component. However, as low-centered images produce a largely distorted projection of the acetabulum, this imaging is not recommended for decision-making and follow-up in hip preserving surgery. The acetabular version is overestimated in low-centered AP pelvic radiographs and substantial acetabular retroversion may even be missed.

- *Axial Cross-Table View*

  The axial cross-table view shows the anterior and posterior aspects of the proximal femur including the head–neck junction. It is typically the second view used for standardized hip evaluation.

  It is performed with the patient in a supine position with the ipsilateral leg in 15° internal rotation to compensate for the femoral anteversion. The contralateral leg is elevated. The X-ray beam is centered at an angle of 45° to the inguinal fold.

- *Lauenstein and Frog-Leg Lateral View*

  Lauenstein view and frog-leg lateral view are alternatives to the axial radiograph to assess the anterior and posterior femoral head–neck junction. The Lauenstein view is obtained with the hip and knee in 30–40° of flexion and the hip abducted at approximately 45°. The heel is rested on the X-ray table. The X-ray beam is centered on the hip. The

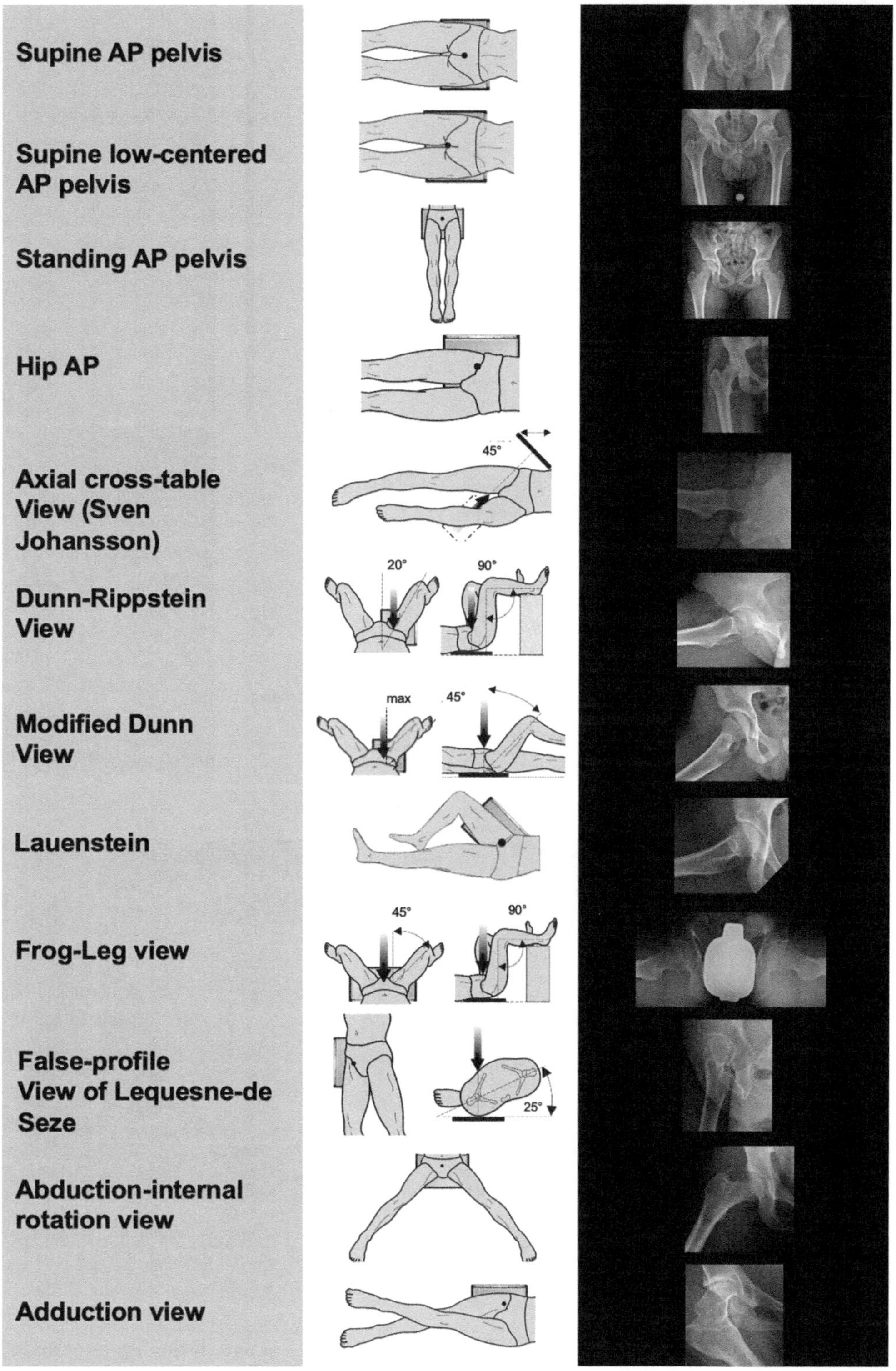

Fig. 2.6 Overview of different radiographic projections and radiographs

frog-leg lateral view is a bilateral simultaneous Lauenstein position with the central beam centered on the pelvis.

- *Dunn–Rippstein and Modified Dunn Views*

The Dunn–Rippstein view was initially developed to assess femoral torsion. The original technique is performed in a supine position with both hips and knees flexed to 90° and the lower extremities positioned on a special holding device that holds the hips in 20° of abduction. This view has become less common as CT-based measurement became the gold standard for the evaluation of femoral torsion due to its higher precision and accuracy while exhibiting fewer errors related to patient malposition.

The modified Dunn view, where the hip is positioned in only 45° of flexion, can be used as an alternative view to

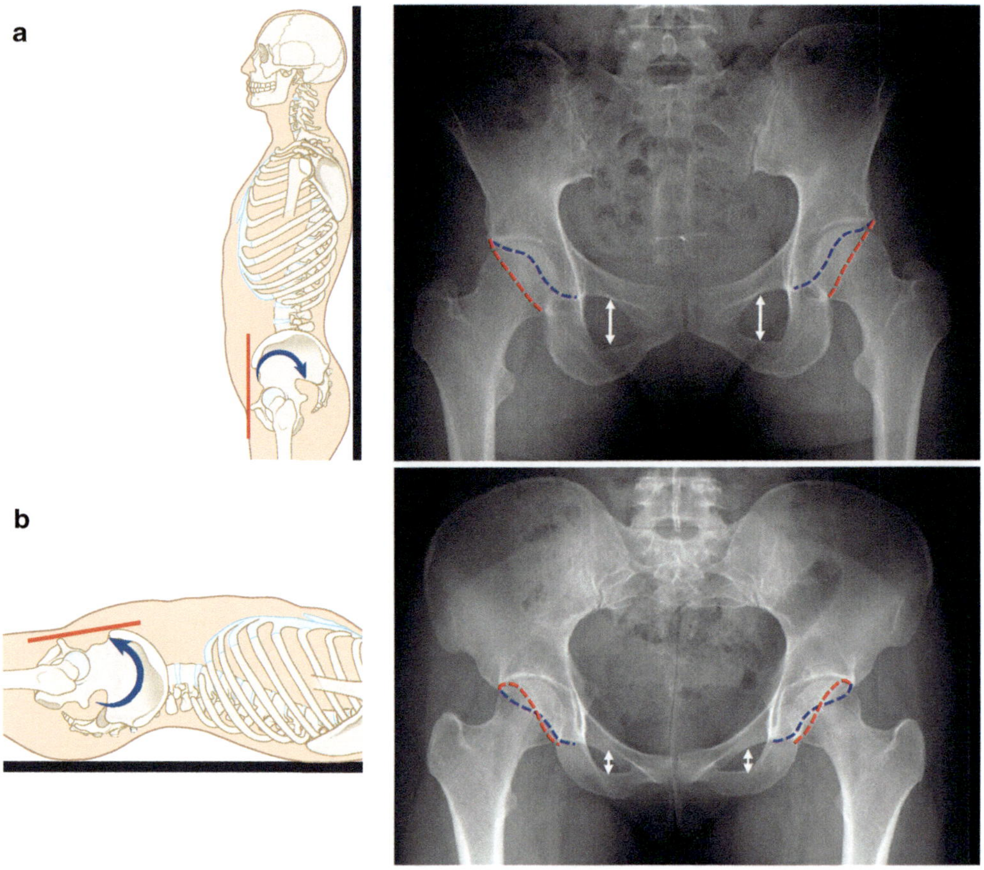

Fig. 2.7 (**a**) In standing position the pelvis tilts posteriorly. A potential acetabular retroversion can be missed because of elevated anteversion. (**b**) In a supine position, the pelvis tilts anteriorly and amplifies the retroversion

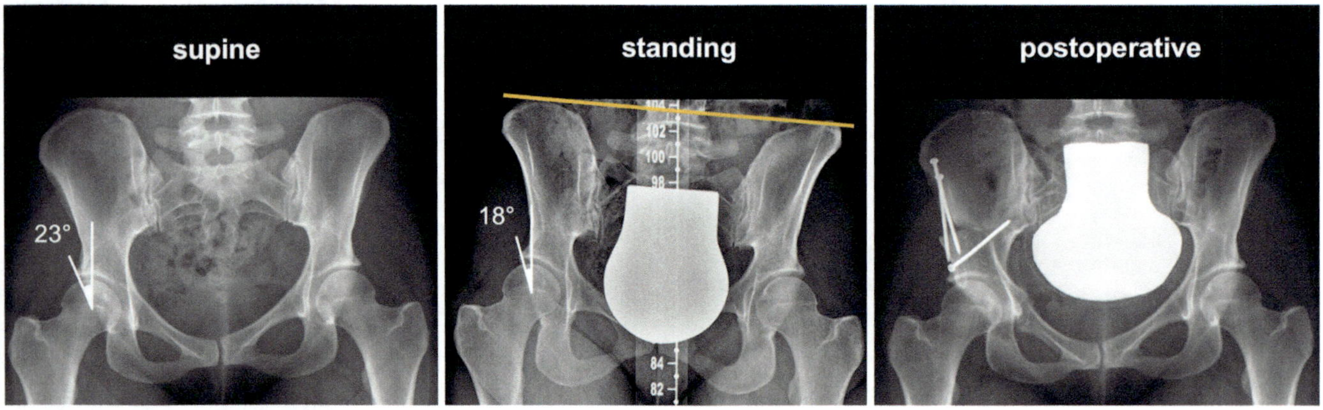

Fig. 2.8 Example of a patient with functional dysplasia. In a supine position, an LCE of 23° angle shows borderline dysplasia. In a standing position, due to a leg length discrepancy, an important dysplasia with an LCE of 18° is visible. Compensation of the leg length with shoe insoles on the left side did not lead to a satisfactory situation, so the patient finally benefited from a PAO

assess the anterior head–neck junction. Typically, the head–neck asphericity in cam-type deformity is located in the anterosuperior portion of the femoral head–neck junction and is best visualized with this view.

- *False Profile View*

A false profile view is performed with the patient in a standing position with the ipsilateral foot parallel to the X-ray film. The contralateral hip is externally rotated 25° away. The X-ray beam is perpendicular to the X-ray film. This view allows assessment of the anterior acetabular coverage of the hip joint and shows any anterosuperior subluxation of the hip, particularly in dysplastic hips or the presence of superior or posterior joint space narrowing in protrusion hips or early superior acetabular degeneration.

- *Functional Views*

Additional functional views are performed in cases such as DDH or Legg-Calvé-Perthes disease to assess joint congruency. Abduction views of the hip can be performed preoperatively to predict coverage following periacetabular osteotomy (PAO) or to support the decision-making process

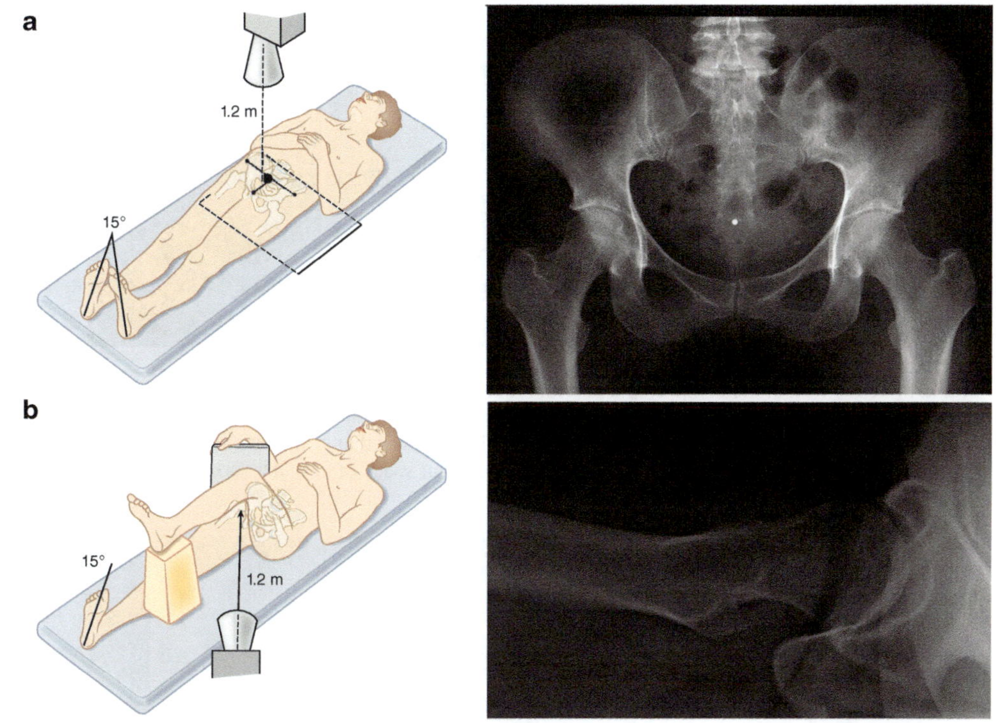

Fig. 2.9 (**a**) Shows the acquisition technique of a standardized AP pelvis radiograph with a film-focus distance of 1.2 m and 15° of internal rotation of the legs to compensate for femoral torsion and the corresponding X-ray. (**b**) Axial cross-table view is performed in a supine position with the ipsilateral leg in 15° of internal rotation and the contralateral leg elevated. The X-ray beam is centered at an angle of 45° to the inguinal fold. On the radiograph, anterior and posterior femoral head–neck junction are easily visible

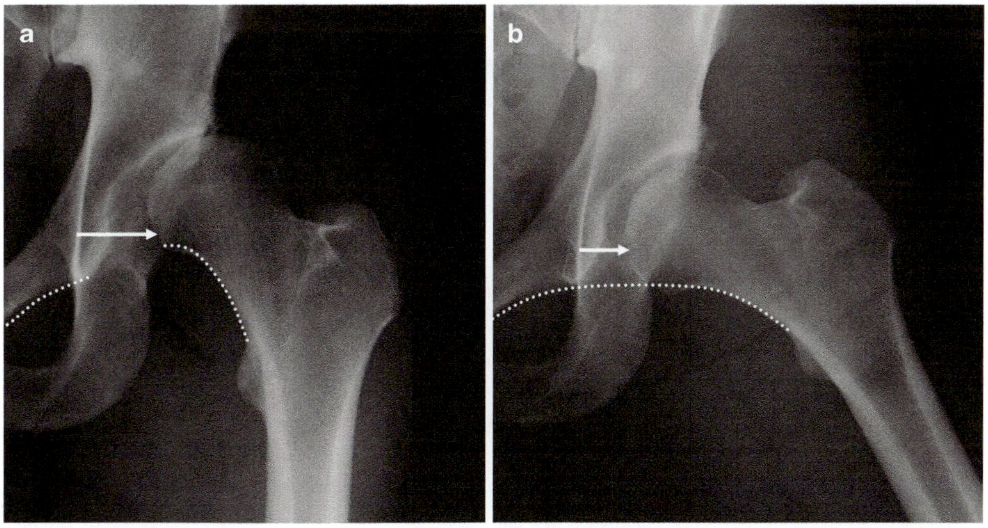

Fig. 2.10 (**a**) This hip with severe hip dysplasia shows lateral joint space narrowing with subluxation of the femoral head. To evaluate if this lateral joint space narrowing is based on the subluxation or cartilage loss due to OA, a hip abduction view is performed. (**b**) The femoral head is re-centered by the abduction of the hip, which leads us to assume that the majority of the articular cartilage is still sufficiently preserved. At the same time, the abduction view also shows us the possible coverage that can be achieved with a PAO

about PAO or proximal femoral osteotomies and joint congruency, especially in cases of Legg-Calvé-Perthes disease.

- *Abduction/Internal Rotation View in Hip Dysplasia (von Rosen View)*: With the abduction view, it is possible to differentiate if lateral joint space narrowing and subluxation of the femoral head are due to joint incongruence or cartilage wear. In the case of subluxation with normal cartilage, the femoral head re-centers in the hip joint with abduction, demonstrating restored congruency (Fig. 2.10). If the femoral head stays subluxated, it is most likely related to cartilage loss, a relative contraindication for hip preserving surgery (Fig. 2.11).
- *Abduction View in Legg-Calvé-Perthes Disease*: Abduction views are useful to evaluate for signs of hinged abduction (Fig. 2.12). In a hinged abduction, the largely aspherical portion of the femoral head provokes a levering out of the hip often producing a vacuum sign. This can be helpful in determining if a PAO will help with joint congruency in Legg-Calvé-Perthes disease. It may be repeated intraoperatively after relative neck lengthening to assess joint congruence.
- *Adduction Views*: In cases of varus hips, an additional adduction view can help evaluate the effect of a valgus osteotomy on the congruency of the hip joint (Fig. 2.13).

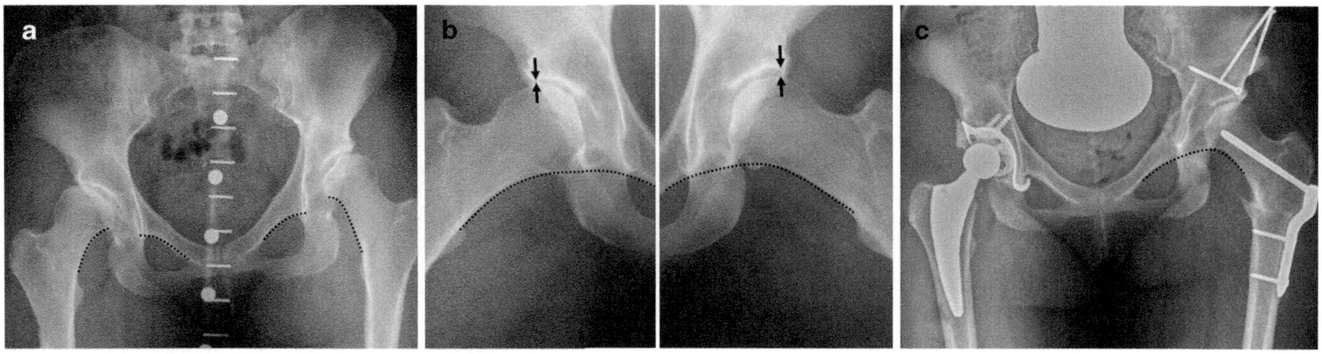

Fig. 2.11 Case with bilateral hip dysplasia with broken Shenton's line (dashed line), which shows a lateral joint space narrowing and lateralization of the femoral head (**a**). The abduction view shows that Shenton's line becomes again harmonic (**b**). The lateral joint space of the right hip stays reduced as a sign of relevant OA. Therefore, the patient was treated with a THA (**c**). The left hip recentered better and the lateral joint space stays open. Hip preservation surgery with a PAO and a varization osteotomy were performed

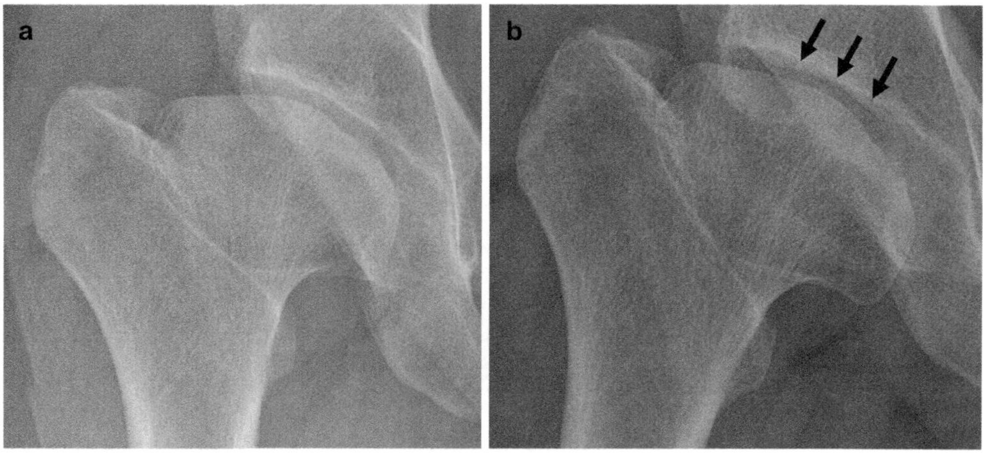

Fig. 2.12 (**a**) Incongruence of the hip joint in a case of Legg-Calvé-Perthes disease with lateral opening of the hip joint. (**b**) Abduction view shows an intraarticular vacuum sign, indicating hinged abduction

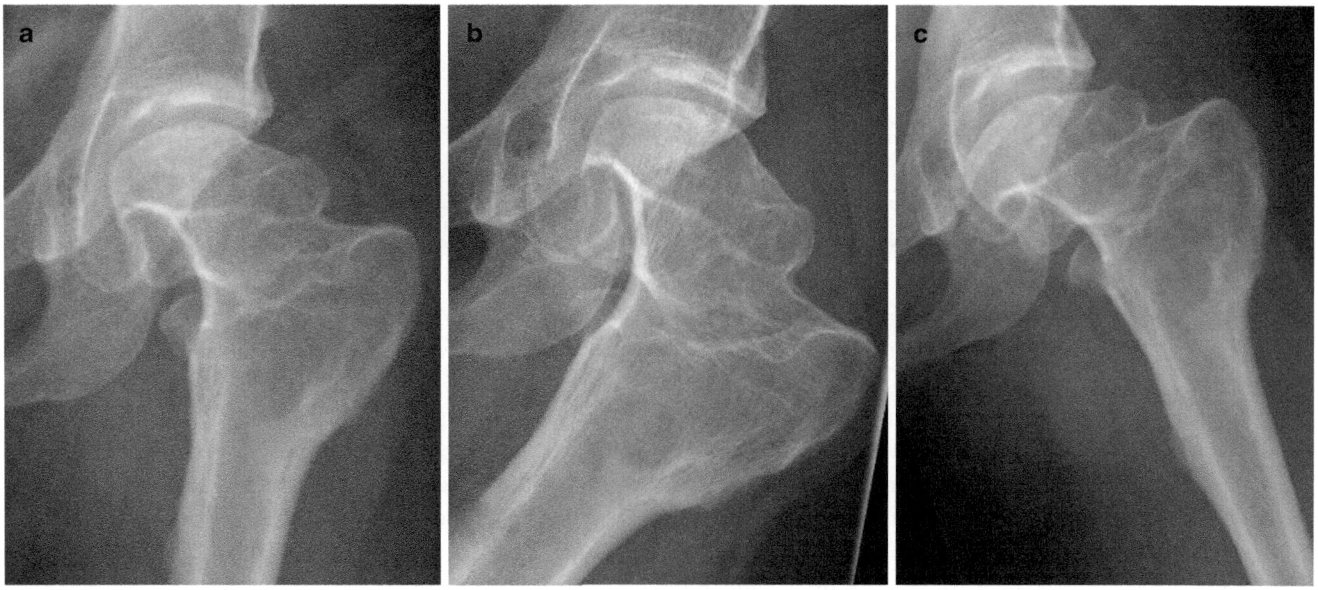

Fig. 2.13 (**a**) Patient with a varus hip post intertrochanteric varus osteotomy during childhood for the treatment of Legg-Calvé-Perthes disease. (**a**) In the neutral position, the lateral joint space appears incongruent and opens. (**b**) With adduction of the leg, the joint appears well-centered and congruent. (**c**) Abduction of the hip provokes an impingement and pathologically increases the joint space

2.4 Radiographic Assessment of Hip Osteoarthritis

An assessment of the presence and degree of hip osteoarthritis (OA) is an important first step in the evaluation of plain radiographs. If significant OA is present, a detailed assessment of acetabular and proximal femoral morphology is not necessary for hip joint preservation surgery.

- *The Tönnis OA Grade*

The Tönnis OA grade characterizes the presence of OA based on several findings including joint space width, sclerosis, and cystic formation (Fig. 2.14). Tönnis Grade 0 has no signs of OA, while Tönnis Grade 1 has sclerosis of the joint with minimal joint space narrowing and osteophyte formation. On the contrary, Tönnis Grade 2 has small cysts in the femoral head or acetabulum with moderate joint space narrowing, and Grade 3 has advanced arthritis with large cysts in the femoral head or acetabulum, joint space obliteration, and severe deformity of the femoral head. Hips with Tönnis 0 or 1 OA grade are typically very viewed as candidates for hip preservation surgery, while those with Tönnis 2 or 3 OA grades are not candidates for hip preservation. It is important to note that the differentiation between Tönnis 0 and 1 grades is difficult and has been demonstrated to have very poor interobserver reliability. Thus, differentiating Tönnis 0 and 1 OA grades is not a good marker of early joint degeneration, since not infrequently, Tönnis 0 hips can show intraoperatively surprisingly large areas of substantial cartilage destruction.

- *Minimum Joint Space Width on the AP Pelvic Radiograph*

Minimum joint space width is an additional useful indicator of joint health. Assessment of minimum joint space width is typically the most reliable as different patterns of hip joint space loss exist (medial vs. lateral joint space width). Philippon and colleagues have demonstrated that a joint space width of less than 2 mm is strongly associated with poor outcomes of hip arthroscopy and higher rates of conversion to THA. However, this threshold is likely somewhat arbitrary and depends on the underlying pathology. For example, dysplastic hips have by nature a larger joint space width compared with other pathologies (Fig. 2.15).

Joint space width less than 3 mm or any loss of joint space width compared with the contralateral hip is often an indica-

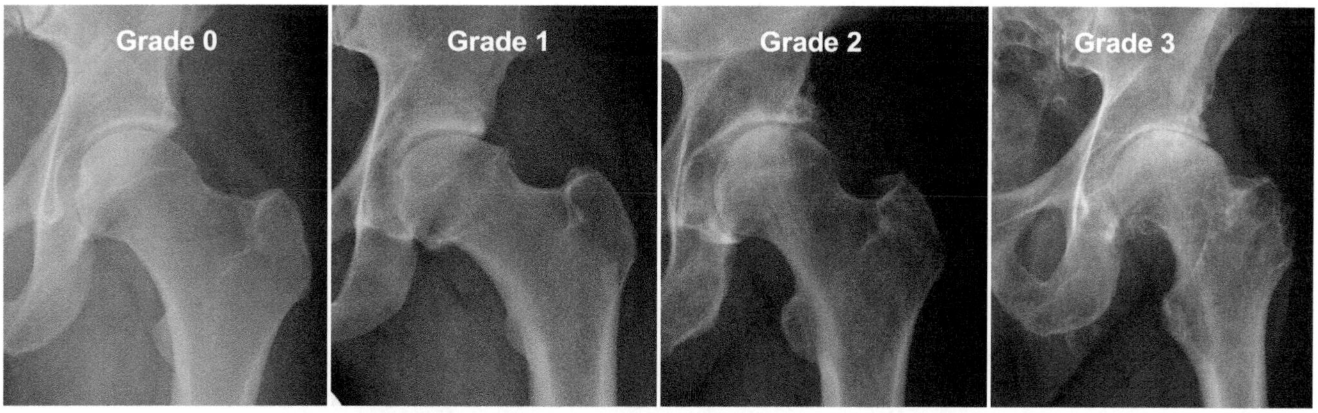

Fig. 2.14 Tönnis classification for OA of the hip joint. From grade 0 to grade 3, the hip joint shows progressive signs of OA

Fig. 2.15 (**a**) Shows an example of a dysplastic hip joint with a wide joint space. In contrast, (**b**) shows a hip with a mixed intra- and extraarticular femoroacetabular impingement with a small joint space. Only the joint space width alone did not predict the cartilage quality

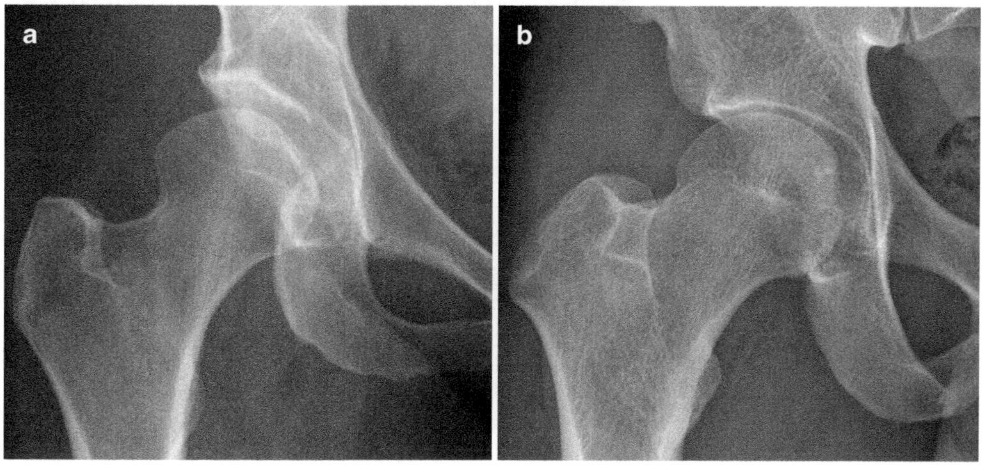

tor of significant OA and deserves careful assessment including on MRI/MRA.

A few additional unique scenarios are important to consider. In the presence of acetabular overcoverage with ossification of the acetabular labrum or an acetabular rim fracture, the overcovered portion of the hip may demonstrate more severe joint space narrowing. When this region would be resected at the time of surgical treatment, it may be appropriate to not consider this region in the overall assessment.

- *Minimum Joint Space Width on Other Projections*

Second, joint space narrowing can also be assessed on other radiographic views, particularly the false profile view. On the false profile view, posterior joint space narrowing may be best appreciated. It is important to note that the normal appearance of the joint space should increase slightly from posterior to anterior because of the variable thickness of the acetabular cartilage in these zones. Similarly, in the presence of subluxation of the joint in severe hip dysplasia, the false profile view can give the appearance of apparent anterior joint space narrowing which is not actually present. In protrusion hips, the false profile view reliably often reveals posterior joint space narrowing while the anterior joint space still is preserved. Finally, in patients with femoroacetabular impingement, superior joint space narrowing is often best noted on the false profile radiograph.

- *Joint Congruency*

Assessment of joint congruency is particularly important in the setting of complex hip deformities. Congruency assessment which is the degree to which the roundness of the femoral head and acetabulum match has been described by Yasunaga et al. as excellent, good, fair, or poor. It is important to recognize that apparent joint incongruity can be due to subluxation of the hip in setting of severe hip dysplasia. Additionally, incongruity can present in the setting of severe femoral head deformity such as residual Perthes disease. Functional radiographs can be utilized to simulate osteotomy corrections to ensure adequate congruency with the planned degree of correction. The von Rosen functional view, or abduction-internal rotation (AIR), is commonly utilized in the assessment of severe acetabular dysplasia to simulate congruency after PAO (Fig. 2.11). Similarly, when femoral osteotomy is planned, congruency after varus correction can be simulated with abduction, valgus correction can be simulated with adduction, and flexion correction can be simulated with hip extension during a functional view (Fig. 2.13).

2.5 Conventional Radiographic Assessment of Hip Instability

- *Broken Shenton's Line*

Cranial subluxation in dysplasia can be detected as a break in Shenton's line (Fig. 2.11).

- *Lateralization of Hip Center*

Lateralization of the hip center, in the absence of true subluxation, can be assessed via the distance from the medial femoral head to the ilioischial line. Assessment of this distance in the lower one-third of the femoral head is most accurate in the setting of a PAO correction (Fig. 2.10).

- *Upsloping Acetabular Sourcil*

Another sign of hip instability on the AP pelvic radiograph is the upsloping lateral acetabular sourcil (Fig. 2.16).

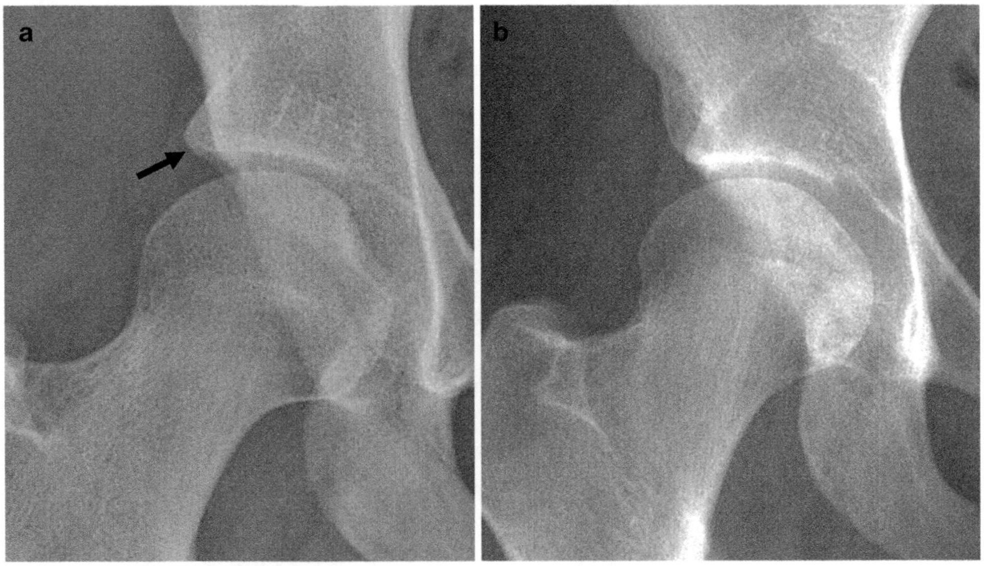

Fig. 2.16 An unstable hip with an upsloping lateral acetabular sourcil (**a**) is shown in contrast to a stable hip with a normal lateral acetabular sourcil morphology (**b**)

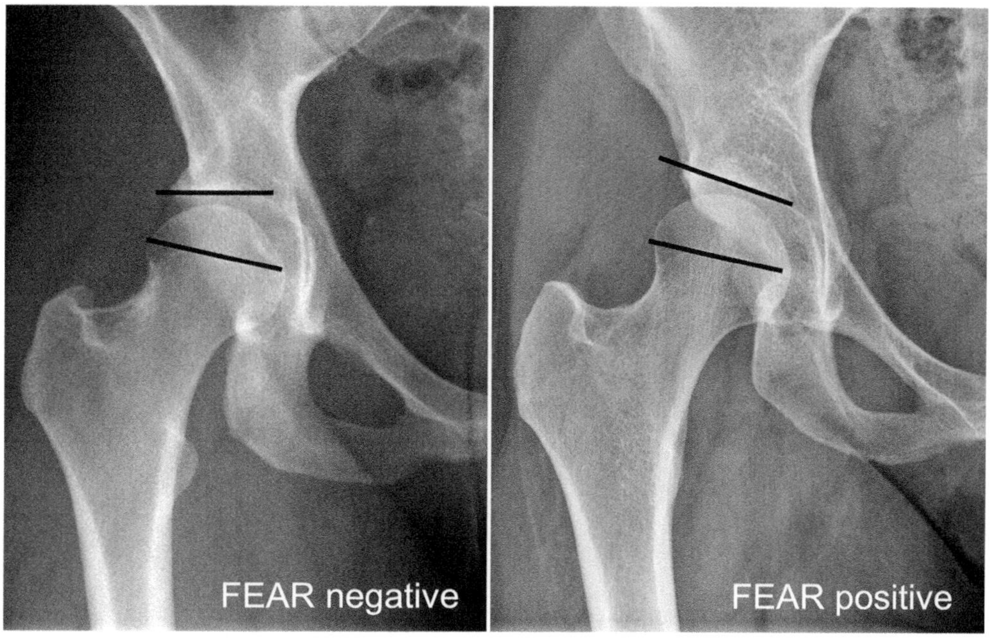

Fig. 2.17 The FEAR index is negative if the angle between the acetabular roof and the central part of the physeal scar of the femoral head is medially divergent, suggesting a stable hip. The FEAR index is positive if the angle is medially convergent, suggesting instability

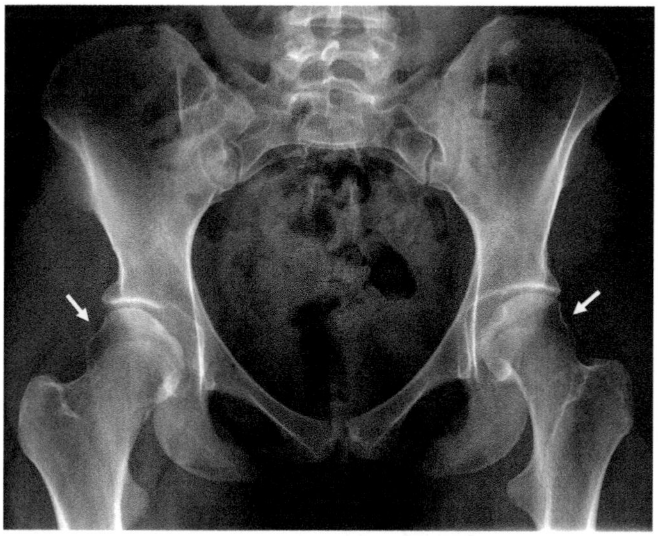

Fig. 2.18 Patient with a bilateral indentation sign (arrows) due to an instability caused by borderline dysplasia associated with a coxa valga et antetorta

- *FEAR Index*

  The FEAR index is another sign of hip instability. If the angle formed between a straight line of the acetabular roof and at the medial third of the physeal scar is laterally directed, the FEAR index is positive (Fig. 2.17).
- *Gluteus Minimus Indentation Sign on the Femoral Head.*

  In some hips with lateral extrusion of the femoral head, a notching of the lateral portion of the femoral head is visible. Beck et al. described it as an indentation of the gluteus minimus muscle which counteracts against the subluxation of the femoral in dysplastic hips (Fig. 2.18).

2.6 Acetabular Morphology

Assessment of acetabular coverage includes assessment of both acetabular depth and acetabular version as these concepts are interrelated. Additionally, it is useful to consider the assessment of coverage in the anterior, lateral, and posterior regions separately. An overview of all relevant coxometric parameters is given in Fig. 2.19 with the definition in Table 2.2 and published reference values given in Table 2.3.

- *Acetabular Depth*

  Historically, acetabular depth has been assessed by the findings of coxa profunda and coxa protrusio. We now recognize these parameters to be inadequate alone. Coxa profunda classically refers to the medial acetabular fossa projecting at or medial to the ilioischial line as a deep acetabulum. It is now recognized that this finding is particularly common in females and even in hips with acetabular dysplasia with an excessively anteverted acetabulum. Thus, it is currently not a particularly useful finding. On the contrary, protrusio defined as the projection of the femoral head at or medial to the ilioischial line remains a useful parameter. Protrusio is a marker of severe hip overcoverage, and can also be seen following fracture or hip OA. Modern plain radiographic analysis of the hip focuses on the detection of much more subtle abnormalities.
- *The Lateral Center Edge Angle*

  The lateral center edge angle (LCEA) remains among the most validated and useful radiographic parameters. The LCEA has a strong association with the natural history of hip dysplasia and its progression to hip OA. The LCEA is a useful assessment of lateral acetabular coverage and is not

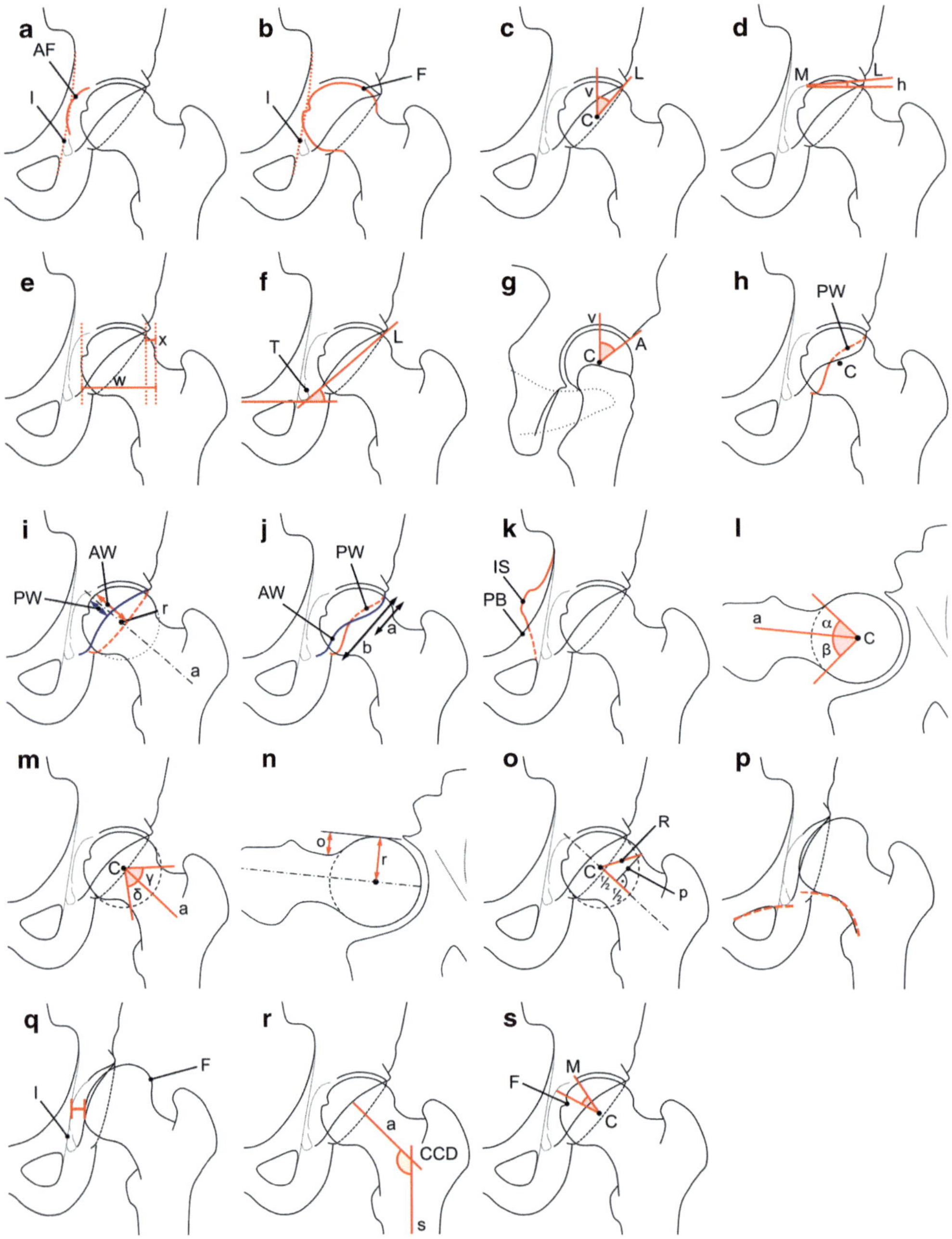

Fig. 2.19 Radiographic parameters to describe the acetabular and proximal femoral morphology. Definitions are given in Table 2.2. (**a**) Coxa profunda, (**b**) protrusion acetabuli, (**c**) lateral center-edge (LCE) angle, (**d**) **AI**, (**e**) EI, (**f**) sharp angle, (**g**) anterior center-edge (ACE) angle, (**h**) posterior wall sign, and (**i**) anterior and posterior acetabular wall index, (**j**) crossover sign with EI, (**k**) ischial spine sign, (**L**) alpha and beta angle, (**M**) gamma and delta angle, (**n**) offset and offset ratio, (**o**) triangular index, (**p**) Shenton's line, (**q**) lateralization of femoral head, (**r**) CCD angle, and (**s**) fovea angle delta

significantly affected by pelvic tilt or rotation. The LCEA is constructed from the center of the femoral head by an angle formed by a line connecting to the lateral acetabular sourcil and a second line utilizing a vertical reference perpendicular to a line connecting ischial tuberosities or tear drops. Several technical aspects of LCEA measurement are important to note. It is important to accurately identify the center of the femoral head, rather than estimating this point, as this can result in variation in the measurement of 2–5° which can be critical, particularly in borderline cases. Second, the LCEA must be measured to the edge of the congruent acetabular sourcil. In cases where the edge of the lateral sourcil flares, measurement to the most lateral portion of the sourcil is not a true estimation of coverage and results in overestimating acetabular coverage. Several different classifications of LCEA measurements have been utilized. Thresholds below which a hip is dysplastic commonly vary from 18° to 22°. We use <22° as our threshold. An LCEA of 22–25° is commonly referred to as borderline acetabular dysplasia. Within this population, there is significant variation in anterior and posterior coverage that results in some hips being truly unstable, while others are not.

A second key parameter of acetabular morphology is the acetabular index (AI), Tönnis angle. AI is the angle between the horizontal reference and a second line connecting the medial and lateral acetabular sourcil. This reflects the obliq-

Table 2.2 Definition of the different acetabular and femoral parameters for coxometry (see Fig. 2.19)

Category	Parameter	Radiograph	Definition
Acetabular depth	Coxa profunda [positive/negative]	AP pelvis	Acetabular fossa (AF) touches or crosses the ilioischial line (I), not very reliable
	Protrusio acetabuli [positive/negative]	AP pelvis	Femoral head (F) touches or crosses the ilioischial line (I), very reliable
Acetabular coverage	Lateral center-edge (LCE) angle [°]	AP pelvis	Angle formed by a vertical line (v) and a line through the center of the femoral head (C) and the lateral edge of the acetabulum (L)
	Acetabular index [°]	AP pelvis	Angle formed by a horizontal line (h) and a line through the medial (M) and lateral edge (L) of the acetabular roof
	Extrusion index [%]	AP pelvis	Percentage of the femoral head width (w) which is not covered by the acetabulum (x)
	Sharp angle [°]	AP pelvis	Angle between a horizontal line (h) and a line connecting the acetabular teardrop (T) with the lateral edge of the acetabulum (L)
	Anterior center-edge (ACE) angle [°]	False profile	Angle formed by a vertical line (v) and a line through the center of the femoral head (C) and the anterior edge of the acetabulum (A)
Acetabular orientation	Posterior wall sign [positive/negative]	AP pelvis	Positive if the posterior wall (PW) runs medially to the center of the femoral head (C)
	Anterior and posterior acetabular wall index [positive/negative]	AP pelvis	Ratio of the width of the anterior (AW)/posterior acetabular wall (PW) measured along the femoral head–neck axis (a) divided by the femoral head radius (r)
	Crossover sign [positive/negative]	AP pelvis	Anterior wall (AW) crosses the posterior wall (PW)
	Retroversion index [%]	AP pelvis	Percentage of the retroverted acetabular opening (a) divided by the entire opening (b)
	Ischial spine sign [positive/negative]	AP pelvis	Positive if the ischial spine (IS) is projected medially to the pelvic brim (PB)
Head–neck sphericity	Alpha (beta) angle [°]	Axial	Angle formed by the femoral head–neck axis (a) and line through the center of the femoral head (C) and the point where the anterior (posterior) head–neck contour exceeds the head radius
	Gamma (delta) angle [°]	AP pelvis	Angle formed by the femoral head–neck axis (a) and line through the center of the femoral head (C) and the point where the cranial (caudal) head–neck contour exceeds the head radius
	Offset [mm]	Axial	Difference (o) between the femoral head radius (r) and the neck radius
	Offset ratio []	Axial	Ratio of offset (o) to the femoral head radius (r)
	Triangular index []	AP pelvis	A perpendicular line (p) is drawn at half the head radius (r). Distance (R) is measured from the femoral head center (C) to the point where p intersects the anterior femoral head–neck contour. The triangular index is positive if $R \geq r + 2$ mm
Joint congruency	Shenton's line [intact/interrupted]	AP pelvis	Interrupted if the caudal femoral head–neck contour and the superior border of the obturator foramen do not form a harmonic arc
	Lateralization of femoral head [mm]	AP pelvis	Shortest distance between the medial aspect of the femoral head (F) and the ilioischial line (I)
Additional findings	CCD angle [°]	AP pelvis	Angle formed by the femoral head–neck axis (a) and the femoral shaft axis (s)
	Fovea angle delta [°]	AP pelvis	Angle formed by a line through the medial edge of the acetabular roof (M) and the center of the femoral head (C) and a line through the lateral border of the fovea capitis femoris (F) and the center of the femoral head (C)

uity of the weight-bearing surface of the acetabular surface and is not directly correlated to the LCEA. It is important to note that variability of the medial sourcil can affect this measurement. Particularly, when the medial sourcil edge is not distinct, this can create some variability in this measurement. AI values of 14° or greater are typically viewed as indicative of dysplasia, while values under 3° may indicate acetabular overcoverage.

- *Extrusion Index*

The extrusion index (EI) is the percentage of the femoral head width which is uncovered by the acetabulum with normal values being recently characterized as 17–27%. However, the EI has a very strong geometric correlation to the LCEA, so it generally provides very little information beyond the LCEA. Another parameter is the Sharp angle, which is the angle between the horizontal reference and a

Table 2.3 Published coxometric reference values for acetabular under- and overcoverage

Category	Parameter	Normal	Hip dysplasia	Overcoverage	Severe overcoverage	Cam impingement
Acetabular depth	Acetabular fossa	Normal or coxa profunda	Normal or coxa profunda	Coxa profunda	Protrusio acetabuli	n.a
Acetabular coverage	LCEA [°]	23–33	<22	34–39	>40	n.a
	MCEA [°]	35–44	>45	34–29	<28	n.a
	Acetabular arc [°]	61–65	<60	66–69	>69	n.a
	AI [°]	3–13	>14	−7 to 2	<−8	n.a
	EI [%]	17–27	>27	12–16	<11	n.a
	Sharp angle [°]	38–42	>43	34–37	<34	n.a
	Anterior center-edge angle [°]	>25	<20	Not described	Not described	n.a
Acetabular orientation	Posterior wall sign [positive/ negative]	Positive	Positive	Positive or negative	Negative	n.a
	Anterior acetabular wall index	0.41	0.28	0.61		n.a
	Posterior acetabular wall index	0.91	0.81	1.15		n.a
	Crossover sign [positive/ negative]	Negative	Positive	Negative	Negative	Negative
	Ischial spine sign [positive/ negative]	Negative	Not described	Positive with retroversion	Positive with retroversion	
Head–neck sphericity	Alpha angle [°]	<50	Often>50	n.a	n.a	>50
	Beta angle [°]	42 ± 7	Not described	Not described	Not described	Not described
	Gamma angle [°]	53 ± 13	Not described	Not described	Not described	Not described
	Delta angle [°]	43 ± 5	Not described	Not described	Not described	Not described
	Offset [mm]	>10	Not described	>10		<8
	Offset ratio[]	>0.20	Not described	>0.20		<0.18
	Triangular index [positive/ negative]	Negative	Not described	Negative	Negative	Positive
Joint congruency	Shenton's line [intact/ interrupted]	Intact	Often interrupted	Intact	Intact	Intact
	Lateralization of femoral head [mm]	Not described	~16	Not described	Not described	Not described
Additional findings	CCD angle [°]	129–135	>135	<129		Not described
	Fovea angle delta [°]	26 ± 10	Not described	Not described	Not described	Not described

line connecting the acetabular teardrop to the lateral sourcil (normal values 38–42°).

- *Anterior Center Edge Angle*

The false profile radiographic view has been historically utilized to characterize anterior acetabular coverage with the measurement of the anterior center edge angle (ACEA). The ACEA is measured similarly to the LCEA but a vertical reference to the upright position and a second line connecting to the anterior edge of the acetabular sourcil. ACEA measurements under 20° have been classified as dysplastic. Assessment of the ACEA is most useful in borderline cases where the LCEA does not definitively dictate the surgical decision-making. This parameter remains to be better validated relative to true three-dimensional coverage.

Modern assessment of acetabular coverage has moved significantly beyond the LCEA, AI, and ACEA.

- *Anterior and Posterior Acetabular Coverage*

The crossover sign is utilized as a measure of the acetabular version on a well-positioned AP pelvis radiograph. A positive crossover sign is present when the anterior rim projects lateral to the posterior acetabular rim as it heads toward the lateral sourcil. Thus, the anterior wall "crosses over" the posterior wall and reverses the normal project of these two structures. The position of this crossover relates to the severity of the acetabular retroversion and can be quantified as the retroversion index (percentage of retroverted acetabular opening divided by the entire opening). However, the crossover sign is not a perfect marker of acetabular retroversion as it has been demonstrated to be present in 15% of asymptomatic hips. A crossover sign also should not alone be viewed as a sign of impingement as it is common in the dysplastic hip, as well as can occur with normal anterior acetabular coverage in the setting of deficient posterosuperior acetabular coverage. Additionally, the crossover sign can be falsely positive in the setting of deformity of the AIIS that can overlap this radiographic projection. A prominent ischial spine sign can be a secondary sign of acetabular retroversion. This is present when the ischial spine project medial to the pelvic brim. The posterior wall sign is additionally critical to evaluate posterior coverage, in combination with the assessment

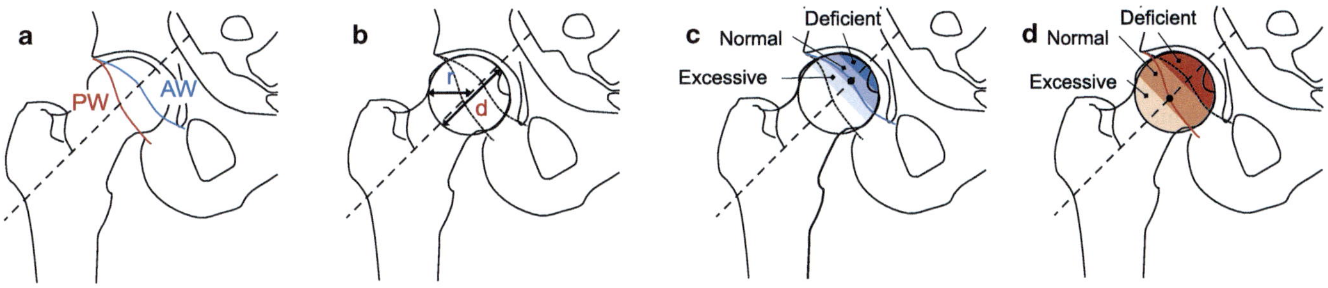

Fig. 2.20 Illustration of the rule of thirds. (**a**) The anterior and posterior walls are depicted, and (**b**) the femoral head radius and diameter are identified. (**c**) For the anterior coverage, the intersection point of the anterior with the femoral neck axis is determined and related to the thirds of the radius. Deficient anterior coverage was determined if the intersection point for the anterior wall was in the medial third of the femoral head radius. Excessive anterior coverage was determined if the intersection point was in the lateral third of the femoral head radius. (**d**) Similarly, for the posterior coverage, the intersection point of the posterior wall with the femoral head diameter is related to its thirds. Deficient posterior coverage was determined if the intersection point for the posterior wall was in the medial third of the femoral head diameter. Excessive posterior coverage was labeled if the intersection point was in the lateral third of the femoral head diameter

of the acetabular version. The posterior wall references the center of the femoral head relative to the posterior wall of the acetabulum. When the posterior wall is medial to the center of the femoral head, the posterior wall sign is positive and is indicative of posterior acetabular undercoverage. In true acetabular retroversion, the crossover sign and posterior wall (and the ischial spine) signs should all be positive.

- *The Acetabular Wall Index*

More recently, quantitative assessments of anterior and posterior coverage have been described and increasingly utilized. The anterior wall index (AWI) and posterior wall index (PWI) utilize an axis along the axis of the femoral neck and calculate the ratio of the width of anterior/posterior coverage of the femoral head to the femoral head radius. Both the AWI and PWI will be affected by any alteration of pelvic tilt or rotation that has previously been discussed to alter the acetabular version assessment. The mean AWI was 0.41 in a normal cohort, compared with 0.28 in dysplasia and 0.61 in overcoverage, while the mean PWI was 0.91 in a normal cohort compared with 0.81 in dysplasia and 1.15 in overcoverage. Threshold-based use of AWI and PWI in a clinical setting can be analyzed using the rule of thirds (Fig. 2.20). The intersection point of the anterior (posterior) acetabular wall and the femoral neck axis is determined and then allocated to a third of the head radius for the anterior wall and the femoral diameter for the posterior wall.

2.7 Femoral Morphology

- *Neck Shaft Angle/Centrum Collum Diaphyseal Angle*

Historically, the basic assessment of the proximal femur was limited to a simple assessment. The neck-shaft angle (NSA) or centrum collum diaphyseal (CCD) is used to quantify the relative varus or valgus orientation of the proximal femur. A normal NSA is generally 129–135°, with lower values indicating a relative varus alignment and higher values indicating a relative valgus alignment of the proximal femur. Additionally, the position of the greater trochanter can be assessed relative to the femoral head as the center–trochanter distance which measures the vertical position of the femoral head center to the tip of the greater trochanter along the femoral shaft axis. Negative values indicate that the trochanter is above the femoral head center, while positive values indicate that it is below the femoral head center. The original description proposed a normal range from −7 to +17 mm.

- *Femoral Sphericity*

The morphology of the proximal femur is now well recognized for its role in the pathophysiology of young adult hip disorders and its association with hip OA. The concept of the cam morphology of the proximal femur was introduced by Ganz and colleagues in 2003. This proximal femoral morphology had previously been recognized as a pistol-grip deformity or tilt deformity as early as 1965 but lacked full development of the understanding of this morphology until many years later. Modern assessments of the cam morphology utilize the alpha angle and head–neck offset ratio as qualitative assessments of femoral-head neck asphericity and decreased head–neck offset. The normal head–neck junction exhibits a seamless transition from the concave head–neck junction to the convex femoral head. The alpha angle is the angle formed between the axis of the femoral neck and a line connecting the center of the femoral head to the point at which the contour of the head–neck junction exceeds the radius of the femoral head. Values less than 50° are typically viewed as normal. Alpha angles above 50° indicate the presence of a cam morphology but are highly prevalent in normal asymptomatic populations as well as patients with acetabular dysplasia. Assessment of head–neck offset is additionally important as decreased head–neck offset can contribute to impingement independently of the alpha angle. Head–neck offset is measured along the axis of the femoral neck and the distance between parallel lines touching the femoral head and the femoral neck. This is commonly expressed as a ratio, head–neck offset ratio, by dividing by the radius of the femoral head. Importantly, the second line in this measurement should be along the femoral neck, rather than the alpha angle point where the diameter of the femoral neck is exceeded. Thus, head–neck offset is a separate concept from the alpha angle and not a simple geometric transformation of the same information. A head–neck offset ratio less than 0.17 is typically viewed as decreased.

The head–neck junction should be assessed on several radiographic views to adequately assess its presence and extent. The AP pelvis view is taken with the feet internally rotated and provides good visualization of the lateral (12:00) head–neck junction. The 45° Dunn radiograph typically visualizes the maximal extent of the cam morphology and corresponds to the anterosuperior region (1:00–1:30), while the frog lateral radiograph visualizes the anterior head–neck junction (3:00). This approach can be used intraoperatively with fluoroscopy as well in six varying positions.

2.8 Summary

Conventional radiographic assessment of the hip requires standardized anteroposterior (preferably supine) and axial X-rays before advanced imaging such as computed tomography and MRI is indicated. Careful evaluation of these images allows the detection of the major pathologies and underlying pathomechanisms based on careful coxometry and subtle radiographic signs.

Further Reading

Castro MO, et al. The Lisbon agreement on femoroacetabular impingement imaging—part 3: imaging techniques. Eur Radiol. 2021;31(7):4652–68.

Clohisy J, Carlisle J, Beaulé P, et al. A systematic approach to the plain radiographic evaluation of the young adult hip. J Bone Joint Surg Am. 2008;90 Suppl 4(Suppl 4):47–66.

Nötzli H, Wyss T, Stoecklin C, Schmid M, Treiber K, Hodler J. The contour of the femoral head-neck junction as a predictor for the risk of anterior impingement. J Bone Joint Surg Br. 2002;84(4):556–60.

Reynolds D, Lucas J, Klaue K. Retroversion of the acetabulum. A cause of hip pain. J Bone Joint Surg Br. 1999;81(2):281–8.

Siebenrock K, Kistler L, Schwab J, Büchler L, Tannast M. The acetabular wall index for assessing anteroposterior femoral head coverage in symptomatic patients. Clin Orthop Relat Res. 2012;470(12):3355–60.

Stetzelberger V, Moosmann A, Zheng G, Schwab J, Steppacher D, Tannast M. Does the rule of thirds adequately detect deficient and excessive acetabular coverage? Clin Orthop Relat Res. 2021;479(5):974–87.

Tannast M, Siebenrock K, Anderson SE. Femoroacetabular impingement: radiographic diagnosis-what the radiologist should know. AJR Am J Roentgenol. 2007;188(6):1540–52.

Tannast M, Fritsch S, Zheng G, Siebenrock K, Steppacher S. Which radiographic hip parameters do not have to be corrected for pelvic rotation and tilt? Clin Orthop Relat Res. 2015a;473(4):1255–66.

Tannast M, Hanke M, Zheng G, Steppacher S, Siebenrock K. What are the radiographic reference values for acetabular under- and overcoverage? Clin Orthop Relat Res. 2015b;473(4):1234–46.

Yasunaga Y, Ikuta Y, Kanazawa T, Takahashi K, Hisatome T. The state of the articular cartilage at the time of surgery as an indication for rotational acetabular osteotomy. J Bone Joint Surg Br. 2001;83(7):1001–4.

Advanced Imaging

3

Christian W. A. Pfirrmann and Young-Jo Kim

3.1 Introduction

The Warwick agreement [1] on femoroacetabular impingement syndrome (FAIS) defines FAIS as a triad of symptoms, clinical signs of impingement, and imaging findings. In Part 3 of the Lisbon agreement of 2021 on femoroacetabular impingement (FAI), recommendations on the selection and use of imaging techniques are provided [2]. Standard radiographs are recommended for the initial assessment. Magnetic resonance imaging (MRI) is recommended as the gold standard for imaging of FAI. The MRI protocol should include a small field of view (FOV) with radial imaging, femoral torsion assessment, and a fluid-sensitive sequence covering the whole pelvis.

3.2 Computed Tomography

The use of computed tomography (CT) is controversial. In the Lisbon agreement on FAI, the role of CT is still not well defined. The main advantage of CT is the capability to produce outstanding 3D imaging. It is therefore very valuable to assess complex deformities and to help plan complex surgery. The 3D datasets of the osseous pelvis from CT may be used for virtual impingement simulation or 3D printing. The CT data may even be used to produce radiograph-like projections that are comparable results to radiographs regarding the standard measurements such as lateral center edge angle or acetabular index. The main problem of CT is the high radiation dose applied to the pelvis in young and therefore sensitive patients. Especially in children and adolescents as well as in young women, CT should therefore be highly restricted to selected, complex cases. With the development of the latest CT detectors and with the recent introduction of tin filtering, ultra-low-dose CT has become available. Ultra-low-dose pelvic CT with tin filtration can be performed at a dose of standard radiographs of the pelvis, with a dose reduction of over 80% [3].

3.3 MR Imaging

3.3.1 General Considerations and Protocols

In recent years, there have been considerable advances in MRI techniques that result in higher image quality. A body matrix phased-array coil or a body matrix phased-array coil in combination with a spine array coil is used for image acquisition. The standard MRI technique for the hip should include small-FOV sequences in three planes focused on the abnormal hip only. These sequences are combined with large-FOV sequences that cover the whole pelvis and the femur for torsional analysis.

Small-FOV sequences focused on one hip provide high-resolution images, which are necessary to assess small structures, such as the labrum and the cartilage. Large-FOV sequences over the whole pelvis are dedicated to diagnosing periarticular abnormalities and addressing the geometry of the pelvis and femur.

The choice of sequences may vary among institutions. The MRI protocol should include fluid-sensitive sequences to depict bone marrow edema, soft tissue edema, and fluid collections. Non-saturated T1-weighted or non-saturated proton density images are useful to assess anatomy, detect fracture lines, and look at muscle quality. T1-weighted sequences with fat saturation are sensitive to gadolinium and are therefore used after administration of contrast material (direct arthrography or intravenous gadolinium administration). With 3D gradient images, thin slices can be obtained, typically to address cartilage and labral lesions or to obtain secondary reformats (for example to reconstruct radial images).

C. W. A. Pfirrmann
MRI Medical Radiological Institute, Schulthess Clinic Zurich, University of Zurich, Zurich, Switzerland
e-mail: cpfirrmann@mri-roentgen.ch

Y.-J. Kim (✉)
Boston Children's Hospital, Harvard Medical School, Boston, MA, USA
e-mail: Young-jo.Kim@childrens.harvard.edu

M. Leunig et al. (eds.), *Surgical Hip Dislocation*, https://doi.org/10.1007/978-3-031-70622-6_3

The following small-FOV sequences are commonly used: coronal T1-weighted fast spin-echo images, coronal proton-density-weighted fast spin-echo images with fat suppression, sagittal intermediate-weighted fast spin-echo images with fat suppression, and transverse oblique 3D water-excitation true fast imaging with steady-state precession images parallel to the long axis of the femoral neck. The transverse oblique images along the long axis of the femoral neck are used for the evaluation of the femoral head–neck junction and acetabular orientation. Large-FOV sequences typically include axial or coronal fluid-sensitive imaging sequences to exclude abnormalities and differential diagnoses that can mimic or coexist with intra-articular abnormalities.

3.3.2 Radial Images of the Femur

Radial imaging of the hip is obtained at angular intervals perpendicular to the surface of the femoral neck with images intersecting through the center of the femoral neck. Radial imaging around the femoral neck axis provides both morphologic imaging of the femoral neck morphology and labral morphology, unlike radial imaging rotating around the acetabular opening axis which only provides optimal imaging of the labrum. The axis of the radial images runs through the center of the femoral neck. Radial images can be obtained as a dedicated radial sequence (using, for example, a proton density fast-spin-echo sequence) or as reformats from a 3D sequence. Radial imaging provides primarily an optimal delineation of the three-dimensional contour of the femoral head and the head–neck junction, especially at the anterosuperior quadrant, where the cam deformity is often most pronounced. Assessment of the alpha angle on oblique axial images only considerably underestimates the alpha angle. Alpha angles are measured between the femoral neck axis and the line that connects the femoral rotation center and the point where the best-fitting circle intersects with the contour of the femur [4] (Fig. 3.1).

Over half of the cam deformities can be missed using standard axial oblique images only [5]. An alpha angle of 60° discriminates best between asymptomatic and symptomatic subjects [6]. Radial cross-sectional imaging helps depict the labrum and articular cartilage of the hip joint limiting the effects of volume averaging.

3.3.3 MR Arthrography of the Hip

For direct MR arthrography, a dilute gadolinium solution is injected into the joint. The gadolinium improves the contrast-

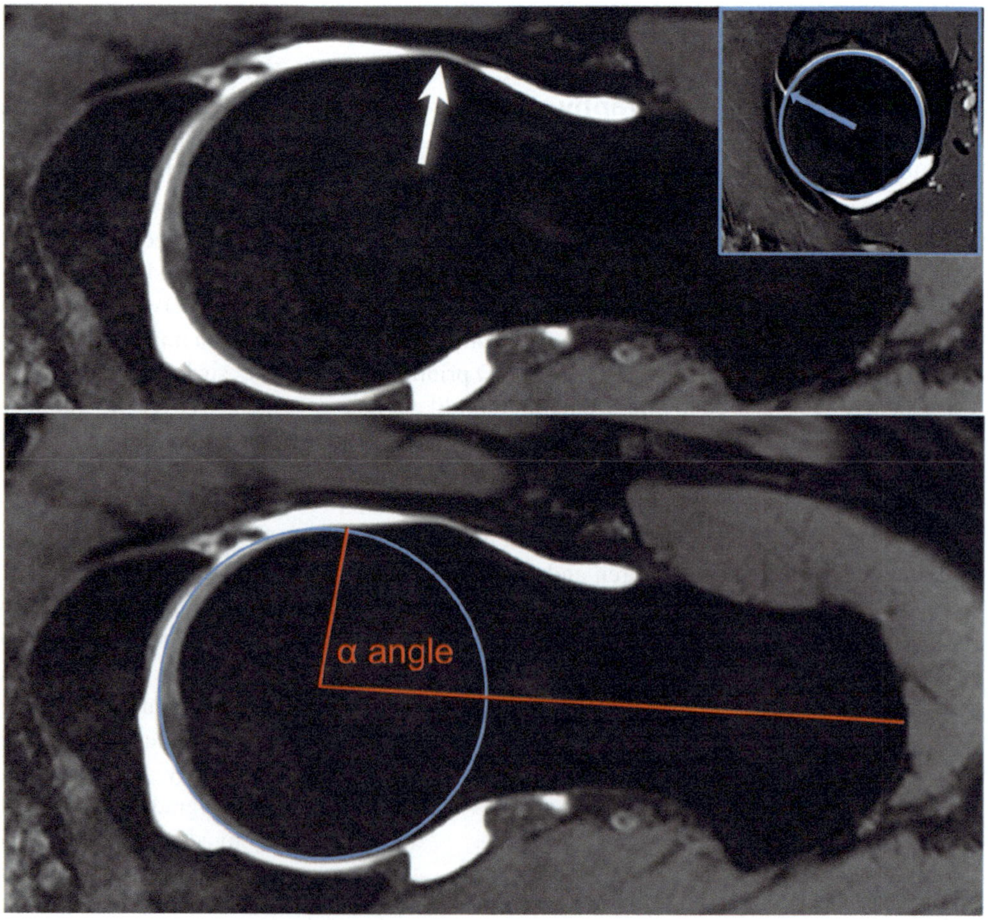

Fig. 3.1 Radial image of an MR arthrography provides optimal delineation of the anterosuperior contour of the femoral head and the head–neck junction. A pronounced cam deformity is displayed (upper image, white arrow). The alpha angle is measured between the femoral neck axis and a line that connects the femoral rotation center and the point where the best-fitting circle intersects with the contour of the femur (lower image)

to-noise ratio of the images. Joint distension optimizes the delineation of the surface of subtle structures of the joint, such as the labrum. Direct MR arthrography may be combined with intra-articular administration of local anesthetics to further characterize the source of pain. The diagnostic performance of MR arthrography is superior to conventional MRI for the diagnosis of labral tears and damage of the acetabular cartilage [7]. For the femoral cartilage lesions, standard, MRI and MR arthrography are similar. The reproducibility of MR arthrography is higher than that of standard MRI [7].

3.3.4 MR Arthrography, Injection Technique

The hip injection is technically not challenging. Several injection techniques for hip arthrography have been described in the literature using ultrasound or fluoroscopy guidance. The proposed techniques include an inferomedial approach (pediatric patients), a lateral supratrochanteric approach, or a straight anterior approach. For the straight anterior approach, using fluoroscopy guidance, targeting either the lateral periphery of the femoral head or the femoral neck is possible. The neck injection technique seems to produce less discomfort but greater extra-articular contrast leakage [8]. MR arthrography is well tolerated [9]. After MR arthrography, temporarily increased joint pain can occur. The volume of the intra-articular injection is between 8 and 12 mL of a 2 mmol/L gadolinium solution.

3.3.5 MR Arthrography of the Hip with Traction

Adding leg traction to MR arthrography of the hip leads to improved visualization of cartilage surfaces. MR arthrography of the hip with leg traction is a safe procedure [10]. The volume of the intra-articular contrast material should be larger than with standard arthrography (25 mL). A weight-adapted axial traction force between 15 and 23 kg is applied [11]. MR arthrography with traction is accurate in identifying central and peripheral intra-articular bodies [12].

3.3.6 MR Imaging of the Labrum

At MR imaging, the normal acetabular labrum is hypointense on all types of sequences, triangular, and firmly attached to the acetabular rim and articular cartilage. Together with the transverse ligament, the labrum forms a complete circle around the acetabulum. Labral damage in FAI typically occurs in the anterosuperior area [13]. Tears of the labrum are characterized by high signal linear changes in the labrum substance. Labral tears can be divided into junction tears and substance tears (Fig. 3.2).

Labral tears are often associated with cartilage damage. Depending on the mechanism, characteristic MR patterns of damage can be observed. In pincer FAI, the labrum is usually small, and small tearing at the base is seen. The associated cartilage damage is limited to the acetabular rim. In Cam

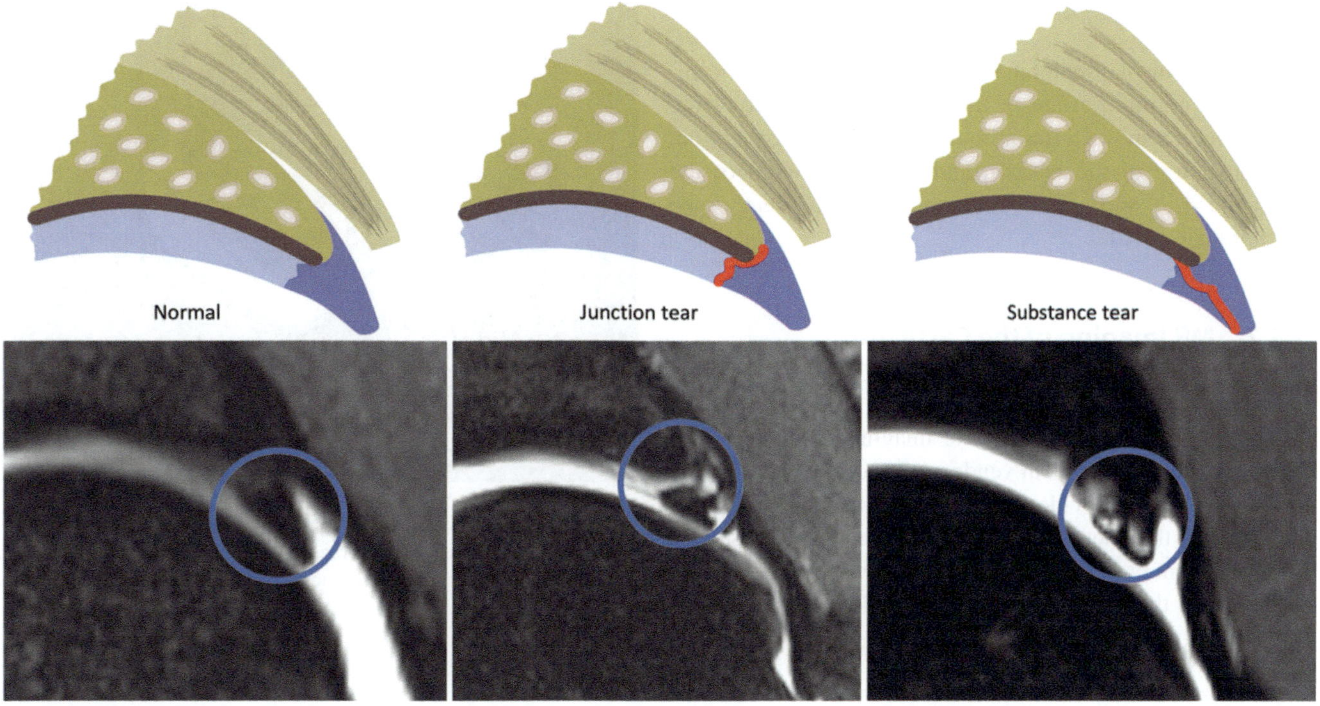

Fig. 3.2 The normal acetabular labrum (left) is hypointense on all types of sequences. The junction tear (center) is characterized as a hyperintense line at the chondrolabral junction. The substance tear (right) is characterized as hyperintense lines/areas extending into the labral substance

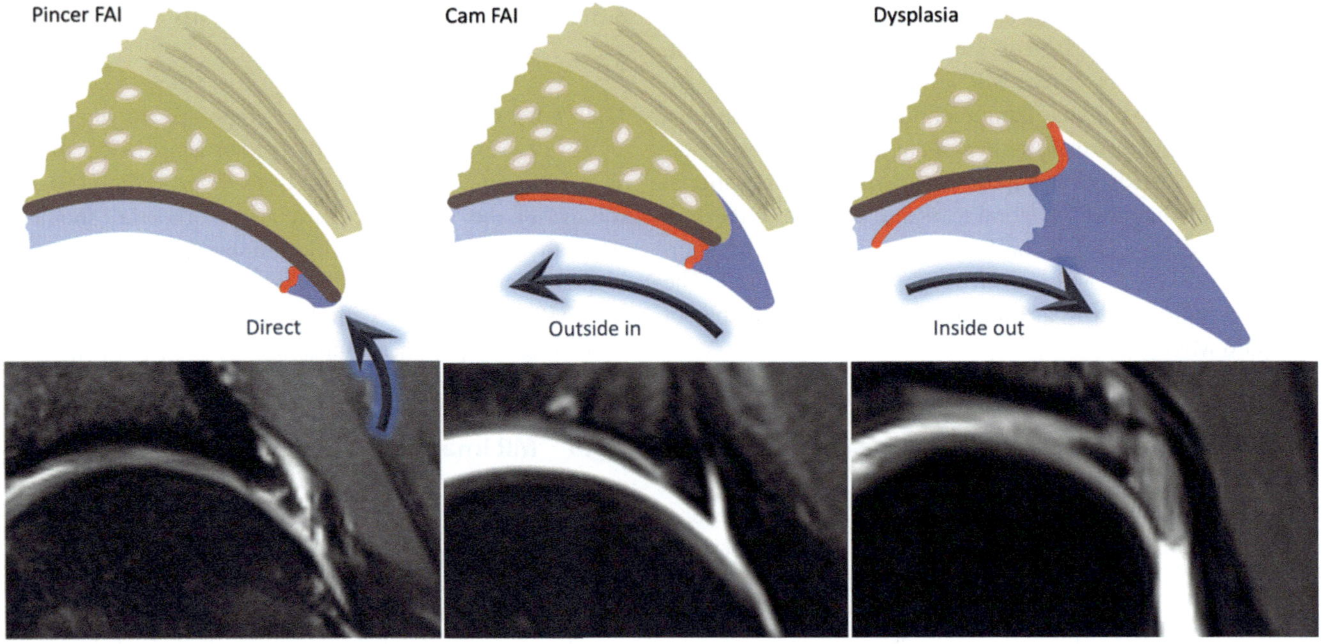

Fig. 3.3 In pincer FAI (left), the labrum is small, and subtle tearing at the base is seen. In Cam FAI (middle), the outside-in shearing force leads to delamination of the cartilage and tears of the labrum. With DDH (right), the pattern of damage is caused by the inside-out shearing force. Note the delaminated acetabular cartilage. The acetabular cartilage is detached together with the labrum. The tear of the labrum extends into the bony attachment at the acetabular rim

FAI, the outside-in shearing force leads to delamination of the cartilage and tears of the labrum at the chondrolabral junction. With DDH, the pattern of damage is caused by the inside-out shearing force. The acetabular cartilage is detached together with the labrum. The tear of the labrum extends into the bony attachment at the acetabular rim (Fig. 3.3).

The labrum may exhibit variants. A recess occurs typically as a normal variant in the anteroinferior part of the joint. A recess shows a linear contrast material interposition, no dislocation of the labrum, and a normal signal of the labrum [14]. A substantial number of labral tears seem to be asymptomatic [15].

3.3.7 MR Imaging of the Cartilage

The articular cartilage of the hip is thin [16]. Many different sequences have been proposed for imaging of the cartilage. The techniques differ from vendor to vendor. Generally, the sequence should provide high-resolution imaging in-plane and in slice thickness [17]. The supraacetabular fossa is a normal variant presenting as a focal zone without cartilage in the center of the acetabulum [18] (Fig. 3.4).

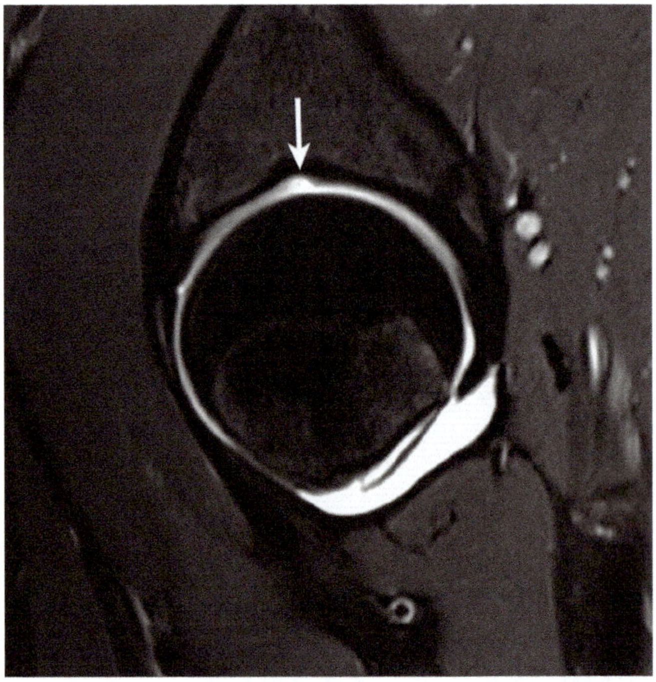

Fig. 3.4 Sagittal MR arthrography image demonstrating a typical supraacetabular fossa. The supraacetabular fossa is a normal variant presenting as a focal zone without cartilage in the center of the acetabulum

The frequency of supraacetabular fossa on MR arthrograms is about 10%. The frequency of the supraacetabular fossa is gradually decreasing with age.

The diagnosis of cartilage delamination at MR imaging is challenging because the cartilage is often realigned onto the subchondral bone without fluid or contrast material interposed [19]. MR arthrography with leg traction improves the differentiation of cartilage layers from 19% to 96% of cases [11] (Fig. 3.5).

FAI-associated focal parafoveal chondral defects have been described. The etiology of these lesions may be related to shearing forces caused by cam deformities or inherent instability of the joint. Parafoveal chondral defects may be difficult to detect and are often missed. The axial oblique imaging plane is often useful to diagnose these defects (Fig. 3.6).

Extensive cartilage damage (more than 2-hour intervals on the clockface) and subchondral acetabular cysts are associated with an increased risk of failure of FAI surgery [20]. It is important to recognize that not all cartilage defects of the hip joint are symptomatic [15].

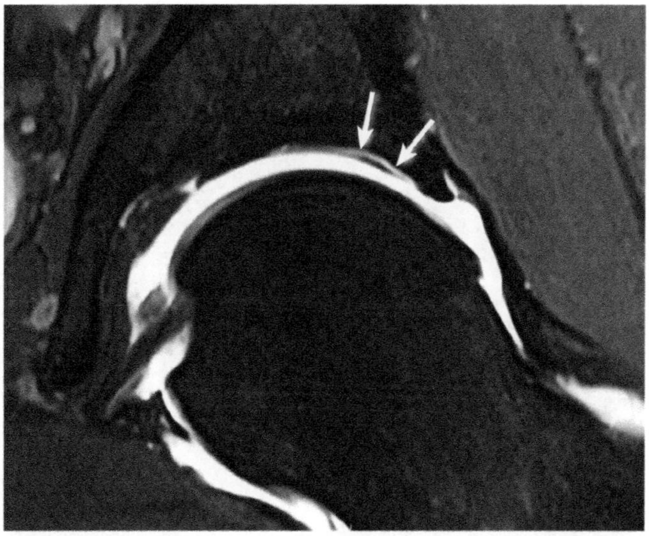

Fig. 3.5 Cartilage delamination is a frequent finding in hips with cam deformities. MR arthrography with traction demonstrates a contrast between the delaminated cartilage and the subchondral bone

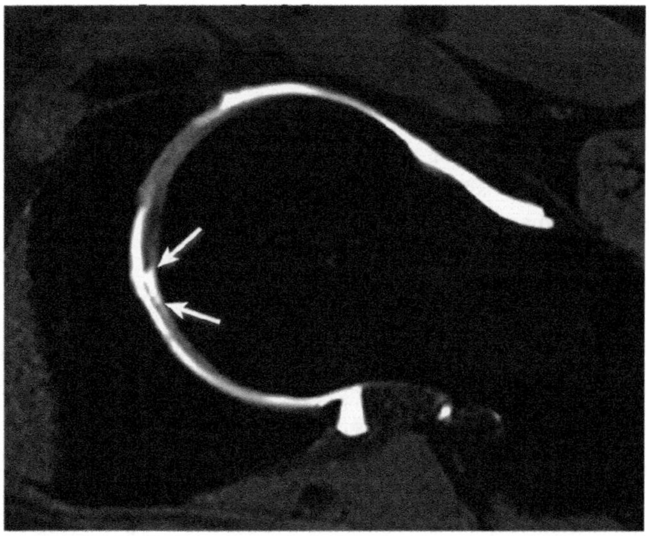

Fig. 3.6 Axial oblique MR arthrography image demonstrating a full-thickness parafoveal chondral defect with focal delamination of the cartilage

3.3.8 Quantitative and Biochemical Assessment of Cartilage

MR imaging has the possibility to assess the biochemical properties of cartilage using techniques such as delayed gadolinium-enhanced MRI of cartilage (dGEMRIC) [21], T2 and T2* mapping, and T1-ρ imaging. Many of the techniques are predominantly used in the research setting. There is increasing evidence that these quantitative imaging techniques may be useful to predict the outcome. In patients with developmental dysplasia of the hip, dGEMRIC can predict failure of periacetabular osteotomies with high accuracy [22] and provides evidence that realignment of the acetabulum can alter the biochemical composition of the articular cartilage [23].

dGEMRIC studies of hips with impingement were performed using a prospective cohort of patients who are at high risk of developing hip osteoarthritis. In hips with cam deformity (alpha angle >60°), lower dGEMRIC values, which indicates cartilage damage, were measured at baseline and there was an association with more joint space narrowing on follow-up radiographs at 5 years, suggesting that compositional MRI such as dGEMRIC has the potential to identify patients that may benefit from early intervention [24]. In a recent study comparing the sensitivity and specificity of standard morphologic MRI and dGEMRIC in detecting cartilage damage at the time of surgery, they found lower dGEMRIC values in clock positions where impingement would occur compared with other locations with the hip. There was also an association of lower dGEMRIC values in hips with cam vs pincer impingement. Furthermore, dGEMRIC was able to detect chondral damage with a higher sensitivity (69%) vs standard morphologic imaging (42%) with a specificity of 83% and an accuracy of 78% [25].

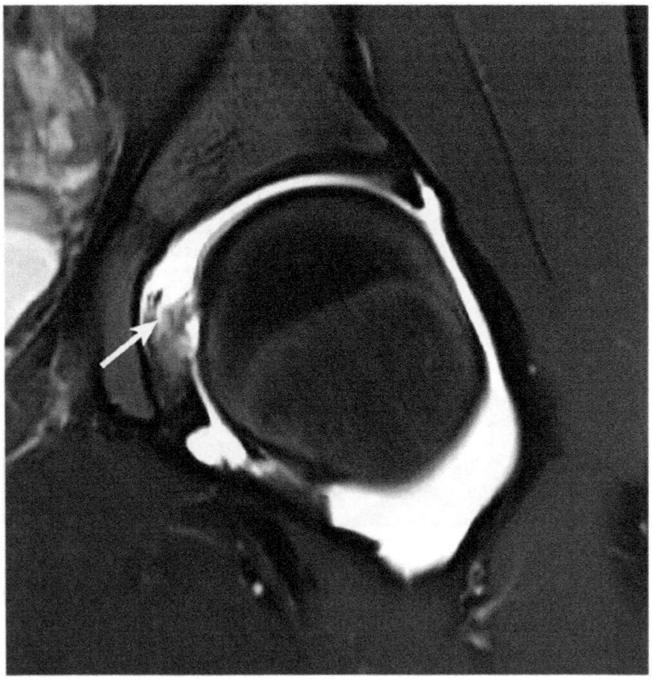

Fig. 3.7 MR arthrography in a patient with a high-grade tear (white arrow) of the ligamentum capitis femoris at its foveal attachment

Attempts have been made to use dGEMRIC as an early objective indicator of joint recovery after impingement surgery. A prospective, nonrandomized, comparative study comparing surgical and nonsurgical treatment for FAI was monitored over a 1-year period by comparing the baseline and follow-up dGEMRIC imaging. In the operative group, despite the improvement in patient-reported outcomes, there was a 96 ms drop in the dGEMRIC values compared with a 16 ms drop in the nonoperative group [26]. Similar findings were noted in a multi-center randomized controlled trial comparing surgical and nonsurgical treatment for FAI. Again, the imaging outcome measure was the dGEMRIC score change from baseline to 1 year. Again, despite an improvement in clinical outcome measures, the surgical group reported a nonsignificant 59 ms decrease in the dGEMRIC values compared with the baseline [27]. Therefore, compositional/biochemical imaging techniques such as dGEMRIC have value in identifying early cartilage biochemical changes and may prove useful in preoperative patient selection. Whether the early changes seen in dGEMRIC after surgery predict long-term outcomes remains to be seen.

3.3.9 Ligamentum Teres

Ligamentum teres tears are a possible source of hip pain. At arthroscopy of the hip tears of the ligamentum teres are often observed (up to 50% of cases) [28]. MR arthrography with traction has a high diagnostic performance to diagnose those tears. Increased articular distraction is observed in patients with complete tears of the ligamentum teres [29] (Fig. 3.7).

3.4 MR Imaging After Surgery

3.4.1 Technical Considerations

At MR imaging, gradient-echo sequences should be replaced by spin-echo sequences or fast spin-echo sequences, because these sequences are less susceptible to metallic artifacts. Spectral fat saturation should be replaced by the Dixon technique or using the short tau inversion recovery technique.

3.4.2 Bone

Bone marrow edema at the site of the osteochondroplasty is normal in the initial phase. Bone marrow edema persisting 3 months after surgery suggests the presence of a stress reaction. Insufficiency fractures of the femoral neck due to bone resection are rare but significant findings [30].

Inappropriate correction of the femoral or acetabular osseous abnormality may lead to persistent symptoms. In post-surgery patients, an α angle of 43° provides impingement-free motion—in subjects without relevant acetabular over coverage [31]. Persistent deformity of the femoral head–neck junction is a common indication for revision hip arthroscopy.

Atypical sites of impingement may persist. For example, arthroscopic correction of the posterosuperior loss of femoral offset is challenging because of the risk of damage to the vascular supply [32]. However, avascular necrosis of the femoral head after arthroscopy is fortunately very rare [33].

After FAI surgery, heterotopic ossification can occur. Heterotopic ossifications are more frequent after surgical hip dislocation than after hip arthroscopy. In a study by Bedi, 5% of the patients developed heterotopic ossification after hip arthroscopy [34].

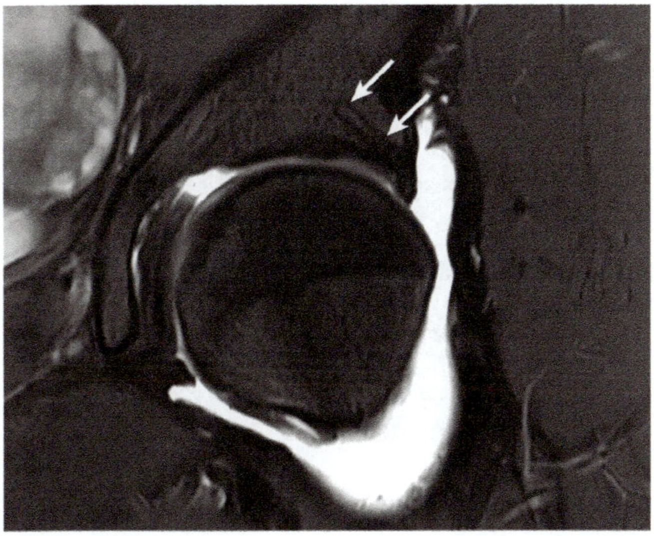

Fig. 3.8 MR arthrography after labral reattachment. The suture anchor presents a hypointense, subtle linear structure (white arrows). The labral reattachment is unremarkable, and no contrast or fluid signal is seen at the base or the substance of the labrum

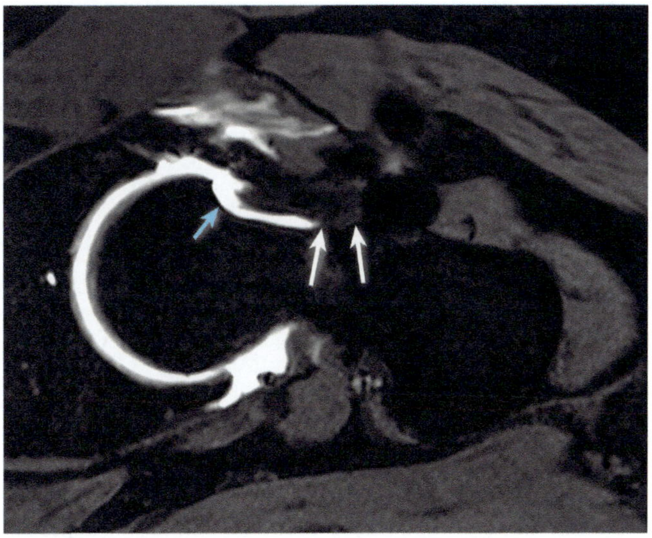

Fig. 3.9 MR arthrography after arthroscopy and osteochondroplasty. Adhesions are seen in the periphery between the joint capsule and the femoral neck (white arrows). Note the contour which is rather excessive with a sharp oteochondral edge of the head–neck junction after the osteochondroplasty (blue arrow). For the diagnosis of capsular adhesions, MR arthrography with joint distention is necessary

3.4.3 Labrum and Cartilage

The suture anchors to reattach the labral after rim debridement or labral repair are placed in the acetabular rim. Depending on the type of material used, the anchor may show different MR appearances. Modern anchors often present as hypointense, very subtle linear structures (Fig. 3.8).

Misplacement of the anchor is rare. A too low position of the anchor may lead to cartilage damage. In the early phase after surgery, fluid and contrast may be seen at the base of the labrum. This should not be overdiagnosed as a tear at least for the first 3 months after surgery.

Ongoing joint degeneration is a reason for persistent pain after surgery. Patients with high-grade cartilage defects had a poor outcome after treatment for FAI after arthroscopic surgery. [35]. Inadequate distraction or forceful entry of instruments may lead to (chondral scuffing) which can be caused by the passage of the arthroscope. The frequency of iatrogenic chondral damage is reported as less than 1% [36].

3.4.4 Soft Tissues

Adhesions tend to occur either between the joint capsule and the osteochondroplasty site at the femoral head–neck junction or between the labrum and the joint capsule [37]. For the diagnosis of capsular adhesions, MR arthrography with joint distention is necessary.

Capsular adhesions at the anterior femoral neck are present in over one-third of asymptomatic and symptomatic patients [35]. Obliteration of the paralabral sulcus is a common asymptomatic finding (Fig. 3.9).

3.5 Assessment of Femoral Torsion

Abnormal femoral torsion affects the biomechanics of the hip joint. Abnormal femoral torsion can aggravate FAI.

Measurement of femoral torsion can be done with CT or MRI. Usually, the measurements are performed on large-FOV transverse MR images over the proximal and distal femur (Fig. 3.10). The reproducibility of femoral torsion using MR imaging is good [38]. However, measurements on oblique images parallel to the femoral neck axis have been proposed as well [39]. Femoral torsion assessment in children is preferably done with MR imaging because of the absence of radiation. Using MRI in children has the advantage that the cartilaginous contours can be used as landmarks [40].

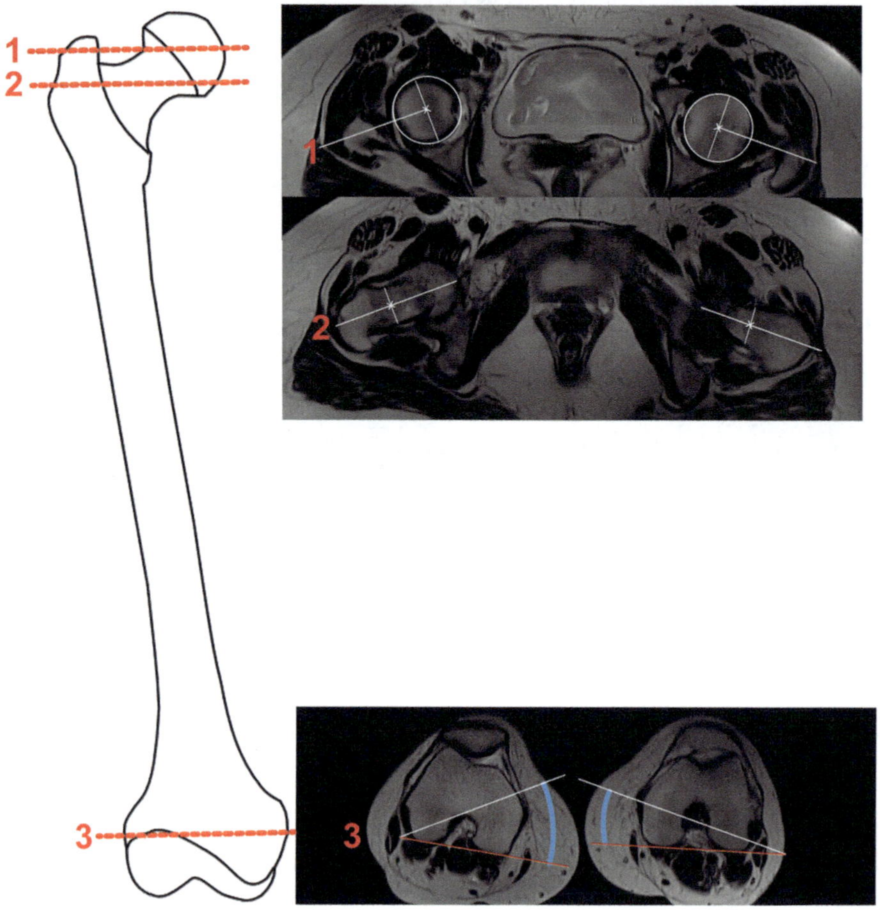

Fig. 3.10 A line connecting the center of the femoral head (1) to the center of the femoral neck (2) is drawn on an image where the anterior and posterior cortices are parallel to each other. A second line is formed by the tangent to the dorsal side of the femoral condyles (3). The femoral torsion is the angle (blue) between these two lines

3.6 Ultrasound

Diagnostic ultrasound is very useful for the evaluation of soft tissues around the hip. The strength lies in the immediate clinical–imaging correlation. The examination can be focused on the painful area. Moreover, dynamic examinations, for example, to evaluate the snapping hip are possible. Functional examinations of vessels and high-resolution assessments of peripheral nerves are possible. Because of the absence of radiation and the comfortable way of its application, ultrasound is preferred in children.

3.6.1 Labrum

The anterosuperior part of the labrum can be well visualized with ultrasound. Diagnosis of labral tears or perilabral cysts at this location is possible using ultrasound [41]. Because a large part of the labrum is not well visualized, the indication to use ultrasound in this regard is limited.

3.6.2 Contour

Ultrasound has been proposed for the evaluation of the anterior head–neck contour to diagnose FAI of the cam type. The detection of a cam deformity is sensitive. However, quantifications, such as alpha angel measurements, were not reliably possible [42].

3.6.3 Postoperative

Ultrasound is rarely used to assess internal derangement. Ultrasound is useful for diagnosing fluid collections and effusions. Ultrasound is useful to guide aspirations.

Recently, dynamic hip ultrasound to assess hip stability and ultrasound-guided diagnostic hip injections have proven very useful in identifying sources of hip pain both in the pre-operative and postoperative setting as well as to identify hip instability post-arthroscopy as well as hips with inherent hip instability that may be a poor candidate for arthroscopic treatment.

Since the inception of hip arthroscopy, the value of diagnostic hip injections has been recognized [43]. A more contemporary study has found that ultrasound assessment and ultrasound-guided hip injection in the setting of atypical symptoms can have high sensitivity (83%), PPV (97%), and accuracy (81%) for cam impingement, 91.7% accuracy for detecting intra-articular abnormality, and 72% sensitivity and accuracy for detection of labral tear compared to arthroscopic assessment [44].

Dynamic hip US is a valuable tool to detect hip instability either due to ligamentous laxity or iatrogenic instability that may be caused by prior hip arthroscopy. When the technique is standardized, the inter- and intra-rater reliability was excellent for the neutral flex (NF), extension and external rotation off the side of the table (EER1), and extension and external rotation off the bottom of the table (EER2) [45] (Figs. 3.11 and 3.12).

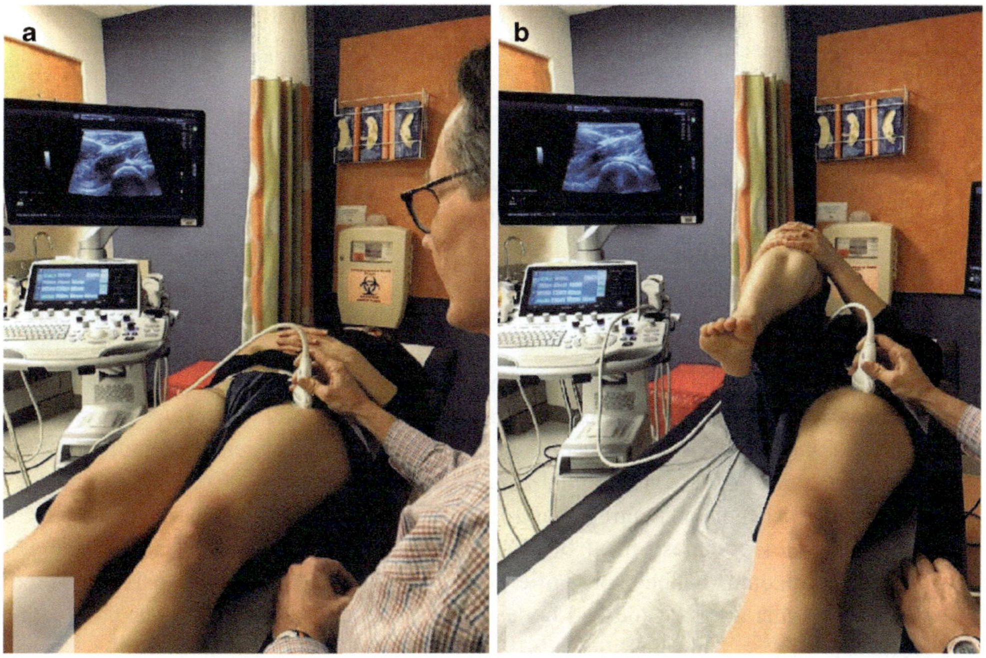

Fig. 3.11 (**a**) Neutral position. (**b**) Neutral flexed (NF) position

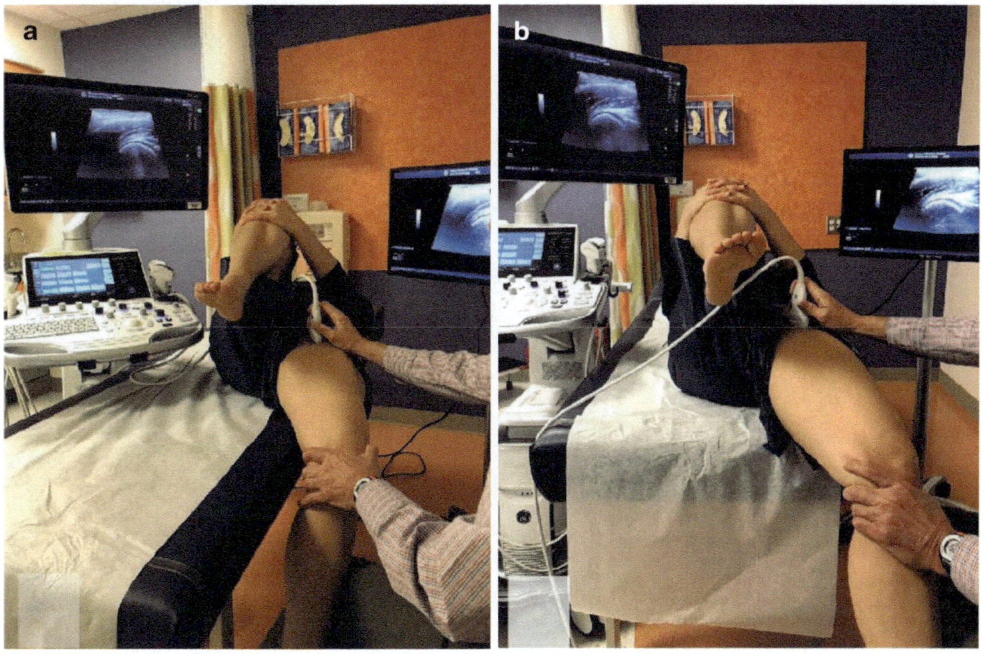

Fig. 3.12 (**a**) EER1-imaged hip held in extension and external rotation by the physician and the contralateral hip held in flexion by the patient. (**b**) EER2-examined hip is held off the bottom of the table by the physician, while the contralateral hip is held in flexion

Using this standardized dynamic hip ultrasound technique, 142 volunteer adolescent dancers (117 females and 25 males) were examined to assess the range of anterior hip translation seen in this population. For female hips, the mean (± SD) translation (EER2-NF positions) of the femoral head was 1.23 ± 2.01 mm, and for male hips, the mean translation was 1.39 ± 2.22 mm [46]. The goal is to better define the normative range as well as to better define the association between ligamentous laxity and femoral head translation. A preliminary study in female dancers with and without hip pain showed increased translation and high Beighton scores in the patients experiencing hip pain [47].

3.7 Characteristic Bone Tumors, Synovial Tumors, and Tumor-Like Conditions About the Hip Joint

3.7.1 Osteoid Osteoma

Osteoid osteoma is a small tumor, typical in young patients, with a peak incidence between 5 and 25 years [48]. Patients present with constant, usually low-level pain and often pain at night. Pain relief with non-steroidal anti-inflammatory drugs is typical. The main imaging feature of the osteoid osteoma is the nidus, which is a local, often rounded radiolucent area. In the center of the nidus, often calcification is found. There is characteristic marked bone marrow edema and soft tissue edema around the nidus. At MR imaging, the nidus may be difficult to detect, especially in peripheral or subperiosteal locations. An additional CT or scintigraphy is often necessary for the confirmation of the diagnosis. The nidus is highly vascularized. Any unexplained marked bone marrow edema in a young patient with night pain should prompt the search for an osteoid osteoma. In the hip, the nidus is often located cortical or subperiosteal. In this location, the osteoid osteoma may manifest as an intense arthritis with marked synovitis [49]. If left untreated, this synovitis will result in extensive, irreversible cartilage damage (Fig. 3.13).

3.7.2 Osteochondroma

Osteochondroma are benign osteocartilaginous tumors. Multiple hereditary exostoses (MHE) is an autosomal dominant disorder. MHE is characterized by multiple osteochondroma. Osteochondroma are typically located near the growth plates at the metaphysis of long bones. Osteochondroma can cause significant osseous deformities and therefore impingement syndromes around the hip. Furthermore, patients with MHE often present with coxa valga. Coxa valga and the presence of an osteochondroma may both reduce the ischio-femoral distance and lead to ischio-femoral impingement [50].

The exostosis is covered by a cartilage cap. In young children, almost the complete osteochondroma is constituted of

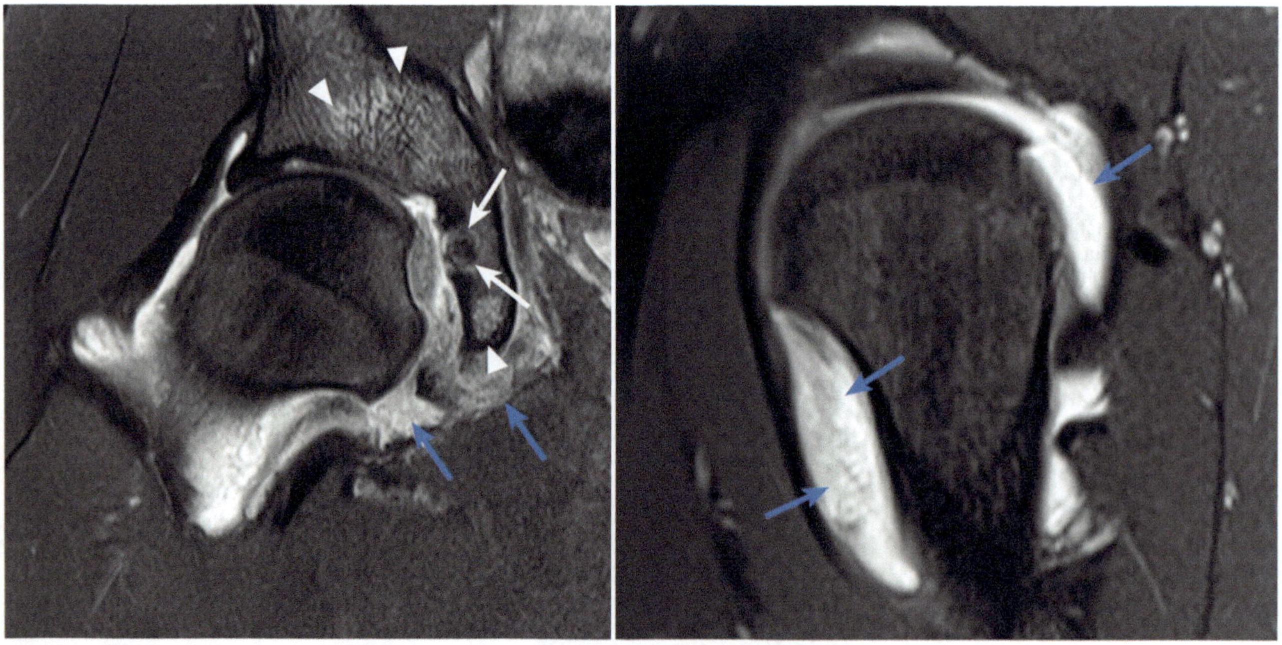

Fig. 3.13 Coronal fluid-sensitive image of a right hip in a 20-year-old man with an osteoid osteoma in the central area of the acetabulum. The nidus is located in the fossa acetabuli (arrows) and leads to extensive bone marrow edema (arrowheads). The osteoid osteoma manifests as intense arthritis with marked synovitis (blue arrows)

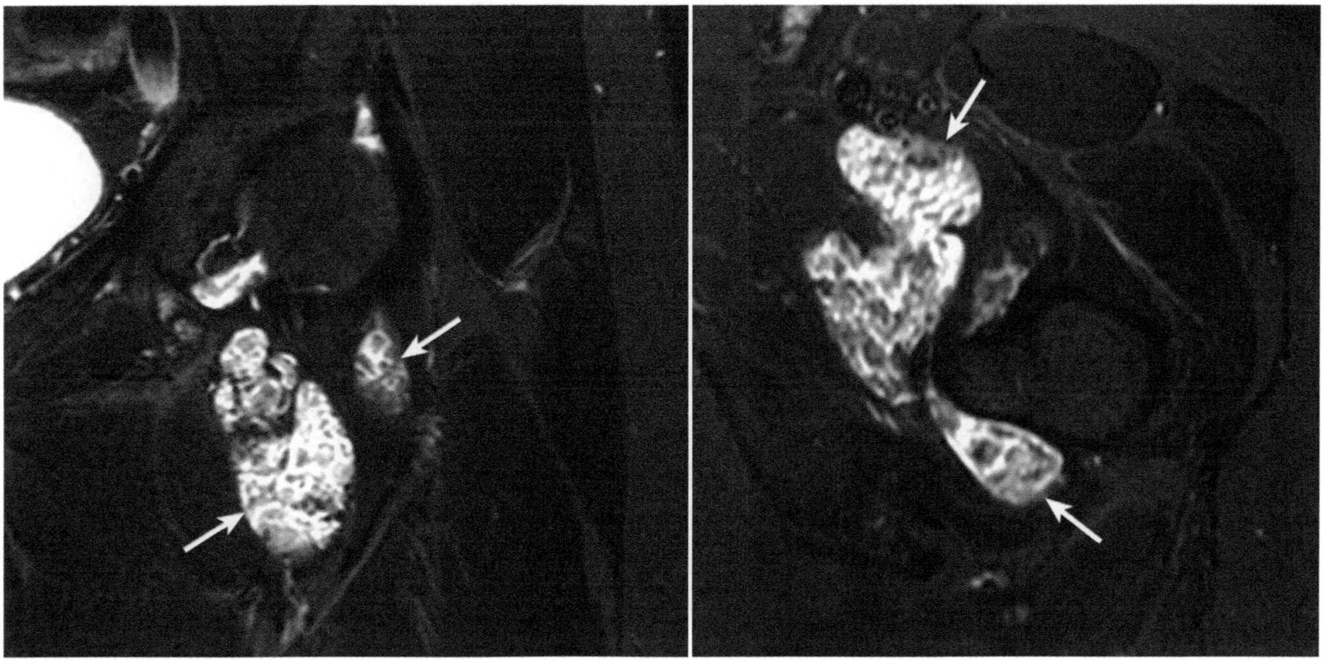

Fig. 3.14 Coronal and axial fluid-sensitive image of a left hip in a 32-year-old man with a primary synovial chondromatosis. Note marked effusion with extensive synovial nodular proliferations

a cartilage. Standard radiographs are the basis for the radiological diagnosis. MRI shows the characteristic continuity from the cortical bone into the mature bone of the exostosis. Ultrasound or MR imaging can detect neo-bursa formation around the tip of the osteochondroma. The exostosis may lead to entrapment of the nerves and vessels, usually diagnosed by MR imaging. Malignant transformation of exostosis in MHE is rare. MRI precisely shows the extent and shape of the cartilage cap. A cartilage cap thickness of greater than 2 cm [51] in a skeletally mature patient is suspicious for malignant transformation with a sensitivity and specificity of more than 95%.

3.7.3 Synovial Chondromatosis

A primary and a secondary synovial chondromatosis are differentiated. The primary synovial chondromatosis is a metaplasia of the synovium. In early primary synovial chondromatosis, there is only synovial reaction without loose bodies. Later uncalcified cartilaginous bodies are formed, which are not visible on plain radiographs. These loose bodies may calcify or ossify; however, one-third of the cases still are negative on radiographs [52]. The synovial chondromas in primary synovial chondromatosis are uniform, numerous, and small. The synovial chondromas primary synovial chondromatosis may completely fill the whole joint cavity. Secondary synovial chondromatosis is secondary to other joint disorders, such as osteoarthritis, avascular necrosis, osteochondritis dissecans, and rheumatoid arthritis. In the hip joint, this may arise from preexisting conditions such as Legg-Calve-Perthes disease or osteochondroma [53] (Fig. 3.14).

3.7.4 Pigmented Villonodular Synovitis

Pigmented villonodular synovitis (PVNS) is a benign intra-articular tumor causing villous, nodular, or villonodular synovial hyperplasia and hemosiderin deposition [54]. Typically, PVNS presents as nodular intra-articular tumors without calcifications. At MRI, the PVNS often shows a typical hypointense signal on T2-weighted images because of the hemosiderin deposition. Signal hypointensity is best visible with gradient echo imaging. The susceptibility artifact causes a blooming effect which indicates the presence of hemosiderin. Contrast enhancement is variable. There is also a diffuse form of PVNS. The PVNS may lead to marginal bony erosions, bony destructions, subchondral cysts, and cartilage lesions. The diffuse form presents as synovial proliferation at imaging and is often difficult to differentiate from inflammatory synovitis caused by arthritis. Often a biopsy is necessary for the diagnosis of PVNS (Fig. 3.15).

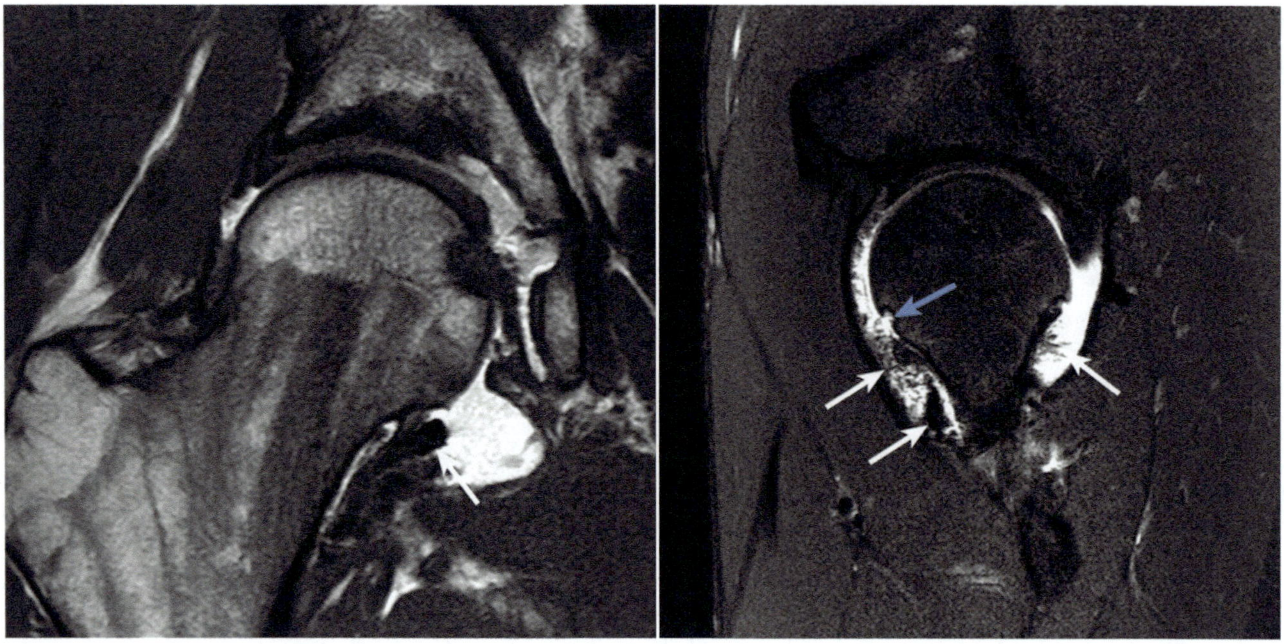

Fig. 3.15 Coronal T1-weighted (left image) and sagittal T2-weighted fluid-sensitive image (right image) of a right hip in a 27-year-old man with PVNS. The PVNS presents as a nodular hypointense signal mass medial to the calcar (arrows). On the T2 weighted image (right image part), the synovial proliferations are markedly hypointense because of the hemosiderin deposition. Note small erosion of the anterior cortex of the femoral neck (blue arrow)

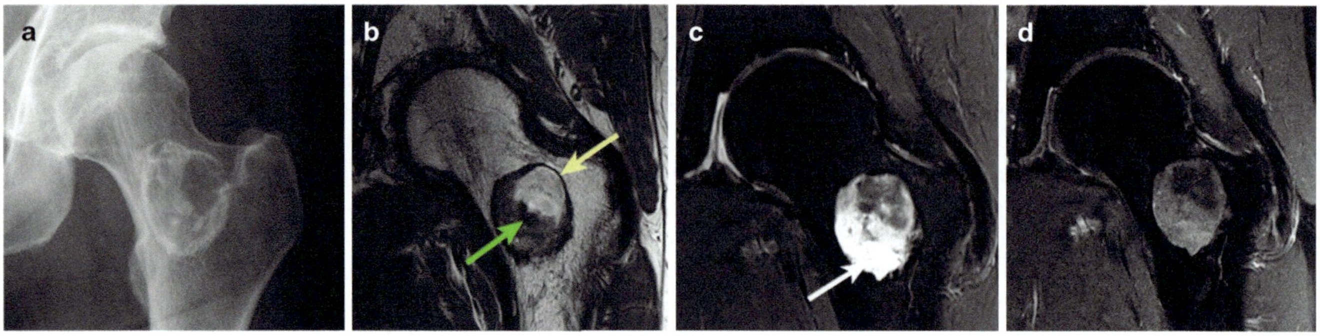

Fig. 3.16 AP-radiograph (**a**), coronal T1-weighted (**b**), coronal T2-weighted fat saturated (**c**), and coronal T1-weighted fat-saturated, contrast-enhanced MR image (**d**) of a left hip in a 64-year-old man with LSMFT of the proximal femur. The tumor shows an osteolysis with a marked sclerotic margin on the standard radiograph. At the T1-weighted image (**b**), fat and fibrous/sclerotic areas are visible. At the T2-weighted fat-saturated image (**c**), myxoid areas are visible. At the coronal T1-weighted fat-saturated, contrast-enhanced MR image (**d**), only a very mild enhancement is seen

3.7.5 Liposclerosing Myxofibrous Tumor

Liposclerosing myxofibrous tumor (LSMFT) is a very typical tumor of the intertrochanteric region of the proximal femur [55]. The fifth edition of the World Health Organization Classification of soft tissue and bone tumors [56] states that the LSMFT should be preferably called "fibrous dysplasia." The tumor presents as an osteolysis usually with marked sclerotic margins. At MRI, the signal is heterogeneous with a prominent fluid-like signal with fibrotic and sclerotic areas. The fatty component can be small or missing. The peak incidence is the fourth decade of life. The tumor is usually nonaggressive; however, malignant transformation has been described. Imaging follow-up is recommended, especially in patients developing symptoms (Fig. 3.16).

References

1. Griffin DR, Dickenson EJ, O'Donnell J. Infographic. The Warwick agreement on femoroacetabular impingement syndrome. Br J Sports Med. 2016;50(19):1179. https://doi.org/10.1136/bjsports-2016-096868.
2. Castro MO, Mascarenhas VV, Afonso PD, Rego P, Schmaranzer F, Sutter R, Kassarjian A, Sconfienza L, Dienst M, Ayeni OR, Beaulé PE, Dantas P, Lalam R, Weber MA, Vanhoenacker FM, Dietrich TJ, Jans L, Robinson P, Karantanas AH, Sudoł-Szopińska I, Anderson S, Noebauer-Huhmann I, Marin-Peña O, Collado D, Tey-Pons M, Schmaranzer E, Padron M, Kramer J, Zingg PO, De Maeseneer M, Llopis E. The Lisbon agreement on femoroacetabular impingement imaging-part 3: imaging techniques. Eur Radiol. 2021;31(7):4652–68. https://doi.org/10.1007/s00330-020-07501-5. Epub 2021 Jan 7.
3. Stern C, Sommer S, Germann C, Galley J, Pfirrmann CWA, Fritz B, Sutter R. Pelvic bone CT: can tin-filtered ultra-low-dose CT and virtual radiographs be used as alternative for standard CT and digital radiographs? Eur Radiol. 2021;31(9):6793–801.
4. Nötzli HP, Wyss TF, Stoecklin CH, Schmid MR, Treiber K, Hodler J. The contour of the femoral head-neck junction as a predictor for the risk of anterior impingement. J Bone Joint Surg Br. 2002;84(4):556–60. https://doi.org/10.1302/0301-620x.84b4.12014.
5. Pfirrmann CW, Mengiardi B, Dora C, Kalberer F, Zanetti M, Hodler J. Cam and pincer femoroacetabular impingement: characteristic MR arthrographic findings in 50 patients. Radiology. 2006;240(3):778–85. https://doi.org/10.1148/radiol.2403050767. Epub 2006 Jul 20.
6. Sutter R, Dietrich TJ, Zingg PO, Pfirrmann CW. How useful is the alpha angle for discriminating between symptomatic patients with cam-type femoroacetabular impingement and asymptomatic volunteers? Radiology. 2012;264(2):514–21. https://doi.org/10.1148/radiol.121.
7. Sutter R, Zubler V, Hoffmann A, Mamisch-Saupe N, Dora C, Kalberer F, Zanetti M, Hodler J, Pfirrmann CW. Hip MRI: how useful is intraarticular contrast material for evaluating surgically proven lesions of the labrum and articular cartilage? AJR Am J Roentgenol. 2014;202(1):160–9.
8. Duc SR, Hodler J, Schmid MR, Zanetti M, Mengiardi B, Dora C, Pfirrmann CW. Prospective evaluation of two different injection techniques for MR arthrography of the hip. Eur Radiol. 2006;16(2):473–8. https://doi.org/10.1007/s00330-005-2865-z. Epub 2005 Aug 16. PMI.
9. Saupe N, Zanetti M, Pfirrmann CW, Wels T, Schwenke C, Hodler J. Pain and other side effects after MR arthrography: prospective evaluation in 1085 patients. Radiology. 2009;250(3):830–8. https://doi.org/10.1148/radiol.2503080276. Epub 2009 Jan 21.
10. Llopis E, Cerezal L, Kassarjian A, Higueras V, Fernandez E. Direct MR arthrography of the hip with leg traction: feasibility for assessing articular cartilage. AJR Am J Roentgenol. 2008;190(4):1124–8. https://doi.org/10.2214/AJR.07.2559.
11. Schmaranzer F, Klauser A, Kogler M, Henninger B, Forstner T, Reichkendler M, Schmaranzer E. Diagnostic performance of direct traction MR arthrography of the hip: detection of chondral and labral lesions with arthroscopic comparison. Eur Radiol. 2015;25:1721.
12. Schmaranzer F, Lerch TD, Strasser U, Vavron P, Schmaranzer E, Tannast M. Usefulness of MR arthrography of the hip with and without leg traction in detection of intra-articular bodies. Acad Radiol. 2019;26(9):e252–9. https://doi.org/10.1016/j.acra.2018.10.008.
13. Ito K, Leunig M, Ganz R. Histopathologic features of the acetabular labrum in femoroacetabular impingement. Clin Orthop Relat Res. 2004;429:262–71. https://doi.org/10.1097/01.blo.0000144861.11193.17.
14. Studler U, Kalberer F, Leunig M, Zanetti M, Hodler J, Dora C, Pfirrmann CW. MR arthrography of the hip: differentiation between an anterior sublabral recess as a normal variant and a labral tear. Radiology. 2008;249(3):947–54. https://doi.org/10.1148/radiol.2492.
15. Tresch F, Dietrich TJ, Pfirrmann CWA, Sutter R. Hip MRI: prevalence of articular cartilage defects and labral tears in asymptomatic volunteers. A comparison with a matched population of patients with femoroacetabular impingement. J Magn Reson Imaging. 2017;46:440.
16. Hodler J, Yu JS, Goodwin D, Haghighi P, Trudell D, Resnick D. MR arthrography of the hip: improved imaging of the acetabular labrum with histologic correlation in cadavers. AJR Am J Roentgenol. 1995;165(4):887–91. https://doi.org/10.2214/ajr.165.4.7676987.
17. Knuesel PR, Pfirrmann CW, Noetzli HP, Dora C, Zanetti M, Hodler J, Kuehn B, Schmid MR. MR arthrography of the hip: diagnostic performance of a dedicated water-excitation 3D double-echo steady-state sequence to detect cartilage lesions. AJR Am J Roentgenol. 2004;183(6):1729.
18. Dietrich TJ, Suter A, Pfirrmann CW, Dora C, Fucentese SF, Zanetti M. Supraacetabular fossa (pseudodefect of acetabular cartilage): frequency at MR arthrography and comparison of findings at MR arthrography and arthroscopy. Radiology. 2012;263(2):484–9.
19. Pfirrmann CW, Duc SR, Zanetti M, Dora C, Hodler J. MR arthrography of acetabular cartilage delamination in femoroacetabular cam impingement. Radiology. 2008;249(1):236–41. https://doi.org/10.1148/radiol.2491080093. Epub 2008 Aug 5.
20. Hanke MS, Steppacher SD, Anwander H, Werlen S, Siebenrock KA, Tannast M. What MRI findings predict failure 10 years after surgery for femoroacetabular impingement? Clin Orthop Relat Res. 2017;475(4):1192–207. https://doi.org/10.1007/s11999-016-5040-8. Erratum i
21. Burstein D, Bashir A, Gray ML. MRI techniques in early stages of cartilage disease. Invest Radiol. 2000;35(10):622–38.
22. Kim SD, Jessel R, Zurakowski D, Millis MB, Kim YJ. Anterior delayed gadolinium-enhanced MRI of cartilage values predict joint failure after periacetabular osteotomy. Clin Orthop Relat Res. 2012;470(12):3332–41. https://doi.org/10.1007/s11999-012-2519-9.
23. Hingsammer AM, Kalish LA, Stelzeneder D, Bixby S, Mamisch TC, Connell P, Millis MB, Kim YJ. Does periacetabular osteotomy for hip dysplasia modulate cartilage biochemistry? J Bone Joint Surg Am. 2015;97(7):544–50. https://doi.org/10.2106/JBJS.M.01233.
24. Palmer A, Fernquest S, Rombach I, Park D, Pollard T, Broomfield J, Bangerter N, Carr A, Glyn-Jones S. Diagnostic and prognostic value of delayed Gadolinium Enhanced Magnetic Resonance Imaging of Cartilage (dGEMRIC) in early osteoarthritis of the hip. Osteoarthr Cartil. 2017;25(9):1468–77.
25. Lerch TD, Ambühl D, Schmaranzer F, Todorski IAS, Steppacher SD, Hanke MS, Haefeli PC, Liechti EF, Siebenrock KA, Tannast M. Biochemical MRI with dGEMRIC corresponds to 3D-CT based impingement location for detection of acetabular cartilage damage in FAI patients. Orthop J Sports Med. 2021;9(3):2325967120988175.
26. Schmaranzer F, Haefeli PC, Hanke MS, Liechti EF, Werlen SF, Siebenrock KA, Tannast M. How does the dGEMRIC index change after surgical treatment for FAI? A prospective controlled study: preliminary results. Clin Orthop Relat Res. 2017;475(4):1080–99.
27. Hunter DJ, Eyles J, Murphy NJ, Spiers L, Burns A, Davidson E, Dickenson E, Fary C, Foster NE, Fripp J, Griffin DR, Hall M, Kim YJ, Linklater JM, Molnar R, Neubert A, O'Connell RL, O'Donnell J, O'Sullivan M, Randhawa S, Reichenbach S, Schmaranzer F, Singh P, Tran P, Wilson D, Zhang H, Bennell KL. Multi-centre randomised controlled trial comparing arthroscopic hip surgery to physiotherapist-led care for femoroacetabular impingement (FAI) syndrome on hip cartilage metabolism: the Australian FASHIoN trial. BMC Musculoskelet Disord. 2021;22(1):697. https://doi.

org/10.1186/s12891-021-04576-z. PubMed PMID: 34399702; PubMed Central PMCID: PMC8369620.
28. Botser IB, Martin DE, Stout CE, Domb BG. Tears of the ligamentum teres: prevalence in hip arthroscopy using 2 classification systems. Am J Sports Med. 2011;39(Suppl):117S–25S. https://doi.org/10.1177/0363546511413865.
29. Cerezal L, Carro LP, Llorca J, Fernández-Hernando M, Llopis E, Montero JA, Canga A. Usefulness of MR arthrography of the hip with leg traction in the evaluation of ligamentum teres injuries. Skeletal Radiol. 2015;44(11):1585–95. https://doi.org/10.1007/s00256-01.
30. Mardones RM, Gonzalez C, Chen Q, Zobitz M, Kaufman KR, Trousdale RT. Surgical treatment of femoroacetabular impingement: evaluation of the effect of the size of the resection. Surgical technique. J Bone Joint Surg Am. 2006;88(Suppl 1 Pt 1):84–91.
31. Neumann M, Cui Q, Siebenrock KA, Beck M. Impingement-free hip motion: the 'normal' angle alpha after osteochondroplasty. Clin Orthop Relat Res. 2009;467(3):699–703. https://doi.org/10.1007/s11999-008-0616-6. Epub 2008 Nov 19. PMID: 19018605; PMCID: PMC2635435.
32. Bedi A, Zaltz I, De La Torre K, Kelly BT. Radiographic comparison of surgical hip dislocation and hip arthroscopy for treatment of cam deformity in femoroacetabular impingement. Am J Sports Med. 2011;39(Suppl):20S–8S. https://doi.org/10.1177/0363546511412734.
33. Harris JD, McCormick FM, Abrams GD, Gupta AK, Ellis TJ, Bach BR Jr, Bush-Joseph CA, Nho SJ. Complications and reoperations during and after hip arthroscopy: a systematic review of 92 studies and more than 6000 patients. Arthroscopy. 2013;29(3):589–95.
34. Bedi A, Zbeda RM, Bueno VF, Downie B, Dolan M, Kelly BT. The incidence of heterotopic ossification after hip arthroscopy. Am J Sports Med. 2012;40(4):854–63. https://doi.org/10.1177/0363546511434285. Epub 2012 Jan 20.
35. Kim CO, Dietrich TJ, Zingg PO, Dora C, Pfirrmann CWA, Sutter R. Arthroscopic hip surgery: frequency of postoperative MR arthrographic findings in asymptomatic and symptomatic patients. Radiology. 2017;283(3):779–88. https://doi.org/10.1148/radiol.2016161078.
36. Sampson TG. Complications of hip arthroscopy. Clin Sports Med. 2001;20(4):831–5. https://doi.org/10.1016/s0278-5919(05)70288-x.
37. Beck M. Groin pain after open FAI surgery: the role of intraarticular adhesions. Clin Orthop Relat Res. 2009;467(3):769–74. https://doi.org/10.1007/s11999-008-0653-1. Epub 2008 Dec 10. PMID: 19082679; PMCID: PMC2635436.
38. Sutter R, Dietrich TJ, Zingg PO, Pfirrmann CW. Femoral antetorsion: comparing asymptomatic volunteers and patients with femoroacetabular impingement. Radiology. 2012;263(2):475–83. https://doi.org/10.1148/radiol.12111903. Epub 2012 Mar 8.
39. Sutter R, Dietrich TJ, Zingg PO, Pfirrmann CW. Assessment of femoral antetorsion with MRI: comparison of oblique measurements to standard transverse measurements. AJR Am J Roentgenol. 2015;205(1):130–5. https://doi.org/10.2214/AJR.14.13617.
40. Rosskopf AB, Agten CA, Ramseier LE, Pfirrmann CWA, Buck FM. Femoral torsion assessment with MRI in children: should we use the bony or cartilaginous contours? Eur J Radiol. 2017;92:153–8. https://doi.org/10.1016/j.ejrad.2017.04.021. Epub 2017 May 1.
41. Billham J, Cornelson SM, Koch A, Nunez M Jr, Estrada P, Kettner N. Diagnosing acetabular labral tears with hip traction sonography: a case series. J Ultrasound. 2021;24(4):547–53. https://doi.org/10.1007/s40477-020-00446-x. Epub 2020 Apr 2. PMID: 32240531; PMCI.
42. Buck FM, Hodler J, Zanetti M, Dora C, Pfirrmann CW. Ultrasound for the evaluation of femoroacetabular impingement of the cam type. Diagnostic performance of qualitative criteria and alpha angle measurements. Eur Radiol. 2011;21(1):167–75. https://doi.org/10.1007/s00330-010-1900-x.
43. Byrd JW, Jones KS. Diagnostic accuracy of clinical assessment, magnetic resonance imaging, magnetic resonance arthrography, and intra-articular injection in hip arthroscopy patients. Am J Sports Med. 2004;32(7):1668–74. https://doi.org/10.1177/03635465042664.
44. Gao G, Fu Q, Wu R, Liu R, Cui L, Xu Y. Ultrasound and ultrasound-guided hip injection have high accuracy in the diagnosis of femoroacetabular impingement with atypical symptoms. Arthroscopy. 2021;37(1):128–35. https://doi.org/10.1016/j.arthro.2020.08.013.
45. d'Hemecourt PA, Sugimoto D, McKee-Proctor M, Zwicker RL, Jackson SS, Novais EN, Kim YJ, Millis MB, Stracciolini A. Can dynamic ultrasonography of the hip reliably assess anterior femoral head translation? Clin Orthop Relat Res. 2019;477(5):1086–98.
46. Jackson S, Whitney KE, Lanois CJ, Yen YM, Owen M, d'Hemecourt P. Ultrasound observation of hip translational motion in adolescent dancers. J Dance Med Sci. 2021;25(2):105–9. https://doi.org/10.12678/1089-313X.061521e. Epub 2021 Mar 29.
47. Scott CP, d'Hemecourt PA, Miller PE, Sugimoto D, Jackson SS, Kobelski GP, Whitney KE, Stracciolini A. Femoroacetabular translation in female athletes and dancers assessed by dynamic hip ultrasonography. BMJ Open Sport Exerc Med. 2021;7(4):e001169.
48. Greenspan A. Benign bone-forming lesions: osteoma, osteoid osteoma, and osteoblastoma. Clinical, imaging, pathologic, and differential considerations. Skeletal Radiol. 1993;22(7):485–500. https://doi.org/10.1007/BF00209095.
49. Chandan N, Paul N, J P, Kaganur R. Intra-articular osteoid osteoma of the hip mimicking as monoarthritis—a case report. J Orthop Case Rep. 2022;12(10):18–21. https://doi.org/10.13107/jocr.2022.v12.i10.3348.
50. Ahn YS, Kim S, Kim WJ, Lim JH, Jung ST. Characteristics of hip impingement syndrome in patients with multiple hereditary exostoses. BMC Musculoskelet Disord. 2021;22(1):153. https://doi.org/10.1186/s12891-021-04021-1.
51. Bernard SA, Murphey MD, Flemming DJ, Kransdorf MJ. Improved differentiation of benign osteochondromas from secondary chondrosarcomas with standardized measurement of cartilage cap at CT and MR imaging. Radiology. 2010;255(3):857–65. https://doi.org/10.1148/radiol.10082120.
52. Knoeller SM. Synovial osteochondromatosis of the hip joint. Etiology, diagnostic investigation and therapy. Acta Orthop Belg. 2001;67(3):201–10.
53. Peh WC, Shek TW, Davies AM, Wong JW, Chien EP. Osteochondroma and secondary synovial osteochondromatosis. Skeletal Radiol. 1999;28(3):169–74. https://doi.org/10.1007/s002560050495.
54. Murphey MD, Rhee JH, Lewis RB, Fanburg-Smith JC, Flemming DJ, Walker EA. Pigmented villonodular synovitis: radiologic-pathologic correlation. Radiographics. 2008;28(5):1493–518. https://doi.org/10.1148/rg.285085134.
55. Kransdorf MJ, Murphey MD, Sweet DE. Liposclerosing myxofibrous tumor: a radiologic-pathologic-distinct fibro-osseous lesion of bone with a marked predilection for the intertrochanteric region of the femur. Radiology. 1999;212(3):693–8. https://doi.org/10.1148/radiology.212.3.r99se40693.
56. WHO Classification of Tumours Editorial Board. Soft tissue and bone tumours. International Agency for Research on Cancer, Lyon, France; 2020. ISBNs 978-9-28-324502-5.

4 Computer Modeling: Collision Models

Moritz Tannast and Asheesh Bedi

4.1 Brief Description

- The hip joint is a complex load-bearing structure with variable degrees of range of motion (ROM) based on proximal femoral and acetabular morphology and soft tissue constraints.
- Femoroacetabular impingement (FAI) secondary to abnormal proximal femoral morphology, acetabular morphology, or both is a leading cause of pre-arthritic hip pain and secondary osteoarthritis of the hip.
- Dysplasia of the hip, typically secondary to decreased acetabular volume and abnormal morphology, results in increased contact pressures and secondary instability.
- Modeling using 3D imaging and collision detection is not without limitations, but can allow for an improved understanding of hip kinematics and mechanical conflict, and may help with preoperative planning for the ideal hip preservation procedure.

4.2 Background

- FAI is usually seen in active, young adults.
- Studies have shown the prevalence rate of cam-type proximal femoral morphology to be 14% in the general population [1].
- The prevalence of FAI is higher in an athletic population. In elite hockey players, the incidence of radiographic cam-type deformity is 69.4%, and in male, elite soccer players, cam and pincer-type lesions were observed in 68% and 26.7% of players, respectively [2, 3].

M. Tannast
Department of Orthopaedic Surgery and Traumatology, Inselspital, University of Berne, Berne, Switzerland
e-mail: moritz.tannast@insel.ch

A. Bedi (✉)
NorthShore Orthopedic Institute, Skokie, IL, USA

- Bedi et al. [4] studied FAI patients and reported that the location of impingement is unique and cannot be predicted without dynamic 3D modeling.
- Computer simulation analysis aids in the visualization of impingement at different limb positions, which can be used in virtual surgical planning and evaluation of improvement in ROM after an idealized virtual correction surgery.
- Image processing software aids in the visualization of 3D models which can be cut, oriented, and scaled in six degrees of freedom.
- Data from different modalities can be fused into a single 3D anatomical model that can aid in better visualization. Complex surgical planning and dynamic simulation of different surgical scenarios can be simulated to plan an optimized surgical resection.
- This simulated model can be later used as a template for computer-assisted surgical navigation with some platforms.
- The research and development in computer models with collision algorithms for simulation is going on for more than a decade. The initial models consisted of analyzing the theoretical ROM and failed to analyze the structural lesions and other anatomical defects.
- The ability to visualize the dynamic location of impingement has improved the surgical planning for FAI surgeries. Currently available clinical models are more sophisticated and aid in better visualization of impingement conflict and aids in patient-specific surgical treatment planning.
- Several commercial software solutions are available such as MIMICS, ZedHip, and 3D slicer which have the capacity to perform segmentation of the acetabulum and proximal femur from computed tomography (CT) scans.
- The individual components of the joint are then imported and simulated with a collision detection algorithm which allows for the motion of the femur in different planes. In the ROM simulation, the proximal femur and acetabulum

M. Leunig et al. (eds.), *Surgical Hip Dislocation*, https://doi.org/10.1007/978-3-031-70622-6_4

are set to collide, and the regions of impingement are predicted.

- Surgical corrections can be simulated virtually to predict the changes in ROM based on osseous conflict but do not account for capsular constraints and the peri-articular soft tissues. The optimum resection is selected based on defined criteria, such as head sphericity and correction of head–neck offset.

4.3 Indications and Rationale

Indications

- Symptomatic FAI in the young, pre-arthritic hip

Relative indications

- Global acetabular overcoverage—profunda or protrusio deformity
- Borderline dysplasia deformity

Contraindications

- Dysplasia with hip instability
- Severe hip arthrosis

4.4 Preoperative Imaging Modalities

- Low-dose computed tomography of the entire pelvis, the proximal femur, and the distal femoral condyles
- Magnetic resonance imaging (MRI) with high bone-soft-tissue contrast covering the entire pelvis, the proximal femur, and the distal femoral condyles

4.5 Reference Coordinate Systems

The following reference coordinate systems and methods for quantification of acetabular and femoral resection have been used for virtual collision detection:

- *Anterior pelvic plane*: Defined by both anterior superior iliac spines and the pubic tubercles. This plane is supposed to be vertical in a standing position.
- *Femoral axis*: Defined by the femoral head center and the knee center and the posterior aspect of the femoral condyles.
- *Acetabular clock system*: Sectoral division of the acetabular impingement zones similar to a clock face with 6 o'clock located at the acetabular notch.
- *Femoral head clock system*: Sectoral division of the femoral head impingement zones with 6 o'clock being located at the calcar.
- *Acetabular resection quantification:* The acetabular segment to be trimmed relative to the acetabular clock system with the maximum resected rim depth in millimeters.
- *Femoral resection quantification:* Millimeter stepwise removal of the non-spherical portion of the femoral head–neck junction (Fig. 4.1).

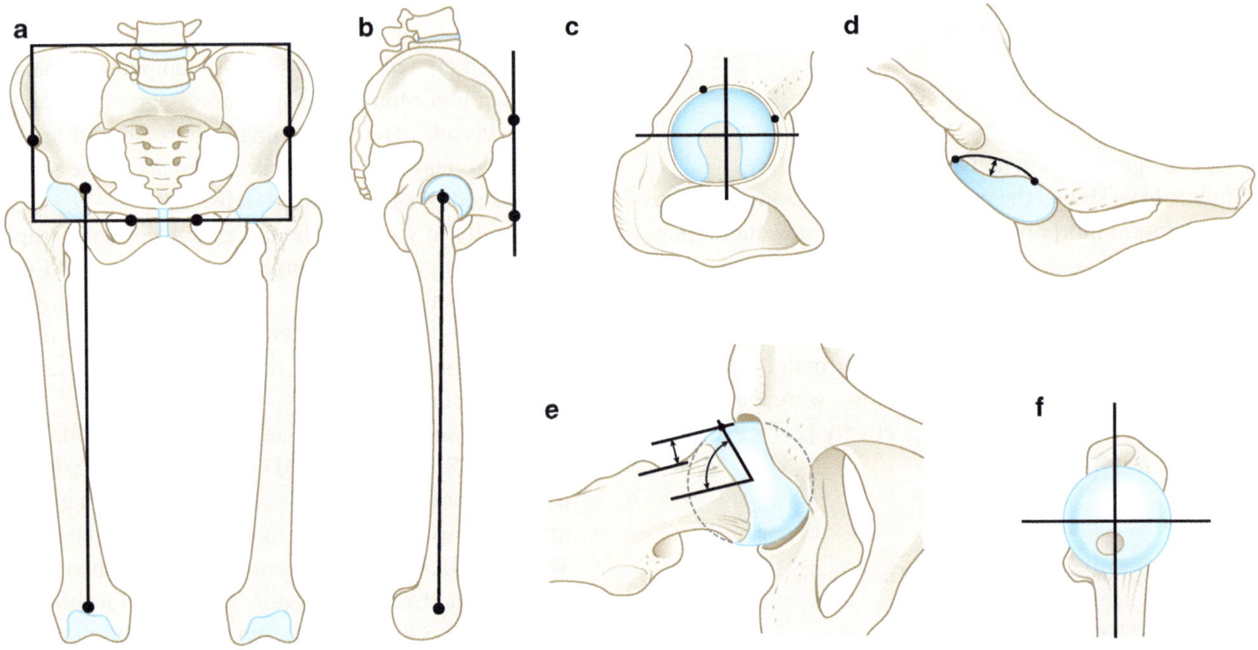

Fig. 4.1 Illustration on the used reference coordinate systems for virtual hip collision detection

4.6 Automated Segmentation

Several algorithms of virtual hip collision detection can be automated allowing a fast and precise virtual hip motion.

- *Automated bone segmentation of the femoral head and the acetabulum*: Several algorithms are present allowing a fully automatic segmentation of the femoral head from the acetabulum.
- *Automated MRI segmentation*: The same three-dimensional (3D) models of the femur and the acetabulum/pelvis can be obtained using MRI without compromising the accuracy of detection of impingement zones or hip amplitudes.
- *Automated detection of landmarks*: Various algorithms are available to automatically detect the anatomical landmarks of the reference coordinate systems.
- *Automated rim detection*: This allows a fast and accurate detection of the acetabular rim which is needed to calculate intraarticular impingement points as well as the two articulating surfaces for the equidistant methods (see below).

4.7 Algorithms for Hip Motion and Collision Detection

From a geometrical standpoint, the native hip joint, unlike the prosthetic hip, is not a perfect sphere. This requires a special algorithm for hip motion in order to precisely detect virtual impingement zones and amplitude of ROM. Four algorithms are known [5]:

- The *simple* method (Fig. 4.2a) uses a pre-defined, fixed, single center of rotation and collects all virtual acetabular impingement zones during motion simulation. This leads to a high number of false positive impingement zones (e.g., between the articular surfaces).
- The *constrained* method (Fig. 4.2b) uses the same pre-defined, fixed, single center of rotation and merely ignores the false positive intraarticular impingement zones by defining a 5-mm detection perimeter around the acetabular rim.
- The *translated* method (Fig. 4.2c) computes a displacement vector according to the detected impingement and subsequently performs an additional translation of the rotation center perpendicular to the detected intraarticular impingement area.
- The *equidistant* method (Fig. 4.2d) determines an equidistant joint space between the femur and acetabulum for every motion step based on the best-fitting spheres of the femoral head and the acetabulum. The best-fitting acetabular opening plane is calculated and allows us to distinguish which parts of the femoral head and the acetabulum are articulating with each other. The resulting additional femoral translation for maintenance of the equidistant joint space is calculated as the vector between the centers of the femoral and acetabular spheres.

In contrast to the other simulation algorithms, the equidistant method can not only be used for mild deformities but also for severely deformed hip joints such as in Legg-Calvé-Perthes disease [6]. It has reportedly been more accurate in terms of the detection of impingement zones and accuracy in the calculation of ROM (Fig. 4.2) [5].

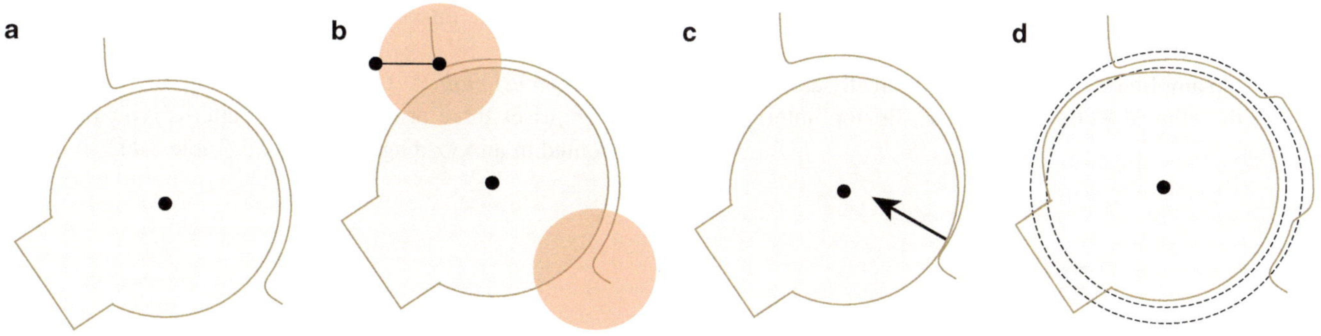

Fig. 4.2 The four different motion algorithms for hip motion are shown. The equidistant method is superior compared with the three others in terms of sensitivity and precision of impingement detection

4.8 Validation

Contemporary dynamic virtual hip joint simulations focus exclusively on bony abnormalities. Structures such as the labrum, the ligamentum capitis femoris, and the joint capsule are usually not considered although they can contribute substantially to hip ROM. As a result, the amplitudes of ROM are typically overestimated with virtual collision detection compared with reality.

The overestimation of ROM depends on the individual motion amplitudes but reportedly ranges from 2 ± 2° in a laboratory setup using sawbones [5], 5 ± 6° in a cadaveric setup [7], and up to 16° in human beings [8].

Despite this overestimation, the location of the individual impingement zones is precise [5] with a specificity of 90% and a negative predictive value of 96%. Thus, it can add substantial clinical information by differentiating between purely intraarticular impingement and impingement that includes extraarticular components. However, the 3D analysis should be only used as an adjunct to the standard clinical and radiographical setup and never as a single diagnostic instrument.

The location of the calculated virtual impingement zones matches exactly the observed degenerative changes of the cartilage and the adjacent labrum [9].

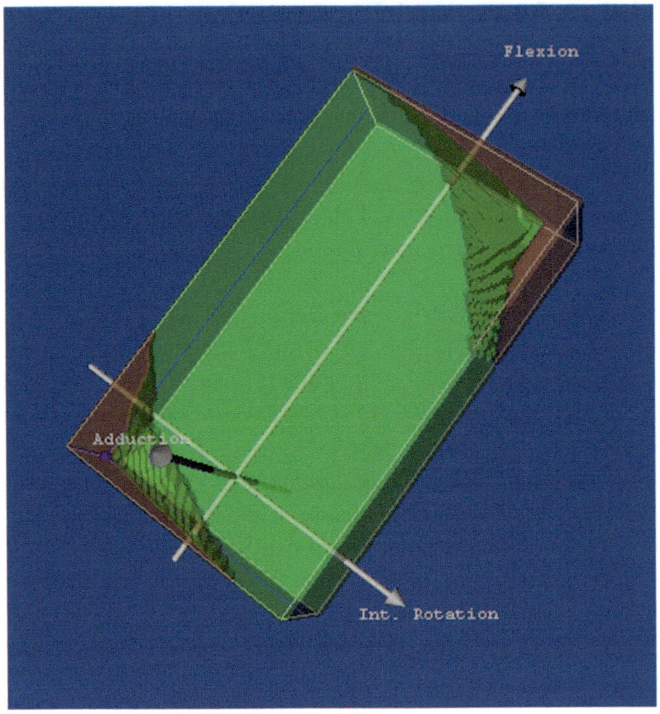

Fig. 4.3 Visualization of a "motion cloud." The cuboid represents the simulated ROM for flexion, adduction, and internal rotation. The green zones represent the impingement-free ROM. The red zones represent the combination of motion where an impingement between the femur and the pelvis has been detected

4.9 ROM: Amplitudes, Motion Patterns, and Motion Clouds

Quantification of ROM can be unidimensional (motion amplitudes), bidimensional (motion patterns), or tri-dimensional (motion clouds).

- *Unidimensional*: Unidirectional hip motion is referred to as "hip amplitude" and comprises typically all amplitudes for the clinical ROM testing (e.g., flexion, internal rotation, etc.).
- *Bidimensional*: Bidimensional hip motion analysis comprises two different motion amplitudes, for example, flexion and internal rotation. The graphical representation comprises a classic xy diagram. This corresponds to the clinical anterior and posterior impingement tests (flexion and internal rotation, extension, and external rotation).
- *Tridimensional*: A tri-dimensional hip motion analysis comprises three or more motion patterns typically represented in an xyz diagram (Fig. 4.3, Table 4.1).

Table 4.1 Overview on the published virtual hip motion amplitudes of different pathologies

Amplitude	Native [10, 11]	FAI (cam-type) [11]	Dysplasia [10]	LCPD	Valgus hip with high antetorsion [12]	Protrusio acetabuli	Acetabular retroversion	SCFE
Flexion	122 ± 16 (103–145)	105 ± 12 (69–142)	148 ± 20 (97–171)	103 ± 40 (26–144)	119 ± 14 (90–140)	104 ± 9 (81–117)	116 ± 6 (102–125)	46 ± 32 (0–113)
Extension	57 ± 20 (12–101)	61 ± 32 (15–129)	24 ± 11 (−3 to 30)	15 ± 27 (−39 to 50)	26 ± 23 (−16 to 50)	27 ± 20 (2–64)	87 ± 10 (64–100)	n.a.
Abduction	63 ± 11 (40–85)	52 ± 12 (13–71)	88 ± 4 (73–90)	22 ± 23 (−18 to 78)	76 ± 15 (56–96)	39 ± 11 (20 − 51)	60 ± 10 (42–86)	n.a.
Adduction	33 ± 12 (4–52)	35 ± 12 (17–64)	41 ± 13 (5–61)	27 ± 15 (8–50)	24 ± 17 (−10 to 50)	20 ± 13 (2–41)	39 ± 10 (17–60)	n.a.
Internal rotation in 90° of flexion	35 ± 7 (11–61)	11 ± 7 (0–29)	39 ± 6 (14–41)	−5 ± 23 (−40 to 40)	59 ± 16 (36–93)	16 ± 12 (−09 to 33)	30 ± 12 (9–48)	−17 ± 18 (−60 to 10)
External rotation in 90° of flexion	103 ± 14 (75–131)	83 ± 34 (1–126)	99 ± 19 (45–125)	59 ± 35 (14–140)	22 ± 21 (−20 to 42)	64 ± 13 (32–82)	92 ± 21 (35–129)	n.a.
Internal rotation in 0° of flexion	111 ± 17 (84–146)	n.a.	n.a.	n.a.	134 ± 9 (114–140)	88 ± 13 (62–105)	109 ± 20 (72–138)	50 ± 27 (0–100)
External rotation in 0° of flexion	38 ± 7 (17–41)	43 ± 13 (18–68)	26 ± 18 (−10 to 41)	12 ± 34 (−51 to 76)	22 ± 21 (−20 to 42)	19 ± 14 (−3 to 42)	56 ± 9 (39–77)	n.a.

4.10 Detection of Impingement Zones

The calculation of impingement zones in an individual is based on all potentially detectable impingement points for a predefined hip motion. Typically, the anterior and posterior impingement tests are evaluated. For the anterior impingement test, the range consists of 70–110° of hip flexion, −20° to 20° of adduction, and internal rotation until osseous contact occurs. Analogously, for the posterior impingement test, external rotation was studied between −5° and 20° of extension and − 20° and 20° of adduction. Depending on the chosen increments (e.g., 1° or 5° of motion), this results in thousands of detected impingement points which can be distributed according to their frequency with regard to the acetabular and femoral impingement zones.

The impingement zones can be further subclassified into:

- *Intraarticular impingement zones:* All impingement zones of the acetabulum and the femoral head–neck junction within the hip joint capsule (acetabular rim, central and peripheral hip compartment).
- *Extraarticular impingement zones*: All impingement zones outside of the hip joint capsule (inferior iliac spine, greater and lesser trochanter, ischium, anterior/posterior intertrochanteric line, femoral shaft).

The different impingement zones have been evaluated for a variety of pathomorphologies of the hip joint. These are summarized in Figs. 4.4, 4.5, and 4.6.

4.11 Clinical Implications of Collision Detection

Although the ROM for collision detection models is generally overestimated, it can be useful to detect the zone of impingement. In turn, this can directly influence the type of surgical treatment.

- *Intra- versus extraarticular impingement*: In cases with reduced femoral version, the impingement zones can be intraarticular, extraarticular, or both. When only a solitary intraarticular impingement is found (most commonly at the zone of the femoral head–neck junction, for instance), hip arthroscopy with femoral osteochondroplasty is indicated (Fig. 4.7). If, however, an extraarticular impingement is found, either alone or in combination with an intraarticular impingement, then open surgical correction with a surgical dislocation would be the appropriate treatment (Fig. 4.8).
- *Resection versus corrective osteotomy*: Simulated surgical correction can help guide toward the correct treatment as well. For instance, a seemingly straightforward anterosuperior intraarticular impingement with cam-type deformity and acetabular crossover (Fig. 4.9) can be virtually corrected with a rim trim and an offset (simulating a common correction that is often performed arthroscopically), only to reveal that the post-resection hip now shows a more complex extraarticular impingement. That same hip having undergone a simulated offset correction and anteverting PAO shows complete resolution of the impinge-

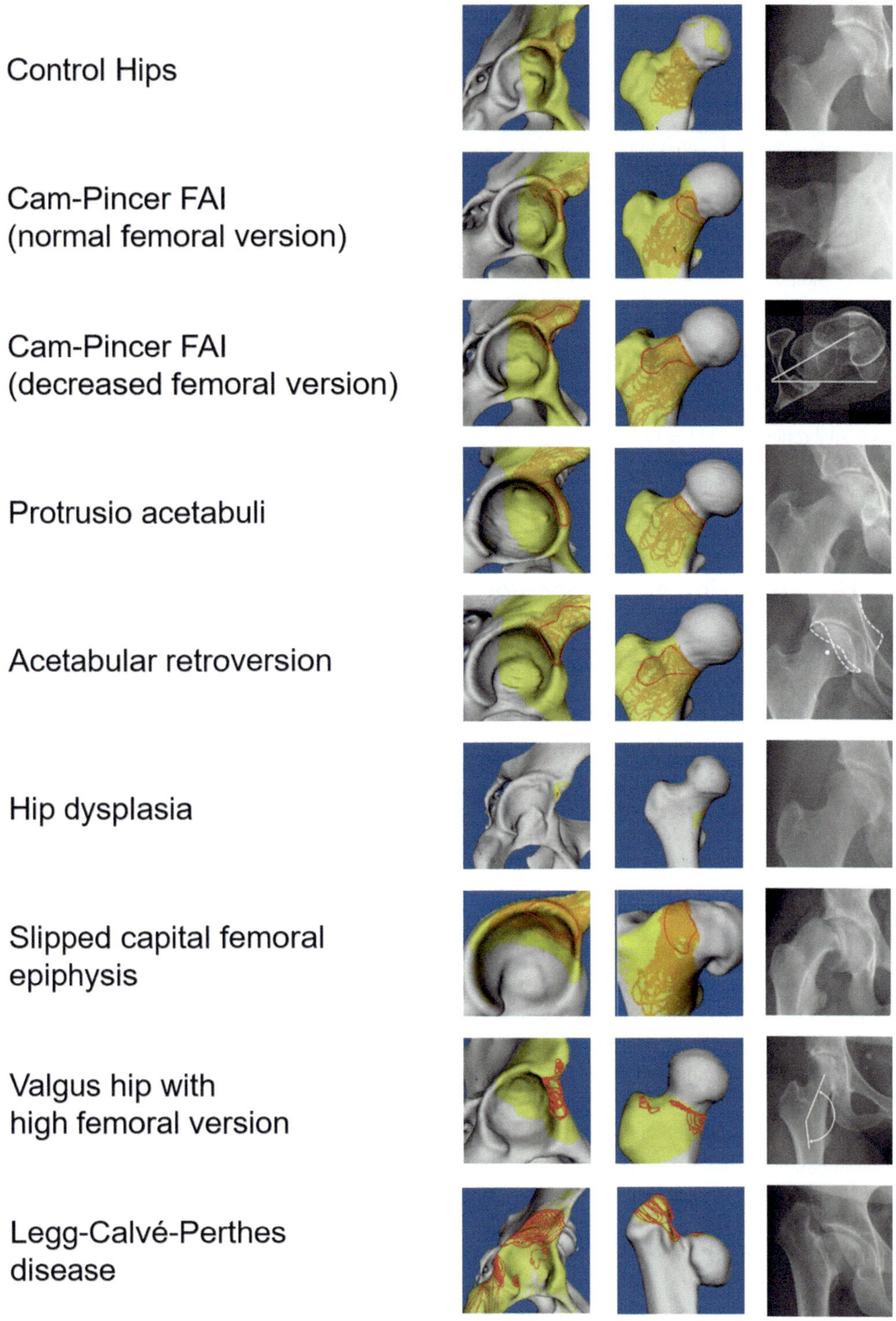

Fig. 4.4 Overview on the detected impingement zones for different hip joint pathologies

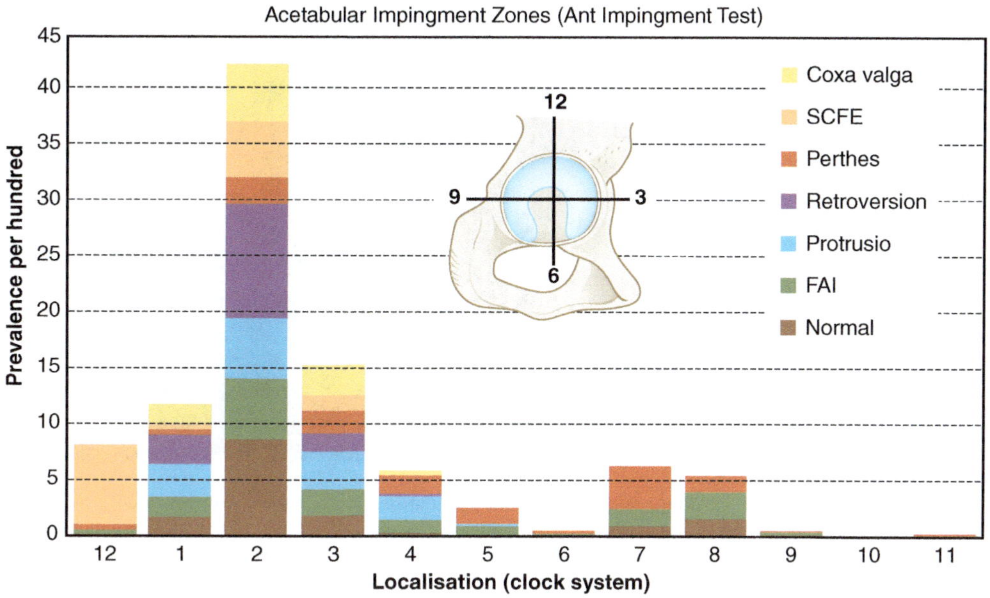

Fig. 4.5 The acetabular impingement zones for the anterior impingement test are summarized for different pathomporphologies

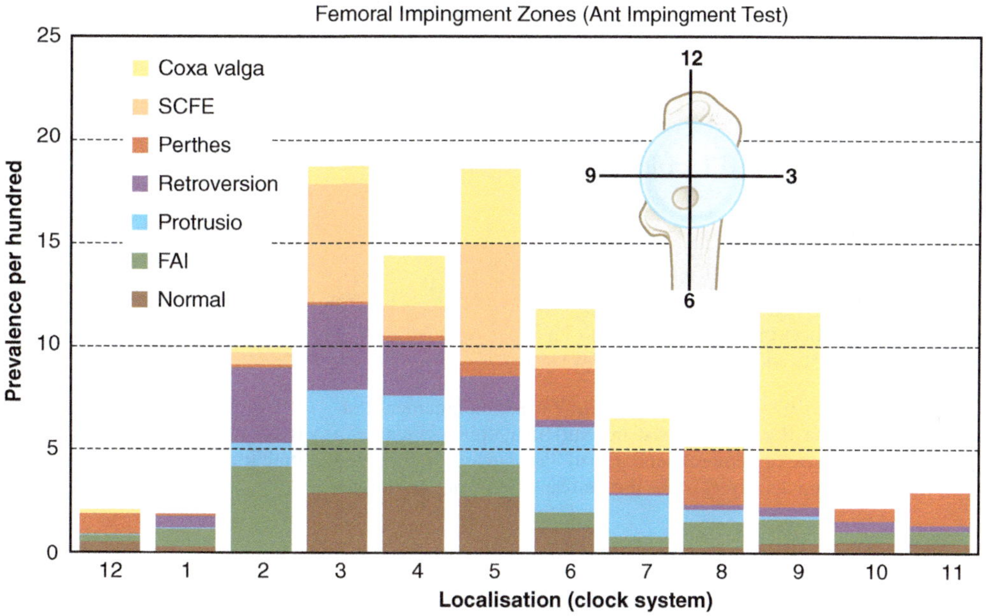

Fig. 4.6 The femoral impingement zones for the anterior impingement test are summarized for different hip pathomorphologies

ments (Fig. 4.10). The simulated corrective osteotomy was then performed (Fig. 4.11).

- *Planning for femoral intertrochanteric osteotomies:* When a corrective osteotomy of the femur is an appropriate indication, virtual impingement testing with simulated surgical correction can not only identify existing impingements but also help avoid unintended postoperative issues. Figure 4.12 shows a patient with a valgus hip and an osteonecrotic lesion that could benefit from a varus intertrochanteric osteotomy. Virtual simulation reveals an existing impingement in the native hip that would remain if only a varus-producing osteotomy was performed (Figs. 4.13 and 4.14). Impingement was confirmed intraoperatively, and therefore the varus osteotomy was augmented with an offset correction (Fig. 4.15).
- *Planning for more complex osteotomies using custom instrumentation:* Because of the complex nature of the hip joint, corrective osteotomies close to the joint, especially on the femoral side, can create unintended consequences. Computer simulation allows the surgeon to plan more complex corrective osteotomies safely. Computer modeling can simultaneously ensure that the primary surgical outcome is achieved while avoiding unintended consequences that could lead to continued pain and dysfunction. In addition, the use of 3D models allows for custom blocks to be created to ensure adequate translation of the surgical plan to its precise execution (see Figs. 4.16, 4.17, 4.18, 4.19, and 4.20).

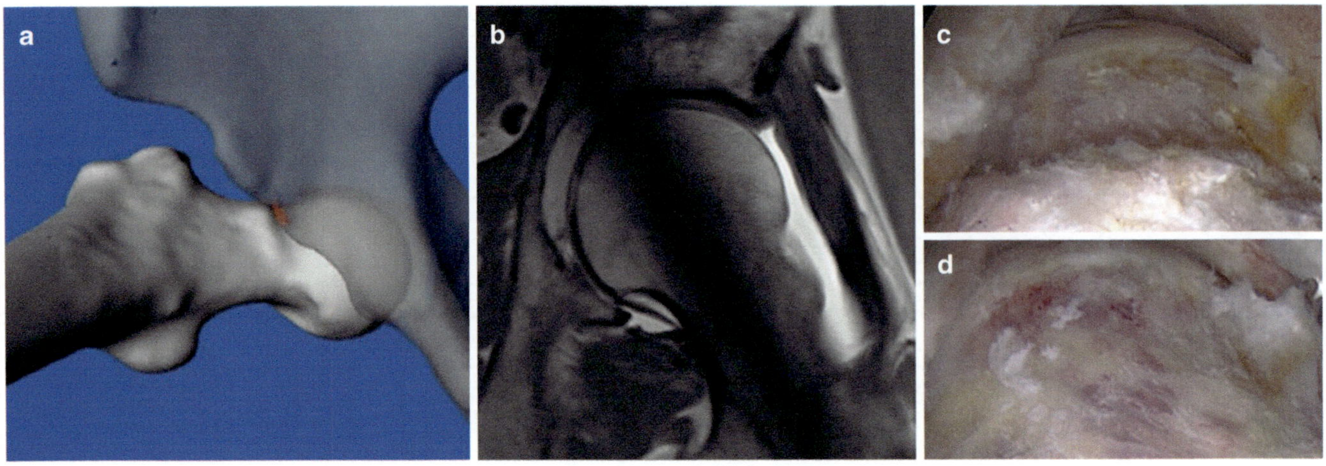

Fig. 4.7 Clinical decision-making using 3D virtual simulation. (**a**) Virtual impingement testing shows an isolated intraarticular impingement between the acetabular rim and the femoral head–neck junction. (**b**) MR arthrogram confirms the location of the offset deformity and shows a concomitant blunted labrum in the predicted impingement zone. (**c**) Arthroscopy is performed to address the solitary intraarticular impingement

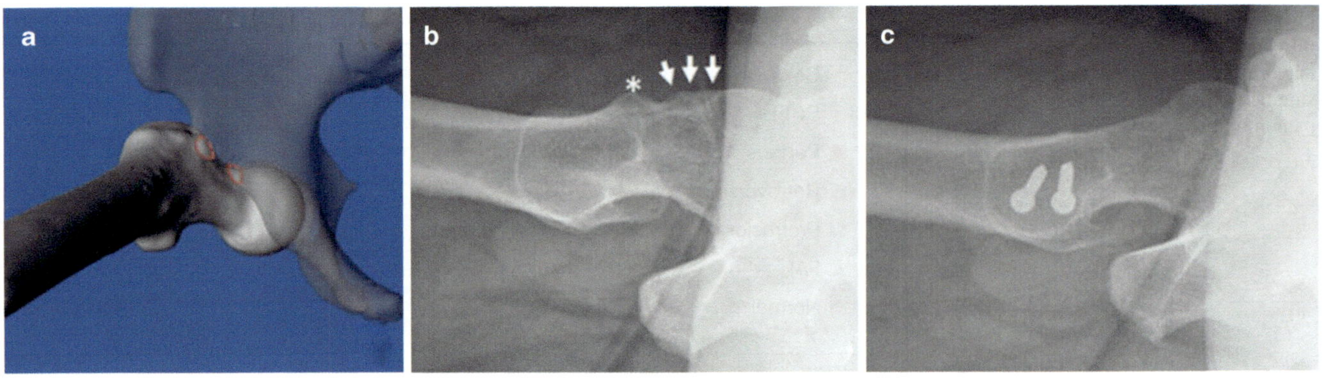

Fig. 4.8 A second 3D virtual simulation. (**a**) Virtual impingement testing shows both an intraarticular and extraarticular impingement in a patient with decreased femoral torsion. (**b**) Preoperative radiograph demonstrates a cam deformity of the femoral head–neck offset (intraarticular impingement) as well as a prominent intertrochanteric massif (extraarticular impingement). (**c**) Surgical dislocation is performed and both impingement sites are treated in one surgical setting

Fig. 4.9 Preoperative AP pelvis and cross-table lateral femoral radiographs show an acetabular crossover sign and a cam-type deformity of the proximal femur

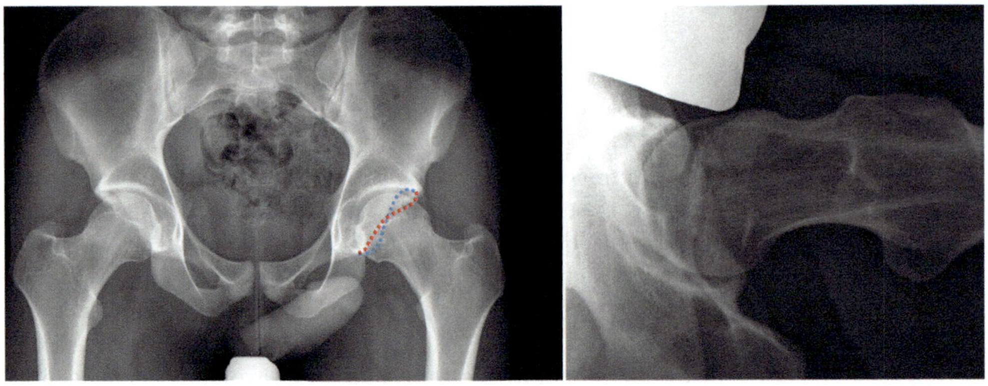

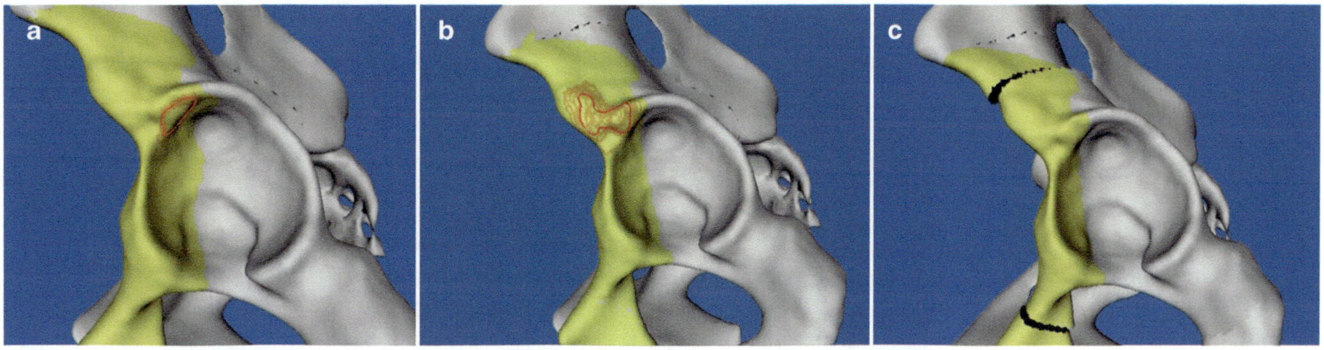

Fig. 4.10 (**a**) Virtual simulation of the case shown in Fig. 4.9 shows a native intraarticular impingement at the anterosuperior quadrant of the acetabulum. (**b**) Following offset correction and rim trimming, the impingement now migrates to the level of the anterior inferior iliac spine. (**c**) When offset correction and anteverting PAO are simulated, however, the impingement completely resolves

Fig. 4.11 Postoperative AP pelvis and cross-table lateral radiographs following corrective osteotomy and offset resection show resolution of acetabular crossover sign and improved femoral head sphericity

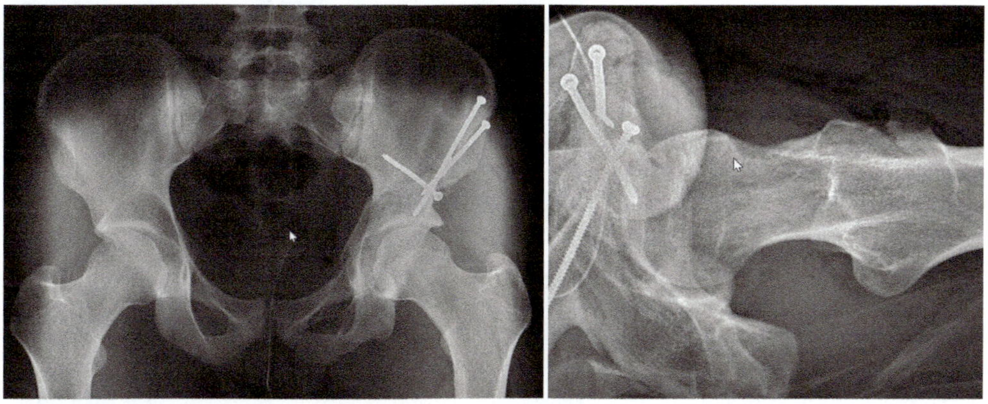

Fig. 4.12 Preoperative AP pelvis and cross-table lateral femoral radiographs show valgus hip in the setting of osteonecrosis of the femoral head. A small offset abnormality can be seen on the cross-table lateral radiograph

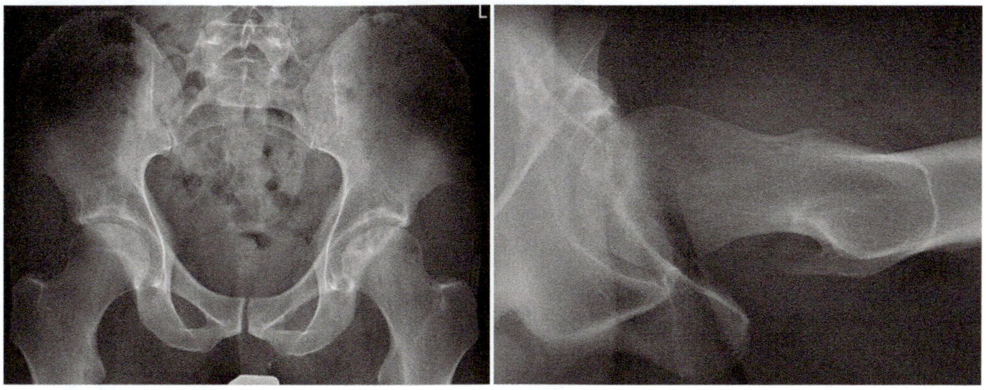

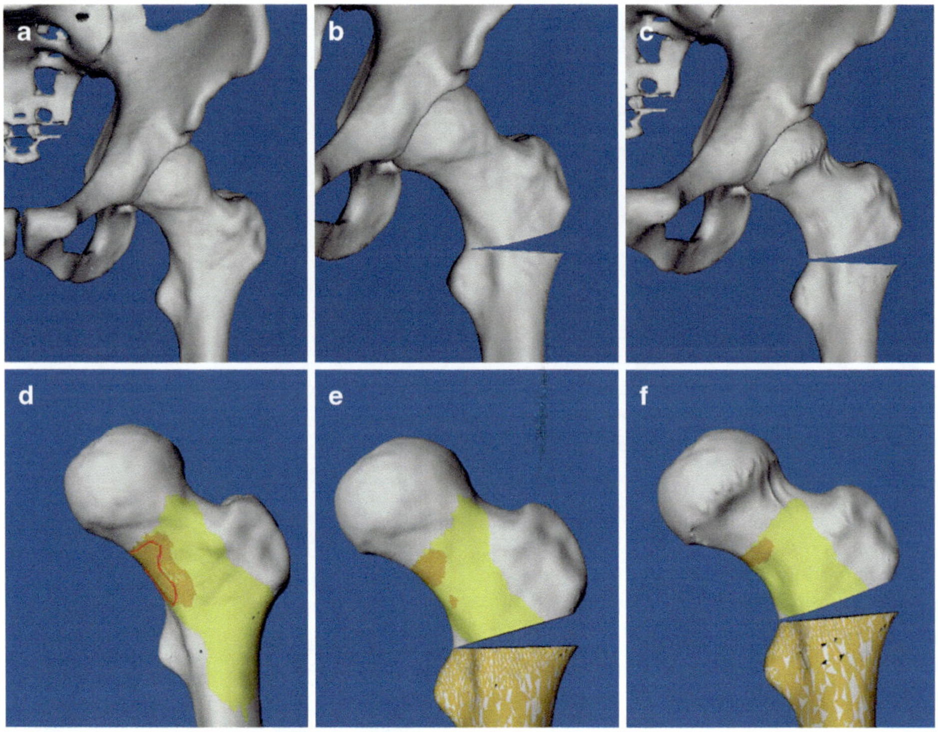

Fig. 4.13 Virtual simulation showing the native hip joint with an impingement conflict on the inferomedial femoral neck (**a** and **d**). With a simulated intertrochanteric varus femoral osteotomy, the inferomedial neck impingement improves (**b** and **e**). Adding an offset correction to the varus osteotomy further decreases the impingement zone (**c** and **f**)

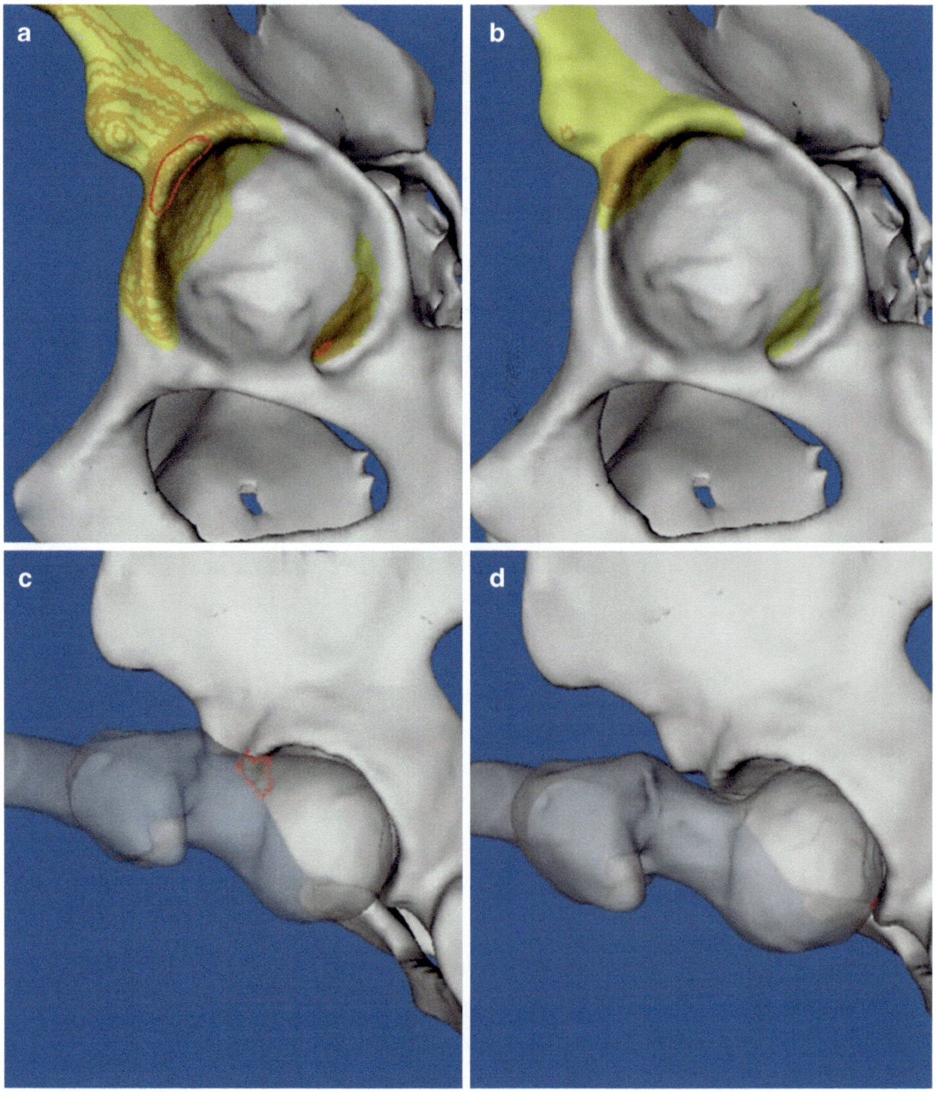

Fig. 4.14 Additional simulation views show persistent impingement on the anterosuperior acetabular rim (**a** and **c**) with varus osteotomy only. This impingement effectively resolves with an offset correction in addition to the varus osteotomy (**b** and **d**)

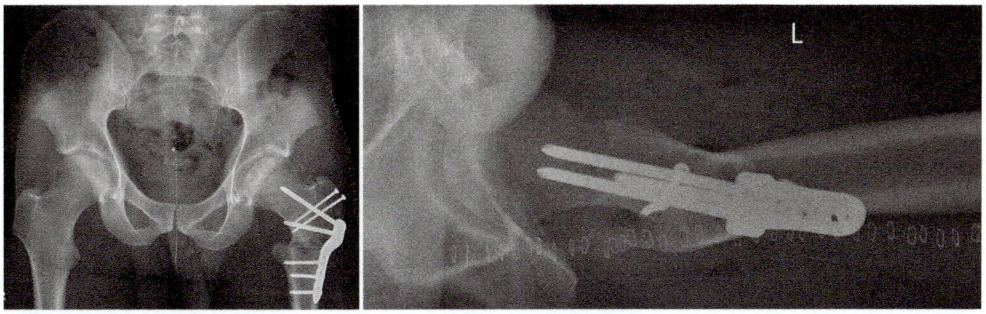

Fig. 4.15 Postoperative AP pelvis and cross-table lateral femoral radiographs show the corrective varus osteotomy of the femur, moving the osteonecrotic lesion out of the weight-bearing zone. The offset abnormality has also been corrected

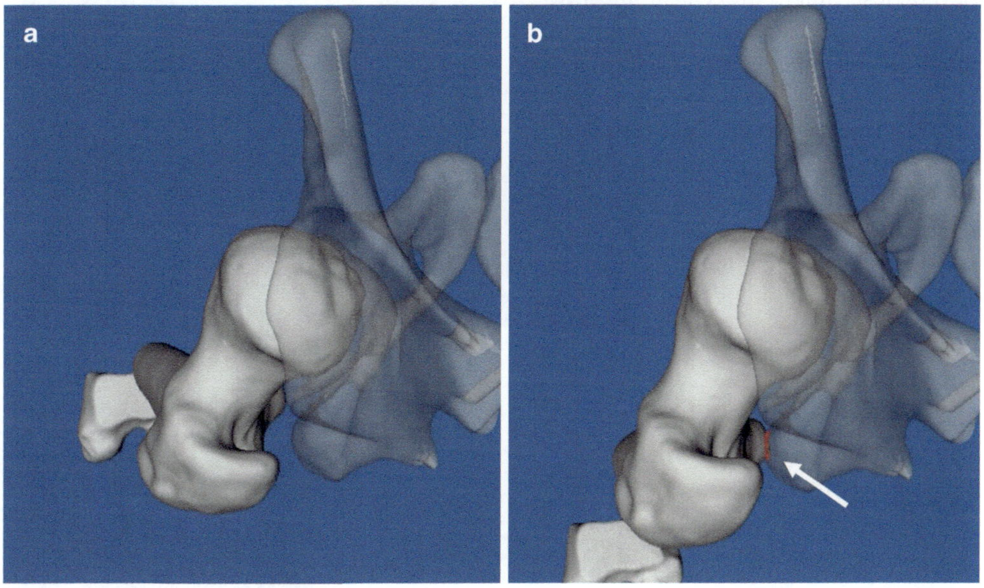

Fig. 4.16 3D simulation of a valgus hip with high antetorsion. (**a**) shows the hip in neutral flexion, adduction and rotation. (**b**) shows a pathological posterior, extraarticular impingement in external rotation and extension

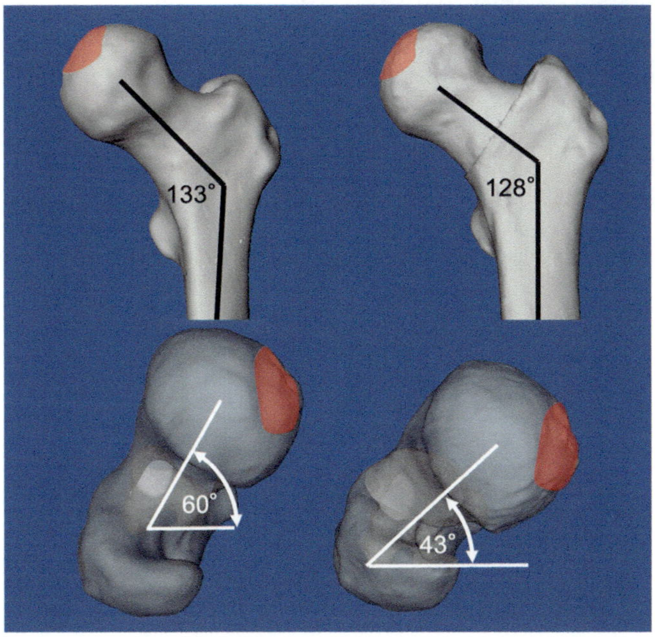

Fig. 4.17 A varus and retrotorsional corrective osteotomy is planned through the base of the femoral neck

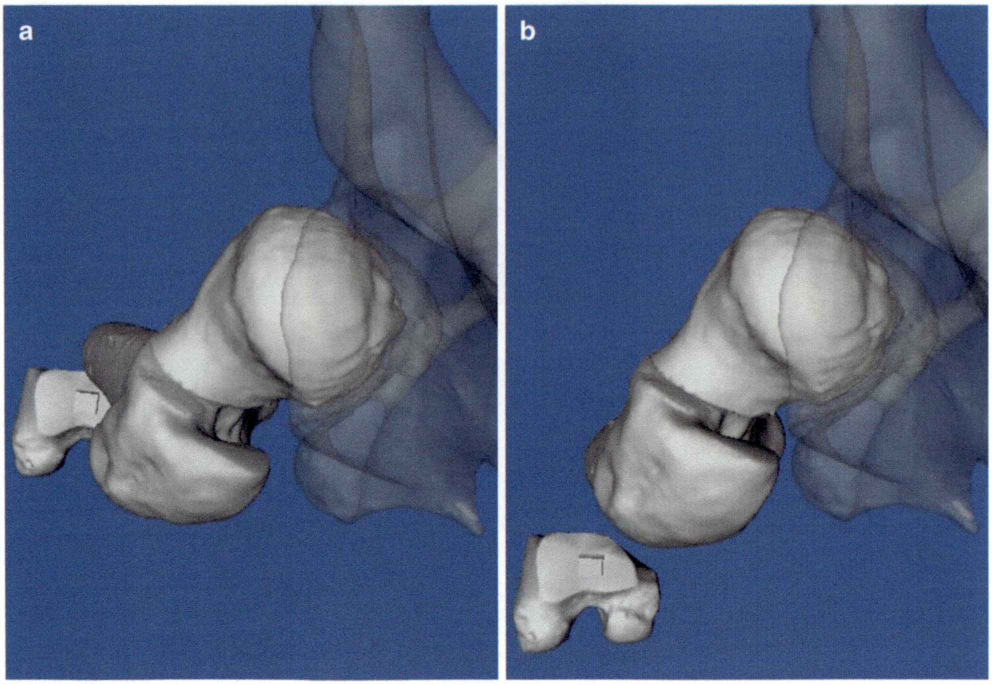

Fig. 4.18 When running the simulation with the corrective osteotomy, the impingement is relieved. (**a**) shows the hip in neutral flexion, adduction and rotation. (**b**) Relief of the extrarticular impingement conflict in extension and external rotation

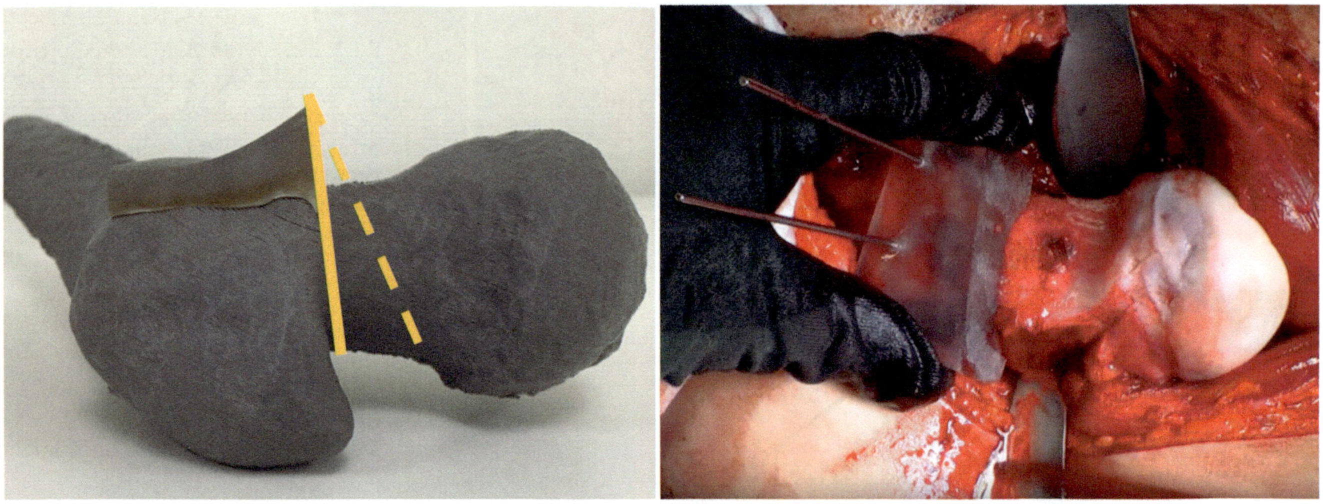

Fig. 4.19 Because of the complexity and precision of the osteotomy, a custom cutting block is created to exactly replicate the computer-simulated correction

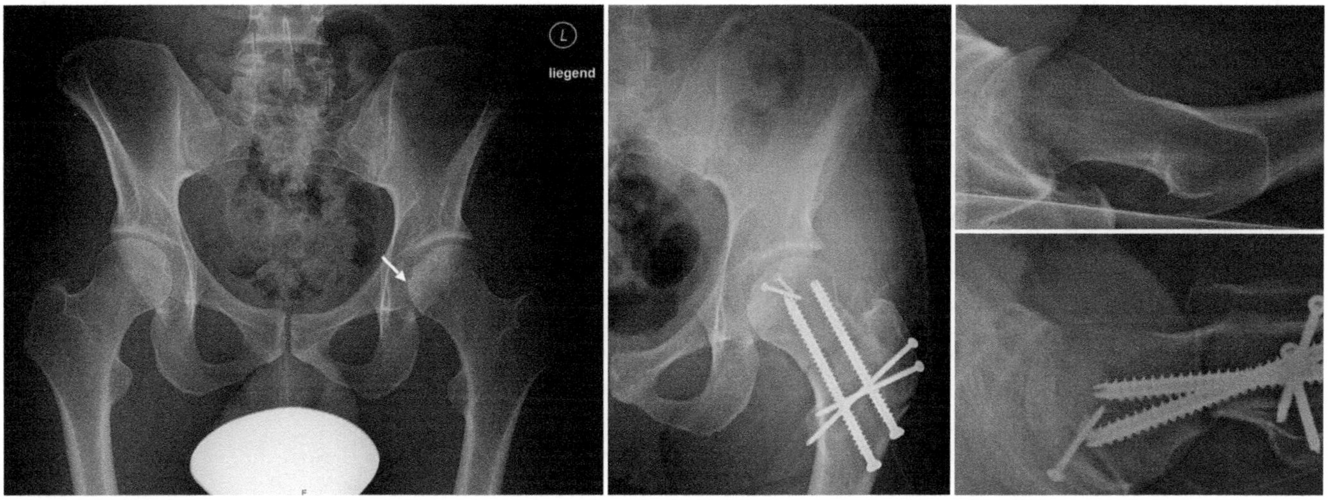

Fig. 4.20 Preoperative and postoperative radiographs following corrective femoral neck osteotomy. Additional screws were placed in the femoral head to treat an osteochondral defect

4.12 Controversies (e.g., Overestimation, Fixed Rotation, Instability, False Positive, Negative, and Lumbar Spine Position)

- One of the limitations of the clinical application of computer-assisted collision model simulation is the potentially high amount of radiation exposure due to CT scanning and fluoroscopic guides for navigation registration. Low-dose protocols have been designed to minimize this exposure, compatible with a hip and pelvis radiographic series.
- Collision models fail to account for the influence of soft tissues such as the joint capsule, labrum, and articular cartilage. These structures are not considered during the simulations and modeling steps, often resulting in an overestimation of ROM. This limitation can be partially addressed with the development of MRI and other visualization techniques including ultrasonography.
- Many collision models assume that the hip joint has a perfect center of rotation, and any translational motion is not accounted for in the model. Accordingly, the locations of impingement may be inaccurate with a collision model, particularly in the setting of joint hyperlaxity or dysplasia.
- The software is not applicable for largely dysplastic hips with shallow acetabulum and hips with advanced osteoarthritis. In these settings, there will be additional femoral head translation which is difficult to predict and simulate accordingly.
- These models also perform measurements and simulations on joints that are not loaded. As joints and tissues undergo viscoelastic deformation due to loading and the biomechanics are load-dependent, this phenomenon is oversimplified in the collision models.
- Lumbopelvic motion is not accounted for in collision modeling, and dynamic changes in pelvic tilt and obliquity may impact impingement location and terminal ROM estimates.

4.13 Future Directions (e.g., Navigation and Augmented Reality)

While computer modeling and virtual surgical planning have grown substantially in the past two decades, there is considerable continued growth in this area. Integration of preoperative plans into surgical execution using navigation, robotic assistance, and/or augmented reality are all in various stages of both development and clinical use. In addition to this, there is the possibility in the future of integrating artificial intelligence more robustly into computer modeling to further facilitate surgical treatment, and there is expanding interest in the use and development of smart instruments.

References

1. Jung K, Restrepo C, Hellman M, et al. The prevalence of cam-type femoroacetabular deformity in asymptomatic adults. J Bone Joint Surg Br. 2011;93-B(10):1303–7.
2. Lerebours F, Robertson W, Neri B, et al. Prevalence of cam-type morphology in elite ice hockey players. Am J Sports Med. 2016;44(4):1024–30.
3. Gerhardt M, Romero A, Silvers H, et al. The prevalence of radiographic hip abnormalities in elite soccer players. Am J Sports Med. 2012;40(3):584–8.

4. Bedi A, Dolan M, Magennis E, et al. Computer-assisted modeling of osseous impingement and resection in femoroacetabular impingement. Arthroscopy. 2012;28(2):204–10.
5. Puls M, Ecker T, Tannast M, et al. The equidistant method—a novel hip joint simulation algorithm for detection of femoroacetabular impingement. Comput Aided Surg. 2010;15(4–6):75–82.
6. Tannast M, Hanke M, Ecker T, et al. LCPD: reduced range of motion resulting from extra- and intraarticular impingement. Clin Orthop Relat Res. 2012;470(9):2431–40.
7. Tannast M, Kubiak-Langer M, Langlotz F, et al. Noninvasive three-dimensional assessment of femoroacetabular impingement. J Orthop Res. 2007;25(1):122–31.
8. Naili J, Stålman A, Valentin A, et al. Hip joint range of motion is restricted by pain rather than mechanical impingement in individuals with femoroacetabular impingement syndrome. Arch Orthop Trauma Surg. 2022;142(8):1985–94.
9. Tannast M, Goricki D, Beck M, et al. Hip damage occurs at the zone of femoroacetabular impingement. Clin Orthop Relat Res. 2008;466(2):273–80.
10. Steppacher S, Zurmühle C, Puls M, et al. Periacetabular osteotomy restores the typically excessive range of motion in dysplastic hips with a spherical head. Clin Orthop Relat Res. 2015;473(4):1404–16.
11. Kubiak-Langer M, Tannast M, Murphy S, et al. Range of motion in anterior femoroacetabular impingement. Clin Orthop Relat Res. 2007;458:117–24.
12. Siebenrock K, Steppacher S, Haefeli P, et al. Valgus hip with high antetorsion causes pain through posterior extraarticular FAI. Clin Orthop Relat Res. 2013;471(12):3774–80.

5 Computer-Assisted Planning and Execution of Joint-Preserving Interventions Around the Hip

Philipp Fürnstahl

5.1 Introduction

The goal of surgical navigation is to enhance the safety, accuracy, and effectiveness of surgical procedures. By combining pre- and intraoperative imaging (computed tomography, CT; magnetic resonance imaging, MRI; and X-ray) with position determination systems, computer methods can create a digital representation of the current situation in surgery. This representation shows the position of surgical tools, instruments, or implants relative to the patient's anatomy. Navigation thus provides the surgeon spatial (three-dimensional, 3D) control in anatomical regions where a direct view during surgery is difficult or impossible to achieve. A surgical execution plan encodes the surgical goals of the relevant steps as target values, allowing measurement and visualization of deviations between plan and execution. In complex surgeries, this execution plan is created as a *preoperative plan* before the operation by incorporating 3D CT or MRI data of the patient. A surgical navigation system must therefore be able to fuse different pre- and intraoperative data of a patient, to interpret them, and to display them to the surgeon in the correct spatial and temporal context. From a technical point of view, the central process here is *image registration*, which allows image data from different modalities to be superimposed and merged.

Alongside neurosurgery, orthopedics was one of the first surgical disciplines to utilize surgical navigation. This early adaption is partly due to the elective nature of orthopedic procedures, allowing sufficient time for preoperative planning. Additionally, the rigidity of the bone anatomy makes the technical processes of preoperative planning, registration, and motion compensation less demanding than in soft tissue surgery. The first clinical trials focusing on the validation of navigation systems in hip and knee prosthetics were successfully conducted in the 1990s. In the early 2000s, the first commercial systems were offered by medical technology companies including Brainlab, Medtronic, and Stryker. In the meantime, a large variety of navigation solutions are available as medical devices, influenced by the technological progress in informatics, robotics, medical imaging, and 3D printing. In addition to the primary application field of endoprosthetics, solutions for the surgical navigation of corrective osteotomies, osteosyntheses, or tumor resections are available.

Despite steady technical innovation, surgical navigation has not yet been accepted as a standard of care in orthopedic procedures. Conservative estimates show that only 5% of all orthopedic interventions are performed with the support of computer technologies [1]. The low acceptance is due to the high costs, lack of insurance coverage, longer operation times, and insufficient integration into the standard surgical workflow. Hip surgery has even lower adaption rates than other orthopedic disciplines because conventionally performed hip prosthetic surgery is safe and effective and delivers very good surgical outcomes. The situation is different for more complex procedures with a higher degree of surgical difficulty, such as corrective osteotomies or tumor resections. These less frequently performed procedures are highly complex in planning and execution. Despite additional costs, this complexity justifies the use of highly individualized surgical navigation based on sophisticated preoperative computer planning. For these specialized procedures, navigation approaches using patient-specific instruments (PSIs) have become widely established [2]. PSIs are customized for each patient and their specific surgery to guide surgical tools such as drills or saws during the procedure. PSIs are designed based on preoperative 3D computer planning and manufactured using 3D printers.

The following sections of this book chapter present the different concepts of and the state of the art in surgical navigation of joint preserving hip surgery. An emphasis will be placed on the description of navigation with PSI (Sect. 5.2), as this technology has been very successful as an effective

P. Fürnstahl (✉)
Research in Orthopedic Computer Science (ROCS), Balgrist University Hospital, University of Zurich, Zurich, Switzerland
e-mail: Philipp.Fuernstahl@balgrist.ch

M. Leunig et al. (eds.), *Surgical Hip Dislocation*, https://doi.org/10.1007/978-3-031-70622-6_5

tool for performing complex corrective osteotomies. Section 5.3 is then dedicated to a principle discourse on navigation by tracking systems. At the end of the chapter, in Sect. 5.4, 5.5 and 5.6, we discuss the advantages and disadvantages of the different methods, provide an outlook on their future development in hip surgery, and summarize the computer-assisted hip approach.

5.2 Surgical Navigation with PSIs

PSIs are mechanical navigation aids tailored to a patient's anatomy and procedure. A PSI is built on a base block designed to fit onto the patient's bone at a location predefined during preoperative planning. Accurate positioning is ensured by the undersurface of the base block, which is molded to exactly match the patient's bone anatomy. For this purpose, anatomically shaped contact points are integrated into the undersurface if the bone anatomy has a sufficient amount of irregularly shaped bony landmarks. Otherwise, if more stability is needed, the entire undersurface of the base block is shaped as a negative of the bone surface.

In the PSI concept, the process of *registering* a preoperative plan to the intraoperative anatomy is accomplished by the shape of the base block itself. Navigation can then be performed relative to this defined reference position. Each step of the preoperative plan is represented by dedicated components integrated into the PSI. Integrated drill sleeves enable navigated drilling, screwing, or the placement of Kirschner wires. Slits align the surgical saw according to a preoperatively defined, 3D cutting plane, and additional attachments ensure navigated reduction of osteotomized bone fragments. Navigation of subsequent surgical steps is achieved by the sequential application of mulltiple PSIs in a modular fashion.

Additive manufacturing processes such as 3D printing are used for the production of PSIs. For biocompatibility and sterility reasons, selective laser sintering based on powder printing is the preferred manufacturing process. In selective laser sintering, the component is built up layerwise by fusing the component's contours on the current layer of the powder bed before adding the next layer. The raw material used for PSI manufacturing consists of biocompatible plastics, such as polyamide 2200, approved for medical use. This ensures that any residual material left in the body is physiologically harmless and does not cause side effects such as inflammation.

PSI, approved as a medical device for navigation of joint-preserving hip surgery, is meanwhile available from various commercial suppliers. For example, the company Medacta (Castel San Pietro, Switzerland) offers the MyPAO and MyOsteotomy systems for correction of the acetabular and femoral components through navigation of the periacetabular osteotomy (PAO) and the femoral head reduction osteotomy (FHRO), respectively [3]. However, performing an FHRO via MyOsteotomy is considered a highly specialized procedure that is only indicated in selected cases where experienced surgeons and specially trained engineers work together. An exemplary FHRO case including pre- and postoperative X-rays along with the 3D surgery planning is given in Fig. 5.1. In the following, we would like to present the approach of PSI-navigated FHRO in more detail in the form of case studies, demonstrating the effectiveness of this navigation technique in very complex osteotomies.

The majority of the PSI manufacturing process is digital and performed preoperatively on the computer. In the first step, a 3D *triangular surface model* (hereinafter called 3D model) of the patient's pathological femur is reconstructed from CT data. Commercial image processing programs such as Mimics Innovation Suite (Materialise, Belgium) or Imfusion Suite (Imfusion GmbH, Germany) provide segmentation capabilities to detect the anatomy in the CT slices, segment them from the rest of the image, and convert them into 3D bone models. The pathological bone model is then imported into computer-aided design (CAD) software specifically developed for surgical planning. The software can simulate the surgical steps to be navigated and is also used to design the PSI (Figs. 5.2 and 5.3).

The simulation is developed through the interaction between a biomedical engineer operating the computer and the surgeon. The latter defines the desired result based on the patient's deformity and anatomical, especially vascular, constraints. The goal of the simulation is to define the osteotomy planes that restore the femoral head's pre-morbid, spherical shape and size while removing the centrally located necrotic area. If healthy, the contralateral side can serve as a remodeling template to approximate this pre-morbid shape. To this end, the contralateral femur model is mirrored and superimposed on the proximal shaft part of the pathological femur by means of surface registration methods. If the contralateral side is not applicable, the femoral head shape can be approximated by a sphere whose center is located in the mechanical hip joint center and whose size is adjusted to the healthy areas of the femoral head (Fig. 5.2a).

The surgeon incorporates MRI findings to decide on the optimal shape and size of the segment to be resected, which is defined by two intracapital osteotomies (Fig. 5.2b). The shape of the segment can be defined by parallel cuts. The segment can also be wedge-shaped, having an anterior or posterior base. Furthermore, a varus or valgus inclination can be included by means of appropriate re-cuts. The intracarpal osteotomies are described by 3D cutting planes in the computer planning. The trochanteric osteotomy is performed freehand and without PSI navigation, requiring only a pro forma simulation—in contrast to the intracapital osteotomies, which need precise cutting plane positioning. The

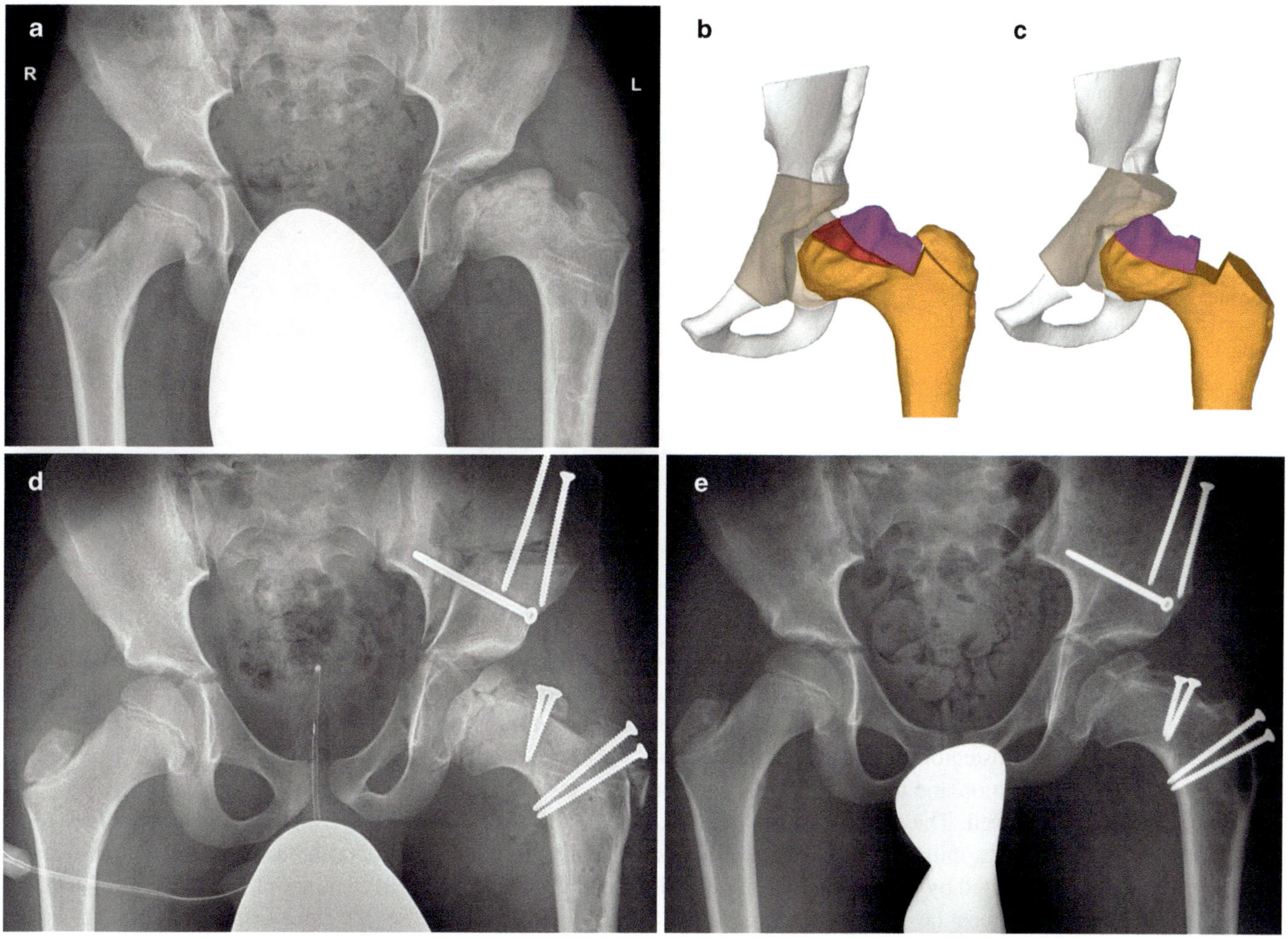

Fig. 5.1 A 10-year-old boy with LCPD, diagnosed 3 years earlier. No improvement of pain and limping after varus intertrochanteric osteotomy. Limited abduction and internal rotation, hinged abduction. (**a**) Coxa magna, slightly shallow acetabulum, head extrusion, subluxation. (**b**) Simulation of osteotomies for achieving the best head size reduction. (**c**) Simulated execution of head reduction followed by PAO. (**d**) Good head reposition and coverage after osteotomy using cutting templates and PAO. (**e**) Excellent radiographic result 2 years after surgery

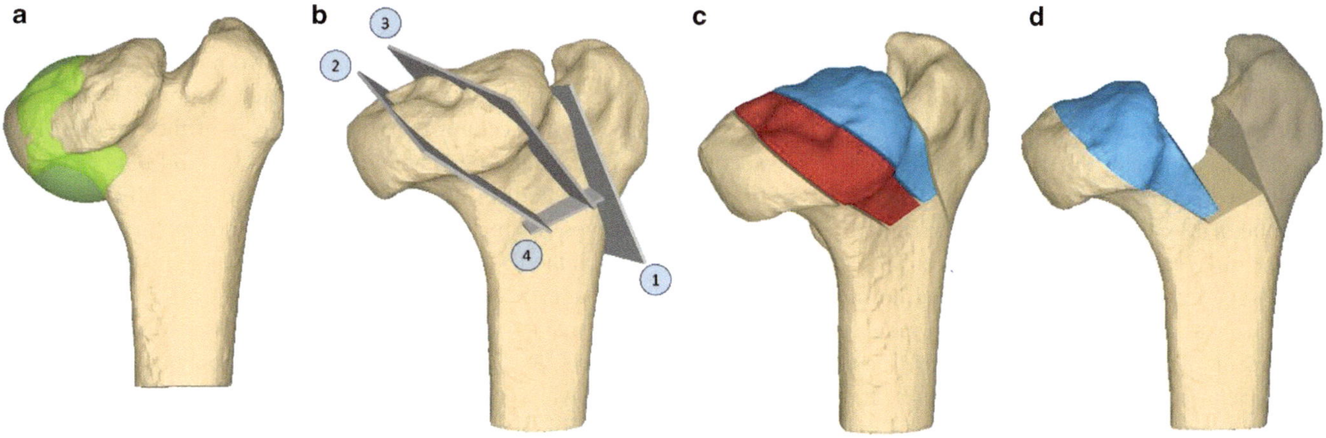

Fig. 5.2 3D computer planning of an FHRO. The 3D models of the patient's anatomy are reconstructed from CT data. (**a**) The remodeling template for the premorbid femoral head is represented by either the mirrored, healthy opposite side or, as here indicated in green, by a sphere. (**b**) Definition of osteotomy cutting planes: intertrochanteric osteotomy (1), medial (2) and lateral intracapital osteotomies (3), and transverse osteotomy (4). (**c**) The intracapital osteotomies define the segment to be resected (red) and the lateral fragment head to be reduced (blue). (**d**) Simulated outcome of the surgery. The form of the resulting head should approximate sphericity, and the size should correspond to the size of the opposite head

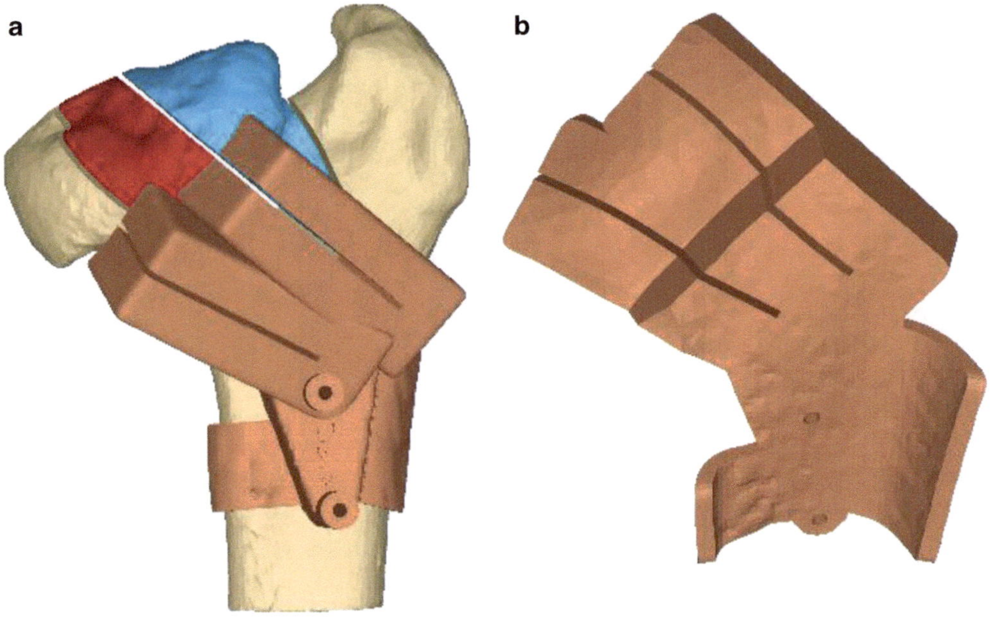

Fig. 5.3 Design of the patient-specific instruments on the computer. (**a**) Based on the preoperative planning, slots are integrated into the PSI to guide saw cutting corresponding to the intracapital osteotomy planes. The integrated drill sleeves are used to place K-wires for the fixation of the PSI. (**b**) The undersurface of the PSI is formed as a negative of the patient's bone surface

medial and lateral cutting planes of the femoral head are positioned at the medial or lateral margin of the central deformation zone, including also parts of or the entire necrosis (Fig. 5.2b). These two osteotomies define the diameter of the stable medial head portion and the size and shape of the central wedge to be removed. The starting point and direction of the osteotomy planes must lie within the dual blood supply of the head represented by the medial and lateral retinaculum. This fine-tuning must be done by the surgeon, who also decides on the diameter of the resulting medial bone pillar. The third, transverse osteotomy of the femoral neck is placed at least 1 cm distal to the head to separate the lateral and central segment (Fig. 5.2c). Afterward, the simulated optimal position of the lateral fragment relative to the medial fragment can be determined by superimposition with the remodeling template. As shown in Fig. 5.2d, the shape of the resulting head should be approximately spherical and in size similar to the contralateral head. However, significant gaps in the surface cartilage must be avoided.

In the computer simulation, the FHRO is considered a multilevel optimization problem with 24 degrees of freedom. A total of 18 parameters describe the centers and inclinations of the three cutting planes (per plane: 3D location and direction vectors for the plane center and normal, respectively), and six parameters describe the 3D reduction of the lateral fragment from pre- to post-operative position (translation along and rotation in three directions each). The first studies on computer-aided FHRO approached solving the optimization problem manually [3] by incrementally refining possible variants of cutting planes and fragment reductions in collaboration with the surgeon. In the meantime, advanced computer methods have largely automated the planning process, which previously took several hours. In particular, artificial intelligence methods enable the calculation of FHRO solutions that can qualitatively compete with those of surgeons and engineers [4].

Based on the computer planning, the PSI for navigating the medial and lateral sections is designed (Fig. 5.3). The main challenge here is to design a base block with a sufficiently large footprint that can be stably and uniquely placed at the anterior neck-head junction of the proximal femur without compromising the inferior-medial vascular supply. Stability is achieved by medial and lateral sidearms that are part of the base block. The contact surface between the PSI and bone is then molded as a negative of the bone surface using CAD functions. In a next step, the PSI is extended proximally towards the femoral head, creating space for the integration of two slots for guiding the surgical saw blade during the medial and lateral head osteotomy, respectively. This part of the PSI has an offset from the bone surface of the femoral head of half a centimeter or more. This distance takes into account the cartilage layer of the femoral head, which cannot be visualized through CT and thus cannot be represented in the bone model. Additionally, two drill sleeves for placing Kirschner wires are integrated through which the PSI can be fixed on the bone to prevent unwanted slippage.

Together with the patient's pre- and post-operative bone models, the PSI model is passed to the manufacturing process, which takes several weeks. The models are fabricated using a 3D printer, verified, cleaned, sterilized, and delivered to the hospital. The application of the PSI in surgery occurs after the femoral head has been presented through the surgical hip dislocation approach as described in Chap. 7, creating sufficient exposure for PSI positioning after careful removal of the periosteum. Correct positioning is verified using the

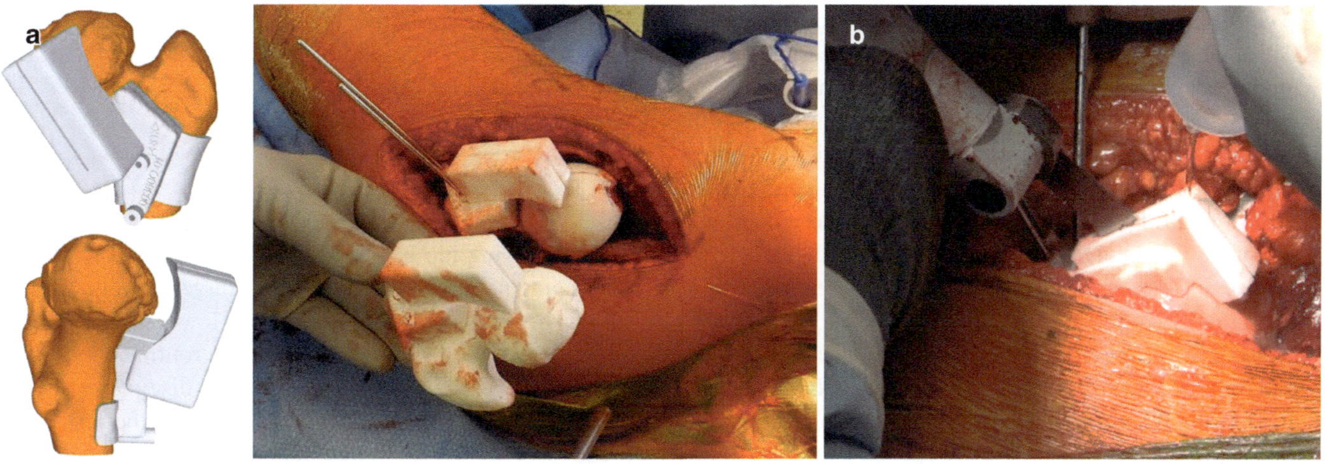

Fig. 5.4 Intraoperative execution of PSI-navigated FHRO. (**a**) Verification of the correct PSI position using 3D prints of the patient's anatomy. (**b**) PSI navigation of the intracapital osteotomies. The cutting slot of the PSI defines the osteotomy and guides the saw blade

3D-printed bone model on which the planned PSI position is marked (Fig. 5.4a). After the PSI has been fixed to the bone with Kirschner wires, the intracapital osteotomies are performed using a surgical saw (Fig. 5.3b and c). Please refer to Chap. 17 to find a detailed description on the surgical technique for intracapital osteotomies including the application of PSIs.

5.3 Principles of Surgical Navigation with Tracking Systems

The localization of surgical tools and anatomical structures in real time is called tracking. Tracking-based navigation systems are capable of visualizing the spatial relationship between tools and anatomy directly in surgery, offering an advantage over the lengthy preoperative manufacturing process of PSI. Currently, two tracking technologies are widely used in clinical applications [1]. By far, the most commonly used is optical tracking [5, 6], followed by electromagnetic tracking [7].

Optical tracking is based on camera systems optimized for the detection of palm-sized instruments called markers. Markers are characterized by a special geometry, which allows measuring their 3D location in all 6 degrees of freedom (position and orientation) only from 2D camera images. Depending on the clinical requirements, different systems with one (monocular), two (stereo), or more cameras can be used, covering various wavebands including those beyond the visible light spectrum. Very precise localization in the submillimeter range is provided by stereo camera systems consisting of two infrared cameras. Reflective, infrared light-sensitive markers are used for localization, which are easily detectable even in difficult lighting conditions or when contaminated by body fluids. The distance between the two cameras, known as the baseline, defines the size of the working volume in which markers can be localized. Systems designed for surgical applications are with dimensions of $50 \times 10 \times 10$ cm relatively large, which, however, allows for a greater distance from the situs and a working volume of more than 1 cubic meter.

The workflow for using optical navigation in surgery can be described as follows. First, a reference marker is attached to the bone anatomy using a clamp or surgical pin. In the case of navigation by intraoperative, 3D imaging, an intraoperative CT image is acquired in the next step. Fusion of the image (anatomy) and camera (instruments with markers) spaces is achieved by calculating the transformation between these modalities, derived from the reference marker visible in both the CT image and the camera. Alternatively, navigation based on a preoperative plan can be performed after determining the positional difference between preoperative and intraoperative anatomy through registration. To this end, the intraoperative position of the anatomy is either determined by conventional fluoroscopy imaging or, if no additional radiation exposure is acceptable, by an approach called surface sampling [5, 6]. In surface sampling, the bone anatomy is scanned and digitized using a pointing device that is tracked by the navigation system. The resulting point cloud of the anatomy is then registered with the preoperative anatomy and the preoperative plan. The joint representation of preoperative plan and localized instruments is shown to the surgeon on a monitor for surgical navigation. The registration process only needs to be performed once, as positional changes of the anatomy are compensated by the reference marker.

Optical tracking systems are unable to locate instruments and anatomy if the markers are not visible to the camera. This problem, called "line-of-sight" issue, occurs frequently during surgical procedures as surgeons, surgical assistants, and equipment interact in close proximity to the surgical site. Electromagnetic tracking systems avoid non-visual sensors within an electromagnetic field to locate instruments in 3D space. In electromagnetic tracking, a sensor attached to the instrument tip measures variations in a magnetic field generated by a field generator. The sensor signal is continuously sent to a control unit where the position and orientation of the sensor are calculated based on the specific geometry of the magnetic field. As in optical tracking, electromagnetic tracking involves attaching reference sensors to the anatomy and using registration methods. Clinically used sensors are wired, but only a few millimeters in size, which makes them suitable for navigation of needle instruments and minimally invasive procedures.

Regardless of the underlying tracking technology, navigation systems require a display unit to present the navigation information. In addition to visualization on conventional monitors, more advanced visualization techniques, especially augmented reality (AR), have increasingly found their way into the operating room in recent years. In AR, the user's visual sensory perception is enhanced by additional computer-generated information. To superimpose information, a so-called head-mounted display (HMD) is employed that is worn on the user's head. Newer generations of HMDs do not require any additional hardware or cabling and use a large number of sensors to localize themselves in space. This capability allows virtual objects to be displayed in real time from the wearer's correct viewing angle, making them perceived as seamlessly embedded in the real environment.

The growing number of preclinical and clinical studies underpins the great potential of AR for intraoperative applications. AR is capable of providing in-situ visualization of preoperative imaging during surgery, especially of anatomical structures, such as nerves or blood vessels, that may be otherwise not visible to the surgeon. Additionally, AR can simplify surgical navigation by displaying directional and positional information from the surgeon's egocentric viewpoint and close to the situs. In the context of hip surgery, AR navigation has been successfully used in PAO [8] and total hip arthroplasty.

5.4 Discussion

Joint-preserving hip surgery is among the most technically challenging procedures in orthopedic surgery, suggesting the use of surgical navigation methods. However, the clinical translation of navigation techniques into routine patient care has been slower than for other orthopedic disciplines such as hand, knee, or spine surgery. One reason is the less widespread use of 3D computer planning for hip procedures, which is limited by the conservative application of CT imaging. The integration of navigation techniques also faces challenges due to the limited space available in the situs and the complex soft tissue situation. Therefore, not all established navigation techniques are routinely used for joint-preserving hip surgery (see Table 5.1). PSIs represent currently the gold standard for the navigation of joint-preserving procedures. Their mechanical instrument guidance is ideal for osteotomies, while not requiring any additional hardware or technology during the surgery. Conversely, navigation through intraoperative technologies such as AR or tracking systems offers more flexibility thanks to the possibility to change or adjust navigation parameters during the surgery.

A key criterion for assessing the performance of surgical navigation methods is the evaluation of surgical execution accuracy. The gold standard measurement method evaluates the 3D angular and positional differences of relevant parameters such as cutting planes, screw trajectories, or bone fragments by comparing the preoperative planning with post-operative CT data. Studies investigating the 3D accuracy of PSI navigation of joint-preserving surgeries were mostly performed for the upper extremities, where an average 3D error of $4.7° \pm 3.5°$ and 0.9 ± 0.5 mm was reported

Table 5.1 Overview of navigation techniques that are established in hip surgery

Technology	Maturity with respect to hip surgery	Advantages	Disadvantages
Patient-specific instruments	In vivo: PAO and FHRO [3], tumor resections, and endoprothetics (all commercially available)	Simple intraoperative use Mechanical guidance of instruments	Long lead time No intraoperative adoption of the planning
Navigation with optical tracking systems	In vivo: PAO (in studies [5, 6]) and endoprothetics (commercially available)	Planning can be adopted	Line-of-sight issues Markers on instruments and anatomy
Navigation with augmented reality	In vivo: endoprothetics Ex-vivo studies: PAO [8]	Planning can be adopted Less line-of-sight issues Egocentric and/or in-situ visualization	Surgeon wears HMD Markers on instruments and anatomy
Navigation with electromagnetic tracking systems	In vivo: extra-articular osteotomies and PAO (in studies [7])	No line-of-sight issues Small sensors replace markers	Small working volume Interferes with ferromagnetic objects or external electromagnetic fields

for intra-articular osteotomies. Due to the higher effective radiation dose in the hip region, the accuracy of PSI-navigated joint-preserving hip interventions has been so far evaluated only on the basis of post-operative radiographs. The only study investigating PSI-navigated FHRO to date [3] measured a radiologically post-operative improvement in femoral head sphericity of 20% and only a 2% deviation in head diameter post-operatively compared with the opposite side. Currently, no studies have been performed on navigating FHRO with electromagnetic or optical tracking systems. In contrast, tracking systems for PAO navigation have already been investigated in patient studies (see Table 5.1). In one of these studies, the combined use of PSI and electromagnetic tracking achieved an average of five times higher accuracy in the reduction of the acetabular fragment compared with the conventionally performed control group [7]. Studies also reported that navigation can lead to shorter operation times, as the use of time-consuming fluoroscopy acquisition can be reduced.

Navigation systems have disadvantages, regardless of the underlying technology used. The use of navigation causes additional costs, most of which are not reimburseable by insurers in the case of joint-preserving interventions. One significant cost factor is 3D preoperative planning, which becomes more labor-intensive as case complexity increases. For example, the cost of preparing an FHRO plan is approximately USD 2000 due to the close collaboration required between engineers and surgeons. Additionally, the costs of 3D printing (in the case of PSI) and the acquisition and maintenance costs (for tracking systems) must be added as well. Another disadvantage is the need for a preoperative CT, which results in additional radiation exposure for the patient. However, new innovations in diagnostic imaging, such as low-dose CT [9], are addressing this issue. Low-dose CT allows high-quality CT images to be obtained with a radiation exposure comparable to that of an X-ray. Due to their high technical complexity, navigation systems can disrupt the standard surgical workflow. This is particularly true for optical tracking systems, where markers and line-of-sight issues can interfere. However, reliance on markers is decreasing due to the development of image-based tracking methods, which are currently under research.

The discussion about the benefits of computer-assisted surgery and its impact on the treatment outcome must be nuanced, also considering future developments. The majority of orthopedic operations are performed without surgical navigation, often achieving excellent surgical outcomes. Literature shows that navigated surgery offers a significantly higher execution accuracy, particularly as the complexity of the treatment increases. However, there is not yet significant evidence for a correlation with a better functional outcome. In complex cases, the greatest added value lies in 3D preoperative planning, which simulates and optimizes each surgical step until the best possible outcome is found.

5.5 Outlook

The development and application of PSIs in surgery show great potential for the future. A key advancement in this area will be the further development of manufacturing technologies. 3D printing already enables the production of patient-specific osteosynthesis implants, but these need to become more cost-effective and faster to manufacture to be regularly used in surgical practice. In the long term, 3D printing of biological tissues will support the customized creation of osteochondral implants and transplants, as well as ligament and tendon reconstruction.

The rapid advancements in diagnostic imaging are a crucial driver for the effectiveness of computer-assisted surgical planning. CT-based imaging technologies now have the ability to measure individual photons and their energy content, resulting in significantly higher image resolution, improved tissue differentiation, reduced radiation doses, and fewer image artifacts [10]. The fusion of CT and MRI images provides important soft tissue information for the surgical planning of FHRO [11] including cartilage structures and blood vessels,

These developments are leading to the replacement of geometric planning with biomechanical planning. In biomechanical planning, range of motion and joint forces can be simulated, which will further enhance the effectiveness and predictive power of computer planning. Surgical navigation, AR, and surgical robotics are increasingly effective tools to assist surgeons in accurately performing procedures according to preoperative plans.

Overall, computer-assisted surgery should be seen as part of digitization in orthopedics, increasingly benefiting from the research advances in artificial intelligence. This interplay with artificial intelligence will help overcome current limitations, such as lack of automation or integration into the surgical workflow, allowing computer-assisted surgery to be used more frequently and efficiently. In turn, computer-assisted surgery will contribute to obtaining quantitative data, allowing data-driven methods to become increasingly effective.

5.6 Summary

The FHRO, combined with periacetabular procedures, has proven to be a safe and effective technique for treating Legg-Calvé-Perthes disease. Computer-assisted planning and PSI-guided execution provide surgeons with optimal preparation and support to perform this demanding operation in a controlled and predictable manner. The PSI technique is pioneering for the precise execution of complex hip surgeries. Despite computer assistance, the procedure remains challenging, requiring solid surgical training, dedicated practice, and a step-by-step approach.

References

1. Joskowicz L, Hazan EJ. Computer aided orthopaedic surgery: incremental shift or paradigm change? Med Image Anal. 2016;33:84–90.
2. Fürnstahl P, Schweizer A, Graf M, Vlachopoulos L, Fucentese S, Wirth S, Nagy L, Szekely G, Goksel O. Surgical treatment of long-bone deformities: 3D preoperative planning and patient-specific instrumentation. In: Computational radiology for orthopaedic interventions. Cham: Springer; 2016. p. 123–49.
3. Fürnstahl P, Casari FA, Ackermann J, Marcon M, Leunig M, Ganz R. Computer-assisted femoral head reduction osteotomies: an approach for anatomic reconstruction of severely deformed Legg-Calvé-Perthes hips. A pilot study of six patients. BMC Musculoskelet Disord. 2020;21(1):1–9.
4. Ackermann J, Wieland M, Hoch A, Ganz R, Snedeker JG, Oswald MR, Pollefeys M, Zingg PO, Esfandiari H, Fürnstahl P. A new approach to orthopedic surgery planning using deep reinforcement learning and simulation. In: International conference on medical image computing and computer-assisted intervention. Cham: Springer; 2021. p. 540–9.
5. Hsieh PH, Chang YH, Shih CH. Image-guided periacetabular osteotomy: computer-assisted navigation compared with the conventional technique: a randomized study of 36 patients followed for 2 years. Acta Orthop. 2006;77(4):591–7.
6. Hooper JM, Mays RR, Poultsides LA, Castaneda PG, Muir JM, Kamath AF. Periacetabular osteotomy using an imageless computer-assisted navigation system: a new surgical technique. J Hip Preserv Surg. 2019;6(4):426–31.
7. Mihalič R, Brumat P, Trebše R. Bernese peri-acetabular osteotomy performed with navigation and patient-specific templates is a reproducible and safe procedure. Int Orthop. 2021;45(4):883–9.
8. Ackermann J, Liebmann F, Hoch A, Snedeker JG, Farshad M, Rahm S, Zingg PO, Fürnstahl P. Augmented reality based surgical navigation of complex pelvic osteotomies—a feasibility study on cadavers. Appl Sci. 2021;11(3):1228.
9. Stern C, Sommer S, Germann C, Galley J, Pfirrmann CW, Fritz B, Sutter R. Pelvic bone CT: can tin-filtered ultra-low-dose CT and virtual radiographs be used as alternative for standard CT and digital radiographs? Eur Radiol. 2021;31(9):6793–801.
10. Marcus RP, Nagy DA, Feuerriegel GC, Anhaus J, Nanz D, Sutter R. Photon-counting detector CT with denoising for imaging of the osseous pelvis at low radiation doses: a phantom study. Am J Roentgenol. 2024;222(1):e2329765.
11. Massè A, Giachino M, Audisio A, Donis A, Secco DC, Limone B, Turchetto L, Aprato A. Ganz femoral head reduction associated with coverage and containment procedures improve radiological and functional outcomes in Perthes' disease. Bone Joint J. 2024;106:40–6.

6 Surgical Anatomy of the Hip

Morteza Kalhor, Christopher L. Peters, and Martin Beck

6.1 Introduction

Knowledge of the local anatomy is of the utmost importance in any successful surgical procedure. This chapter illustrates the normal surgical anatomy of the hip based on a series of fresh cadaveric dissections and with more emphasis on its vascular aspects. The descriptions and illustrations cover the topographic anatomy of the hip applicable to the common anterior through posterior approaches.

6.2 Background

Anatomy is the "Kindergarden" of orthopedics. Only the profound knowledge and appreciation of the surgical anatomy of the hip allows for safe and successful surgical execution of hip preservation surgery. General aspects of the hip anatomy are described in anatomical textbooks [1–3], but successful execution of classical as well as less invasive surgical approaches needs detailed knowledge of the surgical anatomy and the important anatomical structures located in the vicinity of the dissection area. Improved understanding of hip anatomy, especially the vascular anatomy, during the last 2 decades led to the development of new surgical techniques for safe access to the joint and execution of extraarticular and intraarticular procedures [4–9]. Depending on the goal for surgery, the hip joint may be approached from the front, the side, or the back as described in orthopedic textbooks [10, 11]. With a more precise knowledge of the local anatomy, the classic approaches can be customized as needed, allowing for safe and effective practical application. In this chapter, the surgical anatomy of the hip is shown based on a series of cadaveric dissections. The dissections are expanded beyond the classic approaches to demonstrate the important anatomic structures in the vicinity of the surgical field.

The chapter is presented in two parts: first, surgical anatomy of the hip for anterior and posterior approaches and, second, vascular anatomy of the hip with particular reference on femoral head perfusion and surgical implications. The information and illustrations are the results of fresh cadaveric dissections all from white Indo-European origins.

6.3 Surgical Anatomy of Anterior Approaches to the Hip

Anterior approaches to the hip can be focused on either femoral exposure, with the incision distal to the anterior superior iliac spine (ASIS), or iliofemoral with the extension of the incision proximal to the ASIS over the iliac crest, allowing access to the periacetabulum (Fig. 6.1). The ASIS and the iliac crest are the landmarks most frequently referenced in all variations of the anterior hip approaches. Easily palpable at the anterior end of the iliac crest, the ASIS is the site of attachment of the sartorius tendon and inguinal ligament. The tensor fascia latae (TFL) muscle also originates partly from its lateral border (Fig. 6.2). In spite of the variability of skin incisions, dissection for deep layers access, commonly uses the interval between the TFL and sartorius muscle, the so-called internervous or Hueter interval.

Anterior and distal to the inguinal ligament the hip is covered superficially by the TFL and sartorius. The lateral femoral cutaneous nerve (LFCN) emerges from the inside of the pelvis to the thigh medial to the ASIS and usually under the inguinal ligament (Fig. 6.2). Here, it lies anterior to the

M. Kalhor (✉)
Department of Orthopaedic Surgery, Firoozgar Medical Center, Iran University of Medical Sciences, Tehran, Iran

C. L. Peters
Department of Orthopedic Surgery, University of Utah, Salt Lake City, UT, USA
e-mail: Chris.Peters@hsc.utah.edu

M. Beck
Orthopaedic Clinic Lucerne, Hirslanden Clinic St. Anna, Lucerne, Switzerland
e-mail: martin.beck@okl.ch

M. Leunig et al. (eds.), *Surgical Hip Dislocation*, https://doi.org/10.1007/978-3-031-70622-6_6

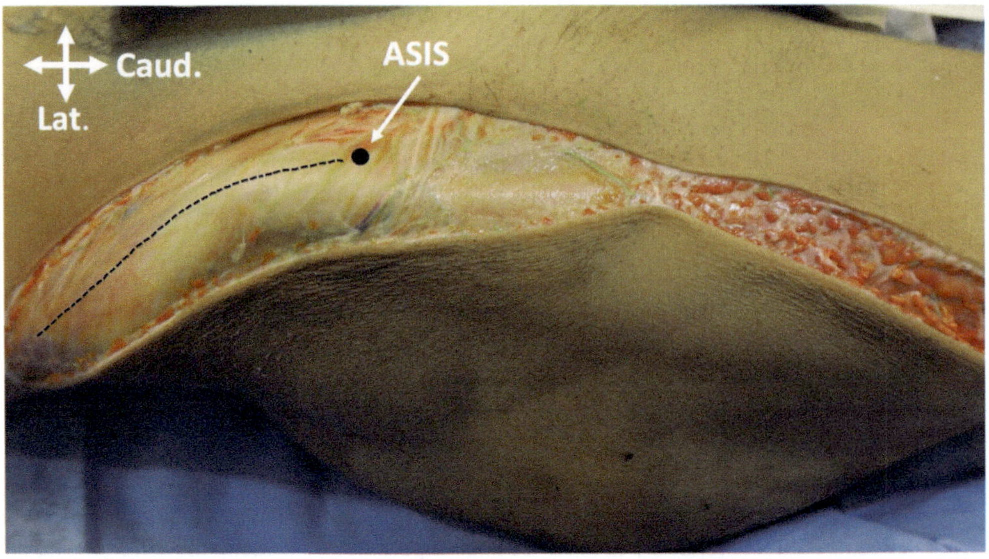

Fig. 6.1 Anterior aspect of the right hip showing the iliofemoral incision for the Smith–Petersen approach. ASIS = anterior superior iliac spine; Caud. = caudad; Lat. = lateral

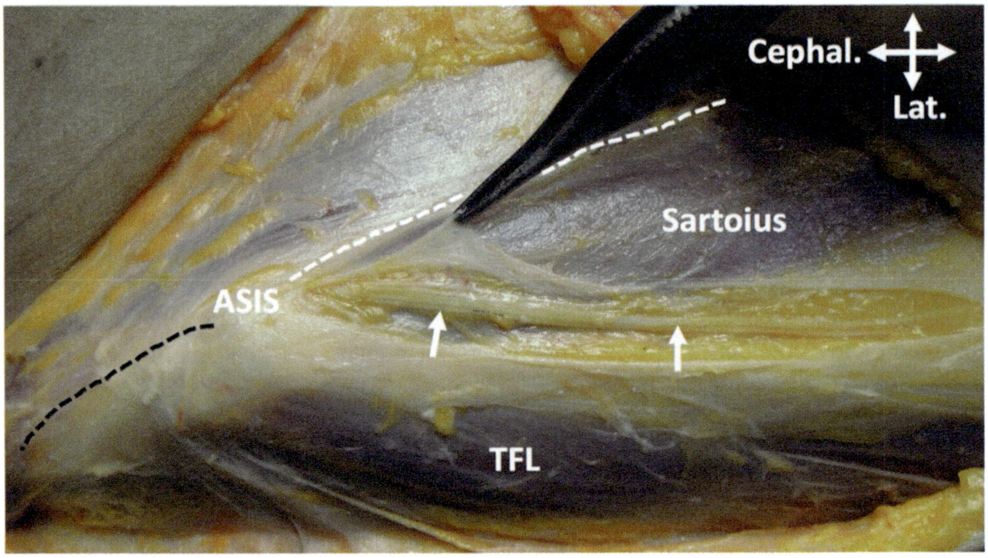

Fig. 6.2 Right hip anterior aspect after skin incision showing the superficial anatomic structures encountered in the Smith–Petersen approach. The black broken line shows the anterior aspect of the iliac crest, and the white broken line shows the inguinal ligament. Arrows indicate the lateral femoral cutaneous nerve. ASIS = anterior superior iliac spine; TFL = tensor fasciae latae muscle; Cephal. = cephalad; Lat. = lateral

tendon of sartorius or sometimes lies more medially and crosses the sartorius fibers obliquely to enter the thigh (Fig. 6.3a). The medialization distance from the ASIS can be up to 5 cm. In their cadaveric study, Rudin et al. found occasional emergence of the cutaneous nerve from over or even lateral to the ASIS crossing the iliac crest [12]. Distal to the inguinal ligament, the nerve runs in the space between these two muscles. In 30% of cases, a branch of the nerve crosses the fascia of the TFL obliquely and often is sacrificed in some anterior approaches [13, 14] (Fig. 6.3b). The emergence and branching pattern of the LFCN have also been described in more detail by Üzel et al. and Rudin et al. in cadaveric studies [12, 15].

Commonly, the space between the TFL and sartorius is opened for access to the deep layers which makes injury of the cutaneous nerve highly likely [15]. Staying more lateral to the interval, by incising the fascia of the tensor, and intrafascial lateral retraction of the muscle fibers, the nerve can be protected from damage in many cases (Fig. 6.4).

The iliofemoral approach extends the femoral exposure proximally, usually with the detachment of the inguinal ligament and sartorius tendon from the ASIS. Osteotomy of the ASIS if pedicled by the sartorius tendon and inguinal ligament can effectively protect the cutaneous nerve during internal iliac exposure [16–18] (Figs. 6.5 and 6.6). After retraction of the superficial muscle layer, that is, TFL laterally and sartorius medially, the origin of rectus femoris is exposed. From this step on and for exposure of the capsule, either the plane medial or lateral to the rectus femoris muscle may be used, depending on the indication for the surgery (Fig. 6.7). More commonly, the lateral plane between the rectus and TFL is used and continued deeply by retraction of

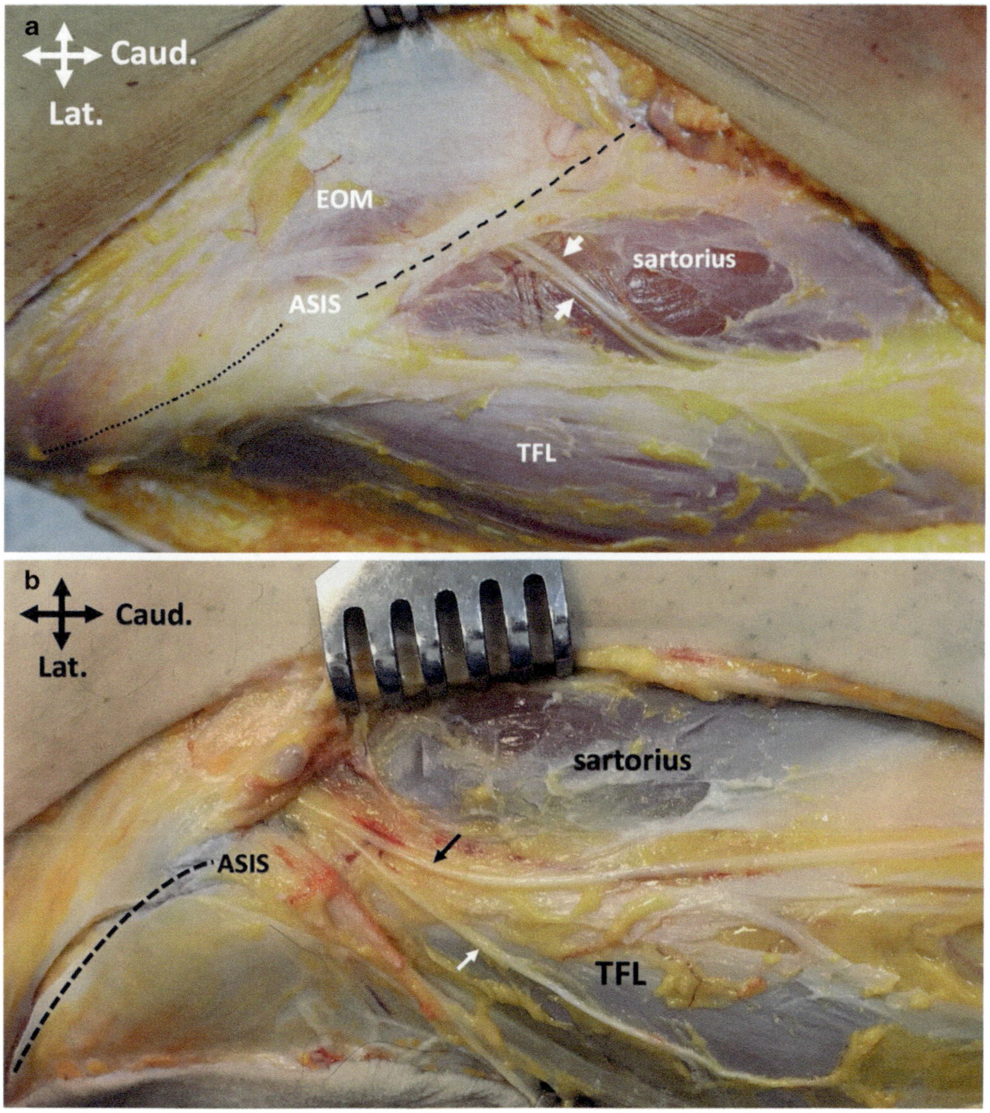

Fig. 6.3 (**a**) Right hip anterior aspect, showing the more medial location of the lateral femoral cutaneous nerve (short arrows). The dotted line shows the iliac crest. The broken line shows the inguinal ligament. EOM = external oblique abdominal muscle; ASIS = anterior superior iliac spine; TFL = tensor fasciae latae muscle; sartorius = sartorius muscle. (**b**) Right hip anterior aspect. Surface anatomy after skin incision showing a normal variation in branching of the cutaneous nerve. In 30% of the cases, a nerve branch crosses the TFL fascia anterolaterally (white arrow). The broken line shows the iliac crest. The black arrow shows the lateral femoral cutaneous nerve. ASIS = anterior superior iliac spine; TFL = tensor fasciae latae muscle; Caud. = caudad; Lat. = lateral

the abductors laterally and the rectus and iliopsoas muscle medially to expose the anterior hip capsule. Medial retraction of the rectus exposes the underlying innominate fascia, which covers the area between the intertrochanteric line and the reflected head of the rectus. In close vicinity of the fascia, runs the ascending branch of the lateral femoral circumflex artery (LFCA) which is the only important anatomic structure encountered in this step of surgery. The artery crosses the undersurface of the rectus transversely to reach the TFL muscle (Figs. 6.5 and 6.8). For wide exposure of the anterior capsule, the reflected and direct heads of the rectus are detached from their origins and retracted medially together with the iliopsoas and iliocapsularis muscles, in continuity with the internal iliac muscle. The small iliocapsularis muscle is located under the iliacus muscle. It originates from the inferior surface of the anterior inferior iliac spine (AIIS) and the subspinous part of the acetabulum [19]. It covers the anterior capsule and its fibers blend distally with the iliacus muscle. More recently, an alternative method for anterior hip joint access was described to allow for the retention of the origins of the rectus femoris muscle. The so-called rectus sparing approach preserves the direct and indirect heads of the rectus, and the anterior capsule is exposed by retraction of the rectus laterally and the iliopsoas medially [20–22] (Fig. 6.9). There is a fascia covering these two muscles. For exposure of the capsule, it is important to divide this fascia in order to separate these two muscles sufficiently. Retracting these two muscles apart for the purpose of intraarticular access, can put excessive tension on the intervening femoral nerve, especially the branch to the rectus muscle [22] (Fig. 6.9). Therefore, the rectus sparing approach cannot be considered an internervous approach as the original approach.

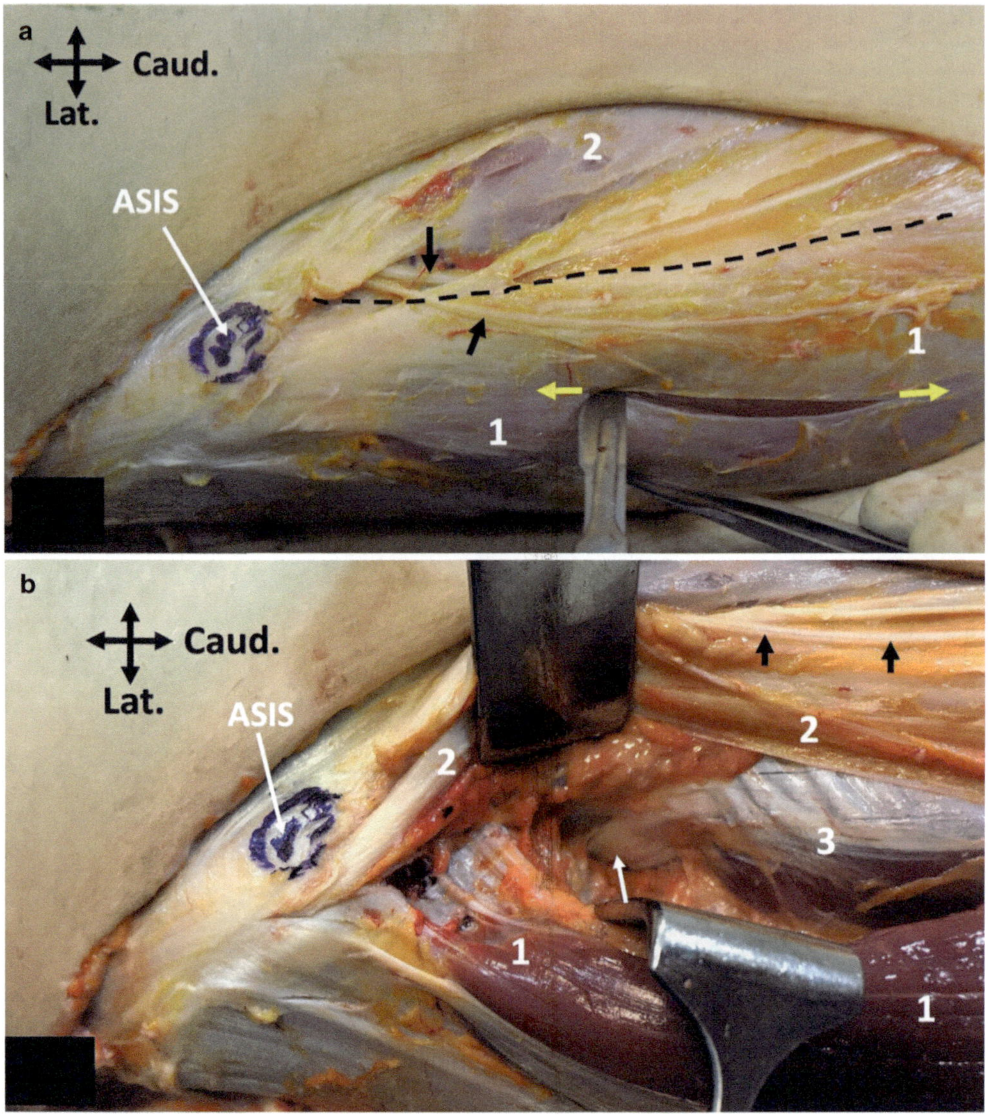

Fig. 6.4 Right hip anterior approach. (**a**) Superficial anatomic structures encountered after skin incision. The classic anterior approach uses the interval between the TFL and sartorius for deep access layers (broken line). Incision of TFL fascia in modified approach for protection of LFCN (yellow arrows). (**b**) Development of the plane between the rectus femoris and TFL showing the reflected head of the rectus as a landmark for the anterolateral acetabular rim. Access to the deep layers is made through the fascia of the TFL to protect LFCN. 1 = TFL; 2 = sartorius; 3 = rectus femoris. White arrows show the reflected head of the rectus. Black arrows show the lateral femoral cutaneous nerve. ASIS = anterior superior iliac spine

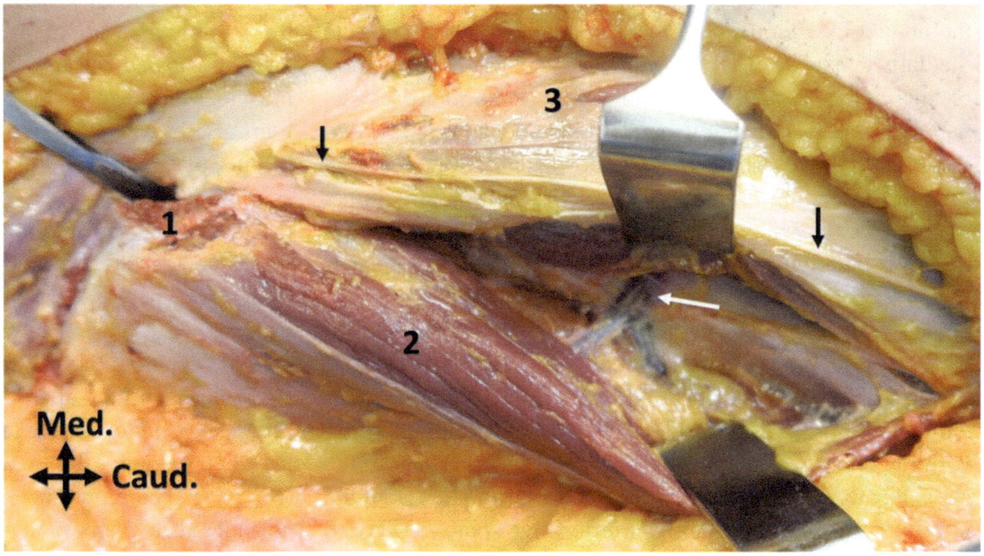

Fig. 6.5 Anterior aspect of the right hip after osteotomy of the ASIS attached to the inguinal ligament and sartorius tendon. Retraction of the TFL and sartorius muscles for access to deeper layers in the anterior iliofemoral approach. The white arrow shows the ascending branch of the LFCA; the black arrows show the lateral cutaneous nerve. 1 = ASIS; 2 = TFL muscle; 3 = sartorius muscle

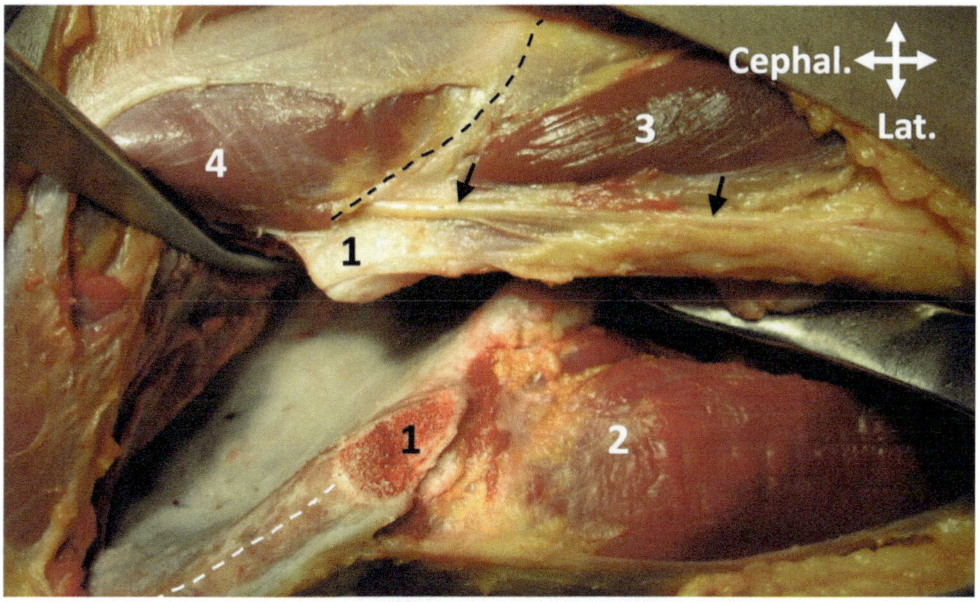

Fig. 6.6 Iliofemoral approach in the right hip. Pedicled osteotomy of the ASIS associated with subperiosteal exposure of the internal iliac surface makes a continuous medial soft tissue flap for protection of the cutaneous nerve proximal to the inguinal ligament. The broken line shows the inguinal ligament. Arrows show the lateral femoral cutaneous nerve. 1 = ASIS osteotomized; 2 = TFL muscle; 3 = sartorius muscle; 4 = oblique abdominal muscle

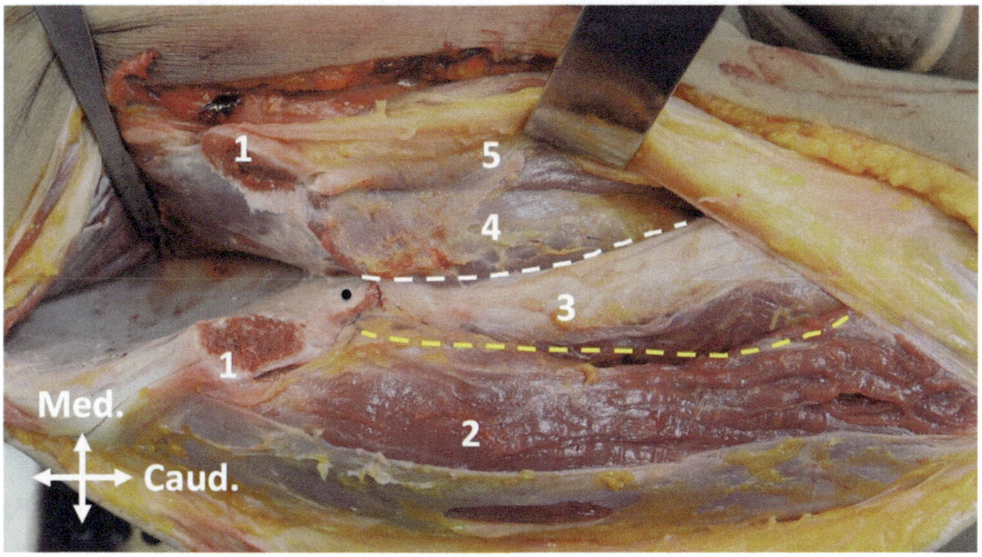

Fig. 6.7 Muscular anatomy of the Iliofemoral approach in the right hip. Pedicled osteotomy of the ASIS associated with subperiosteal exposure of the internal iliac aspect can make a continuous medial soft tissue flap from intrapelvic and extrapelvic muscles to protect the neurovascular structures in anterior approaches. In the classic approach (yellow line), the rectus and its tendons are part of the medial soft tissue flap, but in the rectus sparing approach (white broken line), the rectus is part of the lateral soft tissue flap. The yellow broken line shows the line of the classic approach. The black dot shows the AIIS. 1 = ASIS osteotomized; 2 = TFL muscle; 3 = rectus femoris; 4 = iliopsoas; 5 = sartorius

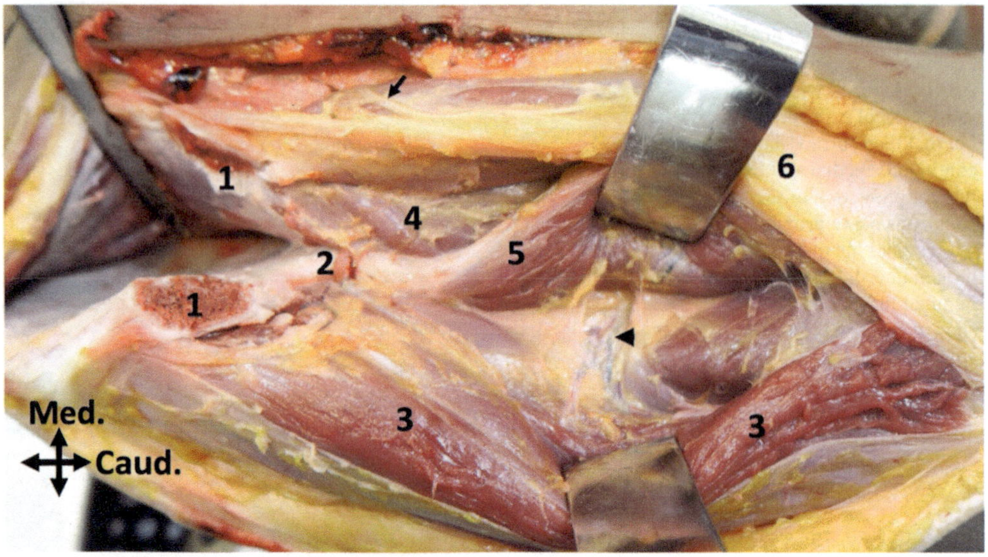

Fig. 6.8 Anatomy and surgical landmarks of an iliofemoral approach showing the anterior aspect of the right hip. 1 = ASIS osteotomized; 2 = AIIS and the insertion of direct head of the rectus femoris muscle; 3 = TFL muscle, retracted laterally; 4 = iliopsoas muscle; 5 = rectus femoris; 6 = sartorius. The arrowhead shows the ascending branch of the LFCA

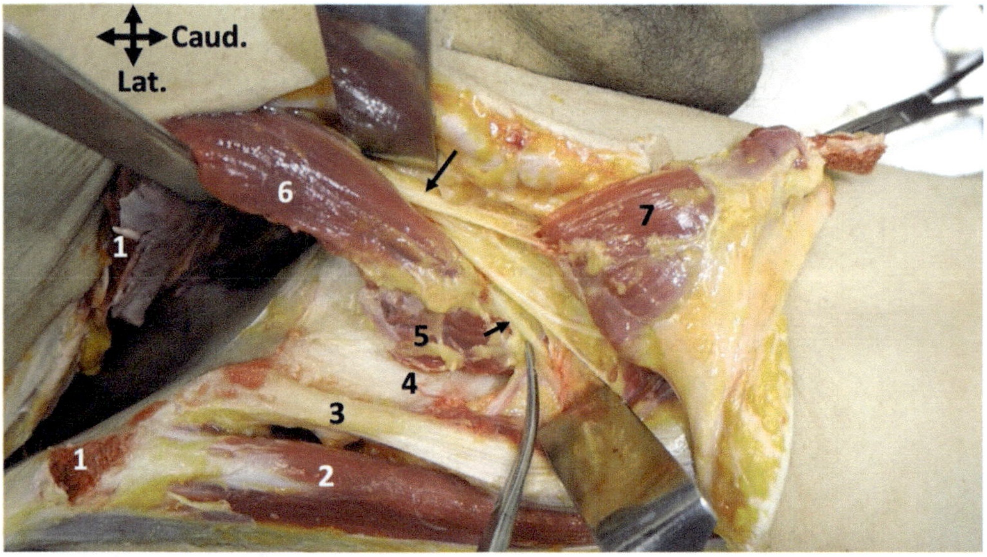

Fig. 6.9 Exposure of the femoral nerve in rectus sparing iliofemoral hip approach. Retraction of the rectus laterally and iliopsoas medially is likely to put excessive tension on the nerve branch to the rectus. Arrows show the femoral nerve (long arrow) and the nerve branch to the rectus (short arrow). 1 = ASIS osteotomized; 2 = TFL; 3 = rectus directed head; 4 = anterior hip capsule; 5 = iliocapsularis muscle; 6 = iliopsoas muscle; 7 = sartorius reflected distally

After full exposure of the anterior hip capsule, a T-shaped capsulotomy is performed with the vertical limb along the anterior aspect of the femoral neck and the transverse limb on the acetabular side. With this technique, there will be minimal or no risk of damaging the femoral head blood supply. The Weitbrecht ligament on the medial aspect of the neck must be protected in order to avoid injuring the inferomedial retinacular artery (or arteries) running on top of the ligament toward the femoral head (Fig. 6.10).

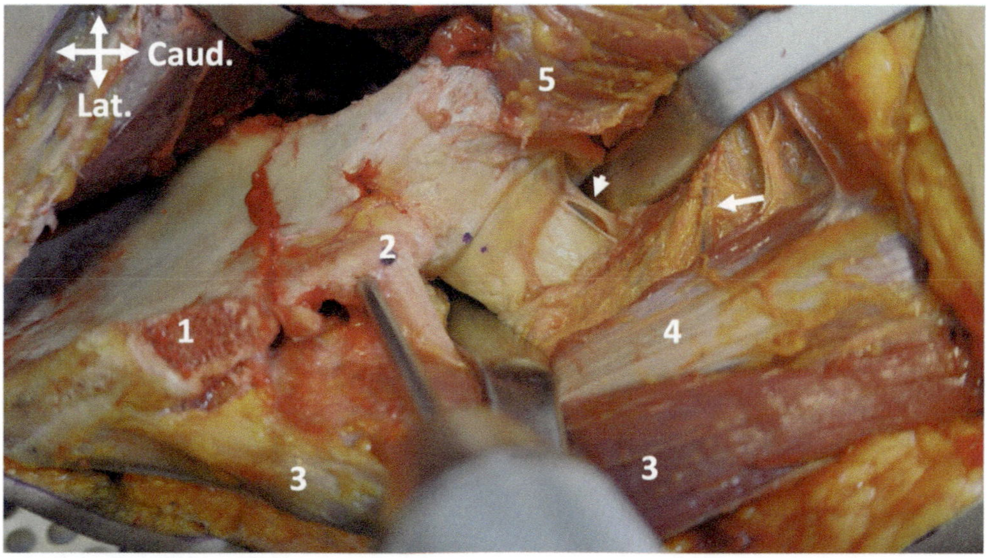

Fig. 6.10 Exposure of the hip through the rectus-sparing anterior approach. Arthrotomy of the right hip through the rectus-sparing approach. 1 = ASIS (osteotomized); 2 = AIIS; 3 = TFL; 4 = rectus femoris; 5 = iliopsoas. Large dot = labrum; small dot = femoral head. The arrow shows the ascending branch of LFCA, and the arrowhead shows Weitbrecht's ligament

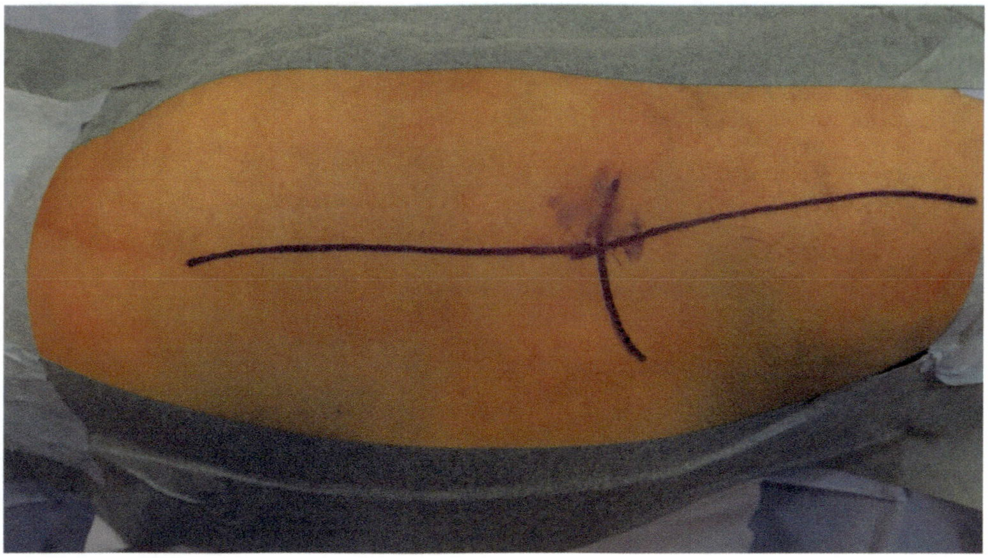

Fig. 6.11 Straight lateral approach centered over the GT. The patient is in a lateral decubitus position with the right side up

6.4 Surgical Anatomy of the Posterior and Posterolateral Approaches

The greater trochanter (GT) is the main and most frequently referenced landmark in posterior and posterolateral approaches to the hip and pelvis. The GT is the site for the insertion of most of the large muscles acting on the hip joint with their origins on the external aspect of the ilium. The entire external aspect of the pelvis from posteromedial to the anterolateral is covered superficially by the gluteus maximus (Gmax), gluteus medius (Gmed), and TFL muscle, respectively [1–3]. These three muscles have no capsular contact. In the deep layer and in attachment to the capsule, are the gluteus minimus (Gmin) and short external rotators (SERs). The gluteus minimus has a wide origin from the external aspect of ilium and is completely covered by the Gmed muscle. It covers most part of the posterior and posterolateral parts of the capsule and converges distally and anteriorly. It attaches to the joint capsule in the area of the iliofemoral ligament and continues to insert into the anterior facet of the GT [23]. The SERs are covered by the Gmax.

The hip can be accessed through lateral, posterolateral, or posterior approaches with the patient in a lateral decubitus position. In this chapter, the anatomy of the posterior aspect of the right hip and pelvis is exposed with the specimen in the lateral decubitus position (Fig. 6.11). A straight lateral incision centered over the GT is used to expose the fascia lata. The incision can be extended proximally and distally as needed for exposure. Proximal to the GT, the fascial incision can be extended along the anterior border of the gluteus maximus muscle (Gibson interval) (Fig. 6.12), or inclined posterosuperiorly toward the posterior inferior iliac spine, as a Gmax muscle splitting approach. The fascia lata along the anterior border of the Gmax delicately blends with the fascia over the

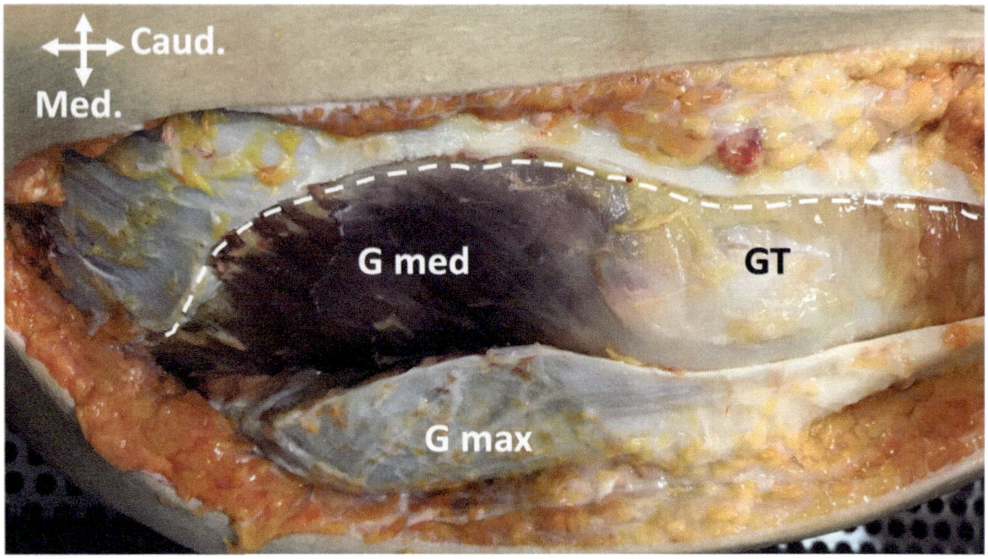

Fig. 6.12 Lateral approach after separation of the anterior border of the gluteus maximus from the fascia lata and gluteus medius. GT = gluteus medius; G med = gluteus medius; G max = gluteus maximus

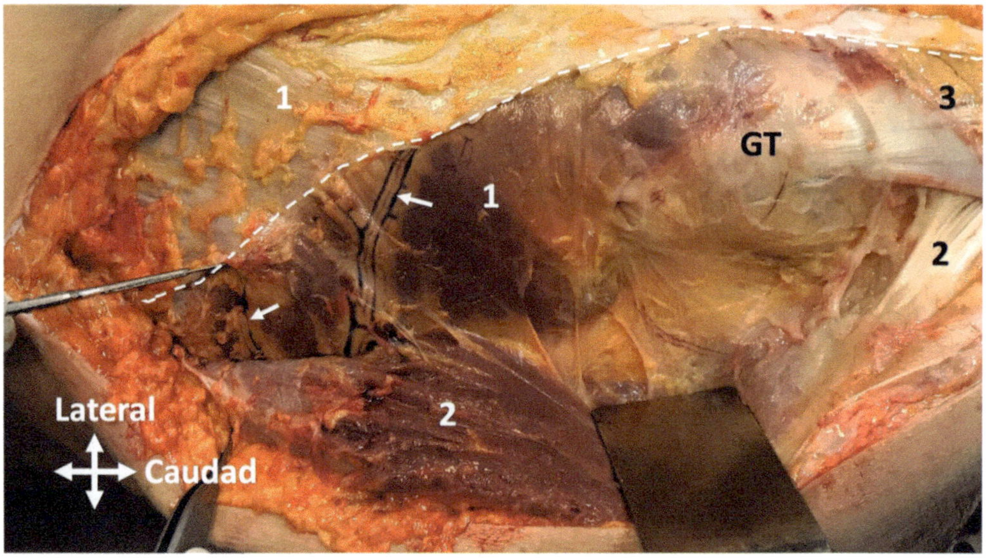

Fig. 6.13 Straight lateral approach to the right hip. Detachment of the anterior border of the Gmax from the fascia lata for exposure of the posterior aspect of the hip. The line can be found using the perforating vessels emerging from the fascia lata along the anterior border of the muscle as landmarks (arrows). 1 = gluteus medius; 2 = gluteus maximus; 3 = origin of the vastus lateralis on the GT. The broken line shows the anterior border of the Gmax

Gmed, so the border is not very well defined. Helpful in delineating this line or interval are a few perforating small vessels emerging exactly along the anterior border of the Gmax (Fig. 6.13). These are usually two and rarely three bundles of vessels originating from the SGA that travel all the way between the gluteus maximus and medius from the posteromedial to the anterolateral surface and finally perforate the fascia lata at the anterior border of the gluteus maximus, to become subcutaneous. The alternate, cosmetically less favorable way to access the deep layers is the Gmax splitting technique. The fascial incision along the anterior border of Gmax can be extended over the GT and vastus lateralis as distally as needed. The Gmax can easily be retracted posteromedially with the fascia along its whole length from proximal attachment to the ilium to its distal tendinous insertion (Fig. 6.13). Retracting the gluteus maximus which is easier with the hip joint held in some extension will allow exposing the Gmed, SERs, and the sciatic nerve (Fig. 6.14).

The gluteus minimus is completely covered by the gluteus medius muscle. Retraction of Gmed proximally and anteriorly with or without osteotomy of the GT exposes the Gmin and also the superior gluteal nerve (SGN) and vessels emerging from the greater sciatic notch. An overview of all deep-layer anatomic structures can be shown by retraction of Gmax medially and Gmed proximally (Fig. 6.15). Underlying Gmed, the Gmin covers most of the external aspect of the iliac bone and posterior capsule. With a wide origin from the external iliac surface, the gluteus minimus converges distally to attach to the anterior facet of the GT (Fig. 6.15).

Distal to the lower border of the Gmin and at the posterior aspect of the hip joint, the SERs are located. The uppermost SER is the piriformis, the main anatomical landmark for the

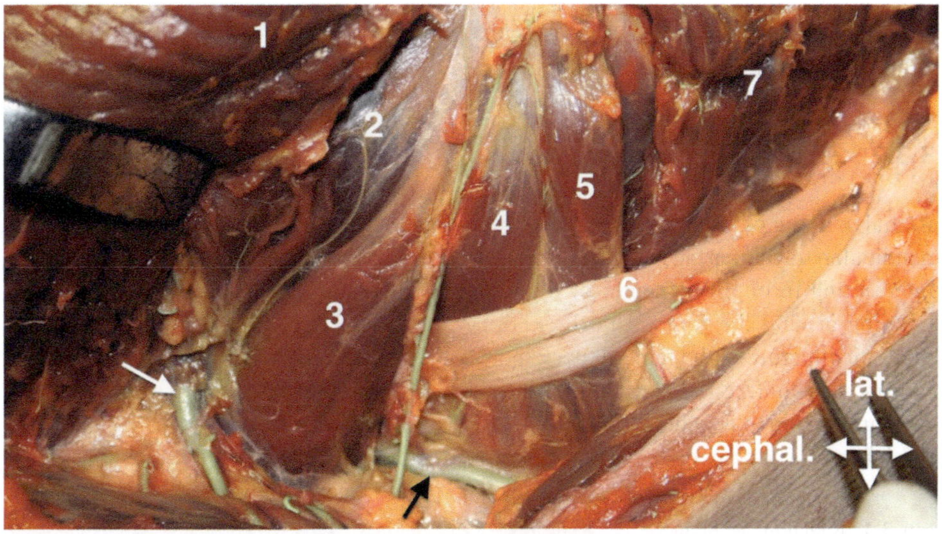

Fig. 6.14 Anatomy of SERs of the right hip. Obturator internus and externus are covered by the neighboring muscles. The white arrow shows the posterior division of the SGA, and the black arrow shows the IGA.
1 = gluteus medius muscle;
2 = gluteus minimus muscle;
3 = piriformis muscle;
4 = gemellus superior;
5 = gemellus inferior;
6 = sciatic nerve;
7 = quadratus femoris muscle

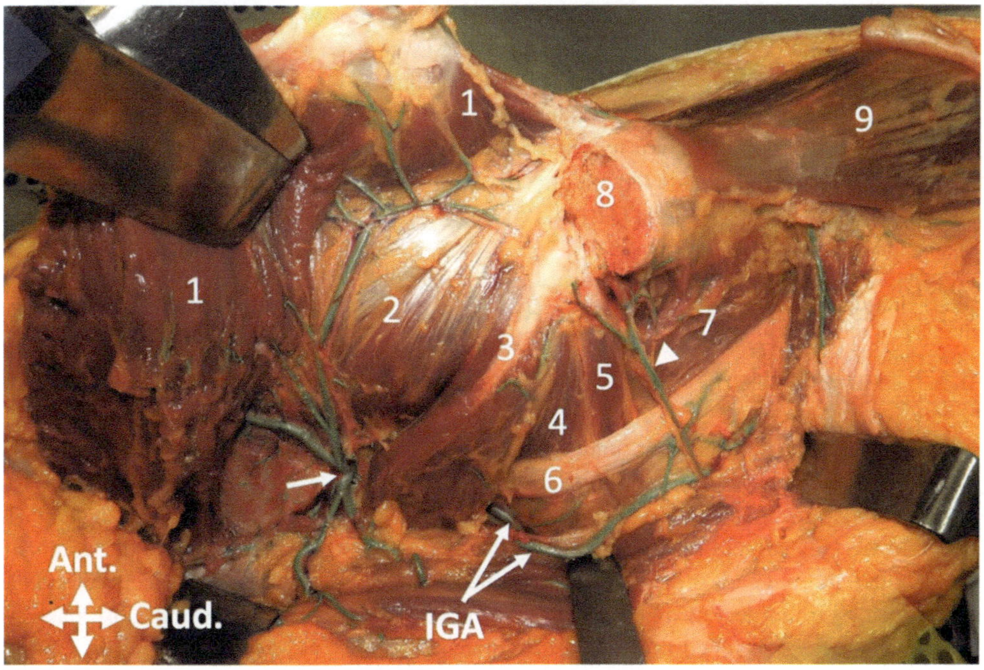

Fig. 6.15 An overview of the posterior aspect of the right hip after GT osteotomy and proximal retraction of the gluteus medius. A single arrow shows the SGA. Arrowhead shows the anastomotic branch of the IGA to the deep branch of the MFCA. 1 = gluteus medius; 2 = gluteus minimus; 3 = piriformis; 4 = superior gemellus; 5 = inferior gemellus; 6 = sciatic nerve; 8 = GT osteotomized; 9 = vastus lateralis

posterior approach hip surgery. Almost all the nerves and vessels emerging from the greater sciatic foramen to the buttock are in close relation to the piriformis muscle. The superior gluteal artery (SGA) and nerve enter the buttock crossing its upper border while the sciatic and inferior gluteal nerve and vessels cross its lower border in most of the cases (Figs. 6.14 and 6.15). The piriformis can be easily identified by its long tendon and the sciatic nerve appearing at its lower border. However, the relation between piriformis and sciatic nerve is variable as occasionally the sciatic nerve runs through or posterior to the piriformis (Fig. 6.16). The piriformis muscle courses obliquely from posteromedial to the anterolateral aspect of the hip, along the inferior border of the Gmin, and inserts to the GT anterior to the so-called piriformis fossa (Fig. 6.15). The other short rotators run transversely from posteromedial to anterolateral overlying the posterior capsule and insert to the posterolateral border of the GT and proximal femur. The lowermost muscle of the short rotators is the quadratus femoris that originates from the ischial tuberosity and inserts on the posterior aspect of the proximal femur in between the two trochanters along the intertrochanteric line.

Between the piriformis and quadratus, and from proximal to distal, are located the superior gemellus, obturator internus, inferior gemellus, and obturator externus muscles. The obturator internus comes out of the pelvis by making a sharp angle around the lesser sciatic notch and is covered by the gemelli. It is not usually visible from a posterior approach unless tenot-

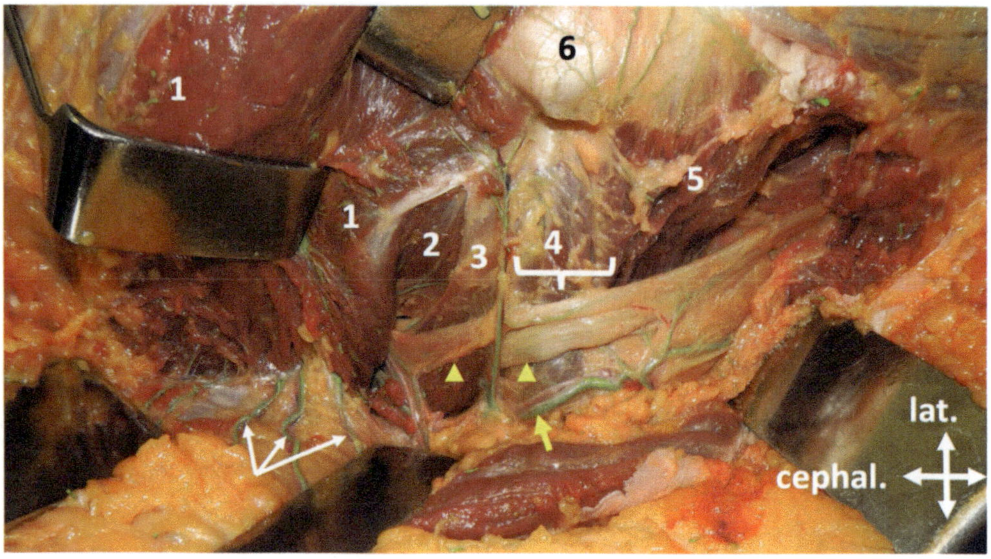

Fig. 6.16 The bisection of the sciatic nerve by the piriformis. White arrows point to the posterior division of the SGA, the yellow arrow shows the distal continuation of the IGA, and arrowheads show the split sciatic nerve. 1 = Gmed; 2 = Gmin, 3 = piriformis; 4 = triceps coxae; 5 = quadratus femoris; 6 = greater trochanter

omy of short rotators is done. The obturator externus is also partly covered by the neighboring muscles and is only partly visible (Figs. 6.14, 6.15, and 6.16). The gemelli and the obturator internus make the conjoint tendon of the triceps coxae that along with the piriformis tendon attaches to the medial surface of the anterior half of the GT [24, 25].

6.5 Vascular Anatomy of the Hip

6.5.1 Introduction

Remarkable recent advances in understanding the surgical anatomy of the femoral head supplying vessels in their extracapsular and intracapsular courses revolutionized the practice of hip preserving surgery [4–7]. The long-standing dogma of iatrogenic femoral head osteonecrosis, as an inevitable complication of hip surgery, was disproven, and new surgical techniques were developed to successfully manage various developmental and traumatic hip entities with minimal or no risk of femoral head avascular necrosis (AVN) [8, 9, 26–32].

The vascular anatomy of the proximal end of the femur has been a subject of interest since many years ago [33–39]. In 1949, Tucker published his article after a vascular injection study and described the MFCA as the main artery supplying the femoral head [33]. In 1953, Trueta confirmed the finding of Tucker in another injection study [35]. Although the general description of hip and femoral head circulation can be found in anatomical textbooks, recently published articles have further emphasized the surgical anatomy of the vessels supplying the femoral head [1–3]. In an injection study, Gautier et al. showed that injury of MFCA during routine hip surgery was the main cause of femoral head AVN [4].

Based on this knowledge, the technique of surgical hip dislocation (SHD) was developed by Ganz et al. in 2001 [8]. The technique provided a comprehensive approach for circumferential access to both sides of the hip and proved to safely preserve femoral head perfusion [40]. Subsequent vascular studies confirmed the results of the Gautier study and added more details to his findings [5–7]. SHD as an appropriate tool for full access to the joint, combined with the recent injectional studies illustrating the intracapsular course of the head supplying arteries, led to the development of various intraarticular procedures including osteotomies around the femoral head and neck with minimal or no risk of AVN [9, 26–32]. The surgical anatomy of the vessels supplying the femoral head and acetabulum in their extra- and intracapsular courses is illustrated in this chapter. The descriptions and illustrations in this chapter are the results of fresh cadaver dissections following arterial injections and have mostly been published as journal articles or book chapters [6, 7, 41–43].

6.6 Origin and Distribution of the Vessels Supplying the Hip

Five vessels mainly provide the articular and periarticular hip circulation outside of the pelvis: medial and lateral femoral circumflex arteries (MFCA and LFCA), from the anterior aspect, the superior and inferior gluteal arteries (SGA and IGA), from the posterior aspect, and obturator artery (OA) from inferiorly. The MFCA and LFCA branch off from the profunda femoris or common femoral artery outside the pelvis, while the SGA, IGA, and OA have intrapelvic origins and branch off from the internal iliac artery [1–3, 6, 7] (Fig. 6.17).

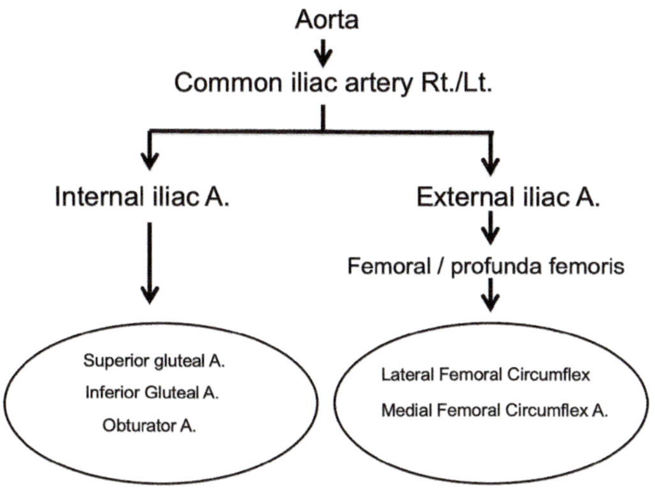

Fig. 6.17 Vascular tree supplying the hip

6.7 Lateral Femoral Circumflex Artery

The LFCA arises frequently from the profunda femoris artery near its origin and occasionally from the common femoral artery itself (about 7–30%) [6, 7, 42, 44] (Fig. 6.18). After division from the main artery, the LFCA courses distally and laterally and, although the branching pattern is variable, gives rise to three branches while underlying the femoral nerve: ascending, transverse, and descending in order of separation. Often the ascending and transverse branches have a common trunk. Only the first or the ascending branch of the LFCA (a-LFCA) takes part directly in the articular and periarticular hip circulation [43]. After division, the ascending branch runs laterally and crosses the undersurface of the rectus transversely toward the TFL. In its way laterally, and deep to the rectus, the a-LFCA sends arterial branches—variable in size and number—to the

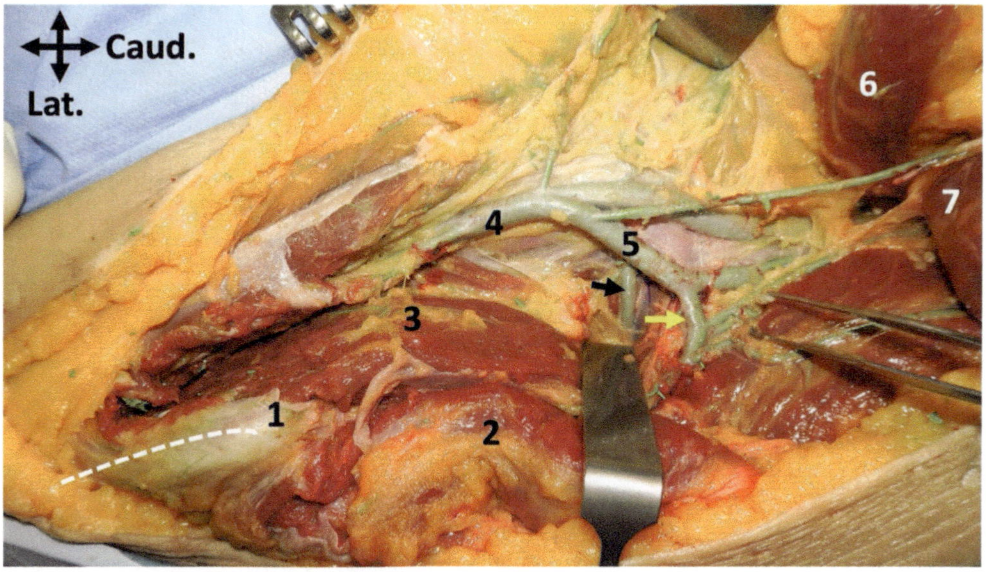

Fig. 6.18 Anterior aspect of the right hip showing the origin of the medial and lateral circumflex femoral arteries. The broken line shows the anterior part of the iliac crest. 1 = ASIS; 2 = TFL; 3 = iliopsoas; 4 = common femoral; 5 = profunda femoris; 6 = sartorius reflected; 7 = rectus femoris reflected. The black arrow shows the MFCA, and the yellow arrow shows the LFCA

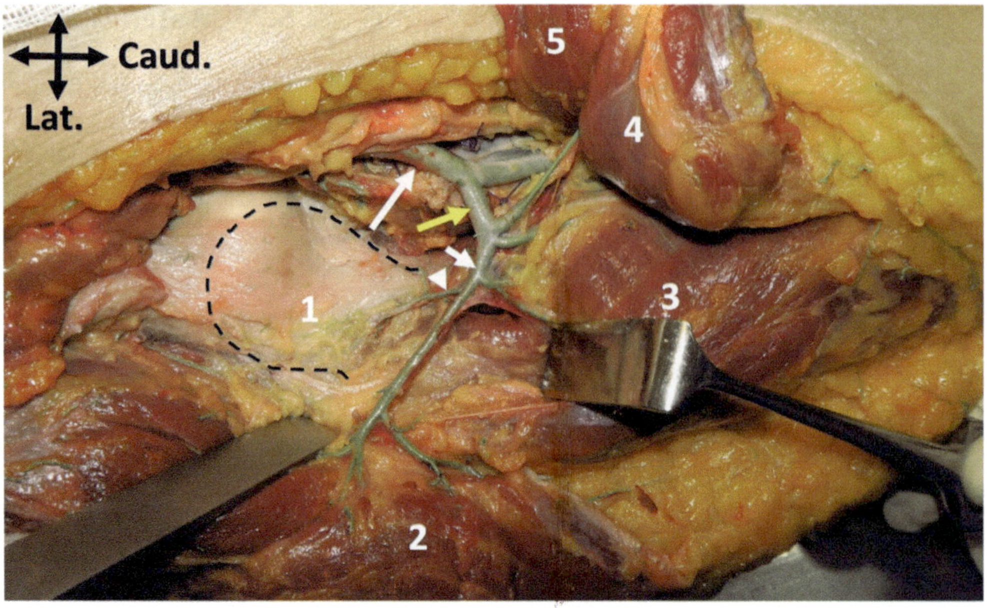

Fig. 6.19 Anterior aspect of the right hip after proximal retraction of the iliopsoas and distal retraction of the rectus and sartorius, showing the course and branches of the ascending branch of the LFCA. The broken line shows the position of the femoral head. A white bigger arrow indicates the common femoral artery. The yellow arrow shows the profunda femoris, the smaller white arrow shows the ascending branch of the LFCA, and the arrowhead shows the capsular branch of the a-LFCA. 1 = anterior capsule; 2 = TFL; 3 = vastus intermedius; 4 = rectus femoris reflected; 5 = sartorius reflected

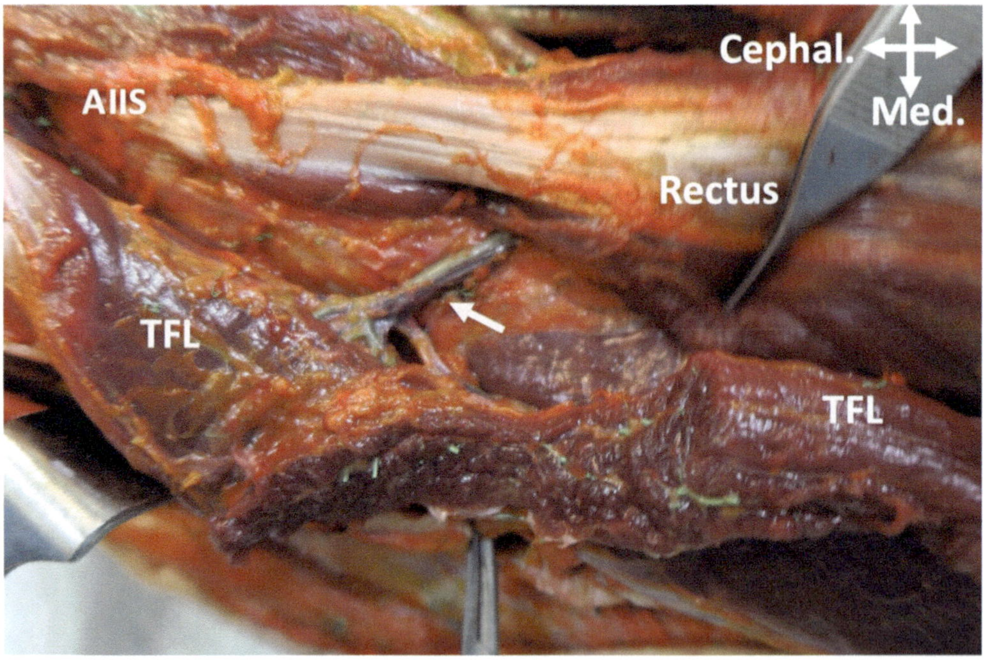

Fig. 6.20 Anterior aspect of the right hip after circumferential exposure of the TFL, showing its vascularization by the a-LFCA, as the main vascular pedicle of the muscle. The stump of the colored cast arteries in the cut surface of the muscle indicates the principal role of the a-LFCA in the perfusion of the muscle

anterior capsule and neighboring muscles, including the rectus [6] (Fig. 6.19). Terminal branches from capsular arteries make variable anastomoses with the vessels coming from the intrapelvic periosteal network. In addition, it sometimes sends one, rarely two small and very fine intracapsular branches that enter the joint from the femoral attachment of the capsule as anterior retinacular artery [6, 42]. After crossing the deep surface of the rectus, the a-LFCA reaches the medial surface of the TFL as its main vascular pedicle (Fig. 6.20). Here it also supplies the most anterior part of the gluteal abductors (Fig. 6.21). The vascular pedicle of the TFL spreads on the deep surface of the muscle and some of its terminal branches perforate the fascia to supply the overlying skin (Fig. 6.22). Before entering the TFL, the a-LFCA gives an arterial branch that turns cephalad and crosses the anterolateral aspect of the capsule proximally to reach the superolateral aspect of the acetabulum (Fig. 6.23). In its course superiorly, the ascending branch gives multiple twigs to the neighboring tissues including the hip capsule. At the superolateral aspect of the acetabulum, the ascending branch finally anastomoses with the supraacetabular branch of the SGA by its terminal branch (Fig. 6.23).

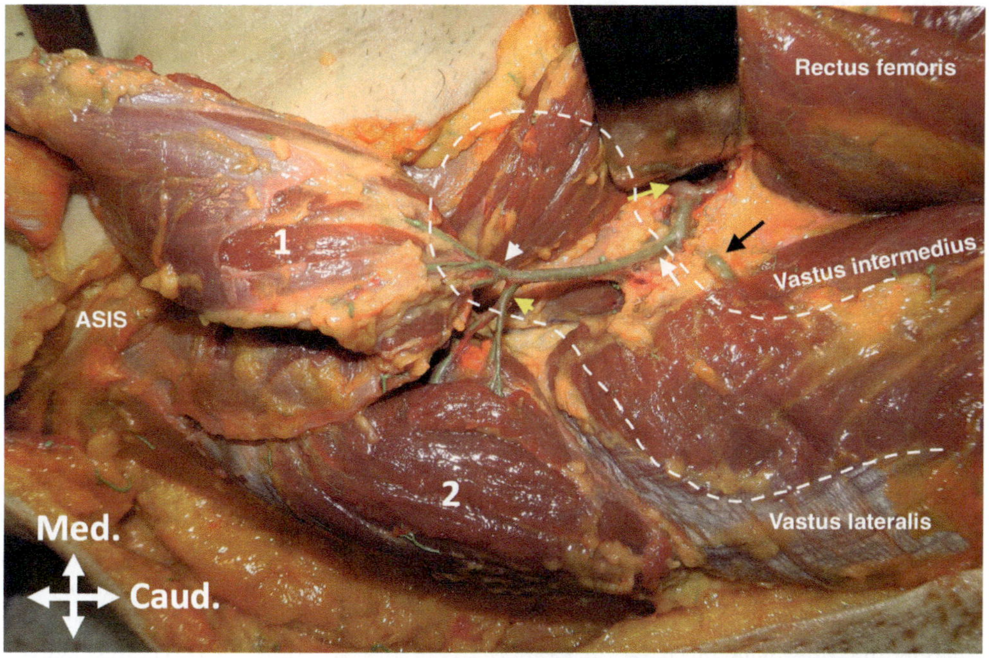

Fig. 6.21 Anterior aspect of the right hip to show the ascending branch (white arrow) supplying the TFL (white arrowhead) and the gluteal abductors (yellow arrowhead) after proximal reflection of the TFL and medial retraction of the rectus femoris. The yellow arrow points to the lateral femoral circumflex artery (LFCA), the black arrow shows the transverse branch of the LFCA. ASIS = anterior superior iliac spine; 1 = tensor fasciae latae muscle; 2 = gluteus medius muscle. (Adapted with permission from [43])

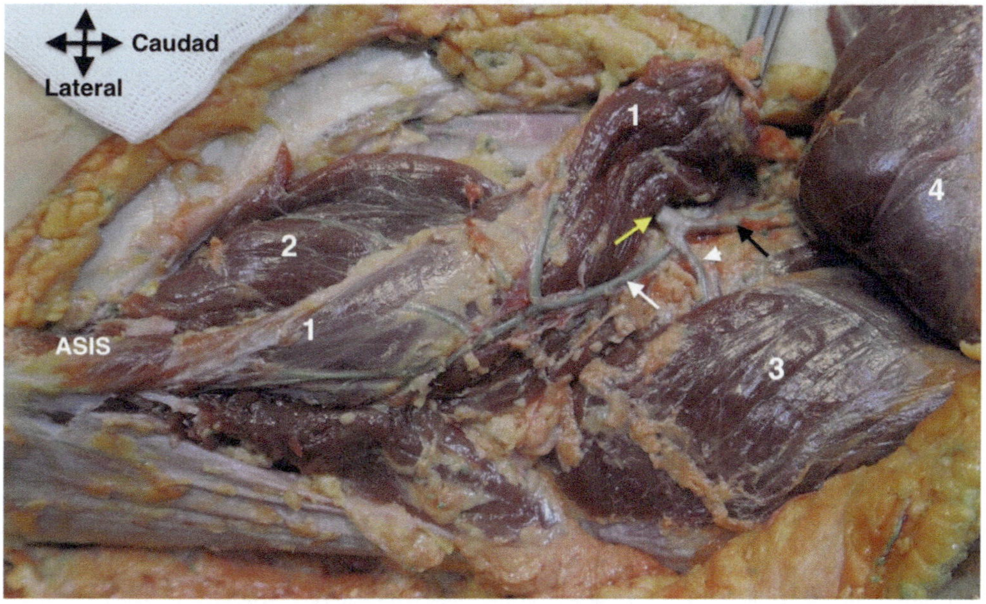

Fig. 6.22 Anterior aspect of the right hip to demonstrate vascularization of the TFL by the ascending branch of the LFCA (white arrow). TFL is freed from its distal attachment and flipped vertically to expose its under surface. The yellow arrow indicates the LFCA, the arrowhead shows the transverse branch, and the black arrow shows the descending branch. 1 = TFL (flipped); 2 = iliopsoas; 3 = vastus intermedius; 4 = rectus femoris (reflected distally); ASIS = anterior superior iliac spine

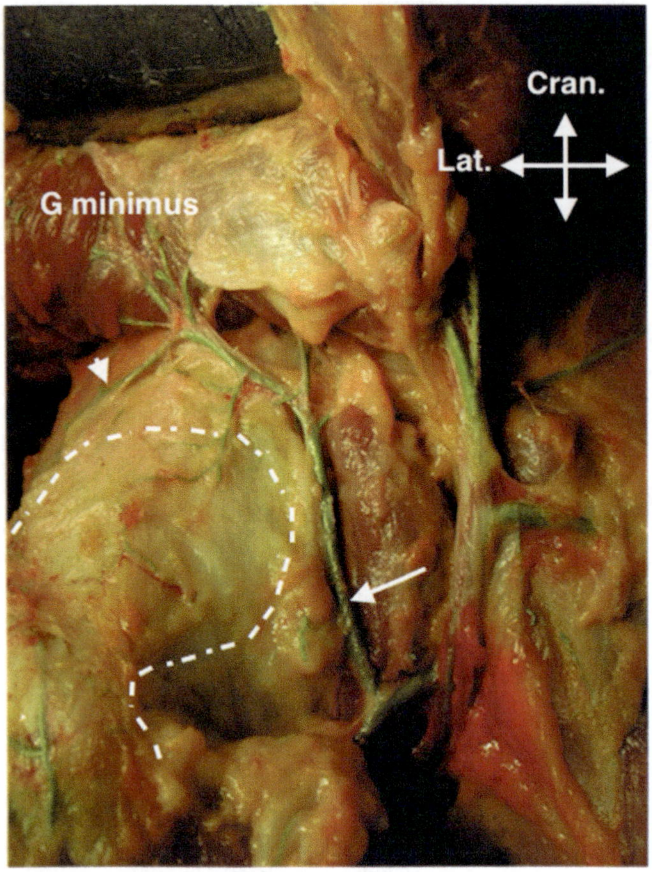

Fig. 6.23 Anterolateral surface of the right hip to demonstrate the anastomosis between an ascending branch of LFCA and the supra-acetabular branch of SGA. The arrow shows the terminal segment of the ascending branch crossing the joint superolaterally. The arrowhead shows the location of the anastomosis. Adapted with permission from [42]

The a-LFCA is the most important supplier of the TFL muscle (Fig. 6.20) and also an accessory supplier of the gluteal abductor in their most anterior aspects (Fig. 6.21).

6.8 Medial Femoral Circumflex Artery

6.8.1 Extracapsular Course

The MFCA originates commonly from the profunda femoris and less often from the common femoral artery itself. After separation from the posteromedial aspect of the main artery, it runs posteriorly between the iliopsoas medially and pectineus laterally [4, 6, 7] (Fig. 6.18). After giving a branch to the adductors, the artery continues posteriorly between the pectineus and medial capsule (Fig. 6.24). Deep to the medial aspect of the capsule and before turning laterally, the artery gives one or commonly two branches that pierce the medial capsule, entering the joint as medial retinacular arteries (Fig. 6.25). These small vessels run toward the femoral head on top of the thickened retinaculum or Weitbrecht ligament. As the deep branch of the MFCA, the artery crosses the posterior aspect of the hip along the inferior border of the obturator externus muscle toward the GT. The deep branch of the MFCA finally emerges between the quadratus femoris and the obturator externus near their attachment to the posterior border of the GT (Fig. 6.26). In its way laterally along the posterior aspect of the hip, it gives some capsular branches that enter the surface of the capsule from its femoral side. Between the quadratus femoris and obturator externus, the artery gives the trochanteric branch that arborizes over the lateral surface of the GT. The trochanteric branch is consis-

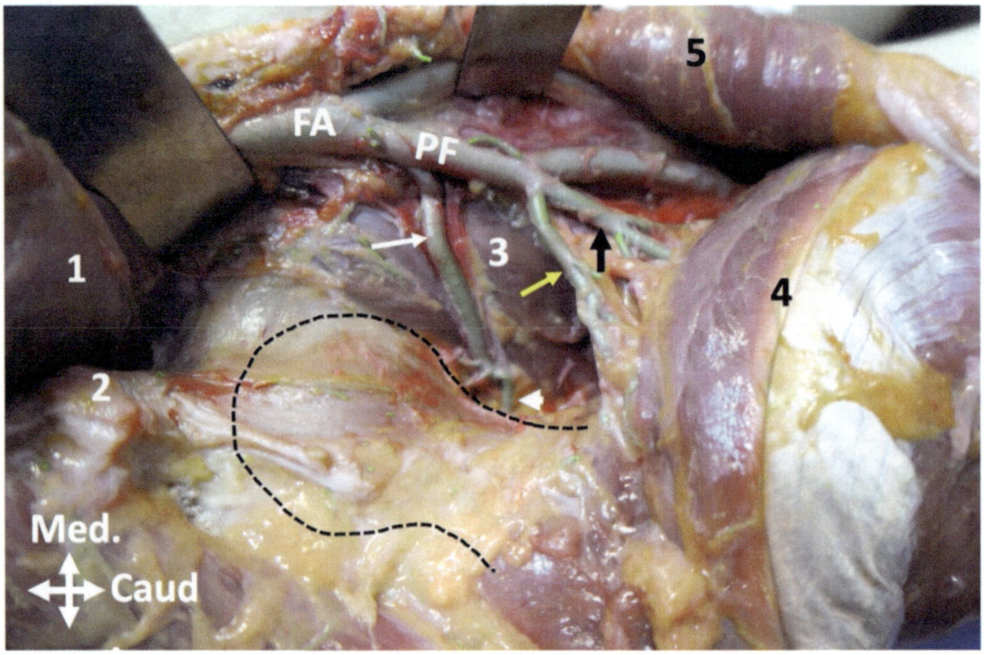

Fig. 6.24 Exposure of the anterior aspect of the right hip capsule after retraction of the overlying muscles showing branching of the femoral artery. FA = femoral artery; PF = profunda femoris artery. The broken line shows the outline of the femoral head. The white arrow indicates the MFCA, the yellow arrow shows the LFCA, and the black arrow shows the descending branch of the LFCA. 1 = iliopsoas muscle (reflected proximally); 2 = AIIS; 3 = pectineus muscle; 4 = rectus femoris reflected distally; 5 = sartorius reflected distally

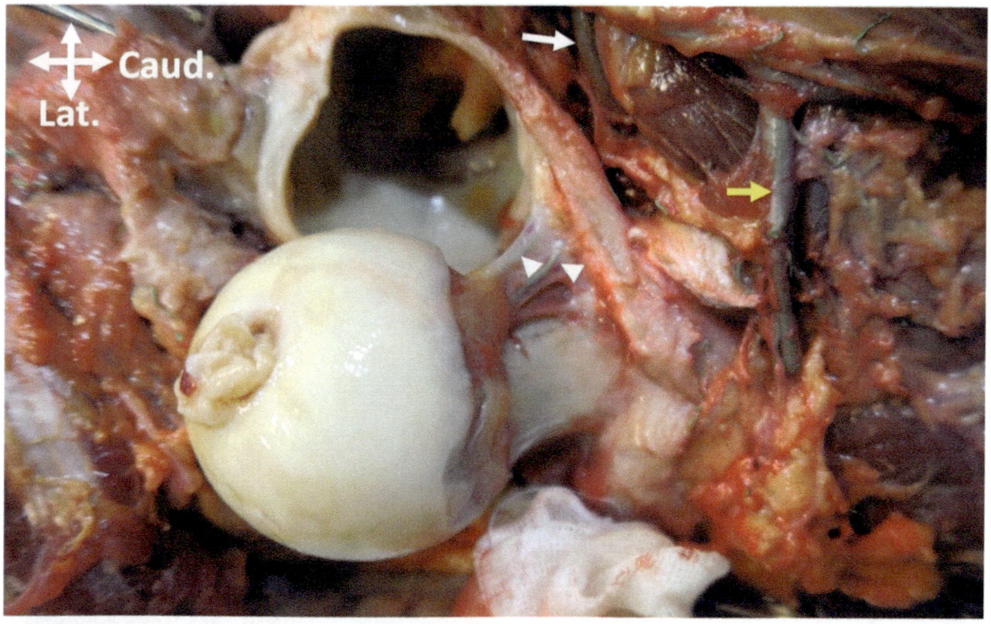

Fig. 6.25 Medial aspect of the femoral neck after capsulotomy and dislocation of the joint showing the medial retinacular arteries originating from the MFCA at the medial aspect of the joint. Arrowheads show the Weitbrecht ligament transferring the retinacular arteries to the medial aspect of the femoral head. The white arrow shows the MFCA, and the yellow arrow indicates the LFCA

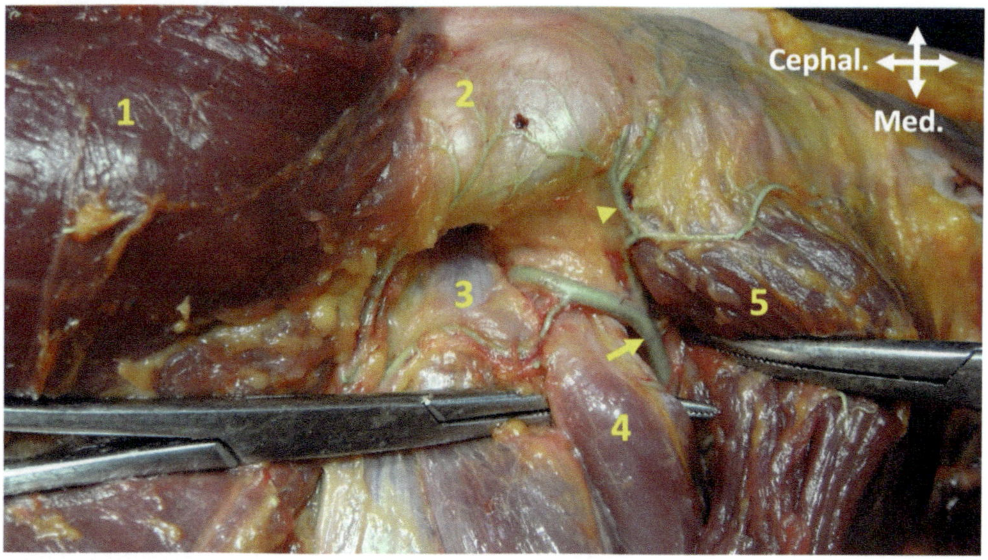

Fig. 6.26 Posterior aspect of the right hip to demonstrate the deep branch of the MFCA in closed contact with the tendon of the obturator externus muscle. The arrow shows a deep branch of the MFCA. The arrowhead shows the trochanteric branch of the artery. 1 = gluteus medius muscle; 2 = greater trochanter; 3 = conjoint tendon; 4 = obturator externus muscle; 5 = quadratus femoris muscle. (Adapted with permission from [7])

tently present and well visible on the posterior and lateral surfaces of the GT. Here also the artery usually receives an anastomotic branch from the IGA that crosses the sciatic nerve posteriorly or sometimes anteriorly and runs along the course of the gemellus inferior to reach the deep branch of the MFCA near the GT (Fig. 6.15). After giving the trochanteric branch, the artery crosses the tendon of the obturator externus posteriorly and cranially, adjacent to the GT and runs anterior to the conjoint tendon of the gemelli and obturator internus (Figs. 6.27 and 6.28). It finally pierces the femoral attachment of the capsule under the conjoint tendon before its attachment to the GT (Fig. 6.29). Of note, MFCA remains consistently distal to the piriformis tendon, which is an important landmark for posterior approaches. Inside the joint, it gives three to five branches that run cranially toward the femoral head as lateral retinacular arteries which are in close contact with the femoral neck and covered by a layer of the retinaculum (Fig. 6.30). Intracapsular connections between retinacular arteries around the neck and between the medial and lateral circumflex femoral arteries are rarely seen.

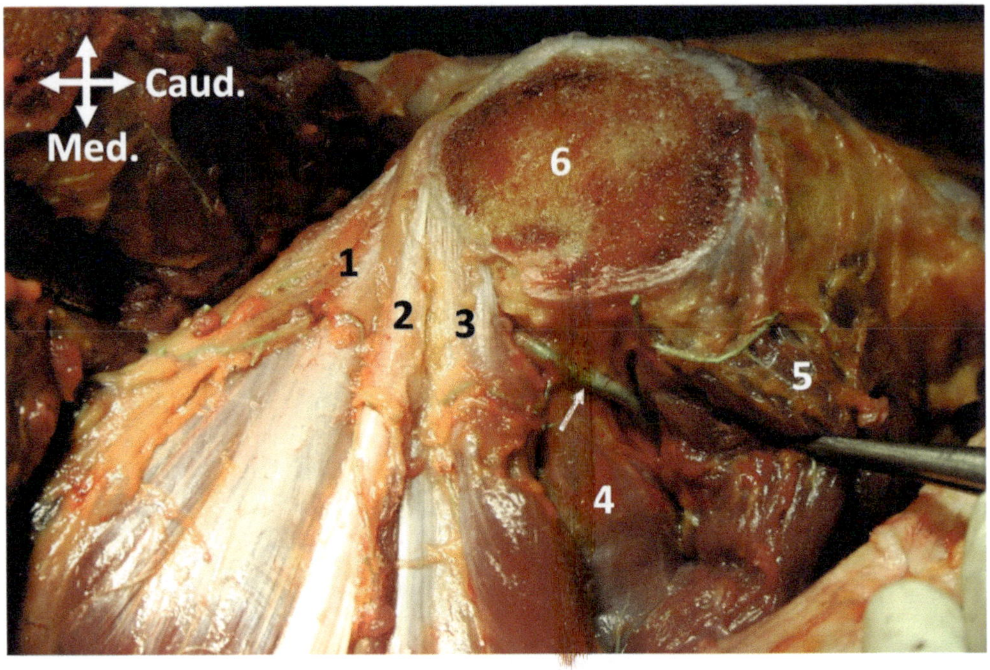

Fig. 6.27 Posterior aspect of the right hip after proximal retraction of the gluteus medius showing the course of the deep branch of the MCFA in close relation to the tendon of the obturator externus and gemellus inferior (arrow). 1 = gluteus minimus; 2 = piriformis; 3 = conjoint tendon; 4 = obturator externus; 5 = quadratus femoris; 6 = stump of the greater trochanter. (Adapted with permission from [42])

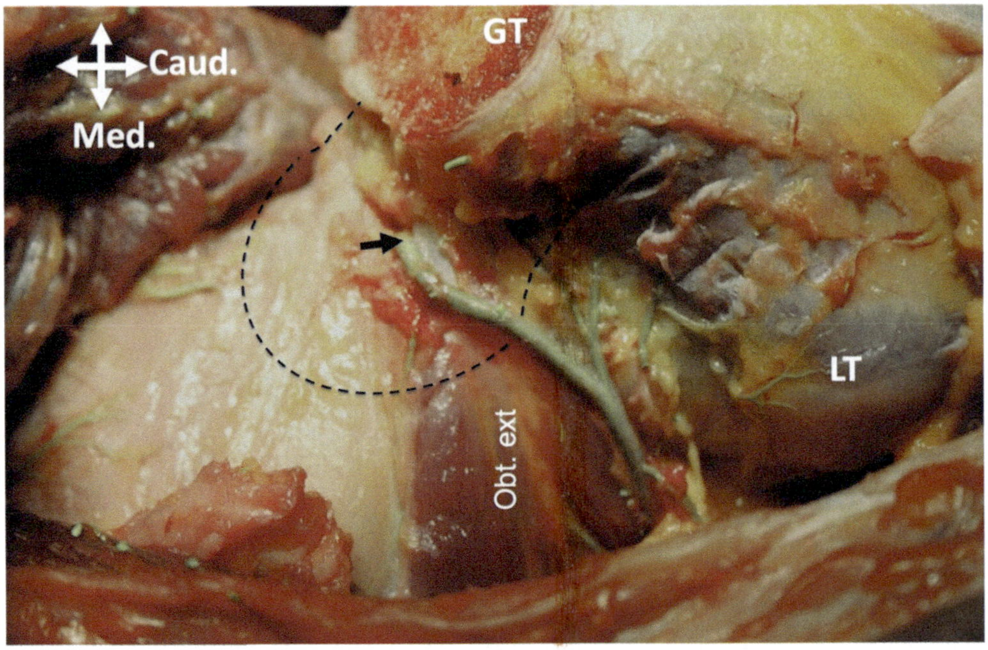

Fig. 6.28 Posterior aspect of the right hip after detachment and retraction of all the muscles except the obturator externus, showing the posteromedial course of the MFCA deep branch and its entry point to the joint. Obt. ext. = obturator externus; LT = lesser trochanter; GT = greater trochanter

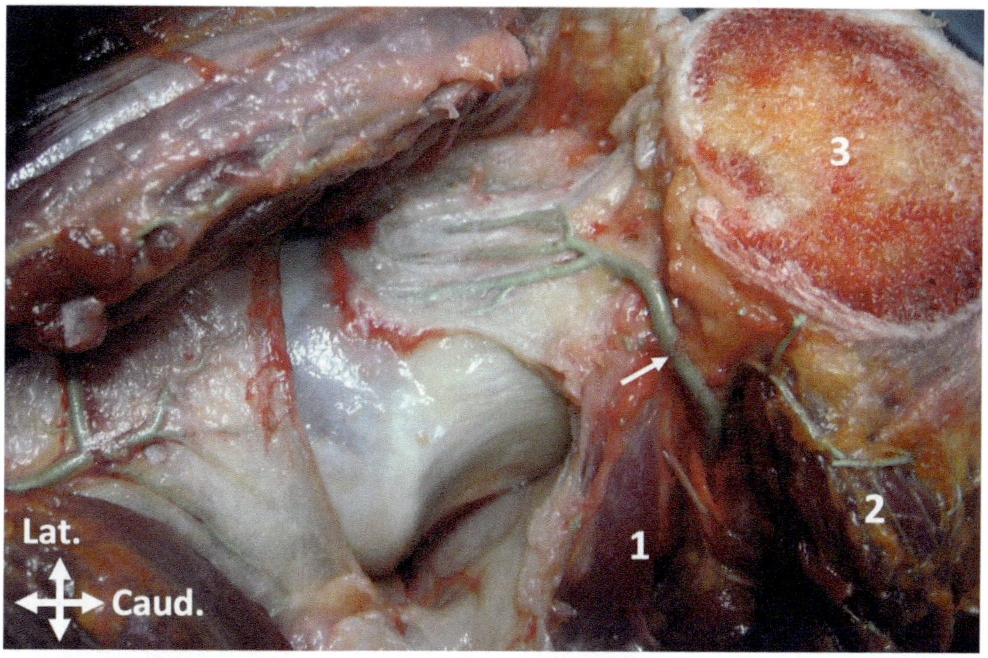

Fig. 6.29 Posterior aspect of the right hip after capsulotomy showing the entrance of the deep branch of the MFCA into the joint. Short rotators proximal to the obturator externus as well as gluteal muscles are retracted to the sides. The arrow shows the deep branch in close contact with the obturator externus tendon. 1 = obturator externus muscle; 2 = quadratus femoris; 3 = stump of greater trochanter after osteotomy

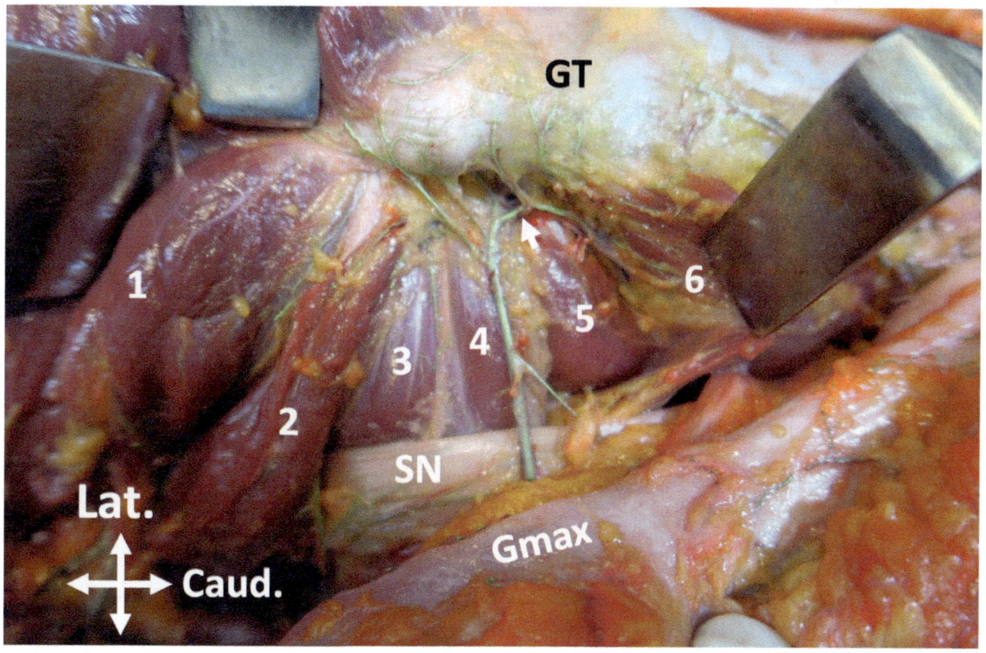

Fig. 6.30 Posterior aspect of the right hip showing the prominent branch of the IGA that crosses the posterior surface of the sciatic nerve to make anastomosis with the deep branch of the MFCA. The arrow shows the site of the anastomosis. GT = greater trochanter; Gmax = gluteus maximus; 1 = gluteus medius; 2 = piriformis; 3 = gemellus superior; 4 = gemellus inferior; 5 = obturator externus; 6 = quadratus femoris

6.9 Superior Gluteal Artery

The superior and inferior gluteal arteries (SGA and IGA) branch from the internal iliac artery and exit from the pelvis through the greater sciatic notch, proximally and distally of the piriformis muscle, respectively (Fig. 6.14). At the roof of the greater sciatic notch, the SGA divides into the posterior and anterior trunks shortly after exit. The posterior trunk goes to the deep surface of the gluteus maximus muscle to supply it. Shortly after entrance to the buttock, the anterior trunk ramifies to two to three branches that go anterolaterally between or through the gluteus medius and minimus muscles to supply them. The most proximal branch turns cranially and enters the deep surface of the gluteus medius to supply the muscle and runs anterolaterally along the long origin of the Gmed. It finally sends some twigs to the TFL near its proximal attachment to the crest. The middle branch travels anterolaterally between the two muscles. It is accompanied all the way from posteromedial to anterolateral by the superior gluteal nerve (SGN). In addition to the more superficial or muscular branches, the supraacetabular and acetabular branches arise from the SGA that run deep to the overlying

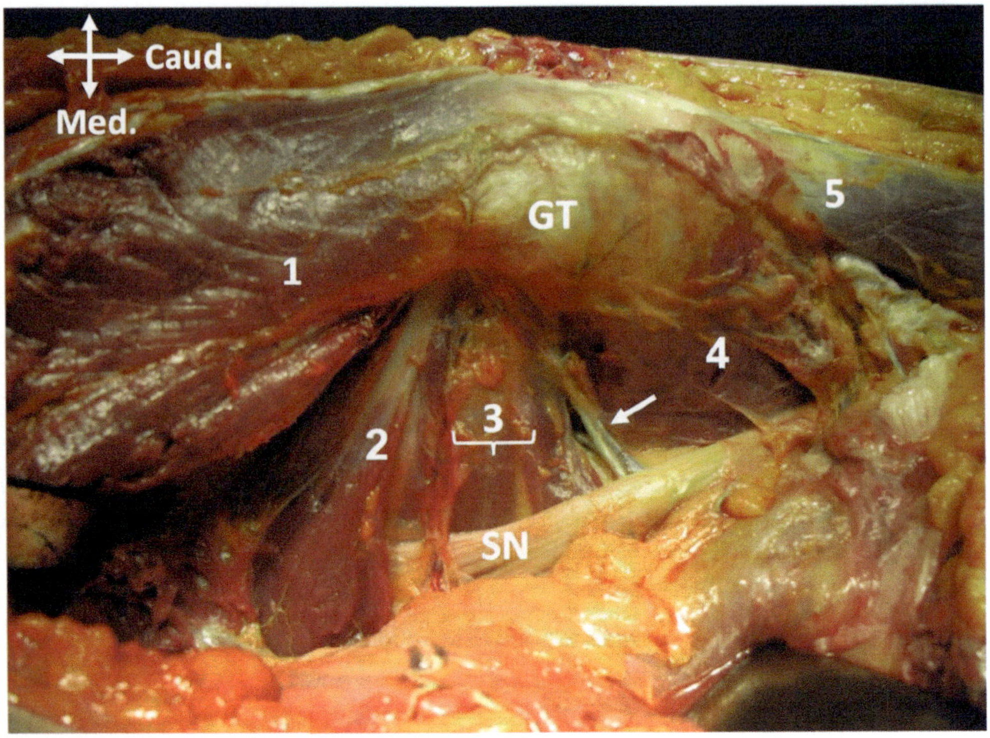

Fig. 6.31 Posterior aspect of the right hip showing the branch of the IGA (arrow) that crosses anterior to the sciatic nerve to anastomose with the deep branch of the MFCA. SN = sciatic nerve; GT = greater trochanter; 1 = gluteus medius; 2 = piriformis; 3 = triceps coxae; 4 = quadratus femoris; 5 = vastus lateralis. (Adapted with permission from [42])

muscles as periosteal arteries. Of notice in length and size is the supracetabular branch, which runs transversely along the posterior and posterolateral aspects of the acetabulum. Its first segment courses through the gluteus minimus and then traverses deeply as a periosteal artery. Variable anastomoses occur between the terminal branches of the SGA and the circumflex femoral arteries either superficially through the neighboring muscles or deeply via the periosteal periacetabular network. The most consistent anastomosis is between the supraacetabular branch of the superior gluteal and the ascending branch of the lateral circumflex artery (Fig. 6.23).

6.10 Inferior Gluteal Artery

The IGA emerges from the pelvis at the inferior border of the piriformis muscle adjacent to the sciatic nerve (Fig. 6.14). It supplies the gluteus maximus and the SER by its muscular and more superficial branches, and the periacetabular bone by its deep or periosteal branches. The IGA almost always takes part in the femoral head circulation by sending an anastomotic branch to the deep branch of the MFCA close to the tendon of the obturator externus muscle. The IGA commonly sends two superficial and two periosteal branches. The proximal superficial branch leaves the artery about the origin of the piriformis and goes deep or superficial to the sciatic nerve, usually along the inferior border of the piriformis muscle, toward the GT (Figs. 6.14 and 6.16). The more constant distal branch sometimes crosses the sciatic nerve superficially (Fig. 6.30) and sometimes deeply (Fig. 6.31) toward the GT and along the inferior border of the gemellus inferior muscle. This is the branch that most commonly makes anastomosis with the deep branch of the MFCA (cruciate anastomosis) and occasionally dominates over the MFCA deep branch in supplying the femoral head from the posterior aspect [5–7].

6.11 Obturator Artery

The OA originates from the internal iliac artery and has an intra-pelvic course. It exits the pelvis along with the obturator nerve through the lateral side of the obturator foramen close to the superior ramus of the pubis. It supplies mainly the hamstring and adductor muscles by its muscular branches. It also consistently contributes to the vascularization of the acetabulum by its acetabular branch. It has no perceptible contribution to the femoral head circulation in adults. The acetabular branch enters the acetabulum through the posterior part of the acetabular notch and spreads in the fossa [41].

6.12 Femoral Head Supplying Vessels

6.12.1 Intracapsular Courses

All mentioned hip-supplying vessels, except for the SGA, have direct connections to the intraarticular circulation, although the femoral head is supplied mainly by the arterial branches that arise from the MFCA. Along its course, and as the main supplier of the femoral head, the MFCA sends intracapsular branches from the inferomedial and posterolateral aspects of the joint (Figs. 6.24 and 6.28). One or more commonly two branches arise from the MFCA at the medial side that enter the joint from or near the femoral attachment of the capsule as medial retinacular artery or arteries. Inside the joint, they course toward the femoral head, on the top of a band or fold of the femoral neck retinaculum called Weitbrecht's ligament (Fig. 6.25).

As the main femoral head supplies the artery, the terminal branch of the MFCA perforates the femoral attachment of the capsule entering the joint from the posterolateral aspect. Here, after crossing the tendon of the obturator externus posteriorly, the artery lies anterior to the conjoint tendon of the gemelli and obturator internus (Figs. 6.26 and 6.27). Inside the joint, the artery divides into two to five branches that run toward the head–neck junction postero-laterally while covered by the retinaculum (Fig. 6.29).

The *IGA* usually contributes to the femoral head as an accessory supplier, by giving the anastomosing branch to the deep branch of the MFCA. In about 15% of the cases, the anastomotic branch of the IGA dominates over the deep branch of the MFCA in size and diameter, taking the main role in supplying the femoral head from the posterolateral aspect [7].

The *LFCA* has an inconsistent and variable contribution to the femoral head only in 30% of cases, by one or sometimes two small and fine arteries that enter the joint from the femoral attachment of the capsule that runs on the anterior aspect of the femoral neck. It may terminate on the neck or reach the head–neck junction as an anterior retinacular artery. Its vascular contribution to the femoral head is inconsistent and negligible [6, 43].

The acetabular branch of the *OA* usually contributes to the circulation of the femoral epiphysis via the ligamentum capitis femoris or teres early in life. It has negligible or no role in the vascularization of the femoral head in adults. Occasional very fine and small arteries seen in the cut surface of the ligamentum teres can supply the ligament itself.

The *SGA* has no direct contribution to the femoral head circulation, but an indirect supplementary contribution through the pericapsular vascular connections is likely.

Femoral head supplying vessels in order of significance are as follows: MFCA, IGA, LFCA, OA, and SGA.

6.12.2 Surgical Implications

Weibrecht's ligament carries the articular branch or branches of the MFCA to the medial part of the femoral head. It is fixed in its two ends and relatively mobile in its middle part (Fig. 6.25). Its mobility gives the medial retinacular artery or arteries a chance to escape from damage in some femoral neck fractures. Also, the Weitbrecht ligament, carrying the medial retinacular artery, usually remains attached to the Pipkin fragment as a vascular pedicle. Perfusion of the fragment can be kept during the reduction and fixation of the fracture if the pedicle is spared. Similarly, knowledge of the intraarticular course of the MCFA makes possible doing some more complex intraarticular surgeries such as relative femoral neck lengthening, epiphyseal reorientation in the slipped capital femoral epiphysis, and femoral head reduction surgery in Perthes disease.

Injury of the deep branch of the MFCA during posterior and posterolateral hip exposure is highly likely if the SERs are taken down from the GT [4–8]. The artery comes to the area of the short rotators in between the quadratus femoris and obturator externus near their attachment to the GT (Figs. 6.26 and 6.27). Here it runs cranially and in contact with the tendon of the obturator externus and the inferior gemellus before entering the joint. It also receives the anastomosing branch here from the IGA (Figs. 6.30 and 6.31). Dissection in the area between quadratus femoris and inferior gemellus can be highly risky because major vessels supplying the femoral head normally or as an anatomic variant, run in this area [4–8]. Therefore, dissection in the area of the SERs distal to the piriformis should be minimized if not avoided. If tenotomies and retraction of the short rotators are absolutely necessary, it should be done about 2 cm from the posterior border of the GT. Any dissection proximal to the tendon of the piriformis is less likely to damage the circulation of the femoral head.

6.12.3 Effect of Capsulotomy on Circulation of the Femoral Head

All femoral head-supplying vessels enter the joint from the femoral attachment of the capsule. The two main entry points are at the posterolateral and inferomedial aspects of the joint. No vessel enters the joint to supply the femoral head from the acetabular side. In this regard, transverse capsulotomy, even circumferential, around the acetabular side has no impact on the circulation of the femoral head. In contrast, distal capsulotomy along the femoral attachment of the capsule can be dangerous if extends to the inferomedial and posterolateral aspects of the capsule. Longitudinal capsulotomy along the anterior and posterior aspect of the femoral neck is unlikely to damage the head circulation [6].

6.13 Periacetabular Vascular Ring

Periosteal branches derived from the superior and inferior gluteal arteries join together to make a periosteal network on the lateral and superolateral aspects of the acetabulum to supply the periacetabular bone. The acetabular branches of the gluteal arteries together with the supraacetabular branch of the SGA form the main structure of the periosteal vascular ring (Figs. 6.32 and 6.33). The MFCA and LFCA make the vascular ring complete, by anastomotic branches from the posteroinferior and anterosuperior aspects of the acetabulum [6] (Fig. 6.34). Some terminal branches from this network continue distally over the capsule, while some others traverse the capsule subperiosteally into the joint to supply the labrum [45] (Fig. 6.32). The distribution of periosteal vessels is not uniform around the acetabulum. They are more concentrated at the posterior and posterolateral aspect of the acetabulum (Fig. 6.32).

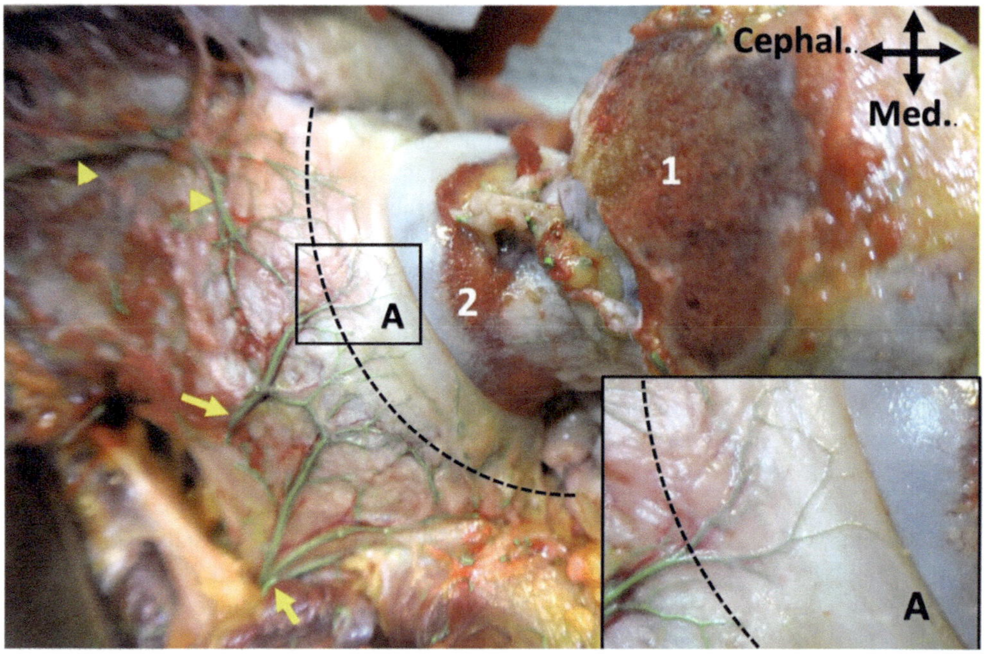

Fig. 6.32 Posterolateral aspect of the hip after retraction of the overlying muscles to demonstrate the formation of the periosteal vascular ring around the acetabulum for vascularization of the acetabulum and labrum. 1 = GT osteotomized; 2 = femoral head. Arrowheads indicate the acetabular branches derived from SGA, and arrows show the part of the periosteal network fed by the acetabular branches derived from IGA. Inset (A) shows vascularization of the labrum by the terminal branches from the periosteal network (the magnified view). The curved broken line shows the stump of the capsular attachment to the acetabulum

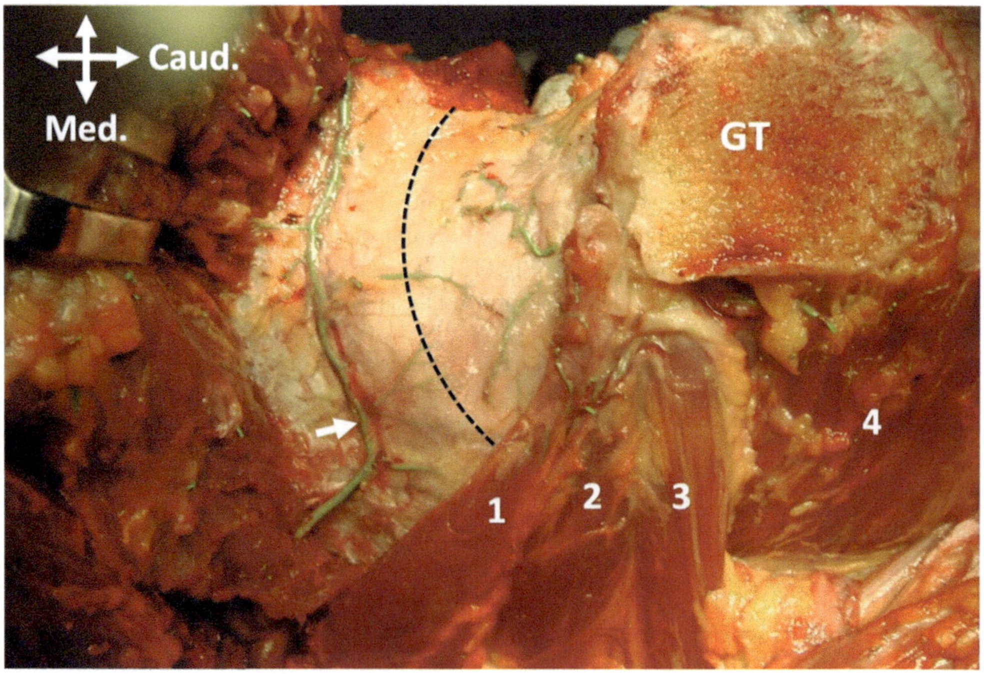

Fig. 6.33 Superior part of the vascular ring fed by the supraacetabular branch of the superior gluteal artery (arrow). Broken line: capsular imprint. GT: greater trochanter; 1 = piriformis; 2 = superior gemellus; 3 = inferior gemellus; 4 = quadratus femoris; GT = stump of the greater trochanter

6.14 Vascularization of the Capsule and Labrum

The hip capsule is supplied by all five mentioned arteries with some variable and inconsistent contributions from the intra-pelvic vessels. The medial and lateral circumflex arteries from the femoral side and the obturator and gluteal arteries from the acetabular side send variable arterial branches on the external surface of the capsule. Anastomoses between these vessels happen on the surface of the capsule. In addition, the capsule receives vascular contributions directly from the overlying muscles and tendons. Capsular vessels are in communication with the periacetabular periosteal network via the bridging vessels (Fig. 6.34).

All vascular communications between the capsule and periacetabular bone take place superficially and through the nonarticular or external surface of the capsule. These vessels bridging between the capsule and the acetabular bone are damaged when the overlying muscle and tendons are dissected away from the capsule for surgical exposure. As a result, capsular contribution to the acetabular perfusion is likely as long as the capsule is not exposed [6].

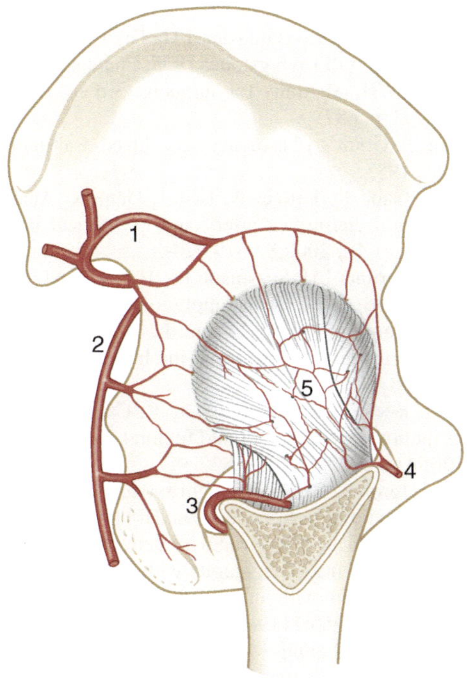

Fig. 6.34 Schematic picture of the right hip viewed from the posterior, demonstrating the periacetabular vascular ring and anastomoses between distal and proximal vessels. 1 = superior gluteal artery; 2 = inferior gluteal artery; 3 = medial femoral circumflex artery; 4 = lateral femoral circumflex artery; 5 = perforating vessels (cut surface). (Adapted with permission from [6])

The acetabular labrum is supplied only by the terminal branches from the periacetabular periosteal network. These vessels traverse the acetabular attachment of the capsule subperiosteally before the entrance to the joint (Fig. 6.32). They run on the nonarticular surface of the labrum while covered by a synovial layer continuous with the synovium of the capsule. Normally, the acetabular labrum receives no contribution from the capsule, synovium, and its bony attachment [45].

6.14.1 Surgical Implications

The role of the normal acetabular labrum in the protection of articular cartilage and the prevention of coxarthrosis has previously been documented [46–49]. Additionally, the role of femoroacetabular impingement as a frequent cause of labral injury has recently been appreciated [49–51]. Currently, repair or refixation of the labral injuries is performed and the importance of labral preservation rather than resection has been emphasized [52–56]. The majority of labral injuries are detachment or cleavage from the articular side of the labrum. A single forceful impact of the femoral head or, more commonly, repeated impact of a cam type of impingement can detach or damage the labrum at its articular attachment. Most often, the vascular layer of the labrum remains attached in spite of labral tear, keeping its healing potential [45]. Theoretically, sparing the vascular membrane of the labrum during surgery, if possible, may improve its healing potential and also reduce the potential for adhesion and scaring following repair and refixation.

6.15 Blood Supply of Acetabulum

The acetabulum and periacetabular bone receive their blood supply from the intraosseous and extraosseous sources fed by the small neighboring arteries. The intraosseous source receives contributions from the numerous nutrient arteries of variable size that enter the periacetabular bone from the internal and external surface of the pelvis and via the vascular foramina. The most prominent and consistent nutrient artery arises from the iliolumbar artery inside of the pelvis near the greater sciatic notch (Fig. 6.35). The artery enters the bone distal to the SI joint and usually anterior to the pelvic brim [41]. The extraosseous source of blood supply to the acetabulum is fed by the periacetabular periosteal network, capsular vessels, and the acetabular branch of the OA. Of the extra pelvic vessels, the supraacetabular branch of the SGA is remarkable in size and length, and by its arcuate shape along the posterolateral aspect of the acetabulum [6, 41] (Fig. 6.33).

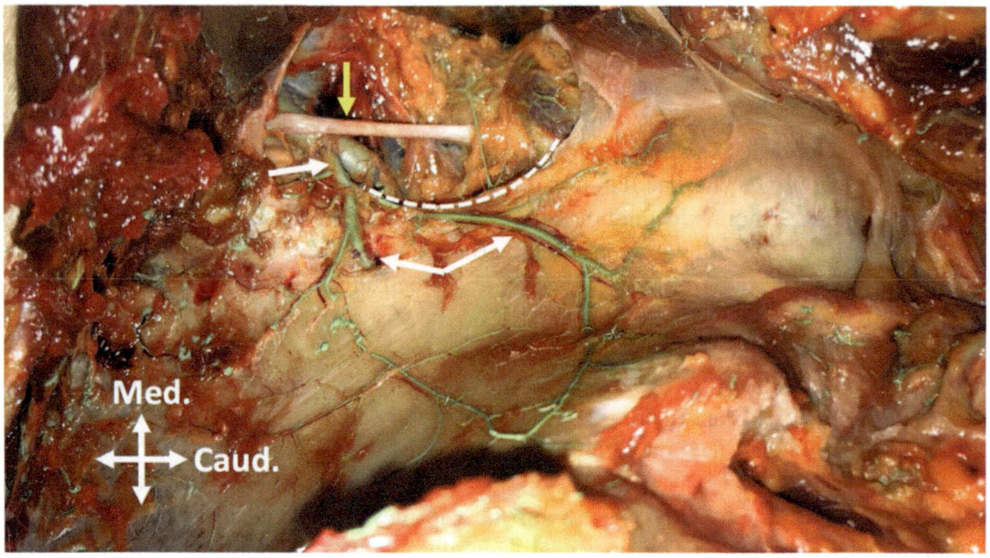

Fig. 6.35 Subperiosteal exposure of the right iliac fossa showing the arterial branches, originating from the iliolumbar artery, supplying the acetabulum. White arrows show the iliolumbar artery and its nutrient and periosteal branches. The yellow arrow shows the obturator nerve. The broken line shows the greater sciatic notch

6.15.1 Surgical Implications

Osteonecrosis of the acetabulum or acetabular fragment can be a potential risk following periacetabular osteotomy (PAO) or acetabular fracture surgery. Hip capsular vessels are believed to contribute blood supply to the acetabular bone provided capsular attachment to the acetabular fragment can be preserved by avoiding capsulotomy during surgery [57–59]. As all vascular communications between the capsule and the acetabulum happen through the vessels running superficially on the non-articular surface of the capsule, any capsular exposure, but not capsulotomy per se, can endanger the capsular contributions to the acetabular perfusion by disrupting these vessels [6].

PAO for treatment of adolescent and adult hip dysplasia may compromise the acetabular circulation by disrupting the intraosseous and extraosseous sources of blood supply. In such instances, the acetabular branch of the OA and capsular vessels remain as possible sources of acetabular perfusion [41]. Variations in acetabular rotational osteotomy techniques may have different vascular impacts. In general, the closer the osteotomy to the capsular attachment, the higher the risk of vascular compromise and potential osteonecrosis. In periacetabular osteotomies performed through wide exposure to the external aspect of the ilium, not only the intraosseous and extraosseous acetabular circulation is damaged, but the bridging vessels running between the capsule and the periacetabular periosteal vessels can also be disrupted [58, 59]. In this regard, spherical and juxtacapsular osteotomies performed through the lateral and posterolateral approaches, with or without capsulotomy [60, 61], carry a higher risk of vascular compromise compared with the Bernese PAO performed through the anterior (modified Smith-Peterson) approach [13, 62, 63]. In addition, experiments by Beck et al. and Hempfing et al. have shown that in the Bernese type of PAO performed through the anterior approach with intrapelvic osteotomy cuts, the remaining periosteal vessels fed by the supraacetabular branch of the SGA sufficiently perfuse the acetabular fragment [41, 63].

References

1. Gray H, Williams PL, Bannister LH. Gray's anatomy. 38th ed. New York: Churchill Livingstone; 1995. Chapter 6: 684.
2. Hollinshead WH. Anatomy for surgeons. 3rd ed. London: Harper & Row; 1982. p. 637–9.
3. Anderson JE. Grant's atlas of anatomy. 8th ed. Baltimore: Williams & Wilkins; 1983.
4. Gautier E, Ganz K, Krügel N, Gill T, Ganz R. Anatomy of the medial femoral circumflex artery and its surgical implications. J Bone Joint Surg Br. 2000;82:679–83.
5. Grose AW, Gardner MJ, Sussmann PS, Helfet DL, Lorich DG. The surgical anatomy of the blood supply to the femoral head: description of the anastomosis between the medial femoral circumflex and inferior gluteal arteries at the hip. J Bone Joint Surg Br. 2008;90:1298–303.
6. Kalhor M, Beck M, Huff TW, Ganz R. Capsular and pericapsular contributions to acetabular and femoral head perfusion. J Bone Joint Surg Am. 2009;91:409–18.
7. Kalhor M, Horowitz K, Gharehdaghi J, Beck M, Ganz R. Anatomic variations in femoral head circulation. Hip Int. 2012;22:307–12.
8. Ganz R, Gill TJ, Gautier E, Krugel N, Berlemann U. Surgical dislocation of the adult hip. A technique with full access to the femoral head and acetabulum without the risk of avascular necrosis. J Bone Joint Surg Br. 2001;83:1119–24.
9. Ganz R, Huff TW, Leunig M. Extended retinacular soft-tissue flap for intra-articular hip surgery: surgical technique, indications, and results of application. Instr Course Lect. 2009;58:241–55.
10. Azar FM, Beaty JH. Campbell's operative orthopedics, vol. 1. 14th ed. Philadelphia: Elsevier; 2021. p. 69–99.
11. Hoppenfeld S, de Boer P. Surgical exposures in orthopaedics: the anatomic approach. 1st ed. Philadelphia: Lippincott Williams & Wilkins; 1984. p. 335–48.
12. Rudin D, Manestar M, Ullrich O, Erhardt J, Grob K. The anatomical course of the lateral femoral cutaneous nerve with special atten-

tion to the anterior approach to the hip joint. J Bone Joint Surg Am. 2016;98:561–7.
13. Ganz R, Klaue K, Vinh TS, Mast JW. A new periacetabular osteotomy for the treatment of hip dysplasias. Technique and preliminary results. Clin Orthop Relat Res. 1988;232:26–36.
14. Hussell JG, Rodriguez JA, Ganz R. Technical complications of the Bernese periacetabular osteotomy. Clin Orthop Relat Res. 1999;363:81–92.
15. Üzel M, Akkin SM, Tanyeli E, Koebke J. Relationships of the lateral femoral cutaneous nerve to bony landmarks. Clin Orthop Relat Res. 2011;469(9):2605–11. https://doi.org/10.1007/s11999-011-1858-2. Epub 2011 Mar 22. PMID: 21424835.
16. Cates RA, Boon AJ, Trousdale RT, Douge A, Sierra RJ. Prospective evaluation of lateral femoral cutaneous nerve injuries during periacetabular osteotomy. J Hip Preserv Surg. 2019;6(1):77–85.
17. Kalhor M, Gharehdaghi J, Schoeniger R, Ganz R. Reducing the risk of nerve injury during Bernese periacetabular osteotomy: a cadaveric study. Bone Joint J. 2015;97-B:636–41.
18. Kalhor M, Collado D, Leunig M, Rego P, Ganz R. Recommendations to reduce risk of nerve injury during Bernese periacetabular osteotomy (PAO). JBJS Essent Surg Tech. 2017;7:e34. https://doi.org/10.2106/JBJS.ST.17.00017.
19. Babst D, Steppacher SD, Ganz R, Siebenrock KA, Tannast M. The iliocapsularis muscle: an important stabilizer in the dysplastic hip. Clin Orthop Relat Res. 2011;469:1728–34. https://doi.org/10.1007/s11999-010-1705-x.
20. Novais EN, Kim YJ, Carry PM, Millis MB. The Bernese periacetabular osteotomy: is transaction of the rectus femoris tendon essential? Clin Orthop Relat Res. 2014;472(10):3142–9.
21. Peters CL, Erickson JA, Anderson MB, Anderson LA. Preservation of the rectus femoris origin during periacetabular osteotomy does not compromise acetabular reorientation. Clin Orthop Relat Res. 2015;473(2):608–14.
22. Kalhor M, Gharehdaghi J, Leunig M, Ahmadloo J, Collado Gastalver D, Ganz R. Surgical anatomy of the rectus-sparing approach for periacetabular osteotomy: a cadaveric study. JBJS Essent Surg Tech. 2021;11(2):e20.00030. https://doi.org/10.2106/JBJS.ST.20.00030.
23. Beck M, Sledge JB, Gautier E, Dora CF, Ganz R. The anatomy and function of the gluteus minimus muscle. J Bone Joint Surg Br. 2000;82(3):358–63. https://doi.org/10.1302/0301-620x.82b3.10356.
24. Ito Y, Matsushita I, Watanabe H, Kimura T. Anatomic mapping of short external rotators shows the limit of their preservation during total hip arthroplasty. Clin Orthop Relat Res. 2012;470(6):1690–5. https://doi.org/10.1007/s11999-012-2266-y.
25. Solomon LB, Lee YC, Callary SA, Beck M, Howie DW. Anatomy of piriformis, obturator internus and obturator externus: implications for the posterior surgical approach to the hip. J Bone Joint Surg Br. 2010;92(9):1317–24. https://doi.org/10.1302/0301-620X.92B9.23893. PMID: 20798456
26. Eijer H, Podeszwa DA, Ganz R, Leunig M. Evaluation and treatment of young adults with femoro-acetabular impingement secondary to Perthes' disease. Hip Int. 2006;16:273–80.
27. Leunig M, Slongo T, Kleinschmidt M, Ganz R. Subcapital correction osteotomy in slipped capital femoral epiphysis by means of surgical hip dislocation. Oper Orthop Traumatol. 2007;19:389–410.
28. Leunig M, Slongo T, Ganz R. Subcapital realignment in slipped capital femoral epiphysis: surgical hip dislocation and trimming of the stable trochanter to protect the perfusion of the epiphysis. Instr Course Lect. 2008;57:499–507.
29. Anderson LA, Erickson JA, Severson EP, Peters CL. Sequelae of Perthes disease: treatment with surgical hip dislocation and relative femoral neck lengthening. J Pediatr Orthop. 2010;30:75866.
30. Leunig M, Ganz R. Relative neck lengthening and intracapital osteotomy for severe Perthes and Perthes-like deformities. Bull NYU Hosp Jt Dis. 2011;69(Suppl 1):S62–7.
31. Albers CE, Steppacher SD, Schwab JM, Tannast M, Siebenrock KA. Relative femoral neck lengthening improves pain and hip function in proximal femoral deformities with a high-riding trochanter. Clin Orthop Relat Res. 2015;473(4):1378–87.
32. Rego P, Mascarenhas V, Mafra I, Oliveira F, Pinto P, Ganz R. Femoral neck osteotomy in skeletally mature patients: surgical technique and midterm results. Int Orthop. 2021;45:83–94.
33. Tucker FR. Arterial supply of the femoral head and its clinical importance. J Bone Joint Surg Br. 1949;31:82–93.
34. Howe WW, Lacey T, Schwartz RP. A study of the gross anatomy of the arteries supplying the proximal portion of the femur and the acetabulum. J Bone Joint Surg Am. 1950;32 A:856–66.
35. Trueta J, Harrison MHM. The normal vascular anatomy of the femoral head in adult man. J Bone Joint Surg Br. 1953;35:442–52.
36. Trueta J. The normal vascular anatomy of the human femoral head during growth. J Bone Joint Surg Br. 1957;39:358–93.
37. Crock HV. A revision of the anatomy of the arteries supplying the upper end of the human femur. J Anat. 1965;99:77–88.
38. Sevitt S, Thompson RG. The distribution and anastomosis of the arteries supplying the head and neck of the femur. J Bone Joint Surg Br. 1965;47:560–73.
39. Wertheimer LG, Lopes SF. Arterial supply of the femoral head. J Bone Joint Surg Am. 1971;53:545–56.
40. Nötzli HP, Siebenrock KA, Hempfing A, Ramseier LE, Ganz R. Perfusion of the femoral head during surgical dislocation of the hip. Monitoring by laser Doppler flowmetry. J Bone Joint Surg Br. 2002;84:300–4.
41. Beck M, Leunig M, Ellis T, Sledge JB, Ganz R. The acetabular blood supply: implications for periacetabular osteotomies. Surg Radiol Anat. 2003;25:361–7.
42. Kalhor M, Ganz R. Vascular anatomy of the hip: an update. In: Ganz R, editor. Modern hip preservation. Cham: Springer; 2022. p. 1–12. https://doi.org/10.1007/978-3-030-91967-2_1.
43. Kalhor M, Gharehdaghi J, Leunig M, Ganz R. Lateral femoral circumflex artery contribution to the articular and periarticular hip circulation: relevance to the anterior hip approach-a cadaveric study. Eur J Orthop Surg Traumatol. 2022;33:1547. https://doi.org/10.1007/s00590-022-03310-2.
44. Zlotorowicz M, Czubak-Wrzosek M, Wrzosek P, Czubak J. The origin of the medial femoral circumflex artery, lateral femoral circumflex artery and obturator artery. Surg Radiol Anat. 2018;40(5):515–52.
45. Kalhor M, Horowitz K, Beck M, Nazparvar B, Ganz R. Vascular supply to the acetabular labrum. J Bone Joint Surg Am. 2010;92:2570–5.
46. Harris WH, Bourne RB, Oh I. Intra-articular acetabular labrum: a possible etiological factor in certain cases of osteoarthritis of the hip. J Bone Joint Surg Am. 1979;61:510–4.
47. Altenberg AR. Acetabular labrum tears: a cause of hip pain and degenerative arthritis. South Med J. 1977;70:174–5.
48. Ferguson SJ, Bryant JT, Ganz R, Ito K. The influence of the acetabular labrum on hip joint cartilage consolidation: a poroelastic finite element model. J Biomech. 2000;33:953–60.
49. McCarthy JC, Noble PC, Schuck MR, Wright J, Lee J. The Otto E. Aufranc Award: the role of labral lesions to development of early degenerative hip disease. Clin Orthop Relat Res. 2001;393:25–37.
50. Ganz R, Parvizi J, Beck M, Leunig M, Nötzli H, Siebenrock KA. Femoroacetabular impingement: a cause for osteoarthritis of the hip. Clin Orthop Relat Res. 2003;417:112–20.
51. Leunig M, Beck M, Woo A, Dora C, Kerboull M, Ganz R. Acetabular rim degeneration: a constant finding in the aged hip. Clin Orthop Relat Res. 2003;413:201–7.

52. Espinosa N, Rothenfluh DA, Beck M, Ganz R, Leunig M. Treatment of femoro-acetabular impingement: preliminary results of labral refixation. J Bone Joint Surg Am. 2006;88:925–35.
53. Kelly BT, Weiland DE, Schenker ML, Philippon MJ. Arthroscopic labral repair in the hip: surgical technique and review of the literature. Arthroscopy. 2005;21:1496–504.
54. Murphy KP, Ross AE, Javernick MA, Lehman RA Jr. Repair of the adult acetabular labrum. Arthroscopy. 2006;22(567):e1–3.
55. Philippon MJ, Arnoczky SP, Torrie A. Arthroscopic repair of the acetabular labrum: a histologic assessment of healing in an ovine model. Arthroscopy. 2007;23:376–80.
56. Philippon MJ, Schenker ML. A new method for acetabular rim trimming and labral repair. Clin Sports Med. 2006;25:293–7.
57. Johnson EE, Matta JM, Mast JW, Letournel E. Delayed reconstruction of acetabular fractures 21–120 days following injury. Clin Orthop Relat Res. 1994;305:20–30.
58. Hsieh PH, Shih CH, Lee PC, Yang WE, Lee ZL. A modified periacetabular osteotomy with use of the transtrochanteric exposure. J Bone Joint Surg Am. 2003;85:244–50.
59. Ko JY, Wang CJ, Lin CF, Shih CH. Periacetabular osteotomy through a modified Ollier transtrochanteric approach for treatment of painful dysplastic hips. J Bone Joint Surg Am. 2002;84:1594–604.
60. Wagner H. Experiences with spherical acetabular osteotomy for the correction of the dysplastic acetabulum. Skeletal dysplasias in childhood. New York: Springer; 1978. p. 131–45.
61. Ninomiya S. Rotational acetabular osteotomy for the severely dysplastic hip in the adolescent and adult. Clin Orthop Relat Res. 1989;247:127–37.
62. Murphy SB, Millis MB. Periacetabular osteotomy without abductor dissection using direct anterior exposure. Clin Orthop Relat Res. 1999;364:92–8.
63. Hempfing A, Leunig M, Nötzli HP, Ganz R. Acetabular blood flow during Bernese periacetabular osteotomy: an intraoperative study using laser Doppler flowmetry. J Orthop Res. 2003;21:1145–50.

Further Reading

Beck M, Kalhor M, Leunig M, Ganz R. Hip morphology influences the pattern of damage to the acetabular cartilage: femoroacetabular impingement as a cause of early osteoarthritis of the hip. J Bone Joint Surg Br. 2005;87:1012–8.

Eppright RH. Dial osteotomy of the acetabulum in the treatment of dysplasia of the hip. J Bone Joint Surg Am. 1975;57:1172.

Ninomiya S, Tagawa H. Rotational acetabular osteotomy for the dysplastic hip. J Bone Joint Surg Am. 1984;66:430–6.

Part 2

Basic Surgical Techniques

Original Technique of Surgical Hip Dislocation (SHD)

7

Michael B. Millis and Reinhold Ganz

7.1 Introduction

The transtrochanteric technique for surgical hip dislocation allows a comprehensive, low-complication approach to the hip joint, enabling dynamic assessment and performance of complex intra-articular and extra-articular procedures that were not previously achievable without frequent major morbidity. The approach requires detailed anatomical knowledge, care in the handling of tissues, and technical precision.

7.2 Background

Before the year 2000, the interior of the hip joint was considered by most orthopedists to be a "black box." The topography of the femoral head blood supply was not well understood. In some anatomic descriptions that are still used today, the anatomy is misleadingly depicted and interpreted. The general opinion persisted for many years that surgical dislocations carry risks, with the daunting complication of avascular necrosis (AVN) of the femoral head being the most important.

On the contrary, intra-articular damage patterns had long been suspected, earlier from evidence on cadaveric bones [1, 2] and more recently in findings from computer simulations [3]. *This stimulated a continuing search for comprehensive surgical access to the hip joint without major morbidity.*

The need for a safe surgical hip dislocation (SHD) technique was emphasized by Crock in 1996 in the preface to his Atlas on the Vascular Supply of the Skeleton and Spinal Cord in which he wrote: "Theoretically, a method is required by which the human hip joint can be dislocated atraumatically in the early stages of disease in such a way that the blood supply to the upper end of the femur is preserved. This would pave the way for the use of new methods of surface replacement of articular cartilage based on developments in tissue culture and molecular biology. Rather than relying on prosthetic replacement of the hip to treat significant intra-articular pathology, a treatment philosophy based on biological and physiological principles could be routinely employed" [4].

Such a beneficial approach for both the surgeon and the patient was already being tested at the time [5]. It was based on the details of the blood supply to the femoral head that were known but had received little attention. Extensive intraoperative perfusion studies [6], followed the detailed dissections of the vascular vessels and their anastomoses, proved that, on the cadaver before first subluxations and later, complete dislocations could be safely performed. The results of clinical experience finally led to the publication of the technique that has remained essentially unchanged in its "classical" form for more than 25 years [7]. Anterior dislocation of the hip can be achieved largely atraumatically via a modified postero-lateral approach according to Kocher-Langenbeck [8] or Gibson [9] using a trochanteric flip osteotomy and later a trochanteric step-cut osteotomy [10]. Access to the interior of the hip joint allows a 360° view of the acetabulum and nearly 360° of the femoral head. Finally, the closure of the capsule and stable refixation of the trochanter allow rapid recovery of function. A number of modifications to the technique allow for novel intracapsular procedures to be performed on the femoral neck and femoral head [11].

7.3 Indications

Fundamentally, SHD is a surgical approach and thus only an adjunct or vehicle to the required surgical therapy. Initially, it was also used to appreciate intra-articular dynamic problems that were not well understood despite contemporary clinical

M. B. Millis
Department of Orthopedics, Children's Hospital, Harvard Medical School, Boston, MA, USA
e-mail: Michael.millis@childrens.harvard.edu

R. Ganz (✉)
Faculty of Medicine, University of Berne, Berne, Switzerland

M. Leunig et al. (eds.), *Surgical Hip Dislocation*, https://doi.org/10.1007/978-3-031-70622-6_7

assessment and imaging. In fact, through the SHD, certain morphological changes of the head and acetabulum that caused cartilage-damaging collisions were observed for the first time. This correlation soon led to the concept and term "femoro-acetabular impingement" (FAI) [12]. Initially, the most common therapeutic indications for dislocation were FAI of the inclusion (CAM) type and FAI of the impaction (Pincer) type, often treated in combination with labral and cartilage surgery. Early success in the open analysis and intra-articular treatment of these conditions was followed by similar treatment of other pathologies such as villonodular synovitis, chondromatosis, exostoses of the head–neck junction, and fractures of the femoral head and certain acetabular fractures. With steadily improving technology, most intracapsular FAI deformities can now be treated arthroscopically. However, certain dorsal and distal marginal deformities and the combination with extra-articular deformities still require SHD.

7.4 Preoperative Analysis and Workup

History/Interview: Symptoms and/or dysfunction severe enough for the patient to consider a surgical intervention. Note. The absence of pain is *not* a definitive contraindication to surgical intervention.

Physical examination: General examination and specific examination of the hip, noting the following: Gait pattern and range of motion compared with the opposite side. Range and arc of painless and painful motion, specific hip tests for impingement and instability, and examination for any hypermobility (Chap. 1).

Radiographs: AP total pelvis, cross-table lateral views, faux profile views, and others depending on the underlying pathology (see Chap. 2). Advanced imaging: CT scans of the entire pelvis, plus slices through the thighs including the knees to calculate the version of the femoral neck and acetabulum, MRI with 3 T, high resolution, with radial sequences, if possible with arthro-MRI (see Chap. 3).

For computational modeling for collision models and cutting templates, see Chaps. 4 and 5.

7.5 Preoperative Planning

- Integration of all available preoperative data should yield or rule out a mechanical diagnosis of the problem.
- Good patient education, including the realistic expected outcome, and patient consent are important prerequisites for the procedure.
- The detailed plan is determined by the intended therapeutic intervention.
- Shared decision-making may play a role.

7.6 Applied Anatomy

Detailed knowledge of the surgically relevant anatomy of the hip—particularly the blood supply to the femoral head, greater trochanter, femoral neck, and acetabulum—is essential (Chap. 6). The approach to hip dislocation is designed so that, if performed correctly, no important nerves, muscles, or vessels are disrupted.

7.7 Special Risks

- Femoral head necrosis is a theoretical risk because the dissection occurs near the course of the medial circumflex femoral artery. Importantly, no necrosis attributable to the SHD approach has been described in the literature to date.
- Sciatic neuropraxia may occur if there are unusual deviations in the course of the sciatic nerve and/or piriformis muscle, or more commonly, if there is scarring around the nerve, which is a consideration after prior posterior hip injury or surgery.

7.8 Type of Anesthesia

General anesthesia with neuromuscular relaxation is routine. The associated muscle relaxation reduces trauma to the surrounding soft tissues during the dislocation maneuver.

7.9 Instruments/Implants

- Special instruments to facilitate exposure include blunt and pointed Hohmann and Langenbeck retractors of various sizes. A pair of long, sharply curved uterine scissors is useful to cut the ligamentum teres, which is the final step before the dislocation maneuver. An oscillating saw and osteotomes of various widths optimize the trochanteric osteotomy. Bone hooks, malets, a long thin periosteal elevator, and curved periosteal elevators simplify the technical execution of the approach (Fig. 7.1).
- Fully threaded screws of 3.5 or 4.5 mm diameter are required for fixation of the trochanter.

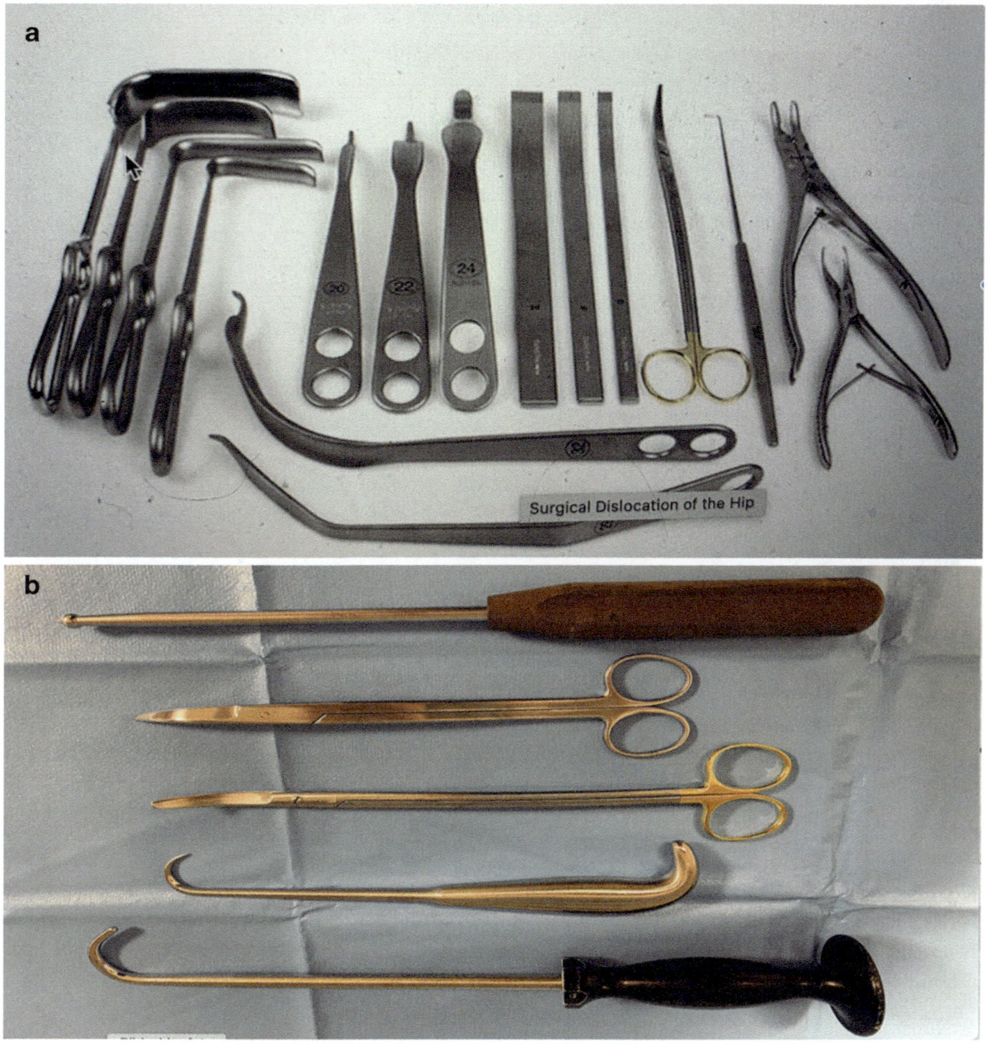

Fig. 7.1 Set of special instruments helpful for the surgical approach in SHD. (**a**) From left: Retractor (R) Hösel, R Kocher (2×), R Dockhorn 80 × 14 mm, R Dockhorn 55 × 14 mm, Bone Lever (BL) Hohmann, 22 cm (2×), BL Hohmann 24 cm (2×), BL blunt 27 cm (2×) *, Lambotte chisel curved 10 mm, 15 mm, 20 mm *, nerve root retractor 10 mm, Scissors curved, blunt, rongeur curved (rc), 24 cm, rc 17 cm. Below: Bone lever deep, bone lever double-angled. *Small blunt Hohmann available. *Straight chisels available. (**b**) Ball with spike, different scissors, and sharp and blunt hooks

7.10 Positioning

- The patient is placed in the lateral position and secured with lateral supports. A long foam cushion with a central channel is ideal for aligning the leg to be operated on horizontally while also protecting the other leg from pressure points. Smaller positioning supports are also useful (Fig. 7.2).
- The leg to be operated on is draped to allow free mobility. On the side of the table opposite the surgeon, a sterile bag is placed so that it can temporarily accommodate the drooping lower leg without loss of sterility.
- The positioning should allow for any necessary intraoperative radiography or image converter control.
- A padded Mayo stand, positioned posterior to the patient, is necessary to enable positioning of the hip in extension which facilitates dissection and exposure.

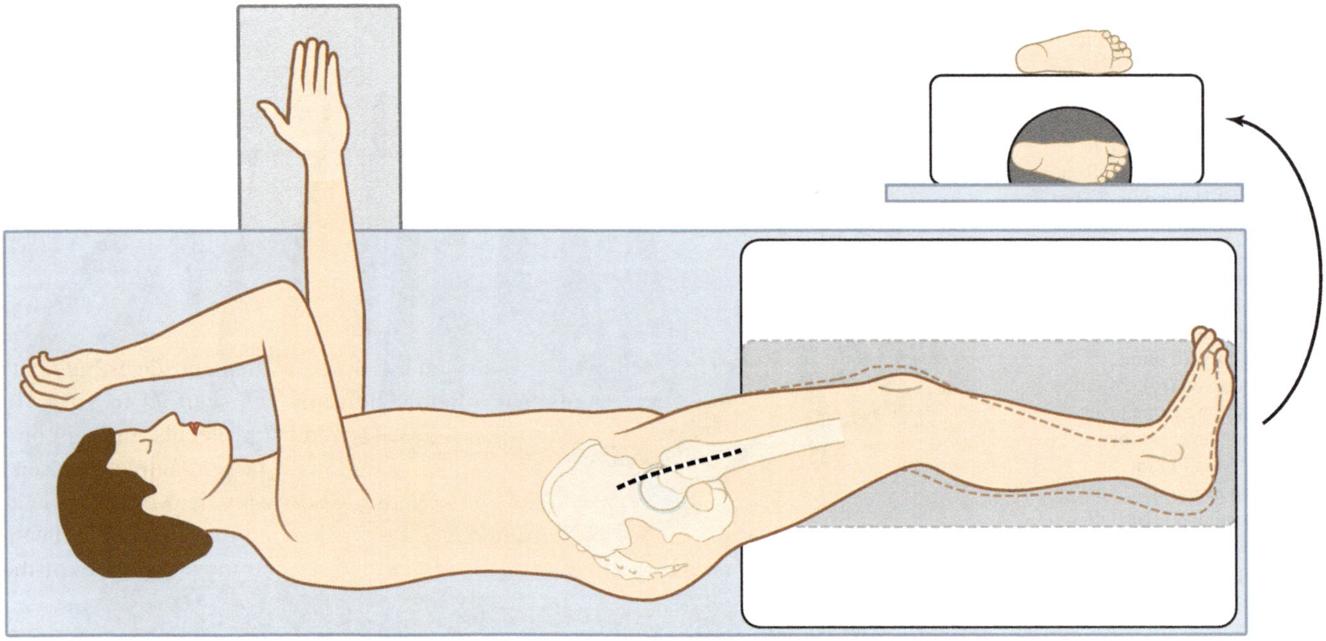

Fig. 7.2 Patient placed in the lateral position with supports for the trunk. Elevated, preferably horizontal, positioning of the freely mobile leg on a foam rubber padding, channeled for the other leg (curved arrow)

7.11 Access

The trochanteric osteotomy should be made deep enough to carry the attachments of the gluteus medius and vastus lateralis during ventral tilt to expose the anterolateral hip capsule for a safe capsulotomy, but superficial enough to leave the piriformis attachment to the stable portion of the greater trochanter intact (Fig. 7.3). This protects the deep branch of the medial circumflex femoral artery and its associated blood supply to the femoral head. The z-shaped capsulotomy provides access to the ligamentum teres, which is transected to allow complete dislocation of the femoral head.

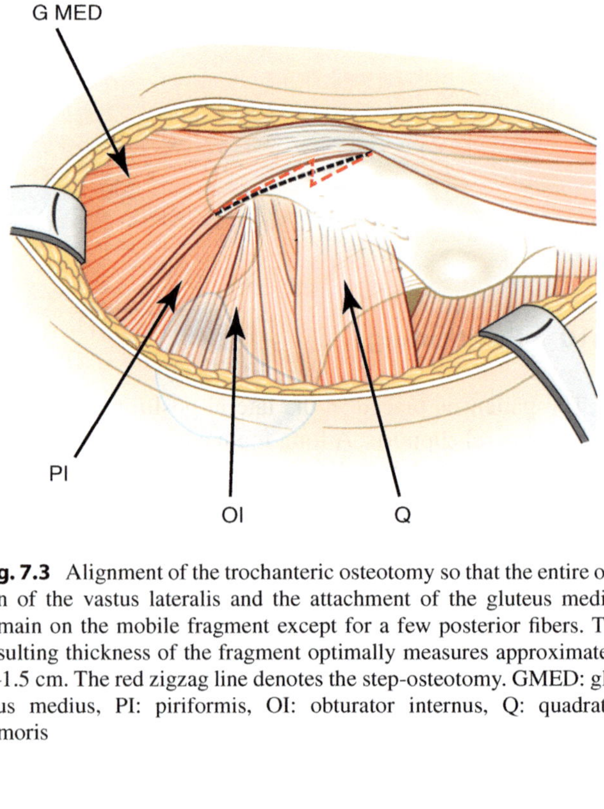

Fig. 7.3 Alignment of the trochanteric osteotomy so that the entire origin of the vastus lateralis and the attachment of the gluteus medius remain on the mobile fragment except for a few posterior fibers. The resulting thickness of the fragment optimally measures approximately 1–1.5 cm. The red zigzag line denotes the step-osteotomy. GMED: gluteus medius, PI: piriformis, OI: obturator internus, Q: quadratus femoris

7.12 Technical Steps

- Drape the freely mobile operative leg, with the lateral skin exposed from the iliac crest to the mid-thigh. Check freedom of movement including trial position of leg in the sterile bag.
- Incision: Kocher-Langenbeck [8], which is proximally posteriorly curved, or modified Gibson [9], which is rather straight.
- Longitudinal incision of the IT band, noting the perforating vessels as a guide for the dissection line proximal to the greater trochanter. Incising the gluteal fascia to enable elevation of the gluteus maximus muscle from the underlying gluteus medius muscle. Exposure of the dorsal edge of the M gluteus medius and elevation along the proximal edge of the piriformis.
- Elevation of the lateral vastus fascia to approximately 5 cm distal to the greater trochanter.
- Identify the trochanteric branch of the MFCA. Define and mark the correct thickness (1–1.5 cm) and location of the trochanteric osteotomy.
- Trochanteric osteotomy with the hip in the internal rotation is made with an oscillating saw. When elevating the trochanteric fragment, some attached dorsal fibers may need to be cut with the scalpel. For a step osteotomy, see Chap. 12.
- Further mobilization and unfolding of the mobile trochanteric fragment, facilitated by slight flexion and external rotation of the leg (Fig. 7.4).
- Entry and dissection of the capsule in the plane between gluteus minimus and piriformis (Fig. 7.5).
- Sharp detachment of the capsular attachment of the minimus tendon, facilitating visualization of the capsule and its subsequent incision.
- The capsulotomy (Fig. 7.5) is best started at the level of the midline of the neck as an anterior longitudinal incision along the anterolateral neck; however, it should be medial to the anterior border of the underlying lateral retinaculum. After extension distally, the incision is carefully continued cranially, avoiding incision of the underlying labrum at the acetabular rim. Completion of the medial flap by incision along the distal-medial capsular attachment.
- The lateral flap is formed with an incision along the cranio-dorsal acetabular rim, taking care to maintain the integrity of the labrum.
- Assess impingement mechanics even before dislocation. Assessment of dislocation distance with subluxation test. In rare instances, transection of the ligamentum teres is not required.
- Placement of the bone hook around the anterior femoral neck, sparing the Weitbrecht's ligament. By raising the hook and simultaneous external rotation, subluxation is achieved, which facilitates the introduction of uterine scissors and allows the tensioned ligamentum teres to be cut.
- With the subsequent positioning of the lower leg in the sterile bag, the femoral head can be exposed anteriorly and the cartilage can be assessed almost circularly by rotating the leg, while the acetabulum becomes fully visible with the use of Hohmann levers (Fig. 7.6).

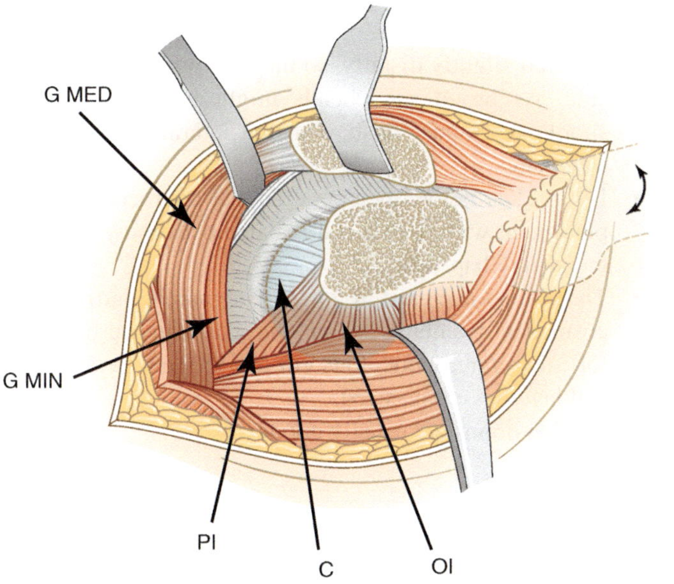

Fig. 7.4 Anterior mobilization of the trochanter including the attached muscles and dissection of the gap between gluteus minimus and piriformis to expose the capsule. G MED: gluteus medius, G MIN: gluteus minimus, PI: piriformis, C: capsule, OI: obturator internus

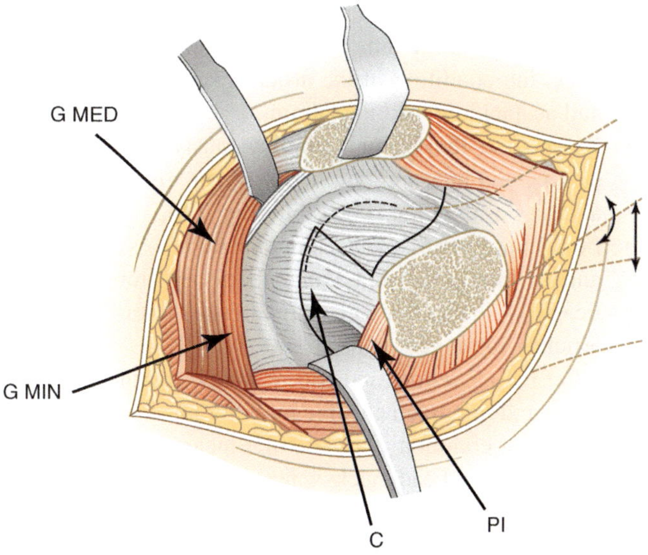

Fig. 7.5 Exposed capsule with z-shaped capsulotomy. G MED: gluteus medius, G MIN: gluteus minimus, C: capsule, OI: obturator internus

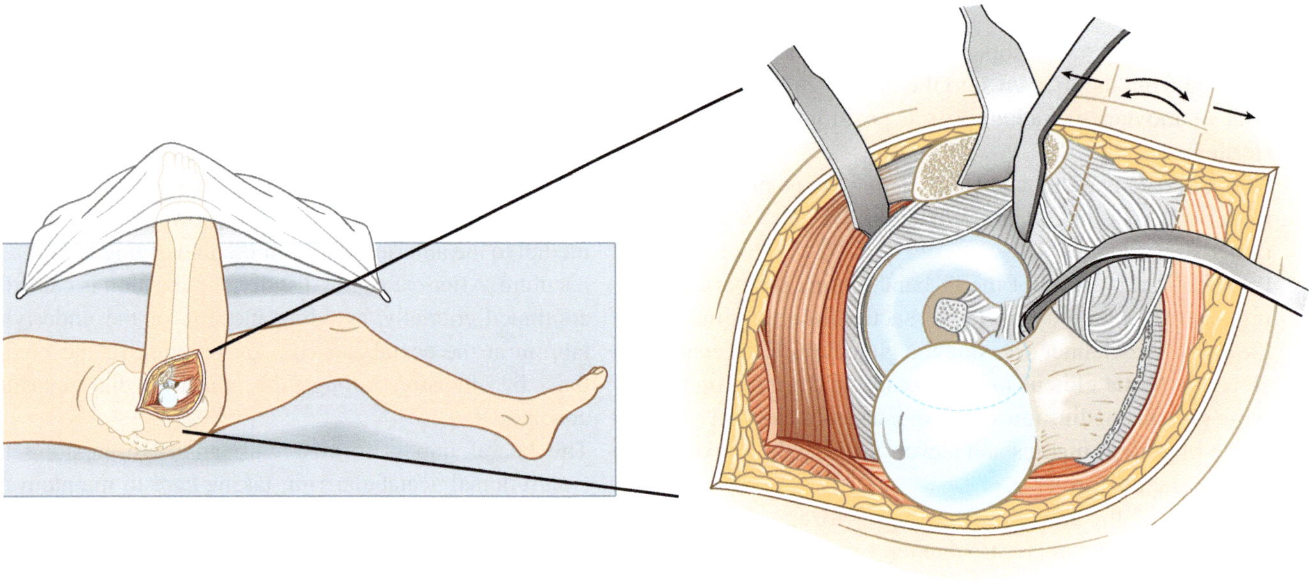

Fig. 7.6 View of acetabulum and femoral head with retractors placed around the acetabular rim. The arrows indicate the range of motion of the leg, allowing all areas of the joint to be seen

- Inspection of the joint begins with resection of the ligamentum teres stump flush with the surface of the head.
- If the visualization is not sufficient, the capsulotomy can be extended. Frequently, the incision of the fascia must also be extended cranially.
- For optimal visualization of the acetabulum, three retractors are placed on the acetabular rim outside the labrum. Most important is a long, thin Hohmann lever that hooks into the acetabular fossa and levers the femoral neck dorsal-distally (Fig. 7.6).
- Intra-articular assessment should look for abnormalities in the shape of the femoral head and the junction with the neck, the condition of the articular cartilage at the head and acetabulum, and the labrum.
- By moving the leg and simultaneously alternating tensioning and loosening of the retractors, visualization into all areas of the joint is possible (Fig. 7.6).
- For dynamic assessment, Hohmann retractors are removed and the joint is reduced. Langenbeck retractors allow sufficient visualization to demonstrate intra- or extra-articular impingement.
- After the procedure and before wound closure, joint stability and impingement-free mobility must be rechecked.
- The most common intra-articular measure is the optimization of the head–neck–waist, a problem that may be primarily antero-lateral. This requires strict attention to the site of attachment of the retinacula. Bleeding from the developing cancellous bone areas is controlled with wax (see Chap. 9).
- The treatment of labral detachments, cartilage detachments, and possibly protruding acetabular rims is described in detail in Chap. 10.
- For the possible treatment of larger cartilage defects of the head, see Chap. 11.
- The capsule should not be closed watertight and under tension because this may occlude the blood supply to the head, as laser Doppler flowmetry studies have shown. Actually, it is only important to approximate the edges.
- Refixation of the trochanter is usually done anatomically. Two, maximum 3, 3.5 parallel aligned fully threaded screws are sufficient. For large dimensions, 4.5 screws can also be used. The tip of the screws should be directed slightly distally, so they are not within the capsule. As proud screwheads might be irritating, they should be almost flush with the lateral of the greater trochanter.
- If it is clear before the operation that no trochanteric displacement will be necessary, a step osteotomy is recommended (Chap. 12).
- The wound is closed in layers. Fat gaps in particular are cosmetically unflattering and they can also cause discomfort; therefore, meticulous closure of the superficial fascial layers is emphasized.
- Suction drains are usually not necessary.

7.13 Postoperative Treatment

- Aftertreatment depends on the complexity of the procedure performed and can range from full weight bearing supported by two crutches and unlimited flexion to partial weight bearing with limited flexion during the first 6–12 weeks.

- Following more complex cases, in bed, the leg is placed in a foam splint in neutral abduction/adduction and neutral rotation for the first few days. A position of slight flexion reduces tension pain and prevents anterior subluxation until muscle activity returns. Some surgeons routinely use a continuous passive motion machine following.
- Passive range-of-motion exercises are initially performed on the first postoperative days. Depending on the procedure, cautious active flexion may also be started. Sitting at the edge of the bed and then standing on two forearm crutches are encouraged as soon as the patient feels able. Initially, the operative leg should only be lifted with the help of the other foot and requires a certain amount of practice. Physiotherapeutic assistance is also useful for the first attempts at ambulation with crutches.
- Medical prophylaxis of heterotopic ossification and deep vein thrombosis is based on individual risk factors.
- A first routine radiographic check is useful after 6–8 weeks. It may also serve as a decision aid to begin active abductor training under appropriate guidance. If a step-cut trochanteric osteotomy has been done, muscle function and weight-bearing may be advanced more quickly. An increase in weight-bearing is routine after 6–8 weeks.
- Recheck X-rays to assess consolidation of trochanteric osteotomy and begin walking with a cane. Walking without a cane should not occur until gluteus medius strength is equivalent to an M5. Resumption of sports activities not before 5–6 months after surgery.
- Screw removal for local discomfort not before 6 months.

7.14 Intra-/Postoperative Complications

- Too limited proximal extension of the fascial incision particularly in athletic patients makes visualization considerably more difficult and can lead to considerable muscle damage due to forceful muscle retraction. As a result, ectopic ossification is not uncommon. The same applies to a lesser extent to capsulotomy.
- Sciatic neuropraxia is a very rare complication and has been observed only in surgical dislocation after extensive scarring, such as that resulting from prior traumatic hip dislocation or posterior pelvic surgery. It can also occur due to entrapment of the sciatic nerve in an altered piriformis muscle [13]; however, this is rare (Fig. 7.7).
- If the exposure of the *interval* between the gluteus minimus and piriformis is extended too far cranially, somewhat into the greater sciatic foramen, injury to the superior gluteal artery and its nerve is possible.
- Insufficient healing of the trochanteric osteotomy with delayed healing and eventual pseudarthrosis can occur following insufficient fixation, poor bone quality, too early and too aggressive abductor training, or after a fall in the early postoperative period.
- Postoperative dislocation has anecdotally been observed but, in each case, could be related to excessive acetabular rim trimming or other surgically created hazards.
- If osteochondral trimming of the femoral neck is performed too aggressively, it can become a risk for a postoperative femoral neck fracture. A postoperative fall is a conceivable cause.
- Overall, however, the SHD technique described here has a very low morbidity [14].

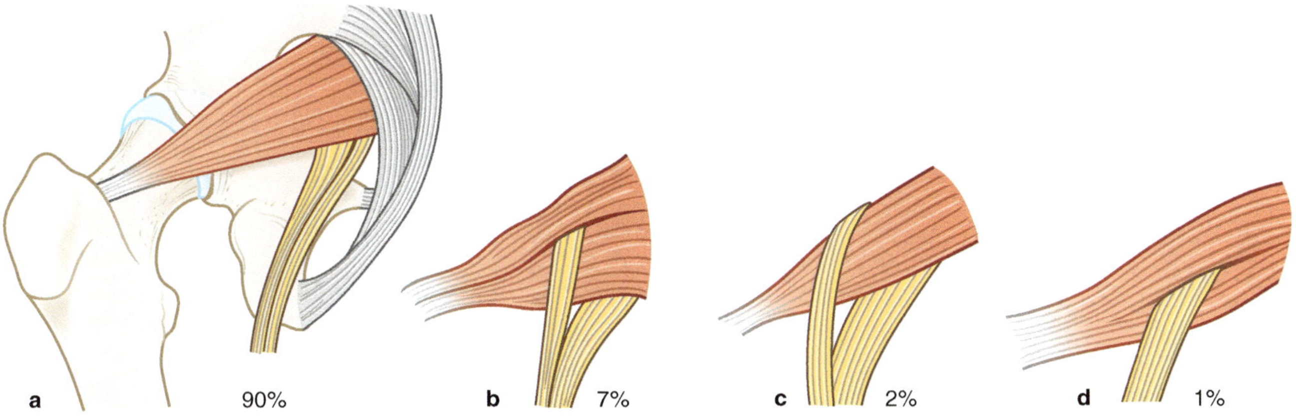

Fig. 7.7 Possible course variants between sciatic nerve and piriformis muscle

7.15 Case Study

As the SHD is the basic technique, case studies are presented in the specific section.

7.16 Controversies

- The decision-making between using arthroscopic and open surgery may continue to evolve especially for the treatment of many cases of FAI that are associated with end ranges of femoral version.
- Transection of the ligamentum teres is repeatedly discussed as a potential cause of loss of proprioception and as a possible cause of subsequent dislocation.

7.17 Results

Follow-up study of the surgical approach in isolation is hardly possible as the results and outcomes are more associated with the therapeutic steps carried out via the approach and can rarely be related to the approach itself. The only study of complications attributable to dislocation was published in 2011 [14]. The procedure is now considered a standard surgical approach to the hip joint with low morbidity.

7.18 Future Directions

- Improve and simplify collision modeling for FAI, with results directly applicable to surgical therapy.
- Consideration for a less invasive procedure while maintaining as much insight into the joint as possible.
- Optimization of indications.
- More prospective follow-up.

References

1. Poirier P. Traité d'anatomie humaine. Vol. 1 embryology (Prenant A) ostéologie, arthrology. Paris: Masson; 1899.
2. Preiser G. Koxarthrosis and its relation to abnormal version of the acetabulum. Dtsch Zeitschr Chirurg. 1907;89:541.
3. Raab GT. The geometry of slipped upper femoral epiphysis: implication for movement, impingement, and corrective osteotomy. J Pediatr Orthop. 1999;19:419–24.
4. Crock HV. An atlas of vascular anatomy of the skeleton and spinal cord. Foreword. London: Martin Dunitz Ltd; 1996.
5. Gautier E, Ganz K, Krügel N, Gill T, Ganz R. Anatomy of the medial femoral circumflex artery and its surgical implications. J Bone Joint Surg Br. 2000;82:679–83.
6. Nötzli HP, Siebenrock KA, Hempfing A, Ramseier LE, Ganz R. Perfusion of the femoral head during surgical dislocation of the hip. Monitoring by laser Doppler flowmetry. J Bone Joint Surg Br. 2002;84:300–4.
7. Ganz R, Gill TJ, Ganz K, Krügel N, Berlemann U. Surgical dislocation of the adult hip. A technique with full access to the femoral head and acetabulum without risk of avascular necrosis. J Bone Joint Surg Br. 2001;83:1119–24.
8. Tosounidis TH, Giannoudis VNK, Giannoudis PV. The Kocher-Langenbeck approach: state of the art. JBJS Essent Surg Tech. 2018;8(2):e18. https://doi.org/10.2106/JBJS.ST.16.00102. eCollection 2018 Jun 27
9. Moed BT. The modified Gibson posterior surgical approach to the acetabulum. J Orthop Trauma. 2010;24(5):315–22. https://doi.org/10.1097/BOT.0b013e3181c4aef8.
10. Bastian JD, Wolf AT, Wyss TF, Nötzli HP. Stepped osteotomy of the trochanter for stable, anatomic refixation. Clin Orthop Relat Res. 2009;467(3):732–8. https://doi.org/10.1007/s11999-008-0649-x. Epub 2008 Dec 9.PMID: 19067094.
11. Leunig M, Ganz R. The evolution and concepts of joint-preserving surgery of the hip. Bone Joint J. 2014;96:5–18.
12. Ganz R, Parvizi J, Beck M, Leunig M, Nötzli H, Siebenrock KA. Femoroacetabular impingement. A cause for osteoarthritis of the hip. Clin Orthop Relat Res. 2003;417:112–20.
13. Beaton LE, Anson AJ. J Bone Joint Surg (Am). 1938;20:686.
14. Sink EL, Beaulé PE, Sucato D, Kim YJ, Millis MB, Dayton M, Trousdale RT, Sierra RJ, Zaltz I, Schoenecker P, Monreal A, Clohisy J. Multicenter study of complications following surgical dislocation of the hip. J Bone Joint Surg Am. 2011;93:1132–6.

Extended Retinacular Flap

8

Ira Zaltz, Michael Leunig, and Reinhold Ganz

8.1 Introduction

The extended retinaculum flap is an application extension of the surgical hip dislocation (see Chap. 7). The combination of both techniques represents the basis for performing intraarticular/capsular osteotomies without compromising the blood supply to the femoral head.

8.2 Background

Because of the proximity of the femoral neck to most deformities of the hip, it would be an ideal site for correction of upper femoral problems while minimizing secondary deformities. Due to concerns about femoral head necrosis from injury to the overlying blood vessels, this region has long been disregarded for correction. The femoral neck has a slightly raised thickening of the periosteum laterally, as well as dorso-medially, called the retinaculum (Fig. 8.1). The medial retinaculum runs on the so-called Weitbrecht's ligament, which freely bridges the waisted bone in the proximal region. Both protect the terminal branches of the medial circumflex femoral artery, the main blood supply to the femoral head This type of blood supply is not completely dual, however, because the supply through the ligament of Weitbrecht safely supplies only the medial half of the femoral head while the supply through the lateral retinaculum can supply the entire head.

Antero-lateral cuneiform neck osteotomies did not sufficiently eliminate problems with epiphyseal perfusion [1, 2], Dunn was the first to reduce the risk of head necrosis by performing local mobilization of the lateral retinaculum before correcting the deformity of the SCFE at its origin [3]. Although the margin gained with his technique is sufficient for small corrections, the risk of overstretching the retinaculum flap increases with the magnitude of correction required. Furthermore, if dislocation of the head is not used, as Dunn did, all surgical manipulations of the neck are further complicated by the inability to control the reduction.

Like the rest of the periosteum, the retinaculum is significantly thicker in children compared with adults and therefore easier to detach without risk of tearing. With an osteotomy of the greater trochanter, a reduction of the remaining portion to the level of the femoral neck, and a subsequent capsulotomy, the lateral retinaculum can be detached from the bone down to the level of the lesser trochanter under visual control. If the trimming of the base of the trochanter is omitted, the dorsal and distal parts cannot be seen, which significantly complicates safe visualization [4].

I. Zaltz (✉)
Department of Orthopaedic Surgery, C.S. Mott Children's Hospital, University of Michigan, Ann Arbor, MI, USA
e-mail: zaltz@med.umich.edu

M. Leunig
Hip Service, Department of Orthopedics, Schulthess Clinic, Zurich, Switzerland
e-mail: Michael.leunig@kws.ch

R. Ganz
Emeritus, Medical Faculty, University of Berne, Berne, Switzerland

M. Leunig et al. (eds.), *Surgical Hip Dislocation*, https://doi.org/10.1007/978-3-031-70622-6_8

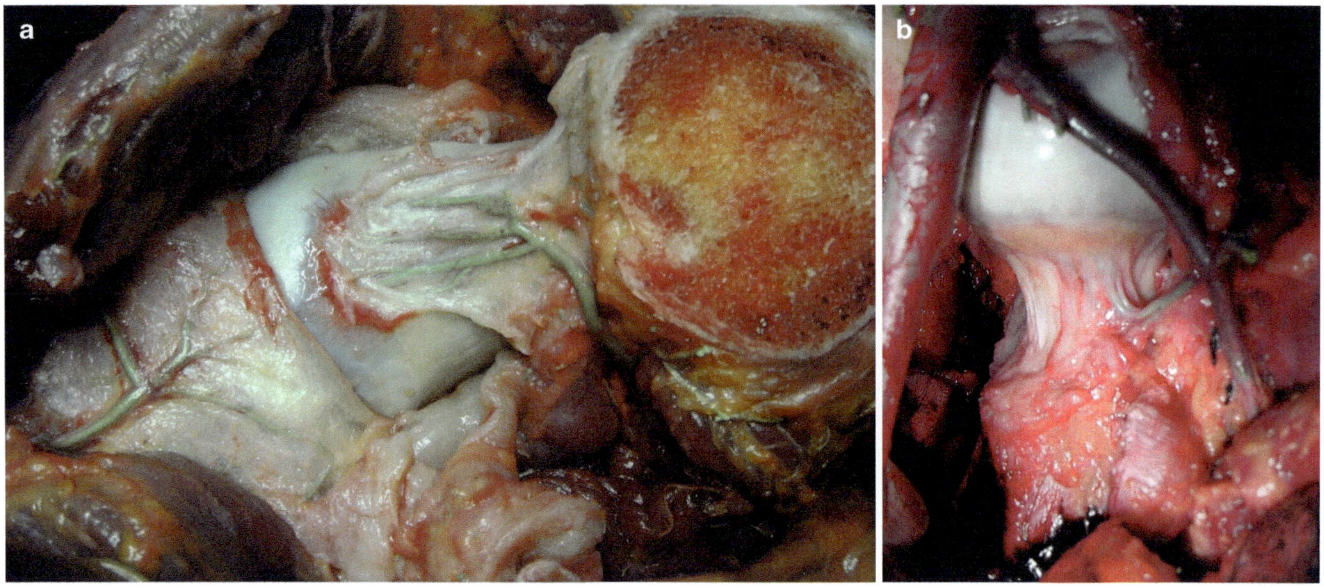

Fig. 8.1 (**a**) Lateral retinaculum with arborization of the deep branch of the MFCA. (**b**) Postero-medial retinaculum with the medial branch of the MFCA on top of Weitbrecht's ligament

8.3 Indications

Indications: In children and adolescents, periosteum and retinaculum are thicker and therefore easier to detach without risk of tearing.

- Intracapital osteotomies in Perthes disease (lateral retinaculum only).
- Subcapital mobilization of the head in epiphysiolysis capitis femoris with open joint (both retinacula).

Relative Indications:

- Femoral neck osteotomies with closed growth plate or in patients >15 years (both retinacula). The tissue layer of the periosteum and retinaculum is thinner in adult individuals and is less easily detached from the bone without tearing.

Contraindications:

- After a femoral neck fracture, scarring of the retinaculum may make detachment without loss of continuity impossible, so this approach should be avoided if possible.
- In very short femoral necks, as in certain Perthes deformities, preparation in the dorsal region of the retinaculum is difficult and requires great experience with the approach.
- In rare head necrosis in young acrobatic athletes, once the flap is dissected, the remaining blood supply in the lateral segment of the head may not be adequate. Supraselective angiography may substantiate or invalidate these concerns.

8.4 Preoperative/Preinterventional Diagnostics

- Pelvic AP as well as Lauenstein or cross-table lateral
- Arthro-MRI of the symptomatic hip
- CT with special sequences for preoperative computer simulation of intracapital osteotomy

8.5 Preoperative Planning/Computer Simulation

Computer simulation allows the surgical steps of an osteotomy to be specified more precisely and the production of cutting devices (see Chap. 5). It has proved particularly useful for head reduction in certain Perthes deformities, especially for the osteotomy direction and the size of the head after correction, and is described in more detail there.

8.6 Applied Anatomy

- A prerequisite for the preparation of the retinaculum soft flap is the fully executed surgical dislocation of the joint [5] (see Chap. 7).
- With the external rotation of the leg, the postero-medially located Weitbrechts' ligament with the medial retinaculum becomes visible. With internal rotation, the laterally located retinaculum at the femoral neck becomes visible. Both contain the vessels from the medial circumflex artery for the blood supply of the femoral head [6]

(Fig. 8.1). Smallest vessel branches from the lateral circumflex artery are insignificant for the head blood supply. The same applies to the artery in the ligamentum rotundum, vessels in the capsule, and vascular branches in the metaphysis of the head–neck transition.

8.7 Special Risks

Disturbance of the blood supply to the femoral head with consequences such as

- Loss of reduction, head collapse, resulting follow-up surgery including joint replacement
- See also Part 4

8.8 Type of Anesthesia

As the procedure is performed in lateral positioning and usually takes more than 90 min, general anesthesia is the recommendation of choice, especially since the patients are mostly children and adolescents.

8.9 Positioning

- Standard operating table
- Lateral positioning with tunnel cushion and lateral bag
- Fluoroscopy and X-ray possibility

8.10 Instruments/Implants

Standard instrumentation for surgical hip dislocation (see Chap. 7). In addition to the instruments required for the surgical dislocation approach, the following special instruments ensure an optimal surgical procedure:

- Two rounded Hohmann retractors, 22 mm;
- One Dockhorn retractor 55/14 mm;
- Curved periosteal elevators, 6 and 14 mm, one each;
- Straight chisel-type Lexer, 5, 10, and 15 mm, one each;
- One metal hammer 300 g;
- Bone hooks small and medium, curved, one each;
- One capsule pliers;
- Bone wax, possibly synthetic;
- One curved hemostasis clamp;
- All cutting instruments should be checked for optimal sharpness prior to surgery.

8.11 Access

- Access for surgical hip dislocation with trochanteric osteotomy (see Chap. 7).

8.12 Technical Steps of Deep Dissection

- *Reduction of the Joint and Internal Rotation*

After completion of the surgical dislocation approach, the lower leg is first removed from the internally sterile bag and the femoral head is reduced back into the acetabulum. For an optimal view of the osteotomy surface of the stable trochanter, especially its posterior edge, the operating table is tilted slightly to the other side and the leg is rotated inward. Full extension of the hip and as little flexion of the knee as possible improve the relaxation of the posterior soft tissue structures.

- *Subperiosteal Development of the Soft Tissue Flap*

First, one to two pointed Hohmann levers hold the mobile part of the trochanter, rotated 180° about the longitudinal axis, with the muscle attachments of gluteus medius, long tendon of gluteus minimus, and vastus lateralis. The periosteum of the femoral neck is then longitudinally notched at the anterior margin of the retinaculum. The notch extends from the cephalic cartilage to the angle between the neck and the trochanter; it serves to prevent an uncontrolled tear in the direction of the retinaculum (Fig. 8.2). Using the various

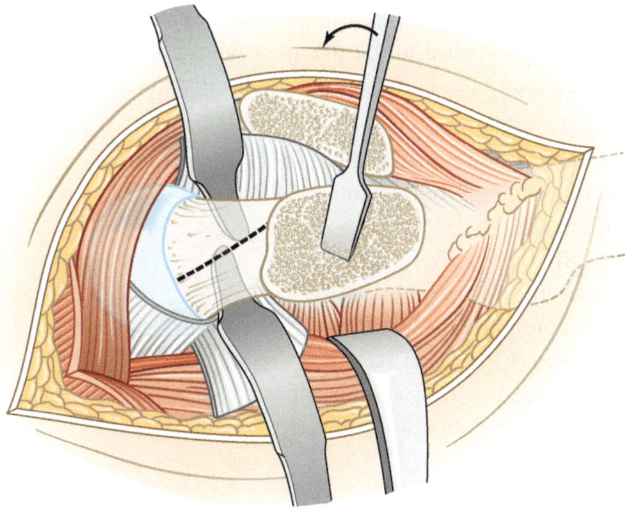

Fig. 8.2 Internal rotation of the leg and reduced head for best presentation of the lateral retinaculum. Periosteal incision of the periosteum anterior to the retinaculum (dotted line). Resection level of the stable part of the trochanter (continuous line). With an open growth line, the segment can be lifted in toto. When consolidated, piecemeal resection is preferred

osteotomes, the trochanteric bone is then gradually reduced in small sections to the level of the neck. During this process, the covering periosteal mantle must be preserved in its continuity. The easiest way to achieve this is to stop the chiseling process just before the perforation and break the bone piece by levering the chisel manually. It is then carefully turned over with bone-grasping forceps and detached from the adhering periosteum with the scalpel. Repeated palpation helps to check progress to the femoral neck level. At the junction with the femoral neck, mobilization of the flap continues as a strictly periosteal elevation. Special care is required to protect the insertion of the flap at the head–neck junction, in the area of vascular penetration into the bone [7]. The distal limit of dissection and mobilization of the flap is at the base of the lesser trochanter. Depending on the requirements of the flap, subperiosteal mobilization may continue well dorsally. At 10–15 cm, the flap is significantly longer and allows visualization into the dorsolateral neck of the femur without risk of overstretching (Fig. 8.3).

- *Re-Dislocation of the Femoral Head to Visualize the Medial Flap*

The best view for dissection of the medial retinaculum flap is with dislocation of the head. With repositioning of the lower leg in the sterile bag, the medial soft tissue package is also relaxed. Even more dorsal overview is possible with an increase in external rotation, but for this, the lower leg must again be removed from the sack. The extent of the medial retinaculum corresponds to the width of the ligamentum Weitbrecht at the postero-medial circumference of the neck. Detachment of the periosteum best begins approximately 10–15 mm ventral to the ligament with a longitudinal incision down to the bone. It extends distally to the level of the palpable lesser trochanter. The gap is first carefully and gradually widened with the 6-mm curved periosteal elevator and a curved hemostasis clamp later with the 14-mm periosteal elevator; not infrequently, the longitudinal incision must be extended further distally. The last step is the connection of the medial gap with the gap of the lateral flap. Strict care must also be taken with the medial flap to preserve the area of vascular perforation into the bone at the head–neck junction. The result is a gutter-shaped periosteal tube with both retinacula; it contains all major blood vessels of the head and allows manipulations of the neck under constant visual control of the tension of the retinacula. Before returning the head to the socket, make sure that the lateral flap is unfolded to its full width.

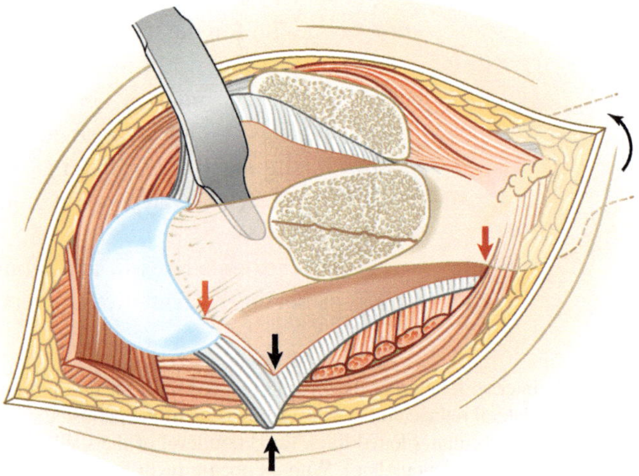

Fig. 8.3 Situation after the dissection of both retinacular flaps resulting in a periosteal half-tube connected with the epiphysis. Lower black arrow: joint capsule, upper black arrow: retinacular flap. red arrows: length of the retinacular flap from epiphysis to lesser trochanter

- *Refixation of the Soft Tissue Flap*

At the end of a procedure, the periosteal tube should never be closed with sutures under tension. To avoid overstretching of the blood vessels, the edges should only be approximated by a few simple sutures. The position of the trochanter can be checked with image intensifiers. If necessary, the lateral cortex of the femur can be flattened to achieve optimal contact with the trochanter. Care must be taken not to crush the lateral retinaculum area when refixing the trochanter. Two, rarely three screws are usually sufficient. When deciding on the entry point of the screws, care should be taken to maintain an optimal lever arm for the gluteus medius muscle, if necessary, with interposition of a bone block, for example, from the remains of the trochanteric reduction.

- *Checking the Head Perfusion*

It is recommended to check the perfusion of the epiphysis during the procedure. Although laser Doppler flow measurement has been shown to provide reproducible results [8], it is too laborious for daily use. Perforation of the epiphysis with a 2-mm drill is practical and easy to use. Leakage of blood may be slight during dislocation of the head and increases after reduction of the head; a continuous outflow of dark blood is sufficient evidence of intact perfusion. When drilling through the fovea capitis, the integrity of the cartilaginous surface remains intact. Perfusion monitoring [8] can be performed before the onset and after the completion of retinacular dissection.

- *Refixation Trochanter*

In nearly all situations where the retinacular flap approach was executed, the trochanter will be refixed with some degree of distal advancement. Care must be taken that its new position does not lead to compression of the readapted retinacular tissue, a mishap which especially may occur during tightening of the screws. Occasionally, a small bone block can hold the tip of the trochanter at the necessary distance.

- *Modifications of the Procedure*

Dissection of the medial retinaculum flap (in addition to the lateral retinaculum) is indicated only for subcapital reorientation of the head in epiphysiolysis capitis femoris and osteotomy of the femoral neck (Chaps. 15 and 16).

In isolated relative neck lengthening, dissection of the lateral retinaculum is sufficient. In an extremely short femoral neck, the very narrow gap to the femoral head places increased demands on the care of the dissection. Provided that no intraarticular measures are planned for relative femoral neck lengthening, it is even possible to refrain from dislocating the joint (Chap. 13).

During reduction osteotomy of the femoral head, the medial retinaculum is also not touched. At most, a circumscribed mobilization of the anteromedial periosteum is necessary for an optimal adaptation of a cutting template (Chap. 17).

If the retinaculum approach is performed together with a peri-acetabular pelvic osteotomy (PAO), it is usually advisable to start with the femoral part. The femoral approach allows the ischial osteotomy of the PAO to be performed under visual control, that is, with optimal control of the sciatic nerve. Overview and visual tissue differentiation of the approach between the inferior gemellus muscle and the obturator externus are clearest when the ischium osteotomy is performed immediately after the trochanteric osteotomy and before the retinacular flap is dissected.

8.13 Postoperative Follow-Up

- *Postoperative Partial Weight-Bearing Depending on the Osteotomies Performed*

Sufficient consolidation of the trochanter with shallow osteotomy can be expected after 6 weeks; however, strengthening of the abductor muscles can begin after 4 weeks. The period of partial weight bearing is determined by the procedure performed. After relative neck lengthening, hip weight-bearing can be increased after 6 weeks, but unrestricted weight-bearing, such as competitive sports, should be postponed until the "new" neck is visibly re-corticated. After subcapital reorientation, weight-bearing can be reduced after 8 weeks and completely discontinued 10–12 weeks after surgery. The process of consolidation is similar after a head reduction osteotomy [9]. Consolidation of the collapsing femoral neck osteotomy takes about 3–4 months; the period of weight-bearing restriction may be even longer for the rarely performed open-wedge osteotomy. Administartion NSAIDS for approximately 10 days for prevention of heterotopic ossifications may be considered and is common practice in many centers.

- *Secondary Procedures*

Screw heads may cause bothersome pain with direct pressure or interfere with iliotibial band gliding; these may disappear after removal of the metal. The tissue adherence of titanium screws may make their removal considerably more difficult.

8.14 Intra-/Postoperative Complications

Complications cannot be readily attributed to the approach with dissection of the retinacula or separated from the osteotomy performed. The rupture of the flap at the base of the head is a possible mishap with the potential for necrosis of the epiphysis. Tight suture closure of the retinaculum-periosteal tube can overstretch the embedded vessels, obstructing blood flow [8]. Finally, crushing of the retinaculum and thus the blood vessels is possible if the greater trochanter is refixed relatively high and without clearance to the neck. In isolated cases, some subperiosteal bone formation between the flap and posterior neck bone has been observed during the healing process; however, no posterior impingement has been demonstrated as a result. In general, the neck maintains a rather slender shape, which may also be related to the circumferential denudation of the neck bone.

8.15 Case Studies

- Not applicable

8.16 Controversies

- The most frequently mentioned counterarguments to the method presented here are related to the treatment of epiphysiolysis capitis femoris and refer to reports from Iowa in the 1980s of good results with "pinning in situ," which is surgically much less complex. This technique convinced many pediatric surgeons because of its ease of performance and its almost certain avoidance of head necrosis. Less read are more recent reports of this procedure showing high rates of poor long-term outcomes with slippage greater than 30° and with more precise examination techniques.
- One response to this has been screw fixation after "gentle manual reduction." There is little literature on the results of this method; the head necroses seen repeatedly are presented as isolated cases. It is difficult to quantify how far a surgeon is willing to go with a "gentle" reduction if the goal is to achieve a better to ideal head–neck relationship. On the contrary, it is known today that even in the case of so-called acute slippage, a callus can already exist dorsally on the neck, which imposes a detour on the retinaculum that can lead to overstretching of the vessels running through it.
- Because of this problem, Dunn [3] recommended circumscribed detachment of the retinaculum with the removal of the dorsal new bone formation and thus achieved a substantial reduction in the risk of head necrosis. The extension of

retinaculum detachment described here has largely eliminated the risk when used correctly. Our own results show that necrosis that can nevertheless be observed is more correctly explained by nonsurgical factors, such as traumatic retinaculum avulsion or too long a perfusion stop.

- Many established pediatric orthopedists object that the technique of extended retinaculum flap as too complex and difficult to learn. Small numbers of cases also make it difficult to gain sufficient experience. The safest alternative is to bundle the cases in centers where the necessary expertise can be developed.
- Correction of established deforimties using intertrochanteric corrections improve the relation between the acetabulum and the head, but lateral projections may reveal persistent subcapital irregularities of the contour and offset [10].

8.17 Expected Outcomes

- Not applicable, as this is covered in the chapters on specific applications of the technology.

8.18 Outlook

- The experience with the long time it took for the acceptance of surgical dislocation suggests that the spread of the extended retinaculum flap will be similarly slow, especially since the indication is much less frequent. An important intermediate step will be for existing centers to publish their experience, especially doing a detailed analysis of the causes of necrosis. More and more new meta-analyses do not contribute meaningfully to any knowledge gains.

References

1. Fish JB. Cuneiform osteotomy of the femoral neck in the treatment of slipped capital femoral epiphysis. A follow-up note. J Bone Joint Surg Am. 1994;76:46–59.
2. Gage JR, Sundberg AB, Nolan DR, et al. Complications after cuneiform osteotomy for moderately or severely slipped capital femoral epiphysis. J Bone Joint Surg Am. 1978;60:157–65.
3. Dunn DM. The treatment of adolescent slipping of the upper femoral epiphysis. J Bone Joint Surg (Br). 1964;46:621–9.
4. Ganz R, Huff TW, Leunig M. Extended retinacular soft tissue flap for intraarticular hip surgery: surgical technique, indications, and results of its application. Instr Course Lect. 2009;58:241–55.
5. Ganz R, Gill TJ, Gautier E, Ganz K, Krügel N, Berlemann U. Safe surgical dislocation of the adult hip. J Bone Joint Surg. 2001;83-B:1119–24.
6. Kalhor M, Beck M, Huff TW, Ganz R. Capsular and pericapsular contribution to acetabular and femoral head perfusion. J Bone Joint Surg Am. 2009;91:409–18.
7. Rego P, Mascarenhas V, Mafra I, Oliveira F, Pinto P, Ganz R. Femoral neck osteotomy in skeletally mature patients: surgical technique and midterm results. Int Orthop. 2021;45:83–94.
8. Nötzli HP, Siebenrock KA, Hempfing A, Ramseier LE, Ganz R. Perfusion of the femoral head during surgical dislocation of the hip. Monitoring by laser Doppler flowmetry. J Bone Joint Surg (Br). 2002;84-B:300–4.
9. Leunig M, Ganz R. Relative neck lengthening and intracapital osteotomy for severe Perthes and Perthes-like deformities. Bull NYU Hosp Jt Dis. 2011;69(Suppl 1):S62–7.
10. Giab M, Hresko MT, Millis MB. Intertrochanteric versus subcapital osteotomy in slipped capital femoral epiphysis. Clin Orthop Relat Res. 2004;427:204–12.

Part 3

Intraarticular Reconstruction/Repair

9 Bone Resection and Reshaping in FAI

Klaus-Peter Günther and Christopher L. Peters

9.1 Introduction

Cam-type femoroacetabular impingement (FAI) is a motion conflict phenomenon wherein the aspherical portion of the femoral head–neck junction produces abnormal contact forces at the articular chondrolabral margin resulting in labral and chondral damage. Pincer impingement can be caused by abnormalities of the acetabulum (i.e., partial or circular bony overcoverage in an otherwise normally oriented acetabulum or excessive anterior coverage of the head in acetabular retroversion), or femoral torsional deformity where the femoral neck impinges against the acetabular rim and labrum. Surgical treatment of FAI aims at restoring normal femoral head–neck offset and/or physiologic acetabular coverage and repair/debridement of damaged chondrolabral tissue. Restoring normal femoral torsion and acetabular orientation by osteotomies may also be indicated to treat FAI.

9.2 Background

Femoroacetabular impingement (FAI) that is predominantly due to abnormal femoral morphology has been termed cam FAI by one of the first publications by Myers et al. [1] reminiscent of the design of a cam shaft in mechanical engineering. An aspherical femoral head produces a motion conflict phenomenon as the femoral head–neck junction enters the acetabulum, most often during flexion and internal rotation of the hip. Typically, the labrum is pushed out of the way by leveraging the aspherical portion of the femoral head, and the underlying articular cartilage-articular labral complex undergoes pressurization or shear that leads to eventual failure, usually in the form of hyaline cartilage delamination and undersurface labral damage [2–5]. The most notable primary radiographic finding in patients with cam FAI is an aspherical femoral head, historically termed as "pistol-grip-deformity" [6–9] by some authors. Secondary findings include fibrocatilaginous lesions ("herniation pit") or cyst formation at the head–neck junction, increased cortical density, ossification of the labrum, and acetabular cyst formation [10–13]. The treatment aims to restore appropriate femoral head sphericity to enhance range of motion, and, when possible, to treat the resulting chondrolabral damage.

The role of physeal stress, particularly associated with early athletic activity, in developing proximal physis during adolescent development appears to be a significant predisposing factor for the development of proximal femoral sphericity.

In 1971, Murray and Duncan described an increased rate of femoral head tilt deformities in a small series of adolescents who participated in a school-based sporting program compared with controls [14]. This report received increased attention after the contemporary description of FAI was proposed by Ganz et al. in 2003 [15]. Subsequently, a number of investigations have demonstrated a link between early and/or vigorous sporting activity and abnormal proximal femoral morphology. Siebenrock et al. have demonstrated increased rates of abnormal proximal femoral morphology in adolescent and elite hockey players and in basketball players [16, 17]. Kapron et al. have shown extremely high (95%) rates of Cam-deformity in collegiate football players, and Larson et al. have similarly shown 75% of collegiate football players an alpha angle greater than 55° [18, 19]. The strong relationship between early sporting activity and abnormal proximal morphology is highlighted in a recent meta-analysis, which showed a statistically significant difference in the prevalence rate of Cam deformity in male athletes (41%) compared with 17% for controls [20]. Agricola et al. used computational modeling to demonstrate the stresses across the physis proving the above observational findings [21].

K.-P. Günther
Center for Orthopedics, Trauma and Plastic Surgery, University Hospital Carl Gustav Carus Dresden, Technical University Dresden, Dresden, Germany
e-mail: Klaus-Peter.Guenther@ukdd.de

C. L. Peters (✉)
Department of Orthopaedic Surgery, University of Utah, Salt Lake City, UT, USA
e-mail: Chris.Peters@hsc.utah.edu

M. Leunig et al. (eds.), *Surgical Hip Dislocation*, https://doi.org/10.1007/978-3-031-70622-6_9

In contrast to CAM deformities, pincer-type deformities do not cause an impingement because of an asphericity of the femoral head. Rather, common features are partial or circumferential bony overcoverge, such as in a deep socket, acetabular retroversion, retro torsional femoral deformity, or a reduced head/neck offset. In these cases, the range of movement of the hip is limited and the femoral neck abuts against the rim directly damaging the labrum. It is compressed between the femoral neck and the underlying bony rim, and the transmission of forces to the acetabular cartilage is mainly restricted to a narrow zone along the acetabular rim. Repeated microtrauma can induce labral tears as well as rim ossifications [2–5]. Contrecoup cartilage lesions are frequently found opposite to the impinging zone, which is mostly the posteroinferior acetabular rim. Typical radiographic patterns of a pincer deformity are an increased CE angle, a positive crossover sign, and partial or even circular labral ossification (see Chap. 10).

A critical feature of FAI is the relationship between proximal femoral shape, acetabular anatomy, and hip motion (see Chap. 4). Indeed, what separates the contemporary FAI description by Ganz et al. from older descriptions of the relationship between abnormal hip morphology and the development of osteoarthritis (such as proposed by Harris, Stulberg, and Murray) is the critical distinction that even relatively small anatomic deviations can result in clinically and pathomechanically significant hip injury when associated with supraphysiologic or extremes of hip motion. With this background, we can understand how an adolescent high-level gymnast can present with hip pain and chondrolabral damage with little morphology alteration just as a collegiate football player presents similarly albeit with severe Cam deformity and limited range of motion.

9.3 Complex Forms of FAI

After the original description and early understanding of FAI, observations during surgical hip dislocation (SHD) revealed that impingement can occur extra-articularly, such as between the greater or lesser trochanter and the pelvis or the anterior–inferior iliac spine.

So-called extra-articular forms of impingement are known to be associated with certain pelvic morphologic patterns including low-lying anterior iliac spines (sub-spine impingement) and femoral morphologies associated with increased proximal femoral valgus with anteversion (ischio-femoral impingement). Additionally, more complex forms of impingement have been recognized in young adults with sequelae of pediatric hip disease such as Perthes disease and SCFE. In these conditions, it is not uncommon to observe both intraarticular impingement during dynamic range of motion due to Cam-like deformity but also extra-articular impingement from reduced femoral neck length and/or abnormal femoral version (usually excessive retroversion).

9.4 Indications

Patients with structural hip deformity and hip impingement can become symptomatic in the second through fourth decade of life. In our practice, the age range for these patients is 14–49 years, with a mean age of 28 years. Patients with classic acetabular dysplasia are more likely to be women and within the age range of 14–35 years, whereas patients with FAI are equally divided in terms of gender and are more likely to be within the age range of 20 years old to the late 40s. Patients typically present complaining of groin pain, which is usually exacerbated by activities. The groin pain can be associated with catching, clicking, or popping in as many as 80% of patients. Associated pain in the buttock, thigh, and lateral hip or low-back region is not uncommon but is usually present with concomitant groin pain. The onset of pain is frequently associated with a traumatic event approximately one-third of the time, although the underlying morphologic abnormality of the hip has usually been present for a longer period of time (see also Chap. 1).

Additionally, it is common for patients who are involved in high-demand and/or impact activities (e.g., martial arts, hockey, dance, gymnastics, soccer, etc.) to have similar symptoms in the absence of gross anatomic abnormalities because supraphysiological motion can induce similar joint injury. Most patients describe exacerbation of the pain produced by sitting, squatting, or activities that involve hip flexion. The duration of pain can range from months to years, with an average duration of 16 months. Most patients have seen multiple prior healthcare providers before an appropriate diagnosis is made and as many as 15–30% of patients have undergone prior surgery for hip pain. Patients with FAI are typically active in moderate to high-level sports activities and over three-quarters of patients report significant impairment in sports activity performance.

The physical examination involves assessment of gait, palpation of the hip and the area surrounding the hip, neurological evaluation, evaluation of the range of motion of the hip, and provocative testing (see Chap. 1). The gait pattern of patients with FAI is nonspecific: a normal gait and slight antalgia are the most common observations. Palpation of the hip and the surrounding area usually results in unremarkable findings. Limitation of internal rotation with the hip positioned in 90° of flexion is the most common physical finding in patients with FAI; it is present in >90% of patients who have FAI and is most pronounced in men who have cam or mixed-type FAI. Many patients with FAI prefer to have the hip positioned in external rotation or extension. In contrast, patients with classic acetabular dysplasia typically exhibit normal or excessive internal and external rotation.

Provocative maneuvers, such as the flexion and internal rotation impingement (FADIR) test and the flexion abduction and external rotation (FABER) test apprehension test, are extremely important in the examination of the adult hip [15, 22, 23]. The FADIR test is positive in over 85% of patients with symptomatic FAI [15, 23]. The apprehension test, performed with the hip in full extension and external rotation, is variably positive and can be indicative of chondrolabral damage in the anterior part of the acetabulum in the absence of instability when the patient's pain is reproduced [22].

9.5 Preoperative/Preinterventional Diagnostics

Imaging of the hip in patients with structural hip deformity includes plain radiographic assessment (see Chap. 2) as well as magnetic resonance arthrography (Arthro-MRI) and computed tomography (CT) to further characterize the state of the femoral and acetabular chondrolabral tissue and determine the true three-dimensional character of the morphologic abnormalities (see Chap. 3). Understanding the plain radiographic findings in patients with symptomatic FAI is the most critical factor in establishing the proper diagnosis and development of a treatment plan. In the author's practice, plain radiographic examination includes the following: an anteroposterior radiograph of the pelvis with symmetrical obturator foramina and a sacrococcygeal-symphysis distance of 1–4 cm, a false-profile radiograph, and a frog-leg lateral and/or modified Dunn radiograph [24, 25]. Pelvic rotation and pelvic tilt can alter the interpretation of the underlying deformity [26, 27]. The following parameters are assessed on the anteroposterior pelvic radiograph: the acetabular index [28], the center-edge angle of Wiberg [28, 29], the relationship of the anterior and posterior walls of the acetabulum as defined by the so-called crossover sign [30–33], the relationship of the center of the femoral head to the posterior wall as defined by the so-called posterior wall sign [34], the presence of a prominent ischial spine [35], and, finally, a characterization of femoral sphericity [6, 36]. The false-profile lateral [37, 38] radiograph estimates anterior acetabular coverage, anterior hip joint cartilage space, and anterior femoral head–neck offset and may reveal a calcified labrum or an os acetabuli. The frog-leg lateral and the modified Dunn radiographs offer the best assessment of femoral head–neck offset, the alpha angle, and secondary femoral signs of impingement, such as herniation pits and cyst formation at the head–neck junction [6, 7, 36].

Advanced imaging with arthro-MRI allows further characterization of femoral and acetabular chondrolabral pathology as well as overall joint morphology. The technique used at our center involves 15 mL of gadolinium injected into the hip joint with a local anesthetic, a field of view of 16–18 cm, and the use of a dedicated torso coil along with surface coil. The following images are acquired: T1-weighted coronal and axial images, proton-density-weighted sagittal images with fat saturation, T1-weighted oblique axial images along the axis of the femoral neck, and T2-weighted coronal images. These sequences facilitate determination of the alpha angle femoral sphericity and the integrity of the femoral and acetabular chondrolabral tissue. Magnetic resonance arthrography has been shown to be sensitive and specific for the diagnosis of labral injury but less so for hyaline cartilage injury [39, 40]. Identification of acetabular hyaline cartilage delamination, a finding present in nearly 50% of men with cam-type FAI, is especially important [41]. Beaule' and Zaragoza described the so-called "inverted Oreo cookie" sign created by high-intensity contrast on each side of low-intensity delaminated acetabular cartilage [42]. We have found that delamination is best seen on sagittal T1-weighted or proton-density-weighted magnetic resonance arthrography with fat saturation [41].

We recommend that a transverse image of the femoral condyles is included in the MRI in order to determine femoral torsion within one examination.

Increasingly surgeons utilize 3D CT imaging to better understand the location and magnitude of femoral and acetabular morphologic abnormalities. This imaging modality can help plan the surgical execution of femoral osteochondroplasty, which is essential in patients with Cam-type FAI. Nowadays, MRI images can also be used for 3D reconstructions of hip anatomy [43].

9.6 Preoperative Planning/Computer Modeling

Recent advancements in digital tools and three-dimensional imaging have enhanced the surgeon's ability to preoperatively plan the correction of femoral Cam deformity and address altered acetabular morphology. Several proprietary software solutions have been introduced that utilize CT data to create a three-dimensional model that can be manipulated in space on a computer screen (see Chap. 4). Typically, these software solutions allow a simulated range of motion to visualize where collision occurs between the proximal femur and the acetabular rim. Simulated proximal femoral and acetabular rim resection or trimming can then be performed and simulated post-operative range of motion improvement can be predicted. Examples of these systems include Clinical Graphics and Dyonics from Smith and Nephew (Fig. 9.1). Meanwhile, MRI data sets can also be used to calculate the virtual hip range of motion and visualize FAI as well as extra-articular impingement [44]. A limitation of all currently available software solutions, however, is that hip collision is not driven by actual patient-specific hip kinematics, and as such, predicted bone resections may not accurately predict the elimination of hip impingement.

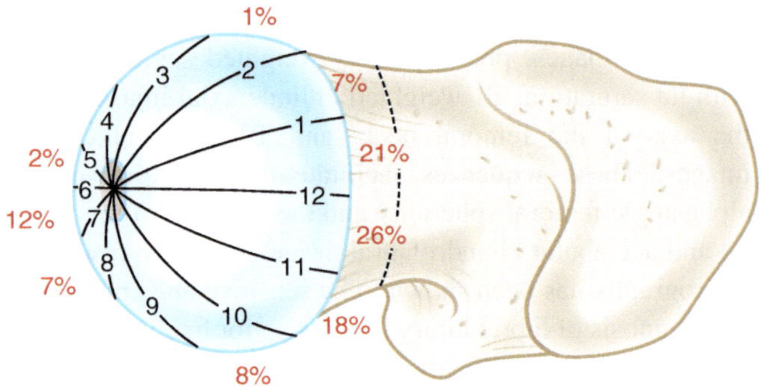

Fig. 9.1 Drawing of a right proximal femur with a clock face system overlying the femoral head. It shows the head/neck transition from superior with a clock system (numbers in black) used to represent the distribution of the vascular foramina. At the head and neck junction area (up to 10 mm from the articular cartilage, dotted line), the distribution of vascular foramina with a diameter of more than 0.5 mm is given in percent (numbers in red). In 80%, vascular foramina enter the femoral head superiorly and only in 20% inferiorly

9.7 Applied Anatomy

Using the SHD (see also Chap. 6) cam and pincer deformities can be treated, which might need to be combined with subtrochanteric osteotomies (Chap. 15). For the treatment of cam deformities, the blood supply to the femoral head should not be compromised. Figure 9.1 shows the head/neck transition from superior with a clock system used to represent the distribution of the vascular foramina. At the head and neck junction area (up to 10 mm from the articular cartilage), the distribution of vascular foramina with a diameter of more than 0.5 mm is shown in Fig. 9.1. Only a few vessels reach the adult femoral head on its anterior aspect, suggesting that surgical procedures on the anterior femoral head and neck can be safely performed by open and closed techniques. Caution should be used, however, when approaching the anterolateral and posteromedial head and neck junction.

During the treatment of pincer FAI, both heads of the rectus femoris (indirect and direct) are close to the area where acetabular rim trimming is performed and should be respected. The supraacetaular branch of the inferior gluteal artery is also close to the area of rim trimming and should be coagulated when bleeding. Moreover, the capsule is thin anterior at the crossing of the psoas tendon. In this area, anchor and suture placement should not be prominent and the rim trim should not cause sharp edges to avoid irritation to the psoas tendon, To avoid direct contact of the psoas to the anterior acetabular rim, the capsule should be closed in this area.

9.8 Specific Risks

When performed by experienced surgeons, SHD has been associated with relatively low complication rates (see also Chap. 7). Potential specific complications associated with SHD include trochanteric non-union, osteonecrosis of the femoral head, femoral neck fracture, disruption of the normal femoroacetabular seal (typically from over-resection of the anterolateral femoral head–neck junction during osteochondroplasty), intracapsular adhesions, heterotopic ossification, and sciatic nerve injury. In a multicenter study of complications with SHD, Sink et al. utilized the Clavien-Dindo surgical complication classification and reported an overall complication rate of 9% in 334 hips [45]. A total of 18 (5.4%) complications were classified as Grade 1 (not clinically relevant and required no deviation from routine post-operative care), and six complications (1.8%) were classified as Grade II (treated on an outpatient basis or with close observation and resolved). There were nine complications (2.7%) classified as Grade III (treatable and resolved with surgery or inpatient management). There was one complication (0.3%) classified as Grade IV (resulting in a long-term deficit). Excluding heterotopic ossification (which was usually clinically insignificant), the complication rate was 16 (4.8%) of 334 [45].

In general, the rate of severe complications including osteonecrosis, femoral neck fracture, and nerve injury is extremely rare (0–2%). Trochanteric non-union has been reported in 1–10% of cases and can be minimized by the step-cut technique described by Notzli et al. [46]. Approximately 10–15% of patients may experience groin pain post-operatively [47], most commonly due to insufficient morphology correction, residual chondrolabral damage, or intraarticular adhesions. Intraarticular adhesions have been noted to occur in up to 60% of patients who undergo revision surgery [47]. Contemporary treatment of adhesions after prior open surgery is usually accomplished with hip arthroscopy.

9.9 Type of Anesthesia

As the patient is in a lateral position during surgical dislocation, the operation is mostly performed under general anesthesia.

9.10 Positioning

The patient is in a lateral position with an operated leg lying on a tunnel pillow and fixation of a sterile bag on the opposite side of the operating table to enable dislocation of the hip joint in the figure-of-four position. Positioning must allow intraoperative fluoroscopy.

9.11 Instruments/Implants

Standard instruments for SHD (see Chap. 8). In order to perform bony resections, the following special instruments are necessary:

- Chisels, osteotomes, and/or a high-speed rotating burr for acetabular rim and cam trimming

- Suture anchors for labral re-attachment
- Templates for assessment of resection area

In case of associated lesions, the following instruments and devices can be necessary:

- Special curettes and shavers for cartilage debridement
- Instruments and devices for cartilage regeneration (i.e., microfracture picks, membranes for autologous matrix-induced chondrogenesis, and autologous chondrocyte transplantation)
- Fluoroscopy unit

Additional instruments for extended osteotomies (proximal femur or intracapsular) are listed in Chaps. 14, 15, 16, 17 and 18.

9.12 Access

The surgical approach follows the exposure of SHD (Chap. 8).

9.13 Technical Steps

- *Inspection of Anterior Femoral Neck and Labrum/ Acetabular Rim (With Range-Of-Motion Testing)* Preoperatively, collision models might be employed to determine the amount of femoral and acetabular resection as well as the necessity for rotational osteotomies (Chap. 4). During the intraoperative examination, the hip is taken through a full range of motion (maximum flexion, maximum possible internal/external rotation in flexion as well as in extension and adduction) in order to visualize impingement. Sometimes even snapping can be recognized, when the hip is subluxing or the suction seal is incompetent.
- *Intraoperative Decision-Making on Bony Resection* Depending on the integrity of labrum and acetabular rim cartilage, the extent of acetabular over-coverage, as well as femoral asphericity and range-of-motion testing, it is possible to determine the necessary extent of bone resection and treatment sequence:
  - In case of mild pincer-deformity without relevant lesions of labrum or acetabular rim cartilage, femoral bone resection is performed, to avoid iatrogenic damage of the chondrolabral complex.
  - In case of significant acetabular over coverage with cartilage or labral damage acetabular rim resection is performed prior to continuation on the femoral side.
- *Acetabular Bone Resection (Pincer FAI)* Acetabular rim resection can be performed with or without temporary labral detachment (Fig. 9.2a and b). In case of already present labral rupture, the detachment can be completed in the area of over coverage. Maximally degenerated parts of the labrum and torn acetabular cartilage are resected. Then the acetabular overhang is reduced with chisels or a burr (Fig. 9.2c). Over-resection laterally as well as anterior and posterior must be avoided in order not to risk instability or iatrogenic dysplasia. A 5-mm resection of the lateral rim equals a CE-angle reduction of about 5° [48]. In case of uncertainty, intraoperative fluoroscopic control is possible, although a valid estimation of the true amount of resection and remaining acetabular coverage without performing an a.p. pelvic radiograph is difficult.
- If the area of necessary trimming is identical to the area of damaged cartilage, it can be removed completely. After bony rim resection, the remaining labrum is re-attached with bone anchors every 10–15 mm (Fig. 9.2d). A resection of maximally degenerated parts of the labrum may be necessary.
- *Femoral Bone Resection* After acetabular rim resection (or if acetabular surgery is not indicated), the area of asphericity and the extent of necessary trimming on the femoral side are determined. The application of a transparent template may be of assistance, especially when assessing the symmetry of offset recreation (Fig. 9.3a). Necessary bone resection can be performed with a chisel or osteotome and/or a high-speed rotating burr (the latter allows very precise and gradual correction). We start re-contouring anteriorly at the head–neck junction (Fig. 9.3b) and continue distally as well as medially and laterally. Lateral and posterolateral bone resection must be performed very cautiously, as any injury of retinacular vessels can result in avascular head necrosis. Medially, the ligament of Weitbrecht should be preserved as part of the medial femoral head is vascularized by the medial retinaculum. In the case of posterior and circular resection, visualization may be impaired. Then additional use of a dentist mirror (Fig. 9.4) or an arthroscope may be of help.
- Bony resection should result in physiologic and homogenic tailoring of the neck without major steps or edges. Repeat control by application of the spheric template may be of help in determining the appropriate amount of resection (Fig. 9.3c). In addition, periodically relocating the hip and examining the motion is very helpful. While it is important to prevent under-resection, it is also important to prevent overcorrection and to avoid excessively large non-physiologic resections. Extensive thinning of the neck must be avoided (risk of fracture with resection of more than 30%) [49]. In the case of fibro cartilaginous lesions, which are often present anterolateral, resection is performed only until a depth, which equals the physiologic femoral neck shape. If the lesions are of a size, which jeopardizes mechanical stability, bone grafting and sometimes even prophylactic stabilization may be necessary [50].
- During head–neck recontouring, it is also critical to avoid scattering bone particles in periarticular soft tissues in order to minimize the risk of heterotopic ossification. This

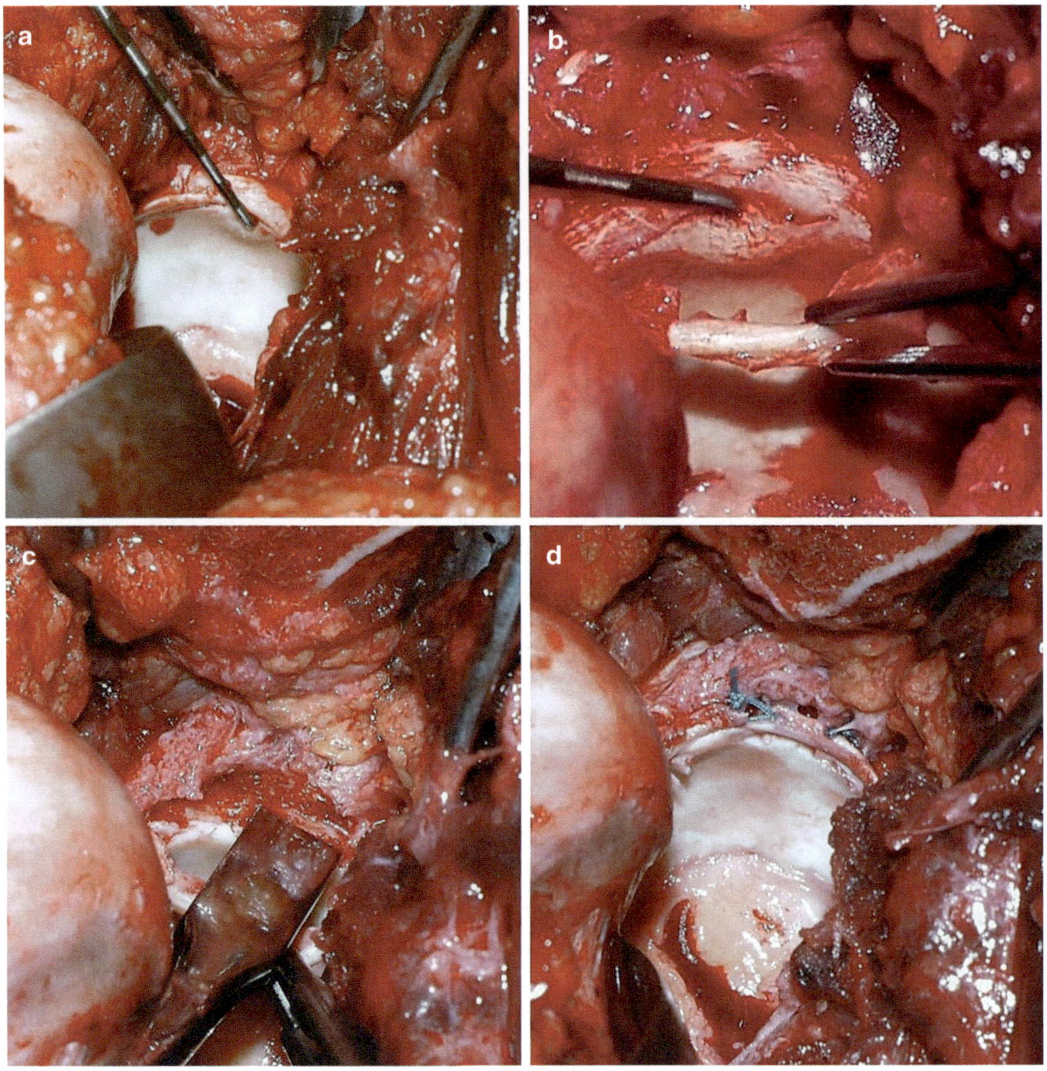

Fig. 9.2 Intraoperative photographs of acetabular rim trimming and labral refixation. (**a**) Probing of the cartilage with a nerve hook followed by (**b**) labral detachment in order to allow for (**c**) rim resection using an osteotome and (**d**) final labral refixation by the use of bone anchors

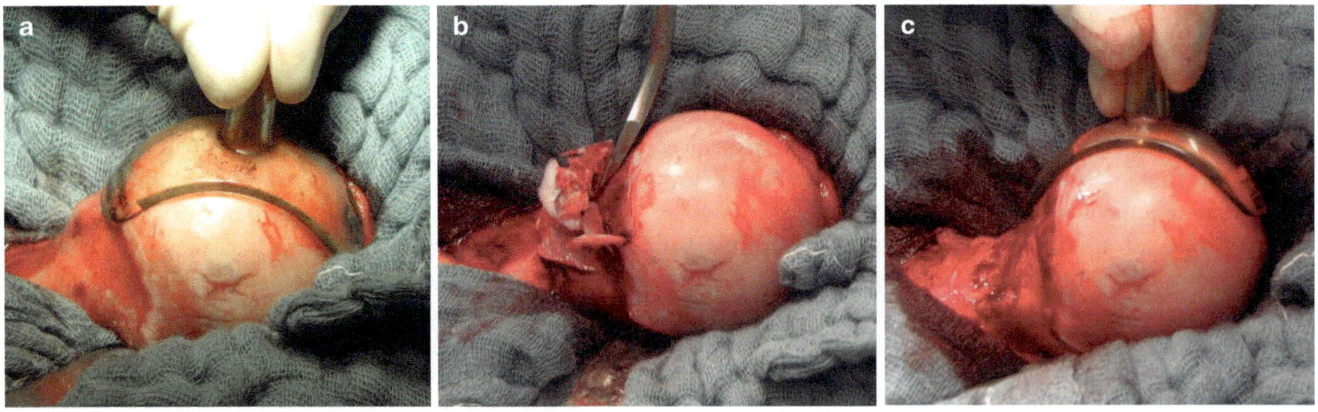

Fig. 9.3 (**a**) Intraoperative view of a left femoral head with a cam-deformity. Spherical templates a helpful in determining the location and severity of the deformity. (**b**) With a curved osteotomy, the excessive bone can be removed. (**c**) Using the spherical template after bone resection again, the sufficiency of bone resection can be assessed

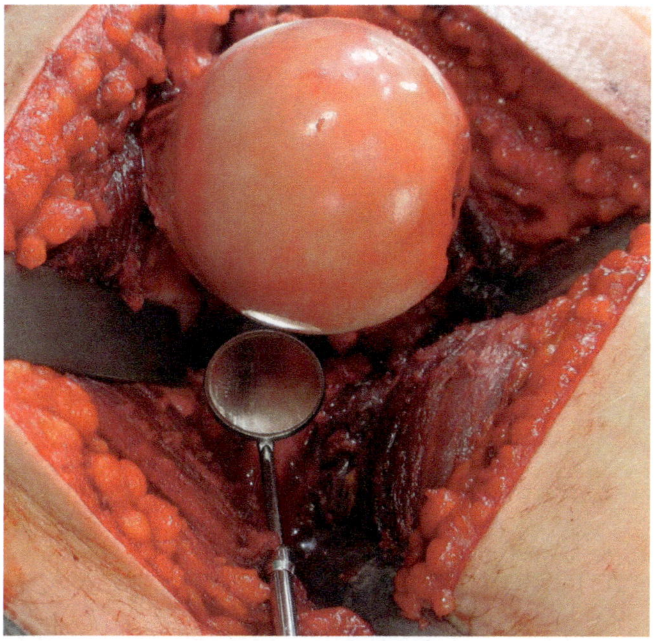

Fig. 9.4 To assess sphericity of the femoral head in areas in which a less accessible dentist mirror or even arthroscope might be used

can be facilitated by the use of preventive coverings and constant irrigation. The latter is mandatory throughout the whole procedure to avoid desiccation and degradation of cartilage morphology [51].

- *Verification of Appropriate Bone Resection* After completed bone resection on the acetabular and/or femoral side, the leg is taken out of the sterile bag and the joint reduced into the acetabulum. Careful reduction is necessary especially after labral refixation, to avoid detachment. After head reduction, the hip is again taken through several cycles of the full range of motion in order to assess appropriate bone resection and impingement-free movement. Although there is no prospective analysis, for most surgeons, it is accepted that a minimum of 20° internal rotation should be reached with 90° of flexion. If necessary, the extent of appropriate resection can be monitored through fluoroscopic control.
- *Additional Treatment in Case of Extra-Articular Pathology* Sometimes FAI is accompanied by extra-articular pathology. If symptoms as well as morphologic abnormalities justify additional treatment, it may be necessary to combine intraarticular bony resections with other procedures. Subspine impingement, for example, may require trimming of the anterior inferior iliac spine; torsional deformities that can be associated with extra-articular impingement may require resection of the anterosuperior trochanter or portions of the posterior intertrochanteric line extending to the lesser trochanter. Additionally, osteoplasty of the femur can be combined with a rotational osteotomy. Rotational osteotomies are most commonly used in patients with femoral retroversion causing pincer-type FAI that cannot be alleviated by a neck plasty.

9.14 Postoperative Follow-Up

No drains are used, and patient immediate mobilization is recommended. Anticoagulation follows hospital standards for major hip surgery. Recommendations regarding prophylaxis of heterotopic ossifications differ between surgeons. We prescribe NSAIDs for 2 weeks. Partial weight-bearing with two crutches is encouraged for 6 weeks, and during this time, flexion of the hip beyond 70° as well as active abduction may be limited. In the following 3–4 weeks, a gradual increase up to full weight-bearing without crutches is advised, while patients perform abductor strengthening exercise programs. Radiographic follow-up depends on hospital and surgeon standards with most surgeons obtaining X-rays at 2 and 6 weeks following the procedure. After acetabular bone resection, the coverage should be documented by a.p. pelvic radiographs before discharge. Return to sport is possible starting 3 months after surgery.

9.15 Intra-/Postoperative Complications

- *General Risks:*
  - Injuries of vessels and/or nerves (i.e., lesion of sciatic nerve through retractor positioning)
  - Thromboembolic events
  - Delayed wound healing and superficial infection
  - Persisting complaints
- *Specific Risks:*
  - Femoral over- or underresection
  - Violoation of retinaculum
  - Acetabular over- or underresection
  - Evertion of the labrum
  - Intraarticular anchor placement
  - Anterior protruding anchor
  - Insufficient deep seating of screw heads

9.16 Case Study

A 27-year-old male presented with hip pain on the right side during walking and sitting. Clinical examination shows reduced internal rotation (about 5°) in 90° of hip flexion. The FADIR test and the FABER test are painful. On the anteroposterior radiograph of the pelvis, a marked cam-deformity is visible on both sides and the frog-leg lateral radiograph also confirms an anterolateral asphericity on the right side (Fig. 9.5). Except a slightly prominent anterior inferior ischial spine, the acetabular coverage is normal. MRI examination reveals a nearly circular asphericity on T1-weighted oblique axial images along the axis of the femoral neck (Fig. 9.6). Neither MRI nor radiographs show significant signs of osteoarthritis. Due to the persisting hip pain, which

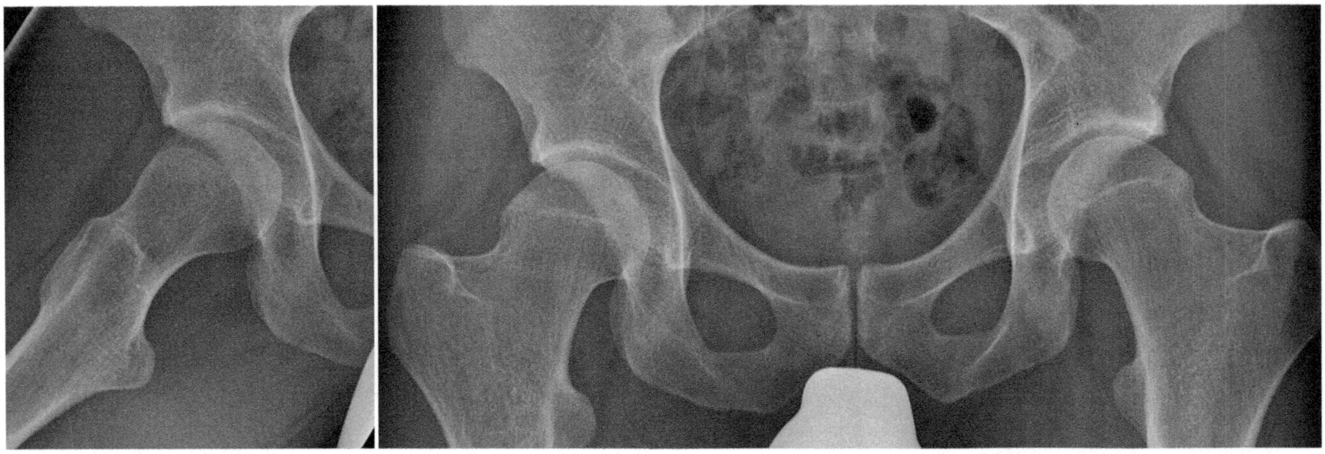

Fig. 9.5 AP pelvic radiograph showing bilateral severe cam-deformities also visible on the frog-leg lateral radiograph right hip confirming an anterolateral asphericity

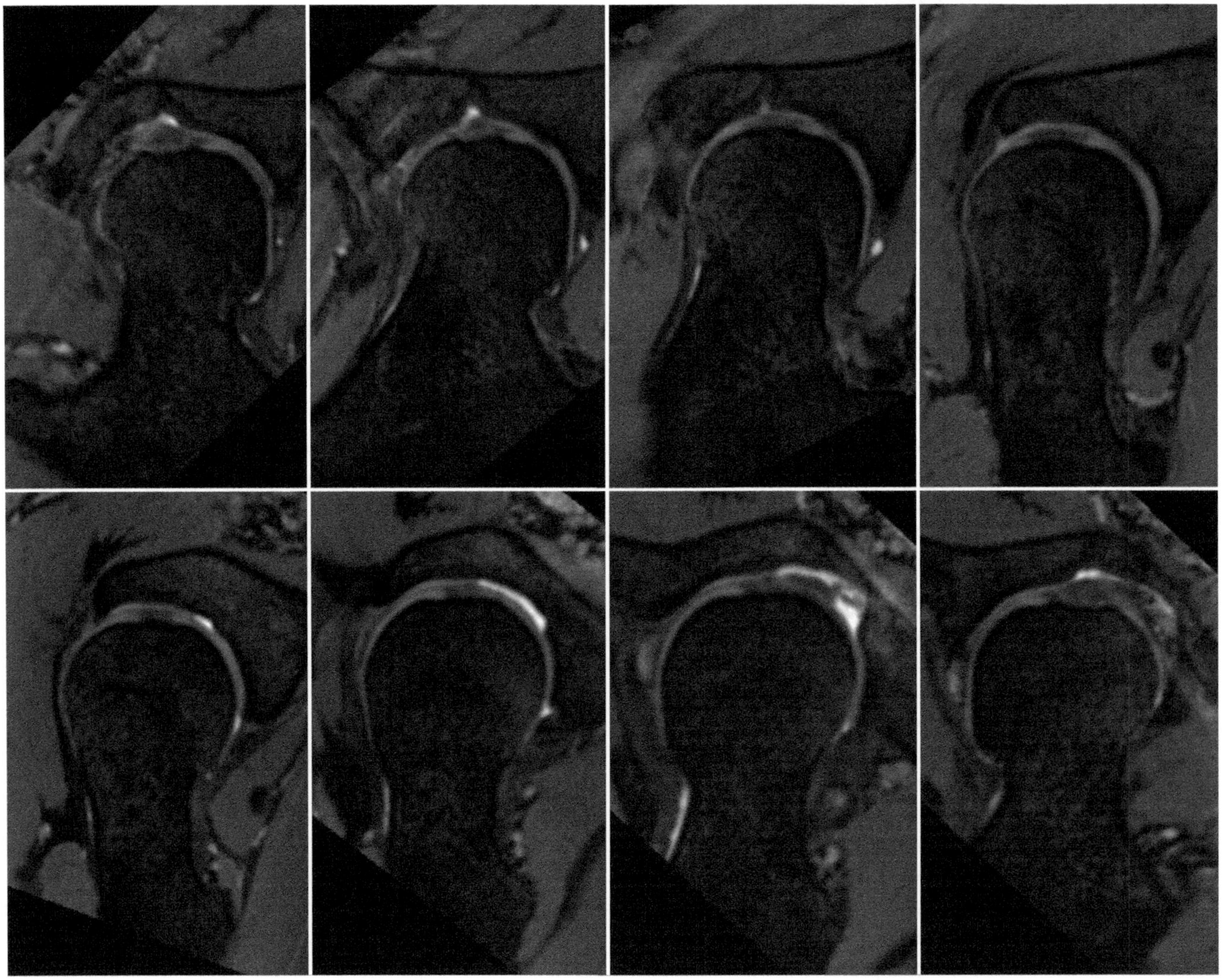

Fig. 9.6 Radial MRI T1-weighted oblique axial images along the axis of the femoral neck confirming the nearly circular asphericity

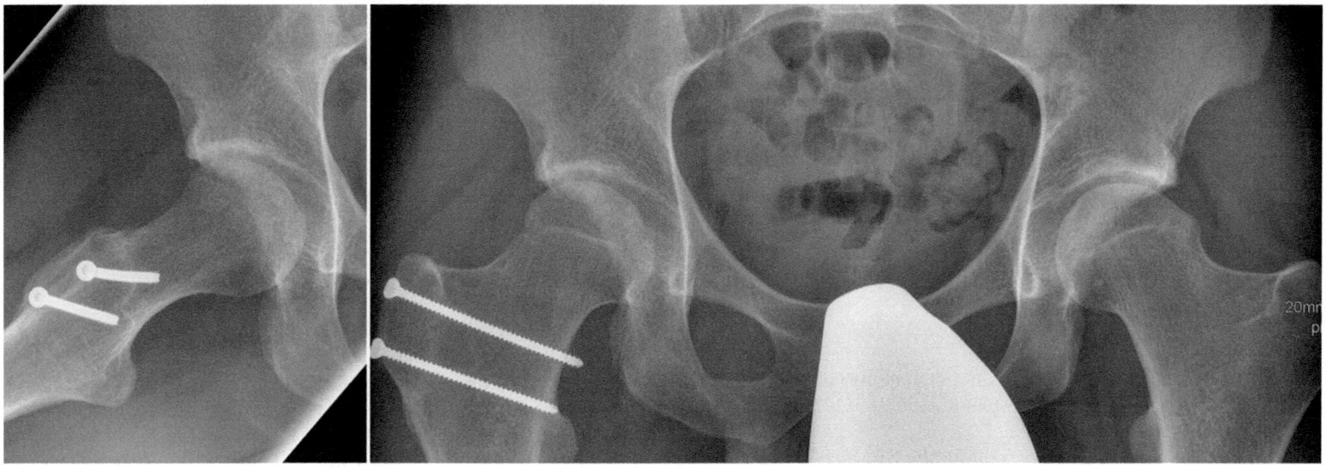

Fig. 9.7 AP pelvic radiograph and frog-leg lateral radiograph at the latest follow-up 3 years postoperatively. Complete removal of femoral head asphericity with the patient being pain-free

is caused by semicircular bone overgrowth at the femoral head–neck junction, offset correction through SHD was recommended. At the latest follow-up 3 years postoperatively, the patient is pain-free and radiographs show physiologic femoral offset (Fig. 9.7).

9.17 Controversies

Perhaps the most controversial aspect of Cam-based FAI pertains to the dilemma that the morphologic abnormality (increased alpha angle and reduced femoral head–neck offset) is variably associated with symptom progression and osteoarthritis development and the relatively silent nature of disease progression. This dilemma leads to the question of when to intervene in the disease process. We know that a Cam-like deformity can be present in as many as 25% of asymptomatic males [15]. We also know that patients present with symptoms (groin pain, activity restriction) relatively late in the disease progression in terms of chondrolabral damage. In addition, recent randomized controlled studies appear to show improved patient outcomes with surgical treatment compared to nonoperative management [52]. Thus, it seems logical that the current data support early surgical intervention at the time of initial symptom presentation in patients with Cam-type FAI. Another controversy is whether to manage CAM-FAI arthroscopically or via an open surgical dislocation. While this text focuses on the technique of SHD, most CAM resections are performed arthroscopically nowadays. The reader should be aware that certain patients are more comprehensively treated with an open approach. These patients may have very large posteriorly extending CAM morphologies associated with femoral retrotorsion.

9.18 Expected Outcomes

Perhaps the most powerful methodology to understand expected patient outcomes and adverse advents is large-pooled data analysis. Addai et al. recently reported on the patient-reported outcome measures (PROM), radiographic correction, and adverse events in 4384 hips in 4094 patients [53]. This systematic review and meta-analysis demonstrated predictable improvement in patient-reported outcomes and alpha angle correction in patients treated surgically for FAI. The authors reported that these improvements occurred regardless of whether the surgical approach was with a mini-open anterior, SHD, or arthroscopic approach. All three groups showed similar rates of revision procedures, but both arthroscopy and SHD had relatively low rates of complications. The results demonstrate that predictable symptom improvement and radiographic correction of Cam deformity can be achieved regardless of surgical approach.

9.19 Future Direction

Surgical treatment of FAI has undergone an evolution over the past several decades. Initial treatment with SHD was invaluable for understanding the pathomechanics and pathoanatomy of the condition. Surgical evolution toward less invasive approaches was a natural progression and has similarly improved patient outcomes. Future improvements are likely to lie in improved diagnostic methods, elucidation of the influence of patient-specific hip arthokinematics, and refinement of surgical execution. Already, quantitative MRI techniques such as D-Gemric, T1-rho, and sodium-based imaging show promise in the identification of early hyaline cartilage deterioration. Translational patient-specific computational modeling techniques combine with patient-specific kinematics from gait analysis or dual-fluoroscopy show promise in improving disease understanding [54, 55]. Finally, robotic technology advancement in other areas such as urology and knee replacement offers promise for the future execution of femoral as well as acetabular bone resection.

References

1. Myers SR, Eijer H, Ganz R. Anterior femoroacetabular impingement after periacetabular osteotomy. Clin Orthop Relat Res. 1999;(363):93–9.
2. Tannast M, Goricki D, Beck M, Murphy SB, Siebenrock KA. Hip damage occurs at the zone of femoroacetabular impingement. Clin Orthop Relat Res. 2008;466(2):273–80. Epub 20080110.
3. Tanzer M, Noiseux N. Osseous abnormalities and early osteoarthritis: the role of hip impingement. Clin Orthop Relat Res. 2004;(429):170–7.
4. Beck M, Kalhor M, Leunig M, Ganz R. Hip morphology influences the pattern of damage to the acetabular cartilage: femoroacetabular impingement as a cause of early osteoarthritis of the hip. J Bone Joint Surg Br. 2005;87(7):1012–8.
5. Johnston TL, Schenker ML, Briggs KK, Philippon MJ. Relationship between offset angle alpha and hip chondral injury in femoroacetabular impingement. Arthroscopy. 2008;24(6):669–75. Epub 20080317.
6. Meyer DC, Beck M, Ellis T, Ganz R, Leunig M. Comparison of six radiographic projections to assess femoral head/neck asphericity. Clin Orthop Relat Res. 2006;445:181–5.
7. Nötzli HP, Wyss TF, Stoecklin CH, Schmid MR, Treiber K, Hodler J. The contour of the femoral head-neck junction as a predictor for the risk of anterior impingement. J Bone Joint Surg Br. 2002;84(4):556–60.
8. Rakhra KS, Sheikh AM, Allen D, Beaulé PE. Comparison of MRI alpha angle measurement planes in femoroacetabular impingement. Clin Orthop Relat Res. 2009;467(3):660–5. Epub 20081127.
9. Neumann M, Cui Q, Siebenrock KA, Beck M. Impingement-free hip motion: the 'normal' angle alpha after osteochondroplasty. Clin Orthop Relat Res. 2009;467(3):699–703. Epub 20081119.
10. James SL, Ali K, Malara F, Young D, O'Donnell J, Connell DA. MRI findings of femoroacetabular impingement. AJR Am J Roentgenol. 2006;187(6):1412–9.
11. Kassarjian A, Yoon LS, Belzile E, Connolly SA, Millis MB, Palmer WE. Triad of MR arthrographic findings in patients with cam-type femoroacetabular impingement. Radiology. 2005;236(2):588–92. Epub 20050621
12. Leunig M, Beck M, Kalhor M, Kim YJ, Werlen S, Ganz R. Fibrocystic changes at anterosuperior femoral neck: prevalence in hips with femoroacetabular impingement. Radiology. 2005;236(1):237–46.
13. Gdalevitch M, Smith K, Tanzer M. Delamination cysts: a predictor of acetabular cartilage delamination in hips with a labral tear. Clin Orthop Relat Res. 2009;467(4):985–91. Epub 20081023.
14. Murray RO, Duncan C. Athletic activity in adolescence as an etiological factor in degenerative hip disease. J Bone Joint Surg Br. 1971;53(3):406–19.
15. Ganz R, Parvizi J, Beck M, Leunig M, Nötzli H, Siebenrock KA. Femoroacetabular impingement: a cause for osteoarthritis of the hip. Clin Orthop Relat Res. 2003;(417):112–20.
16. Siebenrock KA, Behning A, Mamisch TC, Schwab JM. Growth plate alteration precedes cam-type deformity in elite basketball players. Clin Orthop Relat Res. 2013;471(4):1084–91. Epub 20121218.
17. Siebenrock KA, Kaschka I, Frauchiger L, Werlen S, Schwab JM. Prevalence of cam-type deformity and hip pain in elite ice hockey players before and after the end of growth. Am J Sports Med. 2013;41(10):2308–13. Epub 20130802.
18. Kapron AL, Anderson AE, Aoki SK, Phillips LG, Petron DJ, Toth R, et al. Radiographic prevalence of femoroacetabular impingement in collegiate football players: AAOS Exhibit Selection. J Bone Joint Surg Am. 2011;93(19):e111(1-10).
19. Larson CM, Sikka RS, Sardelli MC, Byrd JW, Kelly BT, Jain RK, et al. Increasing alpha angle is predictive of athletic-related "hip" and "groin" pain in collegiate National Football League prospects. Arthroscopy. 2013;29(3):405–10. Epub 20130126.
20. Nepple JJ, Milewski MD, Shea KG. Research in osteochondritis dissecans of the knee: 2016 update. J Knee Surg. 2016;29(7):533–8. Epub 20160817.
21. Roels P, et al. Mechanical factors explain development of cam-type deformity. Osteoarthr Cart. 2014;22(12):2074–82.
22. Holmich P, Dienst M. Differential diagnosis of hip and groin pain. Symptoms and technique for physical examination. Orthopade. 2006;35(1):8, 10-5.
23. Philippon MJ, Maxwell RB, Johnston TL, Schenker M, Briggs KK. Clinical presentation of femoroacetabular impingement. Knee Surg Sports Traumatol Arthrosc. 2007;15(8):1041–7. Epub 20070512.
24. Tannast M, Siebenrock KA, Anderson SE. Femoroacetabular impingement: radiographic diagnosis—what the radiologist should know. AJR Am J Roentgenol. 2007;188(6):1540–52.
25. Fadul DA, Carrino JA. Imaging of femoroacetabular impingement. J Bone Joint Surg Am. 2009;91(Suppl 1):138–43.
26. Tannast M, Zheng G, Anderegg C, Burckhardt K, Langlotz F, Ganz R, et al. Tilt and rotation correction of acetabular version on pelvic radiographs. Clin Orthop Relat Res. 2005;438:182–90.
27. Siebenrock KA, Kalbermatten DF, Ganz R. Effect of pelvic tilt on acetabular retroversion: a study of pelves from cadavers. Clin Orthop Relat Res. 2003 Feb;407:241–8.
28. Mast JW, Brunner RL, Zebrack J. Recognizing acetabular version in the radiographic presentation of hip dysplasia. Clin Orthop Relat Res. 2004;(418):48–53.
29. Wiberg G. Shelf operation in congenital dysplasia of the acetabulum and in subluxation and dislocation of the hip. J Bone Joint Surg Am. 1953;35-a(1):65–80.
30. Reynolds D, Lucas J, Klaue K. Retroversion of the acetabulum. A cause of hip pain. J Bone Joint Surg Br. 1999;81(2):281–8.
31. Jamali AA, Mladenov K, Meyer DC, Martinez A, Beck M, Ganz R, et al. Anteroposterior pelvic radiographs to assess acetabular retroversion: high validity of the "cross-over-sign". J Orthop Res. 2007;25(6):758–65.
32. Bardakos NV, Villar RN. Predictors of progression of osteoarthritis in femoroacetabular impingement: a radiological study with a minimum of ten years follow-up. J Bone Joint Surg Br. 2009;91(2):162–9.
33. Giori NJ, Trousdale RT. Acetabular retroversion is associated with osteoarthritis of the hip. Clin Orthop Relat Res. 2003;(417):263–9.
34. Siebenrock KA, Schoeniger R, Ganz R. Anterior femoro-acetabular impingement due to acetabular retroversion. Treatment with periacetabular osteotomy. J Bone Joint Surg Am. 2003;85(2):278–86.
35. Kalberer F, Sierra RJ, Madan SS, Ganz R, Leunig M. Ischial spine projection into the pelvis : a new sign for acetabular retroversion. Clin Orthop Relat Res. 2008;466(3):677–83. Epub 20080210.

36. Clohisy JC, Nunley RM, Otto RJ, Schoenecker PL. The frog-leg lateral radiograph accurately visualized hip cam impingement abnormalities. Clin Orthop Relat Res. 2007 Sep;462:115–21.
37. Chosa E, Tajima N. Anterior acetabular head index of the hip on false-profile views. New index of anterior acetabular cover. J Bone Joint Surg Br. 2003;85(6):826–9.
38. Lequesne M, de Seze S. False profile of the pelvis. A new radiographic incidence for the study of the hip. Its use in dysplasias and different coxopathies. Rev Rhum Mal Osteoartic. 1961;28:643–52.
39. Petersilge CA, Haque MA, Petersilge WJ, Lewin JS, Lieberman JM, Buly R. Acetabular labral tears: evaluation with MR arthrography. Radiology. 1996;200(1):231–5.
40. Schmid MR, Nötzli HP, Zanetti M, Wyss TF, Hodler J. Cartilage lesions in the hip: diagnostic effectiveness of MR arthrography. Radiology. 2003;226(2):382–6.
41. Anderson LA, Peters CL, Park BB, Stoddard GJ, Erickson JA, Crim JR. Acetabular cartilage delamination in femoroacetabular impingement. Risk factors and magnetic resonance imaging diagnosis. J Bone Joint Surg Am. 2009;91(2):305–13.
42. Beaulé PE, Zaragoza EJ. Surgical images: musculoskeletal acetabular cartilage delamination demonstrated by magnetic resonance arthrography: inverted "Oreo" cookie sign. Can J Surg. 2003;46(6):463–4.
43. Goronzy J, Blum S, Hartmann A, Plodeck V, Franken L, Günther KP, et al. Is MRI an adequate replacement for CT scans in the three-dimensional assessment of acetabular morphology? Acta Radiol. 2019;60(6):726–34. Epub 20180827.
44. Blum S, Franken L, Hartmann A, Thielemann F, Plodeck V, Danowski D, et al. MRI-based static and functional assessment of complex hip deformities in comparison with CT: a validation study. Magma. 2020;33(6):829–38. Epub 20200422.
45. Sink EL, Beaulé PE, Sucato D, Kim YJ, Millis MB, Dayton M, et al. Multicenter study of complications following surgical dislocation of the hip. J Bone Joint Surg Am. 2011;93(12):1132–6.
46. Naal FD, Miozzari HH, Schär M, Hesper T, Nötzli HP. Midterm results of surgical hip dislocation for the treatment of femoroacetabular impingement. Am J Sports Med. 2012;40(7):1501–10. Epub 20120503.
47. Hanke MS, Lerch TD, Schmaranzer F, Meier MK, Steppacher SD, Siebenrock KA. Complications of hip preserving surgery. EFORT Open Rev. 2021;6(6):472–86. Epub 20210628.
48. Philippon MJ, Briggs KK, Hay CJ, Kuppersmith DA, Dewing CB, Huang MJ. Arthroscopic labral reconstruction in the hip using iliotibial band autograft: technique and early outcomes. Arthroscopy. 2010;26(6):750–6. Epub 20100403.
49. Mardones RM, Gonzalez C, Chen Q, Zobitz M, Kaufman KR, Trousdale RT. Surgical treatment of femoroacetabular impingement: evaluation of the effect of the size of the resection. J Bone Joint Surg Am. 2005;87(2):273–9.
50. Günther KP, Hartmann A, Aikele P, Aust D, Ziegler J. Large femoral-neck cysts in association with femoroacetabular impingement. A report of three cases. J Bone Joint Surg Am. 2007;89(4):863–70.
51. Ganz R, Gill TJ, Gautier E, Ganz K, Krügel N, Berlemann U. Surgical dislocation of the adult hip a technique with full access to the femoral head and acetabulum without the risk of avascular necrosis. J Bone Joint Surg Br. 2001;83(8):1119–24.
52. Griffin DR, Dickenson EJ, Wall PDH, Achana F, Donovan JL, Griffin J, et al. Hip arthroscopy versus best conservative care for the treatment of femoroacetabular impingement syndrome (UK FASHIoN): a multicentre randomised controlled trial. Lancet. 2018;391(10136):2225–35. Epub 20180601.
53. Addai D, Zarkos J, Pettit M, Sunil Kumar KH, Khanduja V. Outcomes following surgical management of femoroacetabular impingement: a systematic review and meta-analysis of different surgical techniques. Bone Joint Res. 2021;10(9):574–90.
54. Catelli DS, Ng KCG, Wesseling M, Kowalski E, Jonkers I, Beaulé PE, et al. Hip muscle forces and contact loading during squatting after cam-type FAI surgery. J Bone Joint Surg Am. 2020;102(Suppl 2):34–42.
55. Atkins PR, Fiorentino NM, Hartle JA, Aoki SK, Peters CL, Foreman KB, et al. In vivo pelvic and hip joint kinematics in patients with cam femoroacetabular impingement syndrome: a dual fluoroscopy study. J Orthop Res. 2020;38(4):823–33. Epub 20191114.

Further Reading

Maldonado DR, Monahan PF, Domb BG. Restoration of labral function in primary hip arthroscopy from labral repair to labral reconstruction. Arthroscopy. 2021;37(10):3013–5.

Labrum Refixation/Reconstruction/Augmentation

10

Martin Beck and Rafael J. Sierra

10.1 Introduction

The refixation or reconstruction of the labrum is part of intraarticular work that is done during surgery for intraarticular pathology of the hip. Nowadays, labral surgery is most often performed arthroscopically; however, it can also be performed during surgical hip dislocation (see Sect. 4.1). Correction of the underlying bony pathology is a prerequisite to successful healing of the labrum. Uncorrected structural abnormalities whether impingement or dysplasia will lead to failure of labral refixation.

10.2 Background

The acetabular labrum plays an important role in the structure and function of the hip. Labral tears may be painful, limit activities of daily living including sports, and represent the first step into osteoarthritis of the hip. They may be the first signs of abnormal biomechanics of the hip, including acetabular dysplasia or femoroacetabular impingement, but also more rarely result from an acute hip injury.

The labrum is circumferentially attached to the acetabular rim and connects the anterior and posterior acetabular horns as the transverse ligament. Its shape is triangular and has a variable size, being thickest superiorly and widest anteriorly. The joint capsule inserts peripheral to the labrum. There is a recess between the labrum and joint capsule. The vascular supply and the innervation originate from the capsular side of the labrum. There is a periacetabular vascular ring from the superior and inferior gluteal arteries giving radial branches to the labrum.

M. Beck
Orthopaedic Clinic Lucerne, Hirslanden Clinic St. Anna, Lucerne, Switzerland
e-mail: martin.beck@okl.ch

R. J. Sierra (✉)
Division of Hip and Knee Surgery, Mayo Clinic, Rochester, MN, USA
e-mail: Sierra.Rafael@mayo.edu

The labrum appears to have several physiological functions. Its main function is the sealing of the joint, preventing the extrusion of fluid from the central compartment. This allows pressurization of the fluid layer between the cartilage surfaces, decreasing friction and load transfer [1]. The labrum also contributes to hip joint stability not only by load transfer but also by maintaining an intraarticular vacuum. The labrum varies significantly in size and shape in different hips and how the size variability affects function is not well understood at this time.

Preservation of the labrum results in improved hip function and decreases cartilage degeneration. Labral pathology is quite frequent and clinically asymptomatic. The pathology ranges from simple chondrolabral dissociations, indicating a disruption between the labrum and the cartilage, that most often does not need treatment to the rare traumatic bucket handle tear in the context of major trauma. During degeneration, often degenerative hypertrophy can be observed. The degeneration starts from the base of the labrum and often the peripheral part of the labrum keeps its structure [2]. However, there may be situations where the labrum gradually is ossified from the base and/or atrophies during collision type of impingement. In rare situations, there may be a complete absence of the labrum. However, these two conditions are difficult to distinguish. Another ossification pattern has been described where the acetabular rim gradually overgrows the labrum [3].

Labral refixation is used for conditions where the labrum or part of it can be used to restore the suction seal [2, 4]. Generally, the indication for labral reconstruction is to restore labral-like tissue in the absence of any usable labral tissue [5]. Augmentation can be used to increase the volume of an atrophic labrum, in which the tip is still functional [6]. The concept behind augmentation is to increase the volume and keep the integrity of the labrum with the preservation of the hoop stresses.

A torn or degenerated labrum cannot be repaired back to its original shape and function. Surgical treatment of the labrum results in healing and the formation of a more or less

M. Leunig et al. (eds.), *Surgical Hip Dislocation*, https://doi.org/10.1007/978-3-031-70622-6_10

functional scar [7]. Minor degeneration can be debrided as long the sealing function is preserved. If the quality of the labrum is too poor for reuse, reconstruction of the labrum with a graft can be considered [8]; however, even a reconstruction cannot restore the original shape of the labrum.

10.3 Indications

Indications for Refixation

- In combination with resection of the acetabular rim if the labrum is of good quality
- Hypertrophic degeneration with debridement of degenerated areas
- Unstable labral *tear (bucket handle tear)*
- Resection of labral base ossifications if the labral substance is sufficient for repair
- Resection of osseous overgrowth if the labral substance is sufficient for repair

Indications for Reconstruction

- Ossified or atrophic labrum
- Previous iatrogenic resection of the labrum
- In combination with acetabular rim trimming if a segmental labral defect is created
- Unstable labral tear (bucket handle tear) of bad tissue quality preventing preservation

Indications for Augmentation

- Ossified or atrophic labrum with an intact tip

Contraindications

- Chondrolabral dissociation with the labrum being intact. If the bony anatomy does not need correction, leaving the labrum attached may be advantageous
- Labral pathology in the presence of uncorrected bony deformities

10.4 Preoperative/Preinterventional Diagnostics

- Pelvic AP as well as cross table or lateral Lauenstein view
- Arthro-MRI of the symptomatic hip
- CT to identify the extent of ossification around the labrum

10.5 Preoperative Planning/Computer Simulation

- Preoperative planning includes the analysis of the needed structural correction.
- Is a rim resection necessary to decrease overcoverage?
- Is there hip dysplasia?
- Quality of the labrum?
  - Presence of ossifications of the labral base?
  - Preservation of labrum possible or reconstruction necessary?
- Type of graft?
  - Ligamentum teres
  - Fascia lata autograft
  - Tendon autograft
  - Tendon allograft
- 3D motion analysis to define the area of impingement and planning amount of correction

10.6 Applied Anatomy

- A prerequisite for refixation or reconstruction of the labrum is the fully performed SHD (see Chap. 7).
- The labrum rims the acetabulum circumferentially and bridges the acetabular notch as a transverse ligament. The ligamentum teres originates from the anterior and posterior aspects of the transverse ligament.
- The labrum is firmly attached to the acetabular rim. It is continuous with the hyaline acetabular cartilage without a transitional gap. A gap can be observed at the level of the Psoas-U where the labrum is not firmly fixed to the rim.
- Extensive rim resection will often lead to an increase in the diameter of the acetabular opening, and a segmental defect of the labrum may need to be created requiring segmental reconstructions.

10.7 Special Risks

- Detachment of the refixed labrum during reduction of the hip
- Insufficient reconstruction of the suction seal at subluxing the hip
- Intraarticular penetration of anchors
- Bone anchor placement into the iliopectineal bursa anteriorly causing irritation of the psoas muscle/tendon
  - Too long bone anchor
  - Bone anchor seated too deeply
- Insufficient knot tying with loss of labral refixation
- Secondary dislocation of bone anchors during rehabilitation
- Loss of fixation of the reconstructed labrum/nonhealing of labral refixation tissue
- Risks related to the technique of SHD (see Sect. 4.1)

10.8 Type of Anesthesia

The decision of the type of anesthesia is left to the anesthesiologist and the patient. The procedure can be done with either general or spinal anesthesia. General anesthesia may be preferable in children and adolescents.

10.9 Positioning

- Standard operating table.
- Lateral positioning with tunnel cushion and lateral bag.
- Fluoroscopy and X-ray should be available.

10.10 Instruments/Implants

Standard instrumentation for surgical hip dislocation (see Chap. 7). In addition to the instruments required for the surgical dislocation approach, the following special instruments ensure an optimal surgical procedure:

- 6-mm bur;
- Drill for predrilling bone anchors;
- Short and thin bone anchors;
- All cutting instruments should be checked for optimal sharpness prior to surgery.

10.11 Access

- Access as for transtrochanteric SHD (see Chap. 7).

10.12 Technical Steps

- Visualization of the acetabulum (Fig. 10.1): At subluxation/dislocation of the hip, the presence of a suction seal is observed. The ligamentum teres is cut by a pair of curved parametrium scissors as close as possible to the teardrop to obtain a graft as long as possible. After dislocation, it is resected from the fovea capitis and inspected for possible later use as a transplant if reconstruction of the labrum is needed. First, the knee is lifted, and with a gentle axial push, the head moves posteriorly to visualize the acetabulum. In most cases, three retractors are inserted for exposure. (1) A curved narrow 8-mm Hohmann retractor is placed over the anterior rim between the labrum and the capsule. (2) A narrow 8-mm Hohmann retractor is seated into the bone at the anterosuperior rim, close to the anterior inferior iliac spine (AIIS). (3) An easy rider is placed into the teardrop retracting the femoral head postero-inferiorly giving access to the posterior and inferior parts of the acetabulum. A full 360° view of the acetabulum is obtained. A blunt probe is used to assess the quality of the labrum and the cartilage. The labrum is inspected for chondrolabral dissociation, ossifications, pockets, and hyper- or atrophy.
- Detachment of the labrum: The labrum is carefully detached from the acetabular rim at the injured area with a scalpel trying to obtain its maximum thickness if possible. The area of detachment is determined and depends on

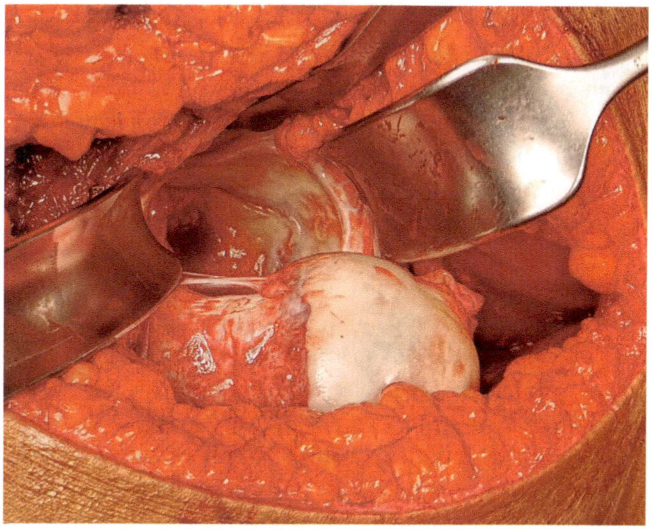

Fig. 10.1 A complete view of a left acetabulum

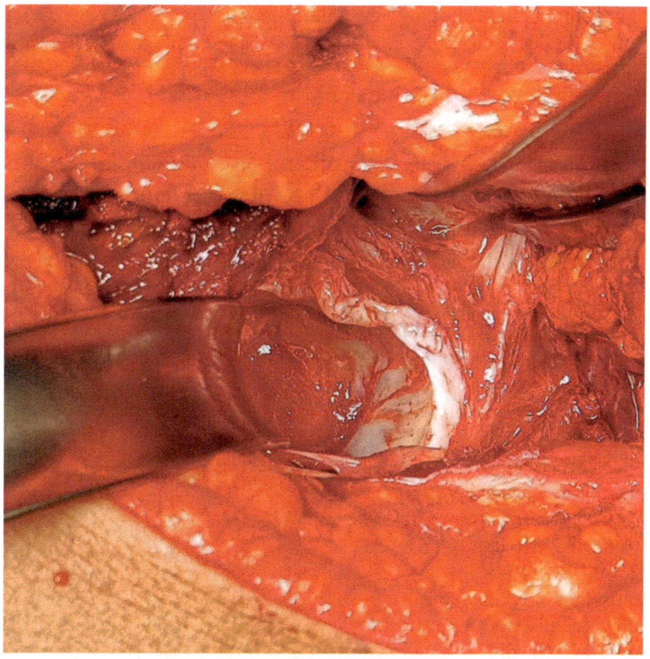

Fig. 10.2 The labrum has been detached from the rim between 11 and the 4 o'clock position (standardized to right hip)

the extent of the pathology that needs to be treated (Fig. 10.2). In the case of global overcoverage, the detachment may be circumferential. In other situations, it may be segmental in the area of degeneration or labral base ossification. If necessary, the degenerated parts of the labrum are removed.

- Resection of the acetabular rim: Using either a curved chisel or a motorized bur, the acetabular rim is resected as planned (Fig. 10.3a and b). Care must be taken that the resection is tangential to the rim. If the chisel is used at a right angle to the rim, the rim may break and cause a segmental defect of the bone and cartilage. This can happen in the postero-superior area because tangential placement of the chisel is difficult in this area. Alternatively, a motorized bur can be helpful, especially in this area. The amount of bony resection is determined by the osseous pathology or ossification of the labrum. In the case of a normal acetabular rim, only as much bone is removed to get a bleeding bony surface.
- Refixation of the labrum: The labrum is reattached with bone anchors (Fig. 10.4). For a circumferential refixation, five to six bone anchors are sufficient. Most acetabular rim lesions are located antero-superiorly and require two to four bone anchors to reattach the labrum. The bone anchors should be thin and short to prevent perforation into the iliopectineal bursa where the psoas tendon could be irritated. Titanium anchors usually are smaller and fit closer to the thin anterior rim. The anchors are positioned about 2 mm away from the bone cartilage interface and directed parallel or slightly divergent from the acetabular surface. Under direct vision, it is hard to drill into the joint, but if the drill penetrates into the acetabulum, it needs to be redirected. The suture is passed through the base of the labrum, the knots being tied on the outer (capsular) surface. This allows the remaining labrum to adapt itself against the femoral head, giving a more anatomic triangular shape (Fig. 10.5). Looping of the labrum has to be avoided because the labral seal will be broken in the area of the indentations by the suture. The need for looping indicates poor quality of the labrum and therefore reconstruction may be considered.
- Reconstruction of the labrum: Replacement of the labrum with an autologous or heterologous transplant is required to bridge circumferential or segmental defects. For short segmental defects, the ligamentum capitis femoris (ligamentum teres) can be used to reconstruct the labrum. For larger defects grafts from the iliotibial band, semitendinosus tendon or an allograft can be used. The transplant is attached to the acetabular rim by means of bone anchors as described above. For segmental reconstruction, the remaining healthy labrum is sutured to the graft with 2-0 Monocryl.
- The ligamentum teres can be variable in length and strength (Fig. 10.6). A thick ligament can be divided longitudinally from one end, leaving a soft tissue bridge of the thickness of the ligament at the other end. This allows duplication of the length of the graft. All synovial tissue is removed, leaving the core of the longitudinal fibers (Fig. 10.7) Bone anchors are placed at both ends of the transplant and in the middle, where both branches can be grasped by the suture.

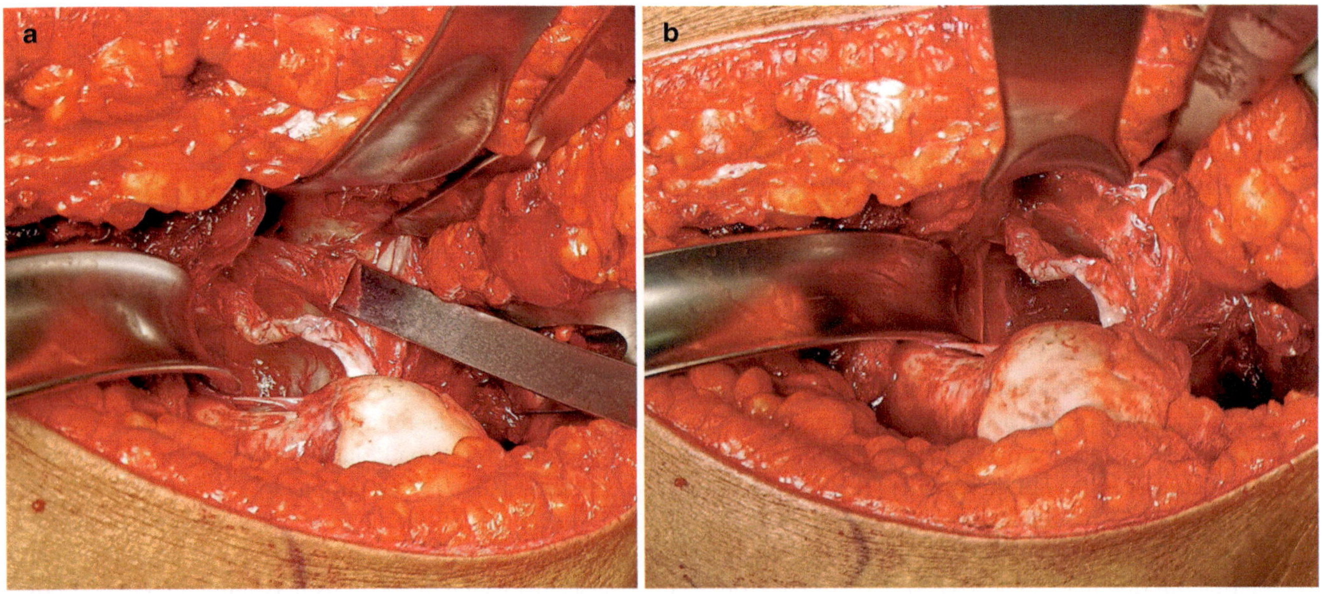

Fig. 10.3 (**a**) Resection of the bony rim with a curved osteotomy, parallel to the acetabular rim. (**b**) After completion of the resection. There is bleeding from the bony surface

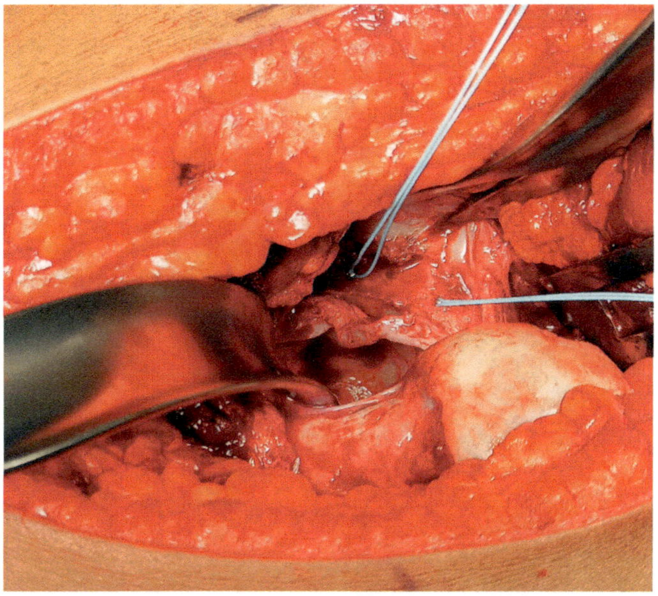

Fig. 10.4 Placement of the bone anchors approximately 2 mm away from the subchondral bone

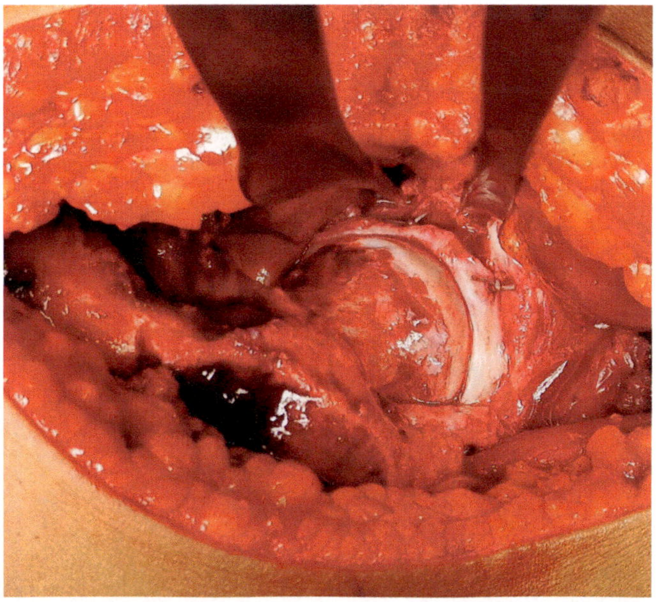

Fig. 10.5 After reduction, the femoral head spans the labrum nicely and labral seal is obtained

- Occasionally, the technique of labral augmentation is helpful. During augmentation, the thin but intact tip of the labrum can be preserved during detachment, but its volume would not allow for a good function. In these situations, a transplant is placed between the acetabular rim and the remaining labrum. This increases the volume and the ability to keep the labral seal by preserving the longitudinal labral fibers. The technique combines the above-mentioned techniques of labral refixation and reconstruction. For improved reconstruction, the labrum and the graft are sutured together in situ with 2-0 Monocryl.

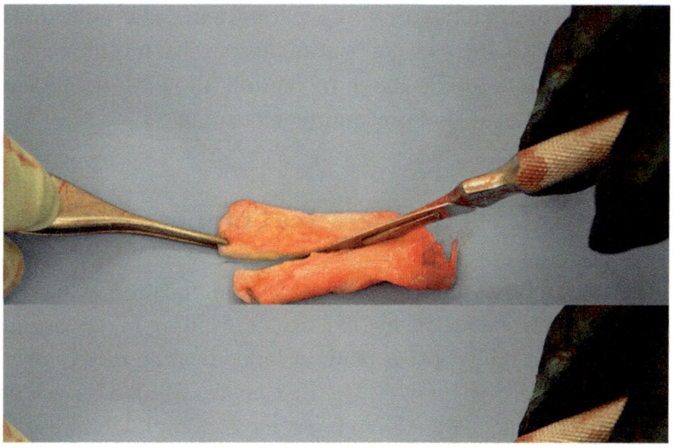

Fig. 10.6 The ligamentum teres has a variable length and thickness. A strong ligament as shown here has to be divided to fit the normal volume of a labrum. If a long reconstruction is required, it is partially divided and then stretched to get a longer implant

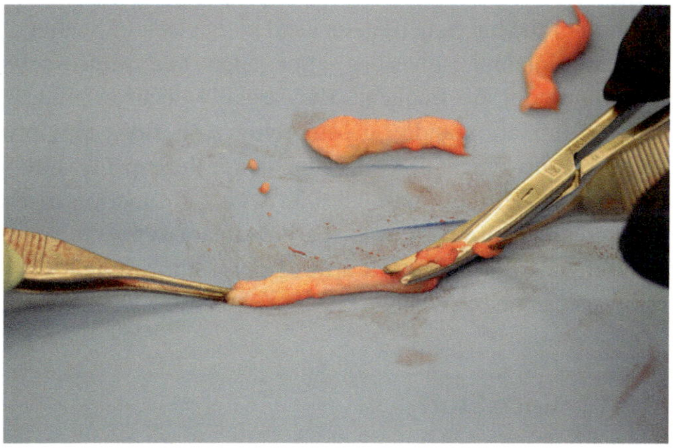

Fig. 10.7 The synovial layer and fat are removed

- Checking for suction seal: After acetabular rim trimming and refixation of the labrum, the acetabulum is irrigated, and all debris is removed. The hip is reduced carefully so as not to avulse the reattached labrum. Once the head is reduced the labrum is spanned nicely. The suction seal is checked by subluxing the femoral head by pulling with a bone hook on the calcar. The suction seal is sufficient if a sucking sound is heard when the femoral head is subluxed.

10.13 Postoperative Follow-Up

The postoperative regime follows the requirements of SHD. Toe-touch weight-bearing for 4 weeks with a gradual increase in weight-bearing thereafter. Early range-of-motion exercises are mandatory to prevent intraarticular adhesions. In these cases, the use of a continuous passive motion device may provide a gentle range of motion allowing healing of the labrum tissue and preventing adhesions.

10.14 Intra-/Postoperative Complications

As noted above, the most common complication would be related to erroneous anchor placement resulting in intraarticular cartilage injury, psoas pain, or failed healing of the labral tissue with persistent pain. The first can be avoided by careful insertion of the anchors into bone and is completely preventable as insertion of the anchors is under direct visualization. Protrusion of the bone anchor can be prevented by measuring the depth of the drill hole and palpating the blind end of the drill hole with a depth gauge or a nitinol wire. It is rare for a well-fixed labral refixation or labral reconstruction not to heal. Persistent pain or mechanical symptoms with a range of motion of the hip may be associated with a lack of healing.

Capsulolabral adhesions after open and arthroscopic labral surgery are frequent. They usually occur around the area of refixation and/or capsulotomy. Adhesions may prevent free movement of the labrum and/or the capsule. If they are too dense, they may interfere with the function of the labrum and cause pain. If the perilabral sulcus is completely obliterated, as seen on MR arthrography, arthroscopic adhesiolysis can be beneficial.

10.15 Case Study

A 45-year-old physically very active and athletic woman, playing badminton at the national level with increasing loss of motion and groin pain. Radiographs showed a severe pincer-FAI secondary to a deep socket with a completely ossified labrum (Fig. 10.8). She underwent a surgical hip dislocation, with osteochondroplasty of the head–neck junction, resection of the ossified labrum (Fig. 10.9), and reconstruction of the labrum with a hamstring allograft (Fig. 10.10). The postoperative ap pelvic radiograph at 6 weeks shows circumferential resection of the ossified labrum (Fig. 10.11). She continued to play badminton at a national level. At 10-year follow-up, she still has a good hip function, although she had to give up playing badminton. The most recent radiographs in 2020 show preserved joint space but progression of the ossifications at the acetabular rim and development of osteophytes at the femoral head (Fig. 10.12) (Courtesy of Michael Leunig).

This case illustrates the evolution of hips with severe pincer impingement, where the labrum has to be reconstructed. Although osteophytes occurred within 2–3 years at the femoral head–neck junction, a good hip function could be preserved for more than 10 years in a highly active patient.

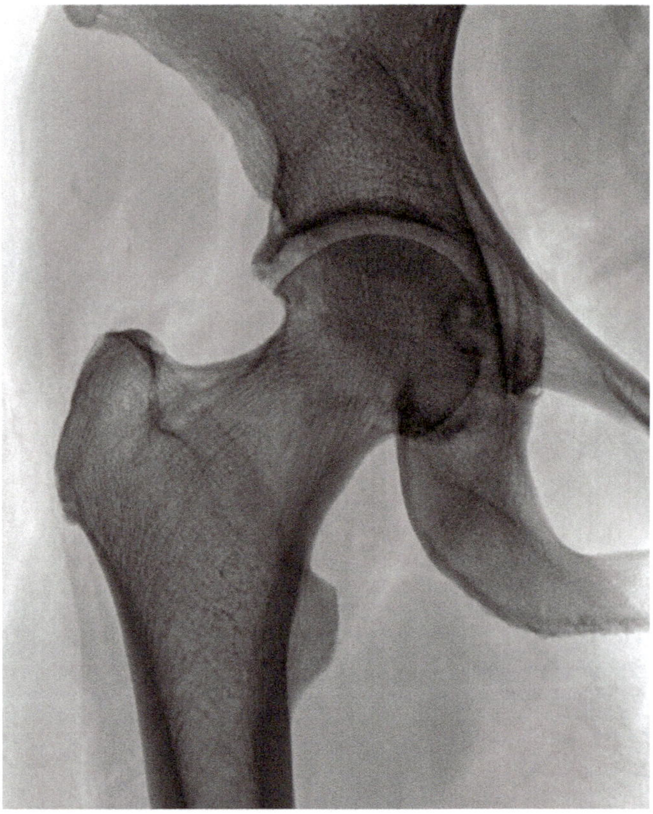

Fig. 10.8 Preoperative radiograph of a 45-year-old athletic female with severe rim/labral ossification and significantly decreased ROM, incapable of continuing her sports

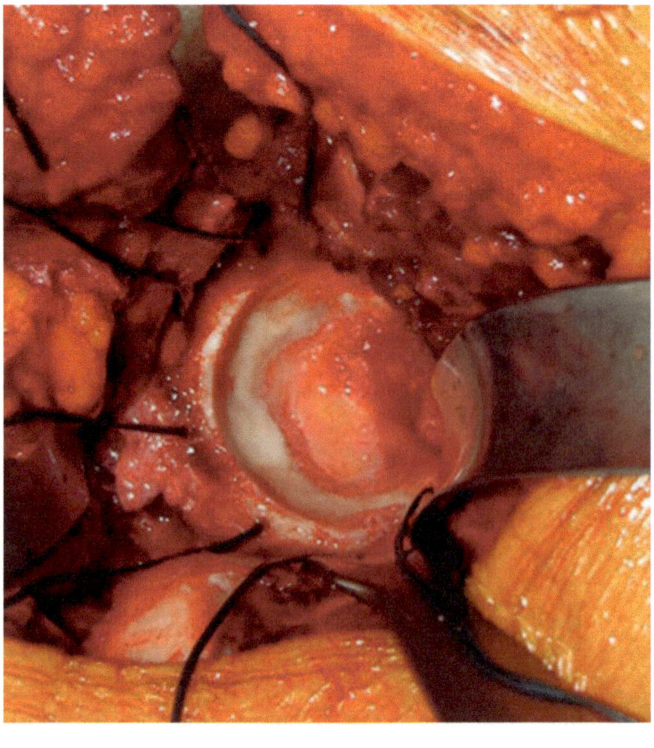

Fig. 10.9 Intraoperative view after resection of the ossified labrum and acetabular rim. The cartilage was not too arthritic. The bone anchors are already placed circumferentially

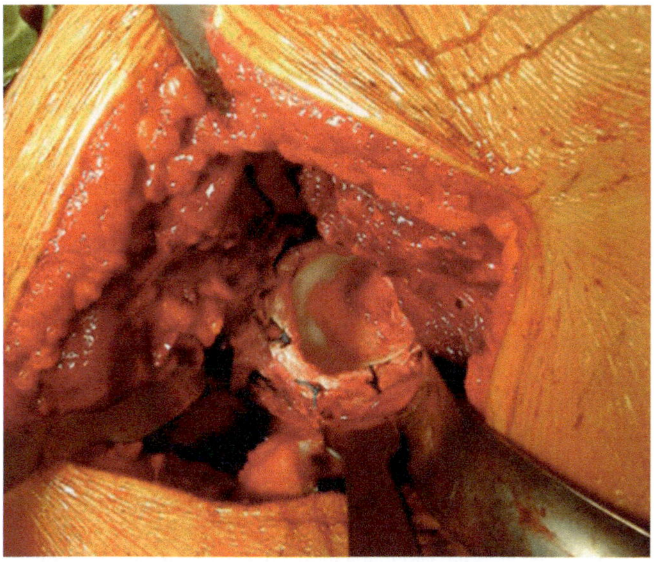

Fig. 10.10 Labral reconstruction using a circumferential hamstring allograft fixed with bone anchors, since the ligamentum capitis femoris was due to the Pincer deformity completely worn out

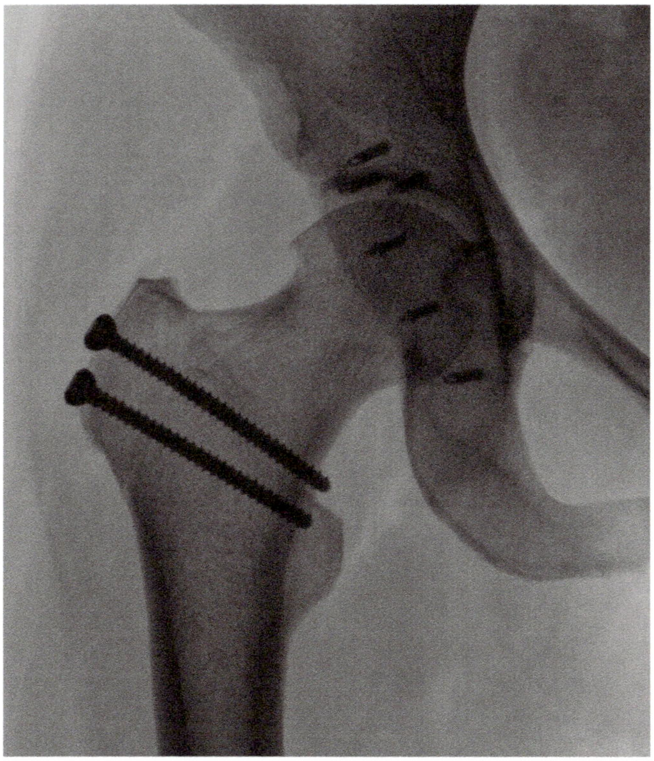

Fig. 10.11 Postoperative radiographs at 6 weeks follow-up. Complete resection of the acetabular rim together with the ossified labrum

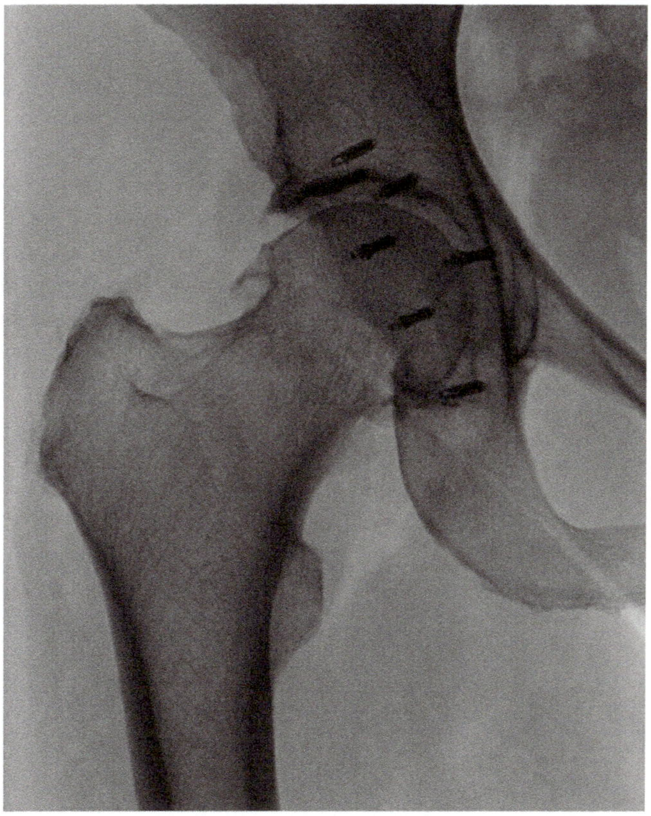

Fig. 10.12 Radiograph 10 years after surgery with a still functioning hip but regrowth of ossifications at the acetabular rim and osteophytes at the femoral head as signs of progressing OA. The joint space remained preserved, and she is still well compensated not requiring THA. This case shows that, despite the progression of OA, a good functional result can be obtained for a long time, delaying the implantation of an HTA

10.16 Controversies

Nowadays, most hips with femoroacetabular impingement are treated arthroscopically. As the experience and technique improve, there is less need to perform an SHD to treat acetabular rim pathology. SHD of the hip currently is more often used for complex deformities not amenable to arthroscopic surgery, and in these situations, open labral surgery is a useful technique.

10.17 Results

There is a large number of publications on segmental and circumferential reconstruction of the labrum using hip arthroscopy [9, 10]. A recent systematic review showed no differences in the clinical outcomes between these two techniques [9]. There are only few publications on open treatment of labral pathology. Labral preservation and reconstruction demonstrate superior results compared with resection of the labrum [11, 12]. Sierra and Trousdale reported on the results of using ligamentum teres in five patients [13]. Out of five patients, four had improvement in symptoms at final follow-up with one patient requiring a THA for persistent symptoms but without radiographic progression. Camenzind et al. compared open reconstruction of the labrum with ligamentum teres in 13 cases to a control group with labral refixation [5]. In this study, open reconstruction yielded excellent results comparable to labral refixation.

10.18 Outlook

With technical advances in hip arthroscopy, the need for open refixation or reconstruction will decrease. However, both, arthroscopic and open techniques are demanding, and circumferential reconstruction of a labrum will remain in the hands of few experts who are able to do it in a good quality. As an adjunct technique during correction of complex deformities of the hip, the open technique will keep its value.

With respect to reconstructions of the labrum, tissue engineering might be able to provide off-the-shelf synthetic graft matching the shape and size of the labrum better than allo- or autografts in the future [14].

References

1. Ferguson SJ, et al. The influence of the acetabular labrum on hip joint cartilage consolidation: a poroelastic finite element model. J Biomech. 2000;33(8):953–60.
2. Ito K, Leunig M, Ganz R. Histopathologic features of the acetabular labrum in femoroacetabular impingement. Clin Orthop Relat Res. 2004;429:262–71.
3. Corten K, et al. Bone apposition of the acetabular rim in deep hips: a distinct finding of global pincer impingement. J Bone Joint Surg Am. 2011;93(Suppl 2):10–6.
4. Espinosa N, et al. Treatment of femoro-acetabular impingement: preliminary results of labral refixation. J Bone Joint Surg Am. 2006;88(5):925–35.
5. Camenzind RS, Steurer-Dober I, Beck M. Clinical and radiographical results of labral reconstruction. J Hip Preserv Surg. 2015;2(4):401–9.
6. Weidner J, Wyatt M, Beck M. Labral augmentation with ligamentum capitis femoris: presentation of a new technique and preliminary results. J Hip Preserv Surg. 2018;5(1):47–53.
7. Su T, et al. The vascularization course of labral autograft and its effect on tissue healing: acetabular labral augmentation versus labral reconstruction in a porcine model. Am J Sports Med. 2022;50(10):2647–58.
8. Costa Rocha P, et al. Circumferential reconstruction of severe acetabular labral damage using hamstring allograft: surgical technique and case series. Hip Int. 2013;23(Suppl 9):S42–53.
9. Maldonado DR, Glein RM, Domb BG. Arthroscopic acetabular labral reconstruction: a review. J Hip Preserv Surg. 2020;7(4):611–20.
10. Scanaliato JP, et al. Hip labral reconstruction: techniques and outcomes. Curr Rev Musculoskelet Med. 2021;14(6):340–50.
11. Anwander H, et al. Labral reattachment in femoroacetabular impingement surgery results in increased 10-year survivorship compared with resection. Clin Orthop Relat Res. 2017;475(4):1178–88.
12. Larson CM, et al. Arthroscopic debridement versus Refixation of the acetabular labrum associated with femoroacetabular impingement: updated mean 7-year follow-up. Am J Sports Med. 2022;50(3):731–8.
13. Sierra RJ, Trousdale RT. Labral reconstruction using the ligamentum teres capitis: report of a new technique. Clin Orthop Relat Res. 2009;467(3):753–9.
14. Santschi MXT, et al. Mechanical and biological evaluation of melt-electrowritten polycaprolactone scaffolds for acetabular labrum restoration. Cells. 2022;11(21):3450.

Techniques for Cartilage Repair

11

Gian Salzmann and Robert W. Westermann

11.1 Introduction

Chondral defects have limited healing capacity and have been associated with worse outcomes in patients undergoing hip preservation surgery. As a result, cartilage repair in the hip is becoming increasingly important. Related to improving surgical techniques and higher frequency of minimally-invasive interventions, the intraoperative technique is of utmost importance as it has the potential to postpone/prevent premature osteoarthritis (OA). The cartilage repair techniques described here are for the treatment of focal, full-thickness cartilage lesions, not generalized OA. The treatment goals for patients with focal cartilage defects are the resolution of pain, restoration of function, return to activity, and prevention of premature OA.

11.2 Background

Chondral as well as osteochondral lesions at the hip joint are frequent [1]. To date, most of the literature, experience, and techniques for treating focal cartilage defects have been for lesions in the knee. Thus, the discussion of recommended therapies and surgical techniques in this chapter is based on the current understanding of cartilage biology in the knee, in combination with what is known about hip biomechanics as well as the limited clinical experience to the present.

Mechanical overload of the cartilage can lead to the death of chondrocytes and damage to the extracellular matrix (ECM). A focal cartilage defect leads to bending and shear forces at the edge of the lesion and to a change in the fluid mechanics in the perifocal region, which is why the lesion can degenerate further due to the increased stress on the chondrocytes at the rim of the lesion. Above a certain threshold-size of a lesion that remains undefined for the hip, it is likely to influence the progression of the disease and adversely affects the surrounding cartilage. Below this size, the surrounding tissue might absorb the increased load caused by the cartilage defect. In the hip, the percent of the total cartilage surface area is likely more important than the absolute size of the lesion (Fig. 11.1a, b). Thus, a cartilage lesion in a female patient with a smaller femoral head may be much worse than the same size lesion in a male with a larger femoral head. Another important and unanswered question is the influence of the concavity/convexity of the surface. For example, would a focal cartilage defect on the acetabulum be less likely to progress than one of the same size on the femur? In addition, the quality of the subchondral bone is different between the acetabulum (relatively harder) and the femoral head (relatively softer). The relevance of this to the likelihood of defect progression or potential therapy has not yet been elucidated.

Specifically with evolving high-resolution MRI techniques such defects are identified more often and, ideally, earlier. A variety of different causes have been associated with chondral injuries of the hip, most notably, femoroacetabular impingement (FAI) as well as trauma, labral tears, arthritis, dysplasia, and osteonecrosis with subsequent osteochondral lesions. The detection and management of chondral injuries of the hip, especially in the younger patient population, is important and treatment may help to prevent or delay hip joint degeneration. Long-term outcomes of cartilage defects within the hip result in pain and early degenerative changes and might result in the subsequent development of arthritis. The severity of these defects occurs along a scale, progressing from superficial or partial-thickness (matrix) disruptions to complex and full-thickness (chondral) defects with the possibility of underlying subchondral bone loss (osteochondral lesions) (Table 11.1). Related to a very limited blood supply, superficial cartilage lesions have a limited capacity to spontaneously heal if left untreated. While this capacity is better among osteochondral lesions, most often

G. Salzmann (✉)
Knee Service, Department of Orthopedics, Schulthess Clinic, Zurich, Switzerland
e-mail: gian.salzmann@kws.ch

R. W. Westermann
Department of Orthopedics and Rehabilitation, University of Iowa Health Care, Iowa City, IA, USA
e-mail: robert-westermann@uiowa.edu

M. Leunig et al. (eds.), *Surgical Hip Dislocation*, https://doi.org/10.1007/978-3-031-70622-6_11

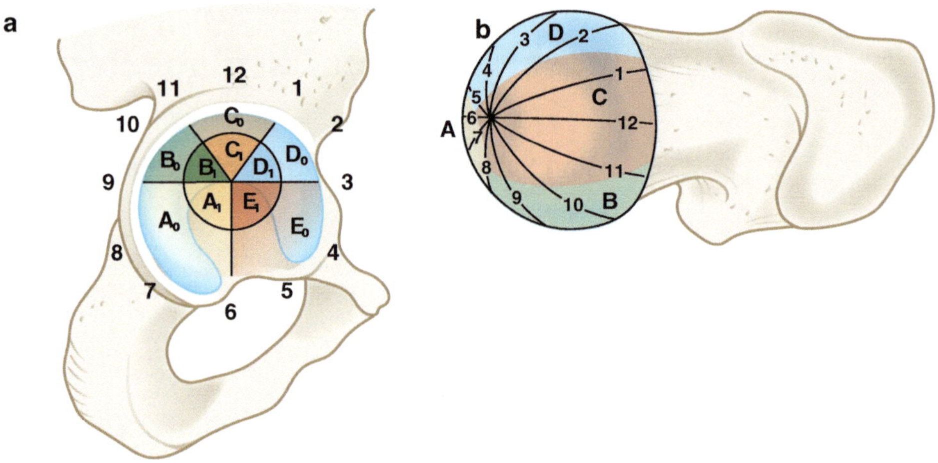

Fig. 11.1 (**a**,**b**) Schematic of acetabular (**a**) and femoral (**b**) cartilage lesions with a sectorial (**a**–**e**) or clock face (1–12) system

Table 11.1 ICRS classification system for cartilage lesions

Stage	Description	Criteria
ICRS classification		
0	Normal	Normal cartilage
1	Nearly normal	Superficial lesions; soft indentation, superficial fissures or cracks
2	Abnormal	Lesions extending down to <50% of cartilage depth
3	Severely abnormal	Defects extending >50% of cartilage depth as well as to the calcified cartilage, but not through subchondral bone. Includes cartilage blistering.
4	Severely abnormal	Cartilage defect that extends into the subchondral bone

insufficient repair tissue will develop within the previously defective area. It is biomechanically not strong enough to withstand the typical loading patterns across the hip joint. Naturally, defects will become larger and deeper over time alongside the progression of clinical symptoms. The management options for an articular cartilage injury have multiplied, including fragment fixation via fibrin adhesive or sutures, microfracture, microfracture plus a biomaterial, autologous chondrocyte implantation (ACI), autologous osteochondral graft transplantation (mosaicplasty), osteochondral allograft (OCA) transplantation, and the use of particulate cartilage. Hip surgeons have to be prepared for spontaneous detection of such lesions since MRI-related sensitivity has been currently reported to be at only approximately 70%. Despite a heavy body of peer-reviewed literature regarding the utility of cartilage repair techniques for other weight-bearing joints, evidence for hip joint cartilage preservation repair remains in its infancy.

11.3 Indications

11.3.1 Indications

Children and adolescents, symptomatic, non-responsive to conservative therapy ICRS grade 3 and 4 chondral and osteochondral lesions. It has to be annotated that patients have to be enlightened that chondral/osteochondral lesions naturally progress and repair is suggested for the purpose of preventing lesion progression, specifically when the underlying co-pathology is being addressed via surgical intervention.

11.3.2 Relative Contraindications

- Asymptomatic ICRS grade 1 and 2 lesions and no underlying co-pathology
- Asymptomatic ICRS grade 3 and 4 lesions with underlying open growth plates and no underlying co-pathology
- Uncontained and bipolar lesions
- Patients unwilling to commit to the required and specific postoperative management
- Lesions associated with generalized systemic inflammatory diseases.

11.3.3 Contraindications

- Osteoarthritis (OA) of the hip joint
- Progressed head necrosis
- Over the age of 60 years (biological age)
- Patients unwilling to commit to the required and specific postoperative management

11.4 Preoperative/Preinterventional Diagnostics

- AP pelvis, false profile, as well as Lauenstein or cross-table lateral.
- Arthro-MRI of the symptomatic hip is useful to measure the size AP and ML diameter of the cartilage injury for femoral head lesions (Fig. 11.1). This can help inform the choice of osteochondral autograft (for smaller lesions <10 mm in diameter) or for osteochondral fresh allograft transfer (for larger lesions >15 mm). For acetabular lesions associated with FAI, the MR is also important to rule out global joint chondral thinning.
- CT with special sequences for preoperative computer simulation of intracapital osteotomy. A 3D CT scan can also be helpful for concurrent FAI correction during surgical intervention.

11.5 Preoperative Planning/Computer Simulation

Cartilage treatment can be generally categorized into palliative interventions (hyaluronic acid, debridement, or lavage), reparative interventions (direct repair, microfracture, and second-generation bone marrow stimulation), and restorative interventions (osteochondral grafting, ACI, and other similar techniques) [2].

For acetabular lesions of significant size, one should be prepared for reparative interventions (direct repair, microfracture, or second-generation bone marrow stimulation) which has demonstrated good results in patients younger than 35 years of age. Microfracture or micro-drilling equipment with acute angles (50–90°) are useful in open or arthroscopic acetabular treatment. Femoral head lesions can be addressed by reparative interventions (direct repair, microfracture, and second-generation bone marrow stimulation), and less frequent restorative interventions (osteochondral grafting, ACI, and other similar techniques) osteochondral autograft (for smaller lesions) or fresh allograft for larger lesions. For lesions >15 mm in diameter, it can often be difficult to restore with head–neck junction autograft. The options at this point would be to obtain autograft from the lateral trochlea of the knee or to use a fresh autograft (typically femoral head or condyle). Chondrocyte viability is best between 21 and 28 days from donor death.

11.6 Applied Anatomy

- Purely chondral defects of the acetabulum can be addressed either open via SHD or arthroscopically assisted using microfracture (and microfracture plus biomaterial), fibrin adhesive, ACI, or particulate cartilage.
- Larger and specifically osteochondral lesions that require cancellous bone plasty have to be addressed via SHD particularly if localized on the femoral head.
- All defective cartilage as well as subchondral bone (if applicable) has to be removed until viable tissue (cartilage and bone) is detected. The underlying bone and subsequent cancellous bone plasty has to be vital, firm, and stable. The defect-surrounding cartilage edges have to be stable and vital.
- Signs of ongoing OA display a contraindication or have to be declared as a salvage procedure, specifically among young subjects.

11.7 Special Risks

- Disturbance to the blood supply to the femoral head (following SHD) with consequences such as loss of reduction, head collapse, and resulting follow-up surgery including joint replacement
- Insufficient cartilage repair stimulation with resulting ongoing pain
- Overgrowth of cartilage repair tissue resulting in ongoing pain and mechanical symptoms
- Continuation/initiation of premature hip joint OA (cyst formation, etc., bone marrow edema)
- See also Sect. 11.14

11.8 Type of Anesthesia

As the procedure is performed in lateral positioning and usually takes more than 90 min, general anesthesia is the recommendation of choice.

11.9 Positioning

- As for SHD (see Chap. 7)
- Standard operating table
- Lateral positioning with tunnel cushion and lateral bag
- Drape with lateral hip set that allows for a sterile pouch for the foot to be placed during dislocation
- Fluoroscopy and X-ray possibility

11.10 Instruments/Implants

Standard instrumentation for surgical hip dislocation (see Chap. 7). In addition to the instruments required for the surgical dislocation approach, the following special instruments ensure an optimal surgical procedure:

- Osteochondral autograft or allograft instrumentation
- Microfracture awl, hip length, angles 50–90°.

- Tissue collector device
- Microdrilling set

11.11 Access

Access for hip joint arthroscopy as well as for SHD with transtrochanteric osteotomy (see Chap. 7).

11.12 Technical Steps of Deep Dissection

Surgical principles (Fig. 11.2) apply for both arthroscopic and open access. It is of utmost importance to address any pathomechanical cause and/or underlying co-pathology most often simultaneously with the indicated cartilage repair procedure (e.g., osteotomy, covered in other chapters of this book). The order of repair is handled differently individually, but most often the cartilage repair step of the surgical procedure is the last step related to its natural fragility. Cartilage treatment can be generally categorized into palliative interventions (not covered in this chapter), reparative interventions (direct chondral flap repair, microfracture, second-generation bone marrow stimulation), and restorative interventions (OAT, OCA grafting, ACI, minced/particulate cartilage repair, and other similar techniques).

11.12.1 Reparative Interventions

Chondral Flap Repair Chondrolabral delamination is commonly faced in hip arthroscopy and is often associated with FAI. Following inspection and probing, the refixation bed is debrided until vital and hereafter the chondral flap is reduced and finally fixed by using fibrin glue, suture anchor fixation, or can be replaced by a scaffold implantation when fixation is not possible. Levinson in 2020 [3] analyzed a total of ten purely chondral acetabular flaps and three non-delaminated control cartilage samples that were resected during surgery. The group concluded that despite the presence of viable chondrocytes with migration potential, the cells resided in a structurally altered ECM and had limited capacity to deposit ECM, leading to question the capacity to produce sufficient ECM within the fibrin sealant for stable long-term attachment of such flaps. Chondral flap fixation seems to be an elegant option within fresh delaminations especially in young subjects (specifically children and adolescents). For chronic flaps as well as among older subjects, a successful fixation is inconsistently effective and must be performed with appropriate expectations.

- *Microfracture:* Depending upon the location within the hip joint, this simple surgical technique should be limited to defect sizes up to 2 cm^2. It remains the current workhorse for cartilage repair due to its simplicity and can be usually done arthroscopically assisted. Clear drawbacks are a violation of the necessarily intact subchondral bone plate (it is contraindicated within osteochondral lesions) and subsequent high risk for the evolution of intralesional osteophytes as well as progressing subchondral pathology (e.g., cysts). First, all nonviable and unstable cartilage around the edges of the defect has to be debrided with a shaver. Using a ringed curette or sharp spoon, loose cartilage has to be scraped away in order to create perpendicular borders around the chondral lesion site. The same should be done to the calcified layer. Once the lesion site is prepared, multiple perforations to the subchondral bone have to be created in order for the bone marrow to settle within the defect site. Such perforations can be performed by using a curved awl. Currently, drilled, smaller diameter (e.g., 1.6) but deeper perforations are recommended with less damage at the intact bone and higher-quality subchondral cell influx. Perpendicular drilling trajectory relative to the bone bed is recommended. Perforations should be started at the periphery of the defect and should be continued towards the center, placing the holes 3–4 mm apart with the idea of avoiding subchondral plate fractures. When using a drill, deep perforations are recommended, while it should be exclusively set on the forward speed in order to reduce the risk of breaking the drill bit. After drilling, the shaver is used to debride any bone that may have accumulated in the joint during drilling in order to prevent inflammatory responses. If successful, initially, a primitive blood clot will evolve within the lesion that will transform into cartilage repair tissue as the patient follows an accordingly tailored rehabilitation protocol in order to protect the maturing cartilage repair tissue.

Augmented Microfracture Augmenting microfracture techniques with biologics [4] could potentially improve and promote hyaline cartilage repair because of a theoretically higher initial repair tissue stability as well as biological support for chondral proliferation and differentiation. However, biomaterials may also theoretically impede chondrocyte migration and proliferation associated with digestion and half-life properties and cause an inflammatory response that is associated with negative consequences to the intraarticular environment. Also, if a biomaterial is sutured to the surrounding cartilage, most often an open approach, the subchondral bone will still have to be violated and the surrounding cartilage may be damaged by the suture place-

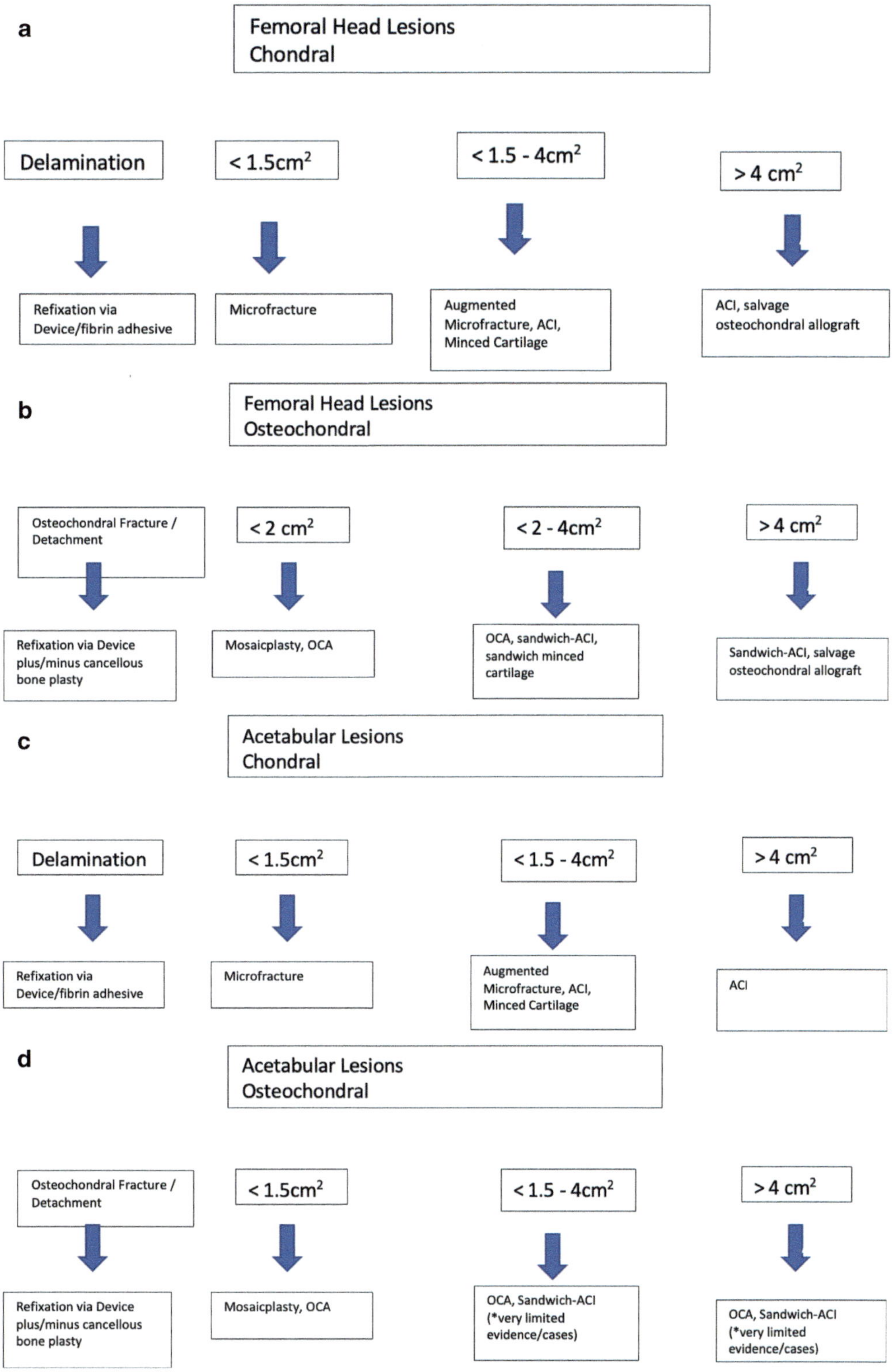

Fig. 11.2 (**a**) Chondral femoral head lesion treatment recommendation according to defect morphology and size (**b**) Osteochondral femoral head lesion treatment recommendation according to defect morphology and size (**c**) Chondral acetabular lesion treatment recommendation according to defect morphology and size (**d**) Osteochondral acetabular lesion treatment recommendation according to defect morphology and size

ment. Generally, the biomaterial can be implanted via an arthroscopic approach, specifically when hydrogel-based materials are applied. Chitosan-based scaffolds or porcine type I/III collagen matrices are usually deployed. Such collagen matrices can be fixed using fibrin glue or sutures. Finally, dehydrated micronized allogeneic cartilage is another scaffold source in development. Micronized cartilage combined with platelet-rich plasma is applied over a microfractured defect: however, biological advantage has to be questioned since, compared with microfracture, healthy subchondral bone is severely violated. Furthermore, biomaterials often impede a natural healing response of the chondrocytes. Ibragimova used a small animal model and a variety of different biomaterials to simulate augmented microfracture, demonstrating that neither the formation of hyaline cartilage nor the presence of chondrocytes or chondroprogenitor cells was not detected in any of the groups, despite observed cellular infiltration into scaffolds present in each group except cellulose. The group concluded that for restoration of hyaline cartilage, scaffolds have to be combined either with cellular therapy or morphogens promoting chondrogenic differentiation.

11.12.2 Restorative Interventions

- Osteochondral autograft transplantation (OAT) also named mosaicplasty allows for the transfer of autogenous, mature, viable hyaline cartilage together with subchondral bone as a cylindrical osteochondral graft to address both chondral and osteochondral pathology. This technique is well established at the talus where bone pathology does play a major role but also addresses osteochondral pathology at the knee joint. Common donor sites include the ipsilateral knee or non-weight-bearing areas of the femoral head–neck junction. It has to be considered that articular cartilage has a highly specific regional topology across the joint—specifically when transplantation across different joints is regarded. Cartilage height and thickness will vary, and the ultrastructure is not the same due to unequal biomechanical load. Also, the architecture of the subchondral bone might be different across locations. Finally, due to varying chondral/subchondral thickness, a mismatch at the cartilage/bone interface at the recipient site may result. Yet, given the replacement of defects with true hyaline cartilage, mosaicplasty has shown superior results in the knee compared with the fibrocartilage scar created by microfracture. In the hip joint, mosaicplasty is indicated in full-thickness chondral defects with subchondral bone damage. The advantages of mosaicplasty include a single-stage procedure and the ability to address damaged subchondral bone. Shortcomings include donor site morbidity as well as the potential for two separate surgical sites. In addition, the use of the anterior femoral head–neck junction may not be a source for physiologically normal hyaline cartilage. Furthermore, transplanting multiple cylinders can be technically demanding in creating a smooth surface intraarticularly. Additionally, femoroacetabular access is often provided via SHD where femoral head vascularity compromise represents a potentially severe complication. Although limited in nature, published mosaicplasty results have, overall, been favorable, including small mid- and long-term studies. Given OAT's ability to address both chondral and subchondral pathology simultaneously, we recommend consideration of mosaicplasty in focal osteochondral defects (<10–15 mm in diameter), particularly when o OCAs are unavailable.
- OCA transplantation involves the patient receiving an allograft of osteochondral tissue, classically obtained from an optimally young deceased donor within 21–28 days of death. In the knee, osteochondral allograft is utilized most commonly for patients aged <40–50 years with an isolated defect of >2–2.5 cm^2 or large subchondral bone loss without generalized OA. Large full-block osteochondral allografts are utilized for primary but most often revision salvage procedures with large diameter and deep lesions that often have no containment. Clear advantages are the off-the-shelf usage with no donor site morbidity, fast return to activity, and the possibility to address both chondral damage and subchondral bone pathology at once. OCA has demonstrated favorable long-term results and 66–69% allograft survival at 20 years follow-up in the knee joint. In the hip, OCA finds rather seldom utilization, while currently published evidence is providing satisfying outcomes.
- OCAs are performed via SHD. The center of the lesion is identified and a perpendicular pin is inserted. A recipient cylindrical reamer is then used here to the depth of the diseased cancellous bone. The depth along each of the four sides of the recipient site is then measured. On the back table, the allograft tissue is placed in a clamp and cut with a donor cylindrical saw. The donor dowel is typically cut 1 mm larger than the recipient for a press-fit fixation technique. If there is instability with the press fit technique, the graft can be secured with a bio-compression screw.
- Furthermore, specifically fresh osteochondral allografts are not available in every country and are often costly. Overall, OCA results may be encouraging, although graft availability, storage, and cost are limitations. Like mosaicplasty, we recommend considering OCA for larger osteochondral defects that are not amenable to OATS or when there are concerns about significant donor-site morbidity. Finally, resurfacing the intraarticular joint anatomy may be surgical challenging. Last, graft survival improves substantially when concomitant anatomically related mechanical abnormalities are corrected simultaneously.
- ACI has become the standard of care across the knee joint for medium-large diameter chondral as well as osteochondral lesions. Regarding its biological potential clinical success and return to sporting activity rates were satisfying. ACI is a two-step procedure where chondrocytes are biopsied from a donor joint surface (most often

low to non-weight-bearing), then expanded, and finally applied to a membrane in the case of matrix-induced ACI (mACI), and subsequently implanted. In the most current fourth generation, ACI cells are already covered by a de novo autologous matrix (in vitro pre-culture phase) or will be mixed (following standard in vitro proliferation phase) with a specific hydrogel just prior to implantation. When specifically using fourth-generation ACI products, an arthroscopic approach is feasible. Oftentimes, the underlying co-pathology may already be addressed during the setting of the initial biopsy. In the hip, biopsy options include the non-articular femoral head–neck junction or around the pulvinar. With few, but generally positive studies available for this technique in the hip, benefits include less donor site morbidity compared with mosaicplasty as well as access in environments where allograft is unavailable. Furthermore, an advantage of ACI over structural grafts (mosaicplasty and OCA) is its utility in concave defects such as acetabular lesions. Given this, ACI can be applied not only for large chondral defects but also for osteochondral lesions where a cancellous bone grafting/plasty has to be generated underneath prior to cell implantation.

- Minced cartilage repair is a procedure that is currently gaining awareness [5]. Very comparable to ACI, the defect is debrided until the edges are stable. A cancellous bone plasty can be installed when required. Hereafter, vital cartilage is either taken from the defect edge or from non-weight-bearing regions. This cartilage is then cut into very small pieces using a knife, specific cutting devices, or designated shaver devices. This particulating process activates the cartilage to proliferate and produce ECM. Finally, the minced cartilage is re-implanted directly into the defect where it will be fixed by using a membrane, fibrin glue, or autologous blood-derived substances [6]. This technique has several possible theoretical advantages; it has a strong biological potential and medium-to-large diameter defects can be covered. However, this surgical technique is novel, especially when used for the hip joint, with little supporting clinical evidence, and, therefore, has to be applied with exceptional care and appropriate patient selection.

11.13 Postoperative Follow-Up

- *Postoperative Rehabilitation and Activity Resumption*

The period of limited weight-bearing is determined by the procedure performed. Most often, hip weight-bearing can be increased after 6 weeks. Continuous passive motion devices can be applied for the time of partial weight bearing—usually three times per week for 30–60 min per session (not underlined by heavy evidence). Following osteochondral transfer (mosaicplasty), weight-bearing can be usually quicker. As most cartilage repair techniques require 9–12 months until the newly grown tissue is fully matured, sport-specific training is not allowed earlier than 4–6 months following surgery starting with a low-level activity and progressing toward full competition at 9–12 months. Return-to-sport assessment tests are valuable and suggested beforehand.

- *Secondary Procedures*

We routinely recommend hardware removal primarily for trochanteric screws that may cause lateral hip pain/trochanteric bursitis and may complicate (screw breakage) future total hip arthroplasty. This is performed 6–12 months postoperatively and unrestricted activity is allowed 6 weeks after screw removal. Trochanteric screw size can affect ease of removal with 4.5 mm having a lower risk of breakage than 3.5-mm screws.

11.14 Intra/Postoperative Complications

Potential intraoperative complications inherent to osteochondral grafting include inappropriate graft height upon final seating/press fit and the absence of a rigid press fit after implantation. The former complication can be mitigated by placing a permanent suture draped into the recipient defect after the graft is implanted if the graft sits too proud or too inset, the suture can be used to extract the graft, and modifications to the recipient socket can be made to assure flush chondral surface after implantation. If the graft is finally impacted and press-fit fixation is not rigid, headless compression screws can be added to augment fixation strength. Both bio-composite and metal headless screws can be useful.

11.15 Case Studies

Case 1 (Fig. 11.3)

Case 2 (Fig. 11.4)

Case 3 (Fig. 11.5)

Case 4 (Fig. 11.6)

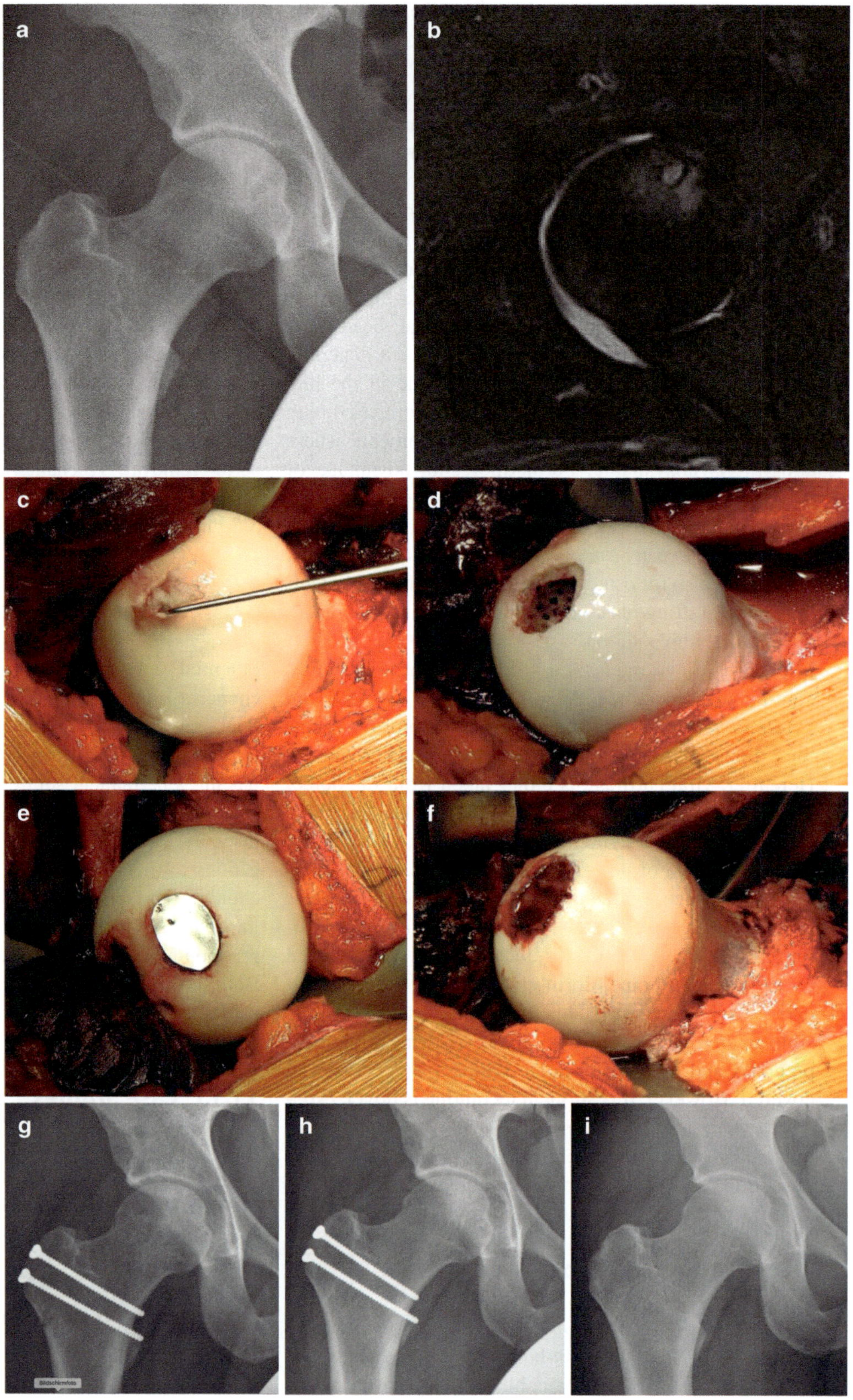

Fig. 11.3 Ap hip radiograph (**a**) taken from an ap pelvic radiograph of a 24-year-old male patient with a history of chronic groin pain. The radiograph shows a mild acetabular retroversion with the suspicion of a femoral head cystic lesion. The MRI (**b**) of the patient confirms the cystic femoral head lesion with a sclerotic margin and bone marrow edema. Corresponding, a femoral head defect on the acetabular side (**c-f**) Intraoperative visualization of the femoral head (**c**) following surgical hip dislocation. Using a small hook, the femoral head lesion is probed (**d**). After debridement of the cyst to the sclerotic margin, the sclerosis was drilled (**e**). An aluminum template matching the size of the defect was taken (**f**). Then, a double-layered collagen membrane was fixed by 6–0 non-absorbable sutures and fibrin glue into the defect, which was previously filled by autologous cancellous bone from the greater trochanter. The trochanteric osteotomy was fixed using two lag screws (**g-I**) Ap hip radiographs at (**g**) 6 weeks postoperative, (**f**) 1 year postoperative, and (**i**) 12 years postoperative (following removal of the two screws) with no signs of early OA. (Courtesy of Michael Leunig)

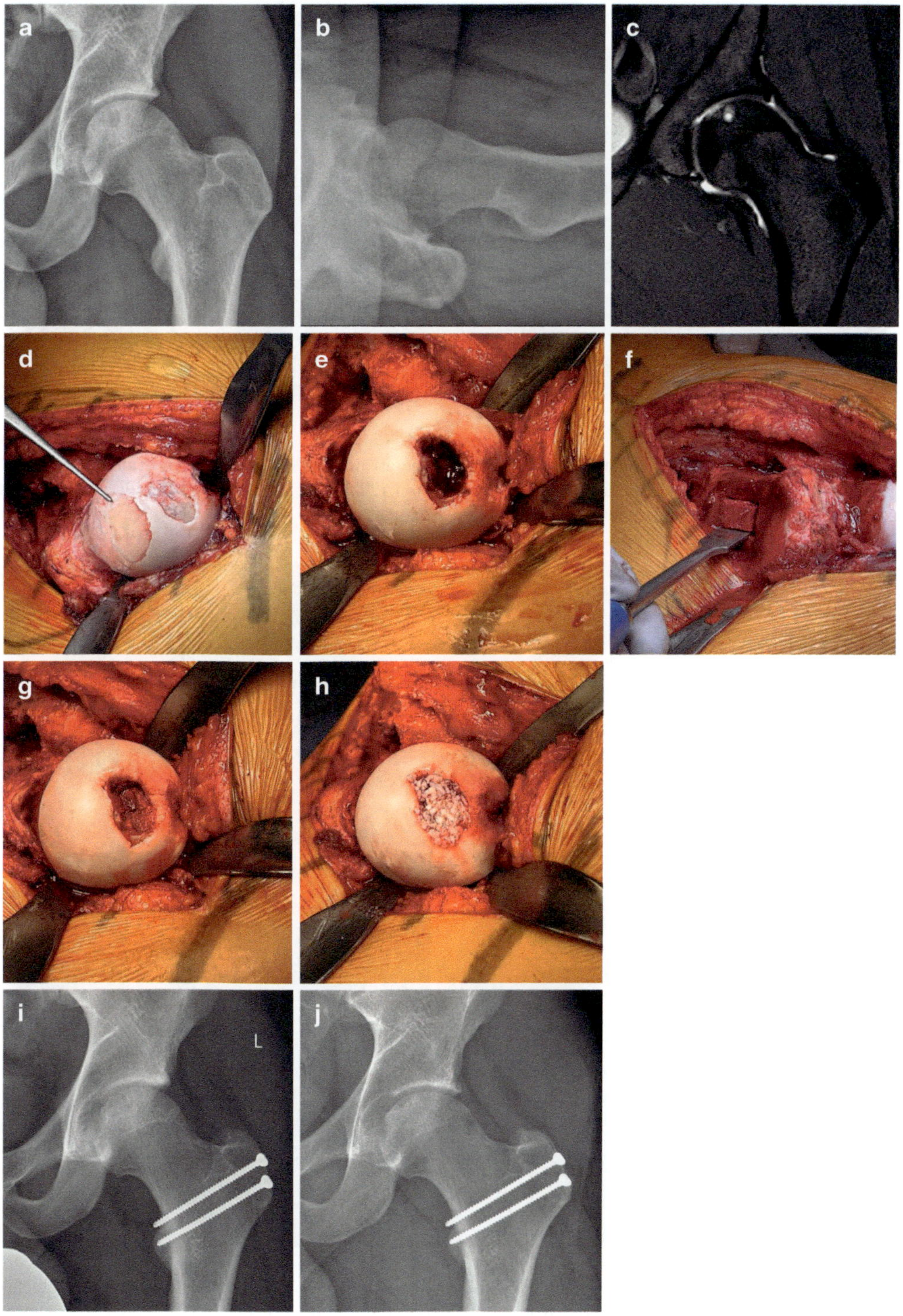

Fig. 11.4 (**a-c**) A 20-year-old sporting active male with chronic left-sided hip pain, presenting a cam deformity in the (**a**) ap hip view (taken from an ap pelvis) with an intact joint space but a cystic lesion at the suprafoveolar region in the femoral head (**b**). The cross-table lateral reveals a flattening of the anterior head/neck junction (**c**). MR imaging depicting a fluid-filled cystic lesion accompanied by a damaged cartilage layer on top of the lesion (**d-f**) During surgery (**d**) and following surgical hip dislocation, the suprafoveolar cartilage was lifted off the femoral head (**e**). Underneath, the bone was altered and debrided to the sclerotic margin of the cyst (**f**). Cancellous bone from the base of the greater trochanter was used to backfill the defect for the concomitant sandwich MCI technique (**g** and **h**) (**h**) After the impaction of the cancellous bone graft in the cyst (**h**), the autologous minced cartilage was used to cover the osteochondral defect. The trochanteric osteotomy was fixed using two lag screws (**i** and **j**) (**i**) 6 weeks postoperative and (**j**) 2.5 years postoperative, the joint space remained normal without signs of premature OA and satisfying bone generation within the previous cystic lesion. (Courtesy of Michael Leunig)

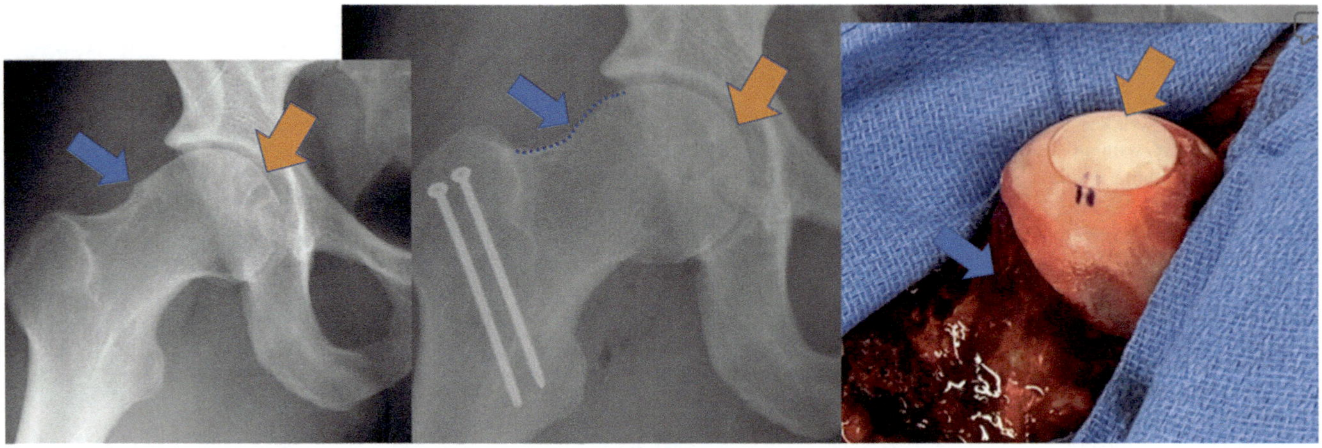

Fig. 11.5 A 32-year-old male with 3 years of progressive hip pain. Preoperative imaging was notable for cam-type FAI (blue arrow) and focal osteonecrosis of the femoral head. This large lesion (22.5 mm diameter, depth 25 mm) was treated with SHD, impingement correction, and fresh osteochondral allograft transplantation with donor dowel cut to 2–3.5 mm and implanted using a press-fit technique. Note that the postoperative radiograph demonstrates the resolution of the cystic changes in the femoral head from the focal osteonecrosis

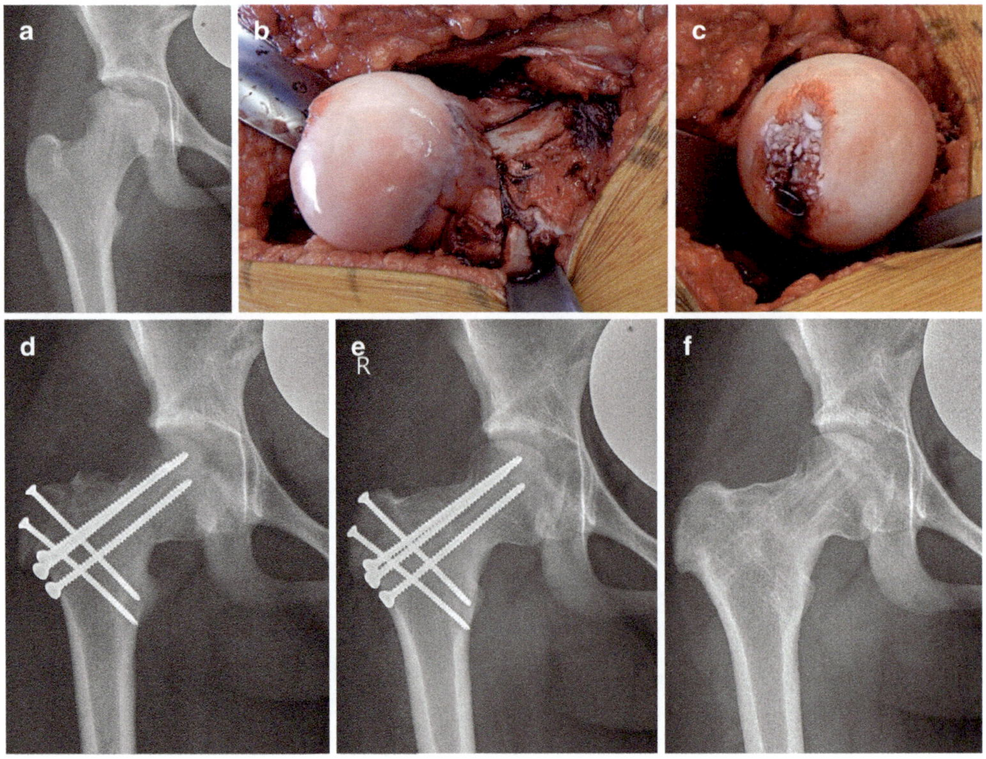

Fig. 11.6 (**a**-**c**) A 15-year-old female athlete with a history of progressive groin pain. The ap hip (**a**) taken from an ap pelvic radiograph shows a cystic femoral head lesion in a valgus-type head/neck configuration with marginal lateral head coverage. The osteochondral lesion might be due to osteochondritis dissecans or epiphyseal dysplasia (**b**). To redirect joint reactive forces, a varus femoral neck osteotomy was performed to unload the defect (**c**). At the same time, the suprafoveolar lesion was repaired by using a sandwich-type osteochondral/minced cartilage procedure using autologous material only (**d**-**f**) Six weeks (**d**), 6 months (**e**), and 2 years (**f**) following varus femoral neck osteotomy combined with sandwich MCI. After hardware removal, the joint space was preserved without signs of early OA. (Courtesy of Michael Leunig)

11.16 Controversies

- Hip preservation techniques are rapidly emerging and are also becoming increasingly available. A large number of varying techniques are available, but many of these do not have a long and robust track record.
- There is a relative paucity of studies available, especially as it relates to prospective, well-controlled, or long-term series studying cartilage restoration.
- Although robust studies are yet to be available, there is a growing body of evidence supporting the use of biological, surgical, and cell-based approaches to young patients with hip cartilage defects.
- Patients who have failed previous repair are a unique population where particular attention should be paid to potential underlying factors that may have led to the failure of previous repair efforts.
- Cartilage repair at the hip joint has the potential to postpone premature OA although complete prevention is unlikely.
- In the aftermath of hip joint cartilage repair, the patient requires a complex and long-lasting rehabilitation protocol that is as important as the intervention itself in order to protect the maturing cartilage and maximize the recovery potential.

11.17 Results

For the treatment of simple intra-articular acetabular and/or femoral cartilage lesions, hip arthroscopy is currently the preferred approach, with microfracture being the most widely used technique. For more complex deformities or larger lesions, open surgery remains the method of choice and provides the option of combining cartilage repair with osteotomies. There is no literature opposing the use of open surgical dislocation in these cases. Most of the current cartilage restoration techniques for the hip have been adapted from those used in knee surgery, though specific indications - such as lesion size and location - may differ. Mosaicplasty remains indicated for osteochondral lesions of the femoral head, particularly in younger patients, with currently limited clinical experience [7]. Recently, we have focused on our experience using AMIC [4, 8], which show promising outcomes for both femoral and acetabular lesions. In addition, emerging techniques such as minced cartilage repair should be considered in future evaluations for cartilage defects [6]. Advances in allogenic cartilage transplantation also hold promise; for instance, recent animal studies have demonstrated significant cartilage regeneration in osteochondral defects when cartilage fragments were applied to an acellular human scaffold in vitro. To establish evidence-based treatment protocols, further comparative prospective studies with larger sample sizes and longer follow-up periods are necessary. However, conducting such studies will be challenging due to the significant variability in case presentations and the complexity of the treatments involved.

11.18 Outlook

Today, there is limited available evidence for the hip regarding the best repair intervention, as most reported techniques lack long-term follow-up. Thus, it is imperative to the cartilage surgeon's practice to be aware of emerging modalities and the science supporting these modalities. When repairing hip joint cartilage, the underlying or co-exiting pathology has to be addressed as well, and the patient has to be educated about long-term rehabilitation protocols.

References

1. O'Connor M, Minkara AA, Westermann RW, Rosneck J, Lynch TS. Outcomes of joint preservation procedures for cartilage injuries in the hip: a systematic review and meta-analysis. Orthop J Sports Med. 2018;6(6):2325967118776944. https://doi.org/10.1177/2325967118776944. eCollection 2018 Jun
2. Cole BJ, Pascual-Garrido C, Grumet RC. Surgical management of articular cartilage defects in the knee. J Bone Joint Surg Am. 2009;91-A:1778–90.
3. Levinson C, Naal FD, Salzmann GM, Zenobi-Wong M, Leunig M. Is there a scientific rationale for the refixation of delaminated chondral flaps in Femoroacetabular impingement? A laboratory study. Clin Orthop Relat Res. 2020;478(4):854–67. https://doi.org/10.1097/CORR.0000000000001135.
4. Leunig M, Tibor LM, Naal FD, Ganz R, Steinwachs MR. Surgical technique second-generation bone marrow stimulation via surgical dislocation to treat hip cartilage lesions. Clin Orthop Relat Res. 2012;470(12):3421–31.
5. Salzmann GM, Ossendorff R, Gilat R, Cole BJ. Autologous minced cartilage implantation for treatment of chondral and osteochondral lesions in the knee joint: an overview. Cartilage. 2021;13(1_suppl):1124S–36S. https://doi.org/10.1177/1947603520942952. Epub 2020 Jul 25
6. Schumann J, Salzmann G, Leunig M, Rudiger H. Minced cartilage implantation for a cystic defect on the femoral head-technical note. Arthrosc Tech. 2021;10(10):e2331–e6.
7. Athanasiou V, Argyropoulou E, Antzoulas P, Lakoumentas J, Diamantakis G, Gliatis J. Mosaicplasty of the femoral head: a systematic review and meta-analysis of the current literature. Cureus 2022;14(11):e31874.
8. Briem T, Stephan A, Stadelmann VA, Fischer MA, Pfirrmann CWA, Rüdiger HA, Leunig M. Mid-term results of autologous matrix-induced chondrogenesis for large chondral defects in hips with femoroacetabular impingement syndrome." Bone Joint J 2024;106–B(5 Supple B):32–39.

Part 4

Specific Applications of SHD

12 Sliding Versus Step-Cut Trochanteric Osteotomy

Paul E. Beaulé and Hubert P. Nötzli

12.1 Introduction

The transtrochanteric approach offers a unique access to the hip allowing for a multitude of intracapsular procedures. Despite the attachment of the vastus lateralis, a slide (flat) osteotomy can sometimes be difficult to anatomically reduce and is less stable and, therefore, prone to malposition, secondary loss of reduction, and, as a consequence, impaired healing. Single-plane osteotomies are associated with inferior rotational stability as primary stability is limited, healing might occur with callus formation, and healing of the osteotomy requires partial weight-bearing for 6–8 weeks with restriction in range of motion (ROM). However, the slide osteotomy may be advantageous, especially when the trochanteric fragment requires substantial advancement. In contrast, in a step-cut osteotomy, the two planes and the step in between neutralize the proximal pull of the gluteus medius and minimus and hence avoid secondary proximal displacement of the trochanteric fragment. In addition, the step improves the rotational stability of the osteotomy and partial weight-bearing can be reduced to 4 weeks without limiting ROM.

12.2 Background

Surgical hip dislocation (SHD) is a technique that can hardly be overrated for its versatility and options to address intraarticular and extraarticular pathologies of the hip. The execution of this approach requires a transtrochanteric approach as introduced by Ganz et al. [1]. Since its original description, a trigastric osteotomy was advocated in order to counteract the forces of the gluteus medius and minimus by the vastus lateralis, and thus the forces on the trochanteric fragment are (partially) neutralized.

To minimize the risk of malreduction and to achieve a higher degree of primary stability, the step-cut trochanteric osteotomy was introduced [2]. The step facilitates the anatomic reduction of the trochanteric fragment. The step also provides a higher degree of primary stability, especially with regard to rotation, and resists proximal translation. The additional formation of an anterior bony ridge further enhances stability. Consequently, rehabilitation can be accelerated. Hardly any restrictions regarding ROM are necessary, and we advocate partial weight-bearing (half body weight) for a period of 4 weeks. By inserting a piece of bone, which can be obtained from the stable trochanter, into the step, the trochanter can even be distalized in a very controlled manner. Proximalization is possible by shortening the step.

12.3 Indications

In children, adolescents, and young adults, trochanteric healing is rarely a problem and a transtrochanteric approach will work well in most cases.

- *Slide Osteotomy:* If a trochanteric advancement is required, a sliding osteotomy might be preferable (easier) over step-cut osteotomy, as there is no obstacle to trochanteric advancement.
- *Step-Cut Osteotomy:* In all other patients and especially in patients with less strong bone (osteopenia), step-cut osteotomies (with/without an anterior ridge) are recommended to enhance primary stability and therefore reduce the risk of secondary displacement.

P. E. Beaulé (✉)
University of Ottawa, Ottawa, ON, Canada

Division of Orthopedic Surgery, Hawkesbury and District General Hospital, Hawkesbury, ON, Canada
e-mail: pbeaule@toh.ca

H. P. Nötzli
Hip Service, Orthopedics Sonnenhof, Berne, Switzerland
e-mail: hubertnoetzli@sonnenhof.ch

M. Leunig et al. (eds.), *Surgical Hip Dislocation*, https://doi.org/10.1007/978-3-031-70622-6_12

12.3.1 Contraindications

- Poor (sclerotic) bone quality at greater tuberosity (GT)
- Partial/complete abductor tear

12.4 Preoperative/Preinterventional Diagnostics

The evaluation begins with a complete physical exam, including determining hip function and ROM, abductor function and strength, leg length comparison, and the localization of any previous incisions.

For the radiographic assessment, the ap-pelvis and the Dunn view are the basic two views obtained for the initial morphologic assessment. Nowadays, MR and/or CT measurements, including torsional assessment, are performed in most cases. In order to perform the osteotomy safely, it is important to recognize anatomical variations and tailor the osteotomy accordingly. In particular, femoral torsion, caput collum diaphyseal (CCD) angle, position and shape of the greater trochanter, and shape and length of the neck are important anatomic features to consider. Residual deformities secondary to childhood hip disease such as Legg-Calvé Perthes, slipped capital femoral epiphysis, or prior childhood surgical procedures are often associated with trochanter deformities and/or abnormal trochanter position which requires careful planning and execution of the osteotomy.

12.5 Preoperative Planning/Computer Modeling

Determining the extent of femoral antetorsion based on either Dunn's view, axial imaging, and/or rotational MRI sections is particularly important because the extent of torsion significantly affects leg positioning for the correct osteotomy plane. For example, high femoral antetorsion carries an increased risk of the osteotomy ending up in the femoral neck, which should be avoided; therefore, the osteotomy should be performed with the hip internally rotated.

The orientation of the trochanter in varus or valgus hips is different, and the osteotomy plane must be adjusted in the transverse plane accordingly. The shape of the trochanter also plays a role. In the case of a diminutive trochanter, the fragment may be less than 1 cm thick at the thinnest point, whereas in the case of a larger trochanter, it may reach a considerable thickness. Due to anatomic variations, intraoperative landmarks are most helpful along with preoperative analysis in order to guide the osteotomy and to avoid any pitfalls.

Collision models, as described in Chap. 6, may be helpful to identify both intraarticular and extra-articular impingement (e.g., pelvic-trochanteric conflicts), to plan possible trochanter reorientation, and to allow for simulation of hip ROM after trochanteric advancement. Furthermore, collision models may help to identify new sites of impingement that can arise due to the gain in ROM.

12.6 Applied Anatomy

The transtrochanteric approach requires the creation of a trigastric trochanteric fragment that includes the attachments of the gluteus medius (except for a small portion of the posterior tendon that is left attached to the stable trochanter and is sharply divided), the gluteus minimus, and the tendon origin of the vastus lateralis. The anterior insertion of the vastus lateralis and the insertion of the piriformis are medial to the osteotomy line, although it should be noted that the piriformis insertion ends much more anterior than described in most anatomy books so that some fibers of the piriformis tendon may stay attached to the trochanteric fragment. One key principle of the approach is the protection of the deep branch of the medial circumflex femoral artery (MCFA), which passes superficial the obturator externus and deep to the short external rotators before it enters the capsule. This MCFA is protected as long as the quadratus femoris and the short rotator tendons remain attached. The lateral and medial retinacular vessels are exposed ventrally. These vessels are located in the connective tissue fibers of the retinaculum, which, inferiorly, is called the ligament of Weitbrecht. The ascending branch of the lateral circumflex femoral artery passes over the anterior base of the capsule and inserts into the posterolateral femoral head. During the procedure, this system is preserved during anteromedial capsular exposure and incision, as well as subsequent femoral neck shaping.

12.7 Specific Risks

Inaccurate position of the osteotomy

Excessively superficial osteotomy with a thin mobile trochanter

Excessive deep osteotomy with damage to the retinacular vessel or risk of femoral neck fracture

Trochanteric bursitis or erosion of the iliotibial band due to prominent trochanteric screws

Difficult hardware removal using 3.5-mm screws (screw breakage)

Heterotopic ossifications

Trochanteric pseudarthrosis/non-union

Femoral head necrosis (iatrogenic damage of the MCFA)

12.8 Type of Anesthesia

Although single shot spinal anesthesia is routine for a surgical dislocation in many centers, due to the lateral decubitus position and the benefits that muscle relaxation provides for exposure and less retraction, general anesthesia with neuromuscular relaxation may be preferable in very musclar patients.

12.9 Positioning

- The patient is positioned in the lateral decubitus position and the pelvis and trunk are secured with padded supports. The posterior support is positioned at the level of the iliac spine and placed low enough so that it does not interfere with the surgical field. The anterior support rests directly on the symphysis and should also not extend too far cephalad so as not to compress the bladder or abdomen. At the level of the rib cage, the trunk is stabilized with two more supports, one anterior and one posterior. The operative limb should be positioned on blanket rolls or a prefabricated tunneled positioner so that the limb is neither adducted nor abducted but neutrally aligned.
- The entire limb, hip, and lateral flank should be included in the sterile field. The leg is then covered starting at the foot with an impermeable stocking up to the transition proximal to the middle third of the upper thigh. The rest of the covering is done with U-shaped drapes over the groin and buttocks and proximal transverse drapes so that the surgical field extends from proximal to the iliac crest to the middle third of the thigh.
- The leg to be operated on is draped to allow free mobility. A sterile bag, placed on the anterior aspect of the patient and on the side opposite the surgeon, is placed so that it can temporarily accommodate the drooping lower leg without loss of sterility.
- The positioning should allow for any necessary intraoperative radiography.

12.10 Instruments/Implants

- An oscillating saw and osteotomes of various widths optimize the trochanteric osteotomy.
- Fully threaded screws of 3.5 mm or 4.5 mm diameter are required for fixation of the trochanter. The screw diameter can be determined by the size of the patient and the trochanteric fragment (Fig. 12.1).

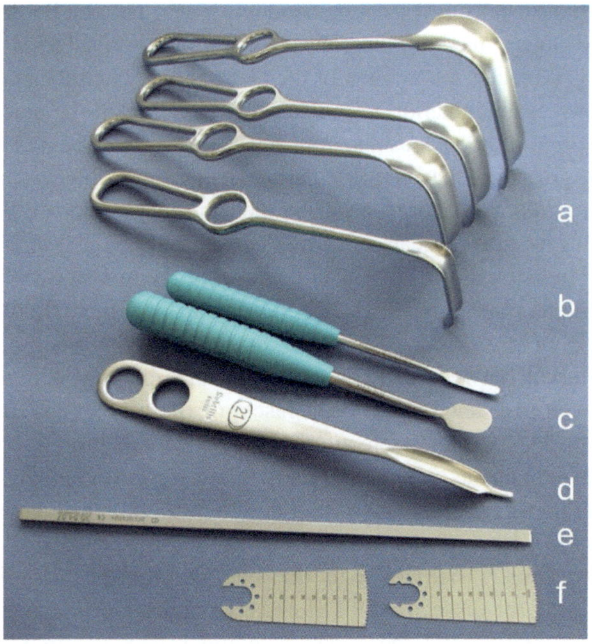

Fig. 12.1 Instruments for the trochanteric osteotomy
a) Langenbeck large and medium with rounded edges to gently hold the muscles away
b) Small Langenbeck for pulling the piriformis tendon distally to visualize the posterior edge of the gluteus minimus
c) Retractors to lift the vastus lateralis distal to the innominate tubercle from the bone
d) Narrow Hohmann to lift the mobilized vastus lateralis before the osteotomy, to lift and tilt the trochanteric fragment after completion of the osteotomy, and to expose the capsule
e) 6 mm osteotome
f) Two 0.6-mm-thick and, 2.7 cm wide and 7 cm long saw blades. The first saw blade is used for sawing. The second is inserted into the first osteotomy and serves as a guide for the 6-mm chisel to complete the step after the second osteotomy has been performed

12.11 Access

With the hip fully extended and slightly rotated inward (15°), a straight, longitudinal, lateral, 15–20 cm skin incision is centered over the greater trochanter. The length of the skin incision depends rather on muscle mass than on body size because muscular male patients require more proximal mobilization in order to minimize the necessary muscular retraction to provide adequate exposure. Approximately one-third of the incision is proximal to the tip of the greater trochanter, one-third is the length of the trochanter, and one-third is distal to it. Slightly less proximal extension is necessary for less robust individuals and for those with more subcutaneous tissue than muscular tissue and therefore more intrinsic mobility. The subcutaneous tissue is split in the same direction. The longitudinal incision of the IT band begins distally over the femur and follows the anterior border of the gluteus maximus muscle proximally, as described by Henry [3]. Typically, the incision of the IT band over the trochanter is between the anterior and middle thirds, although the anterior margin of the gluteus maximus muscle may also be anterior to the greater trochanter, particularly in patients with higher femoral antetorsion. In thin, muscular men, the anterior border of the Gluteus maximus can sometimes be palpated.

Incision of the IT band at the level of the first fibers of the gluteus maximus allows the incision to be adjusted anteriorly or posteriorly, to follow the interval proximally. The interval between gluteus maximus and gluteus medius is developed, leaving the deep fascia of the gluteus maximus muscle with the visible inferior gluteal vessels mobilized on the side of the gluteus maximus. This step is tricky because the gluteal fascia is fused to the gluteus medius just anterior to the gluteus maximus. Pushing the two muscles apart with two fingers helps define the interval during dissection. During the dissection, the gluteus maximus overlies the gluteus medius and the surgeon should reflect the maximus muscle posterior off of the gluteus medius. In athletic patients, the interval between the gluteus maximus and medius often needs to be developed more proximal to reduce tension on the gluteus maximus during dislocation. This extended release can also be done at later stages of the procedure as needed to reduce the soft tissue tension. It is helpful to positioning the hip in some extension while exposing Gibson's interval, many surgeons position a padded stand so that the hip can be slightly abducted and extended during the dissection and exposure.

Once released, the gluteus maximus muscle is retracted posteriorly, and the posterior border of the gluteus medius muscle is identified, mobilized, and elevated anteriorly to expose the piriformis tendon and gluteus minimus. Hip extension, abduction, and internal rotation facilitate exposure at this stage. Dorsally, at the greater trochanter, the bursal tissue is incised longitudinally and pushed away to expose the structures that attach to the posterior aspect of the greater trochanter and to visualize the trochanteric branch of the MFCA. The posterior origin of the vastus lateralis fascia, including usually strong connections to the gluteus maximus tendon and the linea aspera, is transected and the muscle is elevated extraperiosteally from the bone. It is important to maintain an extraperiosteal exposure as the periarticular fat is contiguous with the extraperiosteal space. The insertion of the vastus lateralis at the vastus lateralis ridge remains intact as it is attached to the mobile trochanter.

12.12 Technical Steps

After first using the traditional flat osteotomy, we switched to the step-cut osteotomy approximately 15 years ago [2] because it allows more precise reduction of the trochanteric fragment, facilitates rehabilitation, and is much more likely to heal without problems. The step-cut osteotomy of the trochanter has the same starting and ending points as a slide osteotomy. It begins at the posterosuperior tip of the greater trochanter and ends distally at the base of the innominate tubercle. For reference, the line of a straight osteotomy can be incised into the periosteum with a knife. This results in hemorrhage from the trochanteric end branches of the medial femoral circumflex artery, which are coagulated. The first (proximal) segment of the step osteotomy extends distally from the tip of the greater trochanter by approximately three-fifths of the length of the greater trochanter and ends 3 mm lateral to the plane of a straight osteotomy. The second (distal) segment of the osteotomy begins at the base of the innominate tuberosity, respectively, below the origin of the vastus lateralis, and extends proximally to a point 3 mm medial to the plane of a straight osteotomy and slightly proximal to the first incision. These two incisions are then connected by a third transverse cut, creating a Z-shaped osteotomy with an approximately 6-mm step (Fig. 12.2).

The position of the leg is critical for the osteotomy. When osteotomizing with the oscillating saw, the general plane of the osteotomy is parallel to the lateral surface of the trochanter. Therefore, not only the proximal end of a flat but also the stepped osteotomy (same end) will be more medial than the distal end when the femur is horizontal. This slope from proximal to distal can vary, however, and the plane may be nearly horizontal in patients with valgus neck deformity, while in varus hips, the tilt is much more pronounced.

The plane in the postero-anterior direction depends on hip rotation. To simplify and better control the osteotomy, it is

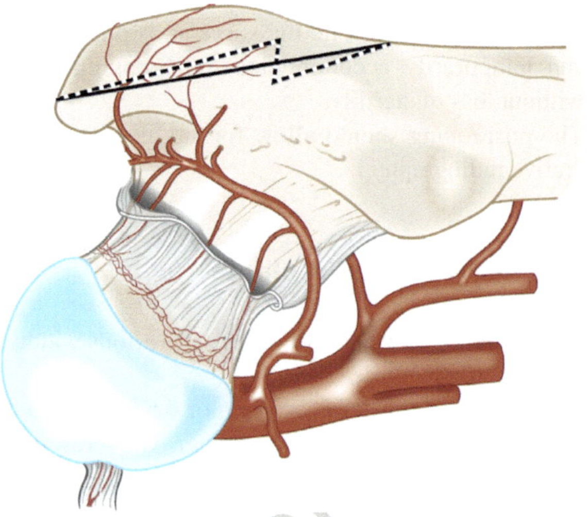

Fig. 12.2 Posterior aspect of the greater trochanter. The flat and the stepped trochanteric osteotomy and their relation to the vessels supplying the femoral head are shown. The angulation of the cut connecting both osteotomies may differ amongst surgeons with respect to its angulation

easiest to adjust the internal rotation of the hip so that the postero-anterior plane of the cuts can be made horizontally. The internal rotation is usually 15–20°, but the higher the antetorsion is, the greater the internal rotation must be to cut parallel to the lateral surface of the trochanter. In obese patients, the soft tissues may not allow a horizontal cut. In such cases, the obstruction caused by the soft tissues can be compensated by greater internal rotation and hip extension with a corresponding anterior inclination of the saw blade. In the case of pronounced retrotorsion, as can occur, for example, in post-SCFE hips, the leg is blocked in external rotation, so the saw cut must be directed from posterior inferior to anterior superior in order to attempt to maintain the intended osteotomy plane. Occasionally, the SHD is performed in conjunction with a femoral osteotomy. In such cases, it is helpful to preposition the plate prior to performing the step-cut osteotomy so that the two parts of the procedure do not interfere.

The thickness of the trochanteric fragment is determined by the size, shape, and curvature of the trochanteric tip and can vary considerably. To protect the deep branch of the medial circumflex artery, the osteotomy must not start medial to the trochanteric tip and enter the trochanteric fossa. Therefore, if the tip is unusually pointed, curved, or hooked, or if antetorsion is high, the proximal portion of the fragment may be only 5 mm thick. A safe landmark is to leave some fibers of the gluteus medius tendon attached to the posterosuperior tip of the trochanter when performing the osteotomy.

After manually incising the intended osteotomy path into the periosteum on the posterior aspect of the trochanter, especially at the trochanteric tip, the osteotomy is performed. For the less experienced surgeon, it makes sense to first mark a straight osteotomy line, followed by the lines for the stepped osteotomy, in which the proximal saw cut ends 4–6 mm lateral to the proximal end of the distal cut. The osteotomy path can be confirmed fluoroscopically using the edge of an osteotome to mark the level and trajectory of the planned osteotomy.

The cuts are preferably made with a thin, flexible saw blade (0.6 mm) which should be approximately 2.7 cm wide. This style of saw blade is easy to control and has a narrow kerf thus resulting in minimal bone loss. When cutting from posterior to anterior, the proximal cut should be angled 25–30° distally (caudally) so that the step tends to be slightly oblique from posterior to anterior. This slant resists the tendency of the fragment to shift anteriorly or proximally. A saw blade is inserted into the distal end of the first cut and serves as an alignment guide for the distal cut, which has its starting point 6 mm more medial proximally and should be as parallel as possible to the proximal osteotomy end. The distal alignment of the osteotomy surface however can be adjusted to match the attachment of the vastus lateralis. The cut should end distal and not within the tendon. The osteotomy is completed by connecting the two incomplete osteotomies with a thin, straight 5-mm osteotome. Once again, the saw blade of the first cut serves as a guide, as the osteotome can simply follow the distal edge of the saw blade up to and through the anterior cortex. Generally, when the connecting osteotomy is chiseled, the fragment lifts off the stable bone by itself. If not, residual bone bridges are cut with another thin osteotome and the fragment is tilted up with wide chisels placed into the osteotomies. Certain surgeons prefer not to osteotomize the ventral cortex and fracture it with the aim of achieving even greater interdigitation during refixation (Figs. 12.3 and 12.4).

The trochanteric fragment is elevated with a Hohmann retractor, and because the osteotomy enters through the tip of the trochanter where the dorsal tendon of the gluteus medius attaches, the tendon attachment must be released longitudinally, leaving the main portion of the tendon attached to the fragment. Bleeding is common from portions of the remaining slip, so vessels must be identified and coagulated. The remaining portion of the tendon on the stable trochanter can be sutured back to the main tendon during closure. An ideal osteotomy leaves the piriformis tendon insertion intact attached to the stable trochanter, but it is common to have some fibers attached to the mobile fragment. The piriformis tender usually inserts much more anteriorly than described in the textbooks, on the femur. The interval between the piriformis and the gluteus minimus is often easier to identify anteriorly. These must be identified and cut so that the fragment can then be fully tilted, but also elevated, when gradually exposing the capsule.

After performing the surgical procedures in and around the joint and closing the capsule, the trochanteric fragment is refixed.

If, during the same procedure, lengthening of the femur or a derotation osteotomy is performed, this should be done prior to fixation of the trochanter. If lengthening of the femur is needed, this should be done prior to fixation of the trochanter with the authors favoring the technique of Cauchoix [4]. The Cauchoix technique is basically a Z-shaped osteotomy with two-cerclage wires placed prior to the osteotomy being completed in order to avoid scissoring of the fragments the length of the longitudinal osteotomy line should be at least twice the length of the lengthening planned (Figs. 12.5 and 12.6).

To refix the trochanter, the leg is placed in the position used for the osteotomy. The osteotomy surfaces are cleared of blood clot and the trochanteric fragment is reduced and held in position. In the stepped osteotomy, the reduction is simple and the correct position is obvious. In the flat osteotomy, the reduction position is sometimes difficult to verify. Refixation is performed with two parallel 3.5-mm self-tapping steel screws angled approximately 45° in a dis-

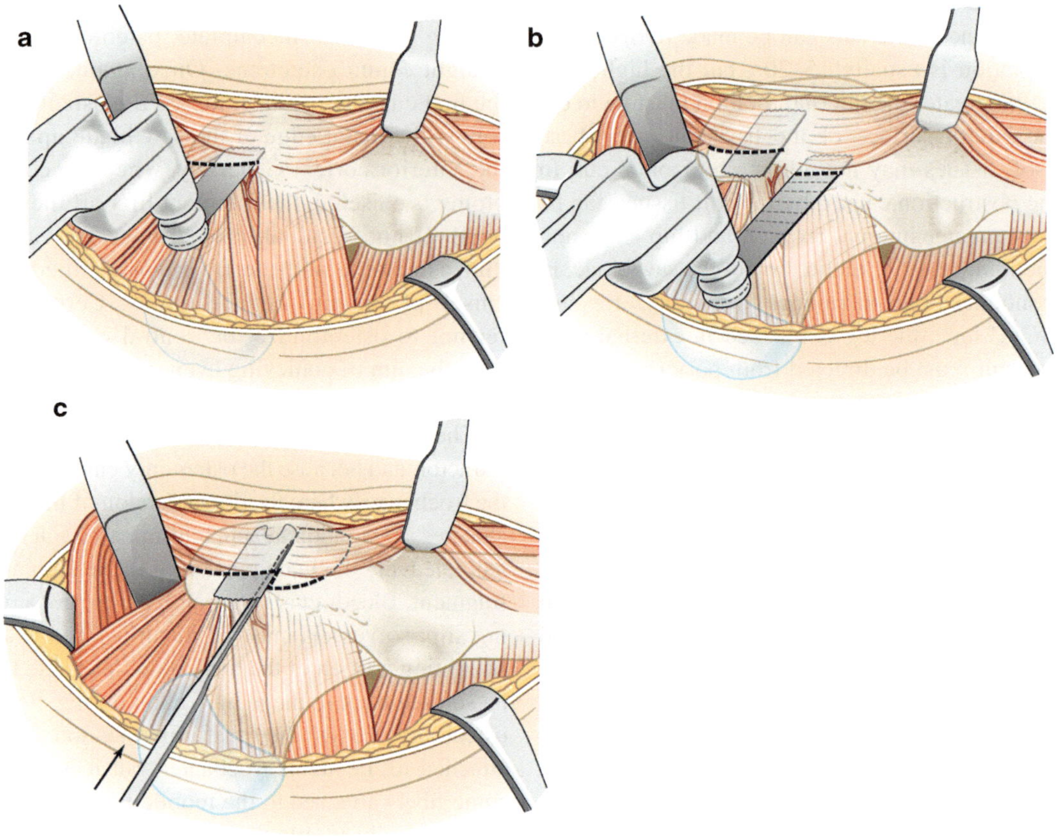

Fig. 12.3 (**a**) Schematic illustration of the first osteotomy starting at the tip of the greater trochanter. The saw cut ends at about three-fifths of the length of the trochanter fragment (**b**) The second osteotomy, starts 6 mm medial to the distal end of the first osteotomy or slightly proximal to it, with the cutting plane parallel to the first osteotomy. A saw blade is inserted into the first cut and serves as a guide to orient the second osteotomy (**c**) To complete the osteotomy, both cuts are connected with a 6-mm osteotome that follows the underside of the saw blade positioned in the first osteotomy

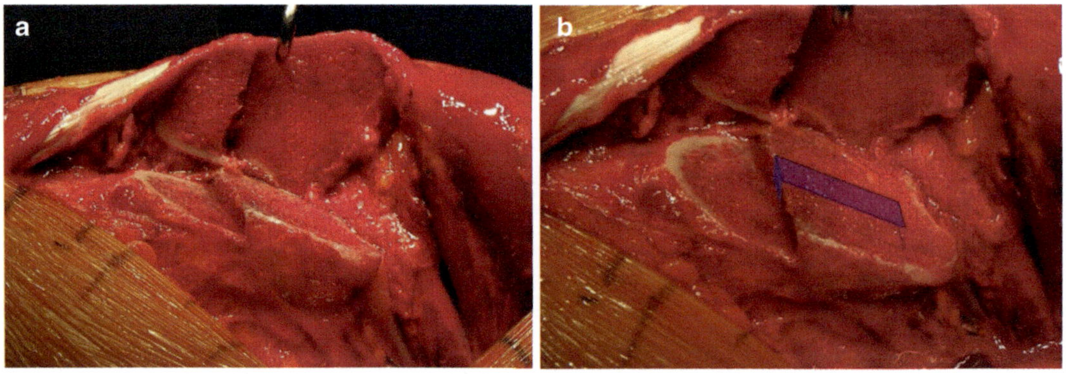

Fig 12.4 (**a**) The trochanteric fragment is flipped anterior, and the osteotomies are entirely exposed, with the gluteus medius and minimus muscles and the vastus lateralis muscle attached to the trochanteric fragment. (**b**) To obtain the bone block for precise distalization of the trochanter, the contour of the bone block is cut with a fine saw to the depth of the lower step, and the block is then undercut with a chisel, lifted out, rotated, and placed against the step before the mobile trochanter fragment is fitted and fixed into the new position

tal and slightly anterior direction to avoid screw placement through the trochanteric fossa. One screw is placed approximately through the center of the proximal osteotomy surface and the other through the center of the distal osteotomy surface. It is helpful to take advantage of the dense bone of the vastus tubercle by inserting the distal screw just proximal to the tubercle. Important in the case of flat osteotomies is that care should be taken to ensure that the screws are spaced sufficiently far apart to provide some stability of rotation to the fragment. Alternatively, 4.5-mm steel screws can be used for fixation which can lower the risk of screw head breakage at the time of removal, especially if screw removal is delayed. As mentioned earlier, the longitudinally split tendon attachment of the gluteus medius is carefully sutured back into place. The detachment of the vastus lateralis from the tendon of the gluteus maximus is also reclosed.

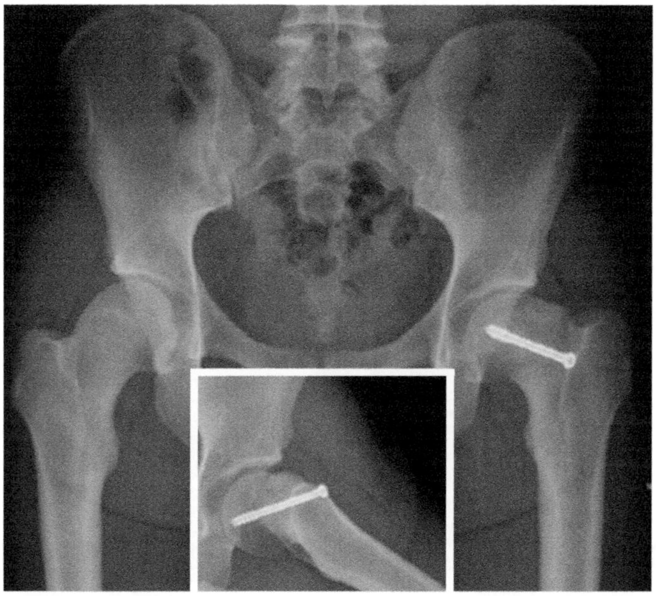

Fig. 12.5 A 19-year-old male with post-slipped deformity and 2 cm leg-length discrepancy

Final hemostasis control is followed by layered wound closure with continuous sutures and suturing of the skin. Drains are not inserted.

12.13 Postoperative Follow-Up

With flat trochanteric osteotomy, weight-bearing is limited to one-quarter of body weight, and flexion is limited to 70° for 6 weeks. Active abduction is not allowed. Transition to full weight-bearing is allowed only after radiographic control and evidence of consolidation.

If the step osteotomy is used, the patient is allowed to bear half body weight immediately following surgery and is permitted to full weight-bearing after 4 weeks without radiographic control. In addition, the joint may be flexed to 90° following surgery. One of our requirements for the patient to leave the hospital is to have achieved at least 70° of flexion with continuous passive motion.

In Europe, low-molecular heparin is administered until the patient is fully weight-bearing (4–6 weeks). In the United States and Canada, aspirin is given for VTE (venous thromboembolism) prophylaxis. To avoid intraarticular scarring, continuous passive mobilization of the hip is started on the day of surgery beginning at 30° of flexion and increasing to 90° as rapidly as possible. Patients are expected to use an ergometer at home three to four times daily for at least 10 min. They are also encouraged to regularly move their legs to the side while seated and to isometrically strengthen the quadriceps and hamstrings in extension. Stretching the quadriceps while standing is also instructed.

Fig. 12.6 2 years after step-cut trochanteric osteotomy, osteochondroplasty of the head-neck junction and subtrochanteric lengthening osteotomy

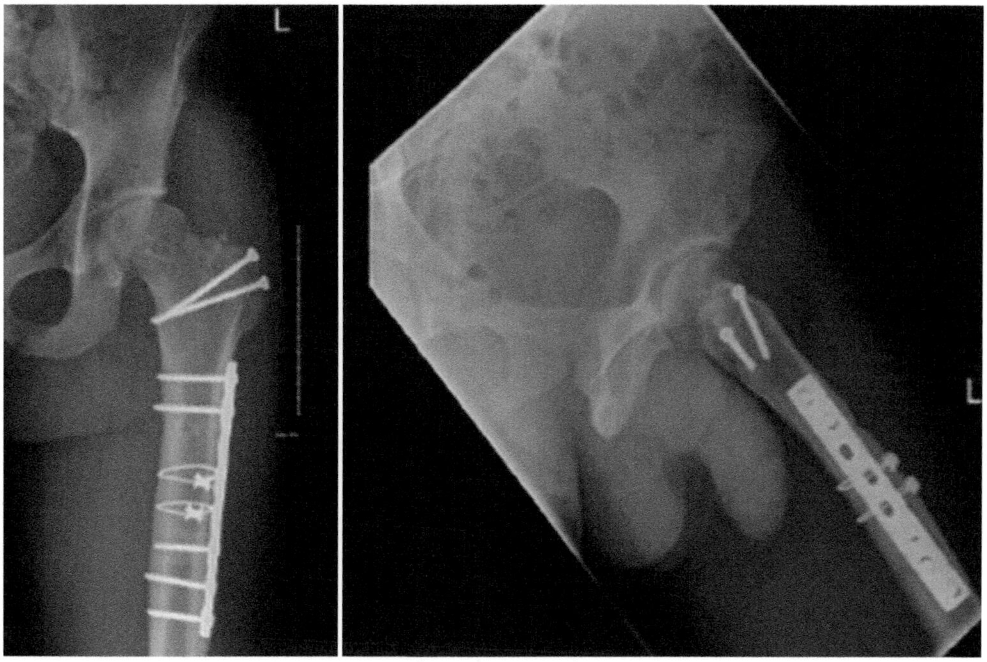

An anti-inflammatory medication (ibuprofen) is prescribed as prophylaxis for heterotopic ossification for the first 10 days postoperatively. On discharge, patients receive a physiotherapy prescription so that they can begin gait training, cane rehabilitation, and abductor rehabilitation from the fifth week.

The first clinical and radiological follow-up is performed after 6 weeks. When consolidation is assured, patients begin unrestricted passive and active movement therapy for joint mobilization and strengthening of the hip abductors as trunk strength. At the same time, sensorimotor exercises to promote neuromuscular control of the pelvis, trunk, and lower extremities are encouraged. A second clinical assessment is scheduled after 12 weeks. In most cases, trochanteric screw removal has been performed as an outpatient procedure by this time.

Some patients are unable to adequately retrain muscles due to irritation in the trochanteric region. Removal of the screws typically provides the necessary relief. We usually remove all screws 2–3 months postoperatively on an outpatient basis under local anesthesia and sedation with a single stab incision under fluoroscopic control. At this time, screw removal, which can be extremely difficult later (risk of screw breakages), is straightforward.

If patients still have limited joint mobility at the time of screw removal, mobilization in sedo-analgesia is highly effective.

12.14 Intra/Postoperative Complications

Intraoperative:

- Unicortical screw placement
- Fragment fracture
- Proud screw heads
- Gap between fragment and stable trochanter
- Too long screws irritating medial structures (Psoas)
- Step on the wrong side
- Too large/small trochanteric fragment

Postoperative:

- Fragment dislocation
- Delayed/non-union
- Ectopic ossifications

12.15 Case Studies (Figs. 12.7 and 12.8)

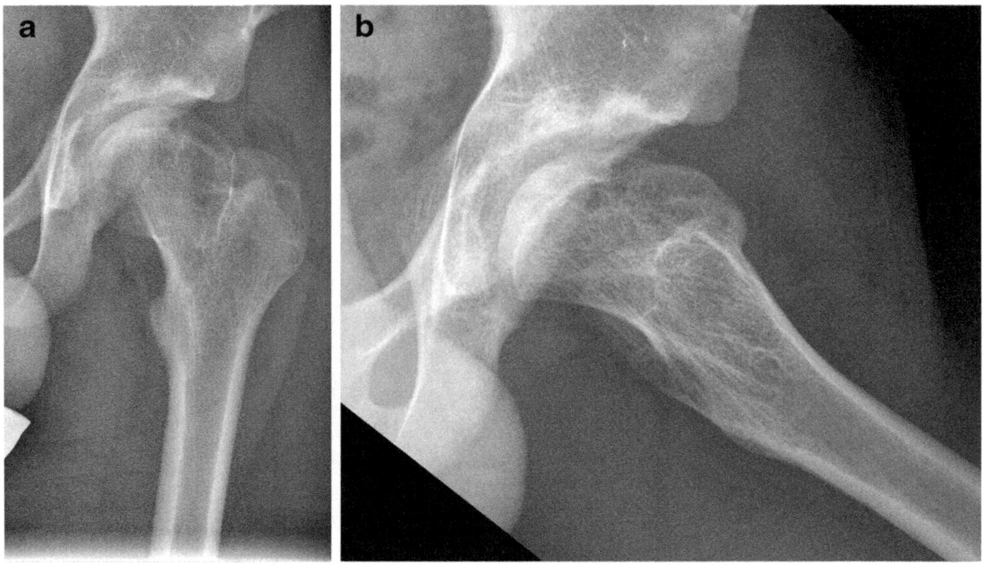

Fig. 12.7 (**a**) A 17-year-old patient with Perthes disease and multiple previous operations including a pelvic osteotomy, an SHD, and epiphysiodesis of the trochanteric growth plate. (**b**) Over 2 years time, a new cam deformation developed

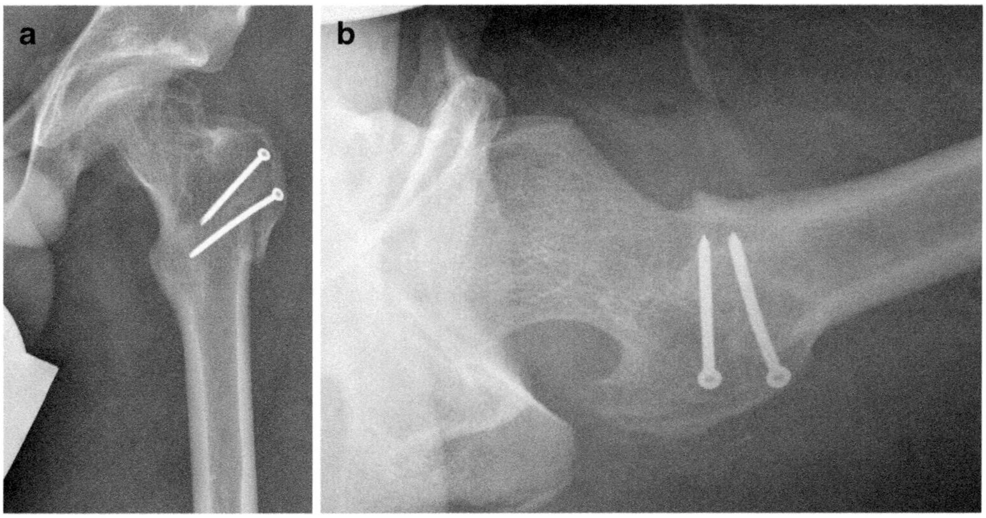

Fig. 12.8 Postoperative X-rays after SHD with plane trochanteric osteotomy for osteochondroplasty of the head-neck junction. 10 mm distalization of the trochanter inserting a 10-mm bone that was harvested from the trochanteric area

12.16 Controversies

In some cases, correction of the preoperative trochanteric position is indicated. With the flat osteotomy, transposition is easily accomplished, although the extent is relatively difficult to estimate. Fluoroscopy is helpful to verify distalization or proximalization. With the stepped trochanteric osteotomy, the correction can be very precise. For distalization, the step is extended distally by inserting a piece of bone of a predetermined size, resulting in the planned distal displacement of the trochanteric fragment during reduction. We obtain the bone piece usually from the trochanter. For the proximalization of the trochanter, the step is shortened by the desired amount using a saw and chisel, resulting in precise proximal displacement of the fragment. If trochanter displacement is planned, the osteotomy cuts are made at right angles to each other and not z-shaped. In addition, in this situation, the two osteotomy surfaces should be parallel.

There exist some technical differences amongst surgeons with respect to the orientation of the step cut (oblique versus orthogonal), the distal extent of the osteotomy (through or below the vastus lateralis ridge), and whether to leave an anterior ridge.

12.17 Expected Outcomes

Complications of SHD were analyzed in a study of 334 cases from eight centers in the United States [5]. Six trochanteric nonunions (1.8%) were reported, all of which healed by refixation. In the original report by Ganz on 213 hips [1], three cases (1.4%) required refixation of the trochanter. At that time, they were all flat osteotomies. In other series of using the flat osteotomy for hip resurfacing arthroplasty, the non-union rate was higher at 8.7% [6].

In a series of 233 cases, there was no osteonecrosis and no trochanteric nonunion with the stepped osteotomy [2]. In our personal series, these numbers are confirmed. Secondary dislocations of the fragment refixation are almost exclusively related to trauma, especially falls, which usually lead to instability or trochanteric displacement, rarely to fractures. The frequency is less than one percent. The osteonecrosis incidence also remained at 0%.

12.18 Future Direction

In the trigastric trochanteric osteotomy, the proximal pull of the gluteus medius muscle is partially neutralized by the distal pulling of the vastus lateralis. With the introduction of the step-cut, anatomic reduction and primary stability have been significantly increased and the risk of secondary displacement is minimized. This allows the hip to be moved postoperatively with only insignificant restrictions and the partial weight-bearing phase to be limited to 4 weeks. Rehabilitation after surgery is thus significantly shortened and patients regain mobility and strength much more quickly. Limited distalization or proximalization is also possible in a very controlled manner. Only in the case of corrections that exceed 1 cm in one direction, it is useful to consider whether a flat osteotomy is more appropriate.

References

1. Ganz R, Gill TJ, Gautier E, et al. Surgical dislocation of the adult hip: a technique with full access to femoral head and acetabulum without the risk of avascular necrosis. J Bone Joint Surg. 2001;83B:1119–24.

2. Bastian JD, Wolf AT, Wyss TF, Nötzli HP. Stepped osteotomy of the trochanter for stable, anatomic refixation. Clin Orthop Relat Res. 2009;467:732–8.
3. Henry AK. Extensile Exposure. Edinburgh: Churchill Livingstone; 1957.
4. Cauchoix J, Morel G, Rey JC, Cotrel Y, Ghosez JP. Single-stage lengthening of the femur. Record of the 1st 100 surgical cases. Rev Chir Orthop Reparatrice Appar Mot. 1972;58(8):753–74.
5. Sink EL, Beaulé PE, Sucato D, et al. Multicenter study of complications following surgical dislocation of the hip. J Bone Joint Surg Am. 2011;93:1132–6.
6. Beaulé PE, Shim P, Banga K. Clinical experience of Ganz surgical dislocation approach for metal-on-metal hip resurfacing. J Arthroplasty. 2009;24(6 Suppl):127–31.

Relative Femoral Neck Lengthening with Advancement of the Greater Trochanter

13

Ernest L. Sink and Martin Beck

13.1 Background

Deformity: There are many different variations in the shape and position of the greater trochanter. A high-riding greater trochanter (GT) or relative overgrowth of the trochanter often is the consequence of:

- Femoral head ischemic necrosis as a complication of conservative treatment of hip dysplasia.
- Consequence of hematogenous osteomyelitis in very early childhood,
- Legg-Calvé-Perthes disease (LCPD).
- Sequela of slipped capital femoral epiphysis (SCFE).
- other rare reasons such as skeletal dysplasia [1]

Deformities with a high-riding trochanter and short femoral neck may lead to extra-articular pelvitrochanteric impingement from the greater and lesser trochanter but also to intra-articular impingement due to the shortened and enlarged femoral neck abutting the acetabular rim. Relative trochanteric overgrowth is the result of a growth disturbance of the capital femoral epiphysis, leading to a shortened neck. The physis of the trochanter usually is not affected and the trochanter grows to its normal size [2]. This chapter focuses on hips with relative overgrowth of the greater trochanter.

Trochanteric development/growth: On the basis of tetracycline studies in pigs, Langenskiöld and Salenius deduced that about half of trochanteric growth can be attributed to growth of the apophysis. The other half is formed by appositional growth at the periphery of the trochanter [3]. This was confirmed clinically by Gage and Cary [2]. Trochanteric growth is present up to the age of 12 in females and 13 in males [4].

Position relative to femur: The trochanter usually is slightly posterior to the axis of the femoral neck but also can be rotated or tilted posteriorly [5]. A posterior rotation and tilt is often seen in low antetorsion and may lead to an increased functional antetorsion with similar effects as in-toeing gait, like in high anatomical antetorsion. At the level of the base of the femoral neck, about half of the trochanter overhangs posteriorly. The posterior overhang continuously decreases until it merges with the femoral shaft at the level of the lesser trochanter.

Muscular insertions: The greater trochanter is comprised of four facets with specific muscular attachments (Fig. 13.1a, b):

- The anterior facet is the location of the bony insertion of the gluteus minimus tendon. The shape of the insertion area can be variable [6]. Medial to it, often a subminimus bursa can be found.
- The posterior facet includes the posterior aspect of the greater trochanter. There is no muscular attachment in this area. It forms part of the visceral side of the trochanteric bursa.
- The posterior-superior facet is the site of the tendinous part of gluteus medius insertion.
- Gluteus medius insertion continues along the distal border of the lateral facet. Piriformis attaches anterior to the insertion of G. medius on the tip of GT. Between piriformis insertion and the insertion of G. medius, a "bald spot" is present that is covered by the subgluteus bursa [7].

Consequences of trochanteric position: A more proximal greater trochanter results in abductor dysfunction secondary to decreased lever arm and shortened acting muscle length with the gluteus medius having a mechanical disadvantage when the insertion is proximal to the center of hip rotation. The most efficient mechanics of the gluteal muscles is when the tip of the greater trochanter is located at the level of the center of hip rotation [8].

E. L. Sink (✉)
HSS Hip Preservation and Pediatric Service, Hospital for Special Surgery, New York, NY, USA
e-mail: sinke@hss.edu

M. Beck
Orthopaedic Clinic Lucerne, Hirslanden Clinic St. Anna, Lucerne, Switzerland
e-mail: martin.beck@okl.ch

M. Leunig et al. (eds.), *Surgical Hip Dislocation*, https://doi.org/10.1007/978-3-031-70622-6_13

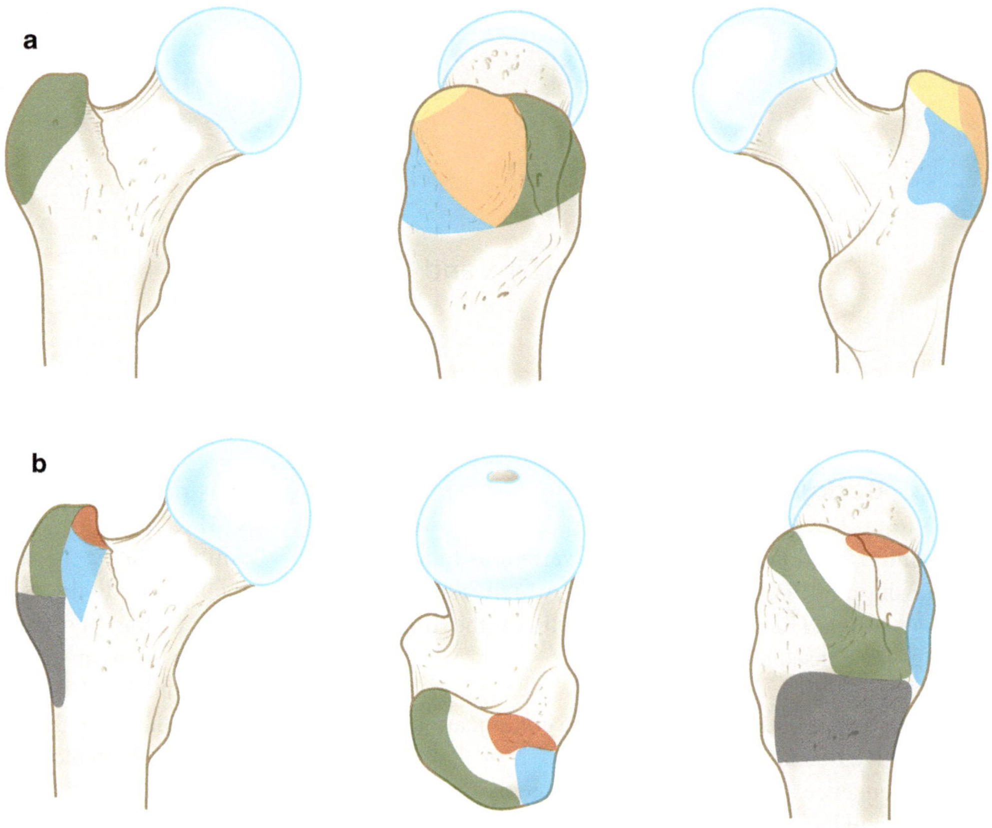

Fig. 13.1 (**a**) The greater trochanter has four facets. Postero-superior (yellow), posterior (blue), lateral (orange) and anterior facet (green) (**b**) Location of the insertion of abductor musculature. The postero-superior facet holds the insertion of the tendinous portion of gluteus medius (green). Along the inferior aspect of the lateral facet the more muscular part of gluteus medius inserts (green). Gluteus minimus (blue) inserts on the anterior facet, which is also covers by a bursa, underlying the tendon of gluteus minimus. Between gluteus medius insertion and the insertion of piriformis tendon (red) there is a bald spot. Vastus lateralis (grey) originated from the lateral femur distal of the vastus lateralis ridge

The best example of a proximal femoral abnormality that limits hip motion and results in extra-articular impingement is LCPD. In LCPD, the relative overgrowth of the greater trochanteric apophysis and distal femoral neck metaphysis relative to the capital portion of the femoral physis results in a short, widened femoral neck and a large, more proximally positioned trochanter, both disadvantageous for lever arm and muscle function. In contrast to is considered a primary trochateric deformity, the growth of the greater trochanter is actually normal while the physis in the femoral epiphysis is abnormal, resulting in a short neck, so that it appears there is "overgrowth" of the trochanter. The proximal, overgrown greater trochanter may limit abduction by impinging on the ilium with abduction. The anterior aspect and facet of the trochanter may impinge on the Anterior Inferior Iliac Spine (AIIS) or the anterior aspect of the acetabular rim with hip flexion and internal rotation. The posterior aspect of the overgrown greater trochanter may impinge on the ischium or posterior/inferior ilium with external rotation. The result of trochanteric impingement is limitation hip abduction, internal rotation, and external rotation. Also, due to diminished lonitudinal growth, the femoral neck is relatively shortened and widened femoral and can cause impingement with the acetabular rim.

In non-LCPD, more subtle variations in the position or the size of the greater trochanter may result in extra-articular impingement even within physiologic range of motion (Fig. 13.2). Variation in femoral neck length can also change the distance of the greater trochanter to the pelvis, potentially impacting the presence of trochanteric impingement with hip motion. Proximal femoral torsion also affects the position of the greater trochanter relative to the pelvis and contributes to extra-articular impingement. In high proximal femoral antetorsion, the greater trochanter may be more posterior and at greater risk of impinging with the inferior ilium or ischium. In retrotorsion, portions of the distal femoral neck or anterior trochanter may impinge on the anterior acetabulum with hip flexion.

Portions of the posterior superior trochanter may also be rotated more posterior and medial. This may be seen in hips with low antetorsion. The retroverted femoral neck may lead to anterior FAI, at the same time the posterior position of the greater trochanter may lead to a functional femoral antetorsion, forcing the hip into internal rotation [5]. There is the potential impingement of the greater trochanter against the ischium in external rotation and extension. This may potentiate anterior hip instability and compression sciatic nerve symptoms. Three-dimensional evaluation of the acetabulum should also evaluate for concurrent acetabular anteversion.

There may also be a prominent anterior facet of the greater trochanter. This may result in impingement against the anterior acetabulum or region of the AIIS.

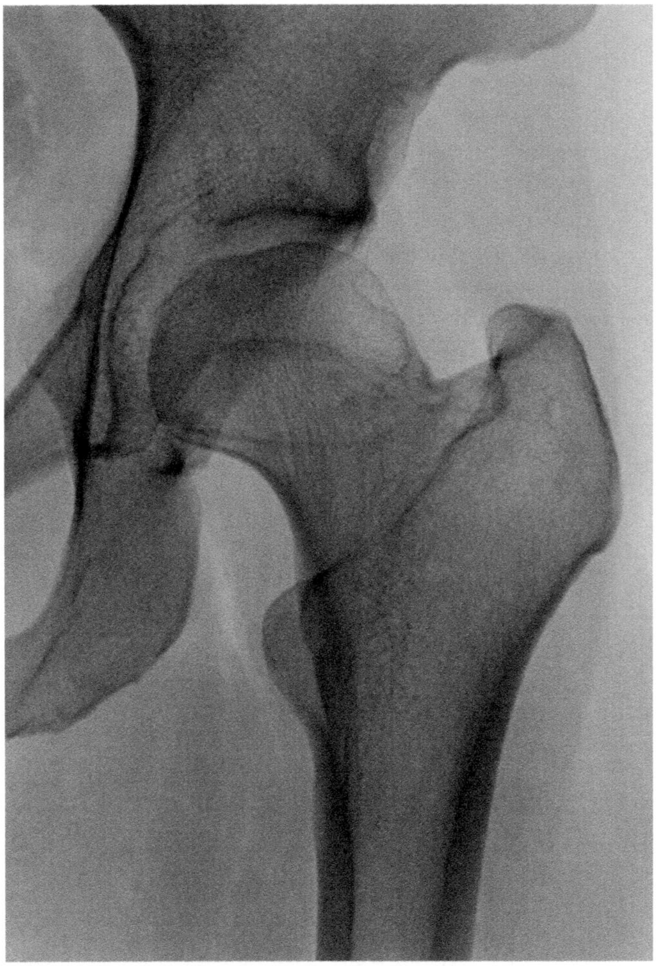

Fig. 13.2 Deformity of the proximal femur resulting from arrest of the lateral proximal femoral physis with a high positioned greater trochanter may result in extra-articular impingement, limited range of motion and poor abductor function, and a wider, shorter femoral neck causing intra-articular impingement

Ideal Position of the Greater Trochanter The optimal position from a mechanical perspective is when the tip of the greater trochanter is level with the center of hip rotation [8]. When the greater trochanter is too proximal, it can alter the mechanics of the abductor muscles particularly the gluteus medius. The gluteus medius muscle is a large fan-shaped muscle that has anterior, posterior, and central components. In flexion the anterior segments shorten and the posterior segments lengthen while the central component remains isometric. During extension the opposite occurs where the posterior fibers shorten and the anterior fibers lengthen. Alteration of the position of the greater trochanter will disrupt the muscle balance of the gluteus medius [9]. For example, too much distalization results in the isometric point moving more anterior resulting in less active muscles for flexion, and the opposite occurs with distalization. Too much distalization will increase the passive tension of the gluteal muscles but may result in loss of muscle strength due to excessive sarcomere length. Clinically, this may result in abductor muscle fatigue and discomfort. In the frontal plane, both proximal and distal positioning of the greater trochanter can alter lateralization which may impact the abductor lever arm. While lateralization may not affect the balance of the muscles, and is debated how muscle function is affected by increasing the lever arm of the muscle, it may lead to increased pressure from the overlying iliotibial band that can cause bursitis.

13.2 Indications for Surgery and Relative Neck Lengthening

Many patients with proximal femoral alterations may have compensated any muscle dysfunction and have no symptoms or limitations, and, therefore, seldom require surgical treatment. Those patients that do have symptoms of muscle insufficiency and/or pain at the greater trochanter with distal radiation should first receive physical therapy to improve the gluteal muscle strength. If nonoperative treatment is not successful, surgery is considered. First, many patients with Perthes-like deformity may have significant arthrosis as early as their 30 s, so evaluation with imaging and MRI should rule out osteoarthritis (OA). Common physical exam findings are the following:

- Limited abduction, limited and painful internal and external rotation [1]
- Positive Flexion, Adduction, Internal Rotation Test (FADIR)
- Positive apprehension test
- Signs and symptoms of impingement, positive FADIR, and pain with rotation but no significant cam deformity may indicate impingement from a shortened femoral neck or alterations of the trochanter resulting in extra-articular Femoroacetabular Impingement (FAI).
- This technique can also be used to transfer a malunited greater trochanter after fractures of the proximal femur. The osteotomy and resection of the base of the trochanter are executed in the same fashion with reattachment of the trochanter at its anatomic position.

13.2.1 Contraindications to Surgery Include

- OA based on X-ray or MRI.
- Age > 40 years is a relative contraindication

13.3 Preoperative/Preinterventional Diagnostics

- Anterior-posterior (AP) radiograph of the pelvis as well as Lauenstein or Cross table lateral view
- AP hip view in abduction to confirm impingement and/or leverage.
- MRI of the symptomatic hip
- CT with 3D reconstructions to identify anatomy and position of the greater trochanter, version, and femoral head and neck shape.

13.4 Preoperative Planning

- Surgical Hip Dislocation (SHD) enables the surgeon to asses intra-operative observation with range of motion. Even following osteotomy of the greater trochanter, the conflict between the trochanter and pelvis is visible. This will allow direct observation of extra-articular FAI from regions of the greater trochanter. Any articular impingement from the wider metaphyseal region and intertrochanteric line can also be assessed.
- With SHD the surgeon should also be prepared to perform any of the following procedures that can be done concurrently:
  - Extended retinacular flap [10, 11]:
    - Exposure of the complete femoral neck to the lesser trochanter is not always necessary, but the concept is similar.
    - Distalization (advancement) of the trochanteric fragment. Careful preoperative planning should be used to calculate the distance that the trochanter should be advanced so that the proximal tip of the trochanter is located at the center of hip rotation.
    - Anterior placement or rotation of the fragment.
  - Femoral osteotomy in cases of torsion extremes.
  - Periacetabular osteotomy.
  - Resection of the anterior or posterior/superior facet of the greater trochanter.

13.5 Applied Anatomy

- A prerequisite for performing a relative neck lengthening is the fully performed SHD (see Chap. 7).
- The deep branch of the medial femoral circumflex artery (MFCA) runs close to the medial wall of the greater trochanter. In the normal hip, this branch runs posterior to the tendon of obturator externus and continues anterior to the tendon of obturator internus and then onto the femoral neck (see Chap. 6). In hips with growth disturbance of the femoral head and neck (relative overgrowth of the greater trochanter), the exact course of the deep branch of the MFCA is highly variable. However, the insertion of the obturator externus is proximal to the growth plate of the greater trochanter (Fig. 13.3) and is consistently located even in hips with high-riding trochanter (Fig. 13.4). Since the anatomic relationship is consistent, even in distorted growth, one can conclude that the deep branch runs as in normal hips posteriorly over the obturator tendon and from there "down" to the femoral neck.
- The greater trochanter has a threefold vascular supply [12]. Preserving it as much as possible improves healing of the osteotomy:
  - The internal iliac system via G. medius and minimus
  - Transverse branch of the Lateral Femoral Circumflex Artery (LFCA)
  - Descending branch of the LFCA (via V. lateralis)
- The size of the greater trochanter is not significantly different in normal hips and hips with growth disturbance of the femoral head and neck. The trochanter-to-trochanter distance (TTD) remains similar [1].

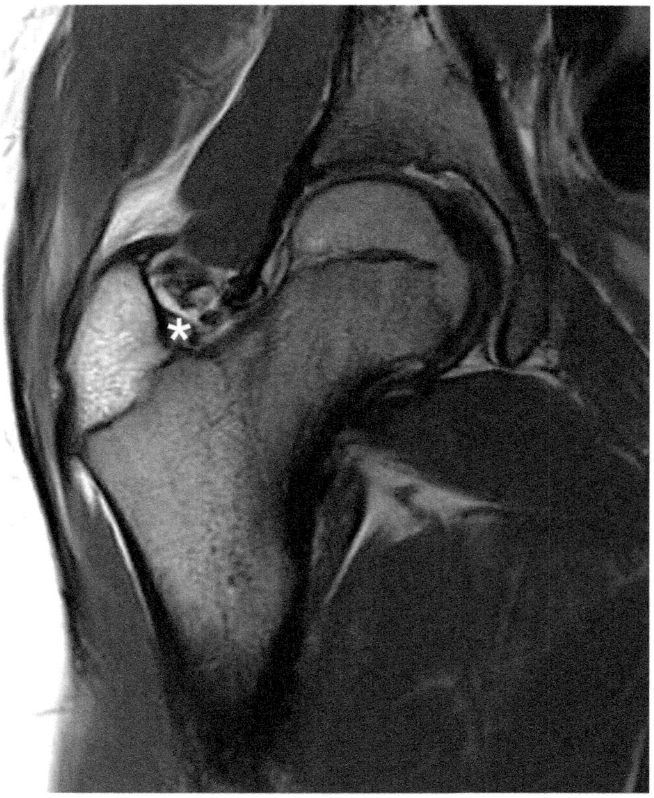

Fig. 13.3 MRI image of a proximal femur. The insertion (*) of the obturator tendon is proximal to the growth plate of the greater trochanter, at the base of the femoral neck

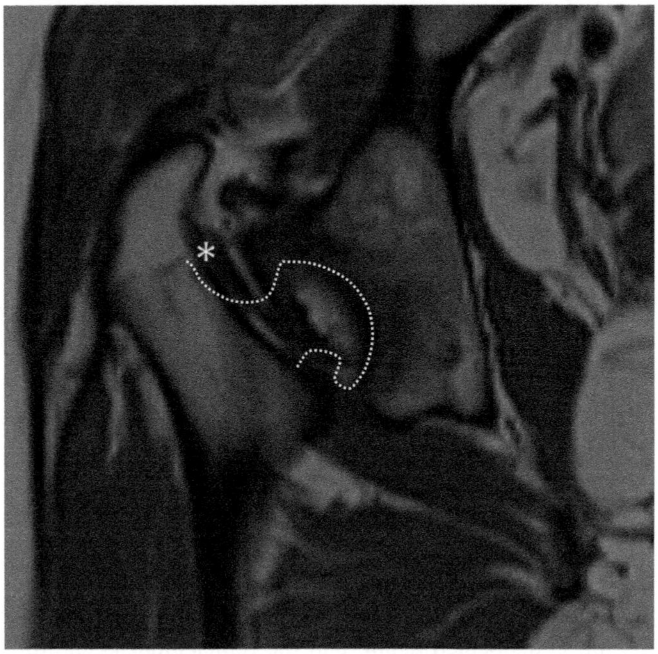

Fig. 13.4 MRI image of a patient with a high-riding trochanter. The Insertion of obturator externus (*) remains proximal of the trochanteric growth plate, being now high above the base of the femoral neck. The projection of the femoral head and neck is outlined with the dotted line

13.6 Special Risks

- Risks related to the technique of SHD (see Chap. 7)
- Damage to the deep branch of the MFCA with avascular necrosis of the femoral head
- Nonunion of the greater trochanter
- Dislocation of the greater trochanter
- Fracture of the greater trochanter
- Intertrochanteric fracture if trochanteric fragment is too big
- Over or under translation of the greater trochanter

13.7 Type of Anesthesia

The procedure can be done with either a general or spinal anesthesia. A general anesthesia may be preferable in children and adolescents. Good relaxation may make it easier to advance the greater trochanter.

13.8 Positioning

- Standard operating table.
- Lateral positioning with tunnel cushion and anterior sterile bag (see also Chap. 4.1).
- Fluoroscopy should be available.

13.9 Instruments/Implants

Standard instrumentation for SHD (see Chap. 7). In addition to the instruments required for the SHD, the following special instruments ensure an optimal surgical procedure:

- Curved and straight Lambotte-type chisels 10 mm 15 mm.
- 1 metal hammer 300gr.
- Strong forceps or small Luer.
- All cutting instruments should be checked for optimal sharpness prior to surgery.
- For refixation of the trochanter usually 2 or 3 3.5 mm or 4.5 mm are necessary.
- Osteotomy plates in case of additional osteotomy of the proximal femur.

13.10 Access

- Access as for SHD (see Chap. 7).

The osteotomy of the GT is performed as in a SHD mostly with a slide and occassionally a stepped osteotomy if minor distalization is needed (Chap. 12).

13.11 Technical Steps

- Flat osteotomy, starting at the tip of the GT and extending to the vastus lateralis ridge. A step-cut osteotomy is usually not suitable, because the trochanter rquired greater than 1 cm of advancement. Anatomy and future position of the trochanter must be taken into consideration, and the osteotomy may have to be adapted accordingly. As the trochanter is normally sized and shaped, the same consideration about thickness and length need to be made as in a standard SHD. Sometimes it may be helpful to extend the osteotomy more distal to get a larger contact area of the osteotomy to facilitate consolidation. It is helpful to preoperatively template the desired position of the greater trochanter and to outline the osteotomy using intraoperative fluoroscopy.
- If internal rotation is limited, performing the trochanteric osteotomy might be more difficult with an increased risk of an anteriorly deeper and intra-articular osteotomy course.
- The dissection of the interval between M. piriformis and G. minimus is frequently more difficult because the piriformis muscle/tendon rather runs cephalad, overlapping the interval between these two muscles.
- Because the femoral head and neck are shortened, the distances are usually very short and dissection of the joint capsule can be difficult especially in hips with previous childhood surgery.

- Once the capsule is prepared, the capsulotomy is performed. As a general rule, it is performed as in a regular SHD. The shape is Z-like with the longitudinal limb starting at the acetabular rim posterior of the iliofemoral ligament, aiming to a point at the base of the femoral neck, anterior to the base of the trochanter. It then continues distally along the intertrochanteric line. Proximally the capsule is detached from the acetabular rim in an anterior to posterior direction. In a situation with a very short neck and therefore very prominent trochanter, it may be necessary to first remove the base of the trochanter to get access to the acetabular rim.
- After the capsulotomy is completed, the hip is dislocated. The leg is positioned in the anterior sterile bag that is attached to the operating table, and the head is dislocated. When present, The Lig. teres is divided; however, often the Lig. teres is already ruptured. Some hips may have had previous surgery (i.e., open reduction, resection of the Lig. teres, etc.), and there may be extensive scaring between the fovea of the femoral head and/or Lig. of Weitbrecht. This scar tissue has to be released carefully before dislocation may be possible. Once the hip is dislocated, it can be inspected for cartilage damage, labral pathology and femoral torsion, etc.
- The hip is relocated and internally rotated such that femoral part of the trochanter is well exposed. Following the preoperative planning, the trochanter is then removed in a piecemeal fashion down to its base (Fig. 13.5a). Sometimes this step has to be performed prior to the dislocation to get access to the superior capsule. The technique is identical to the development of a lateral retinacular flap (see Chap. 8). Starting at the tip of the greater trochanter, a fragment of about 10 × 5 mm is osteotomized. The osteotome is not driven completely through the bone but stops short of the medial cortex adjoining the soft tissues in the piriformis fossa. The weakened bone is fractured with the thumb or by levering the osteotome (Fig. 13.5b). This technique avoids uncontrolled penetration of the osteotome into piriformis fossa with the potential to damage the deep branch of the MFCA. The blood vessel runs in areas only 2–4 mm away from the medial cortex and can be damaged. The mobile fragment is everted with a sturdy forceps or a small Luer such that the soft tissues on the inner side can be dissected off with a scalpel (Fig. 13.5c). If the fragment is too small, it is difficult to hold with an instrument and if it is too big it may not be possible to evert it.
- This is repeated from proximal to anterior and proximal to distal until the base of the femoral neck is reached. The hip is dislocated again, and the retinaculum is carefully mobilized from the anterolateral neck with a blunt periosteal elevator. This exposes the base of the femoral neck. The neck now can be trimmed with a curved osteotome and shaped as required.
- Intra-articular work is done as planned and the capsule is closed.
- The trochanter is positioned based upon preoperative planning typically in a distalized and slightly anterior position. The tip of the trochanter should be approximately at the level of the center of the femoral head and

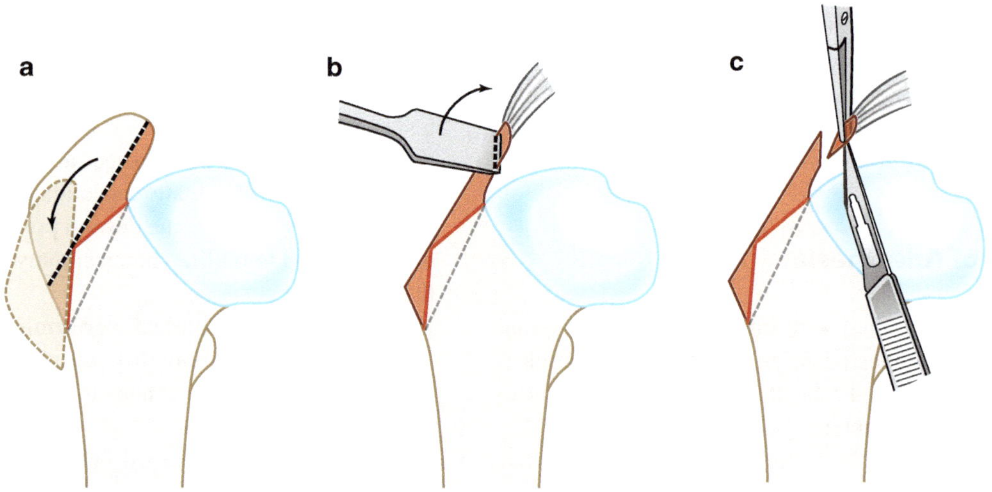

Fig. 13.5 (**a-c**) Drawings illustrating the careful excision of the stable part of the trochanter for the relative neck lengthening (area between the two black dotted lines). (**a**) Preoperative planning of the resection and future position of the greater trochanter. (**b**) The osteotome is driven into the bone without perforating the medial cortex. It is then levered to break the fragment to protect the soft tissues including the blood supply on the inner aspect of the trochanter. Sometimes the bone is fractures with a push with the thumb. (**c**) The fragment is peeled off the soft tissues with a scalpel. Further resection of the reddish area and down to the dotted line in a piece meal technique, carefully respecting the periosteum and retinaculum

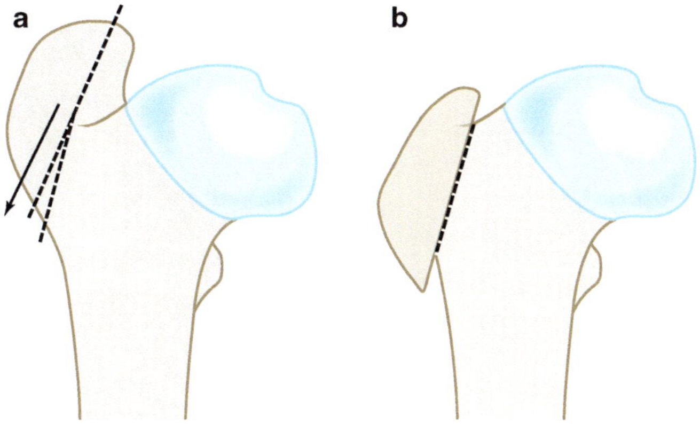

Fig. 13.6 (**a**, **b**). Advancement of the trochanter including attached musculature. (**a**) Short dotted line indicates eventual additional osteotomy to lateralize the tip of the trochanter. (**b**) Definitive position of the trochanter with relative lengthening of the postero-lateral neck, increasing the pelvis-trochanteric clearance

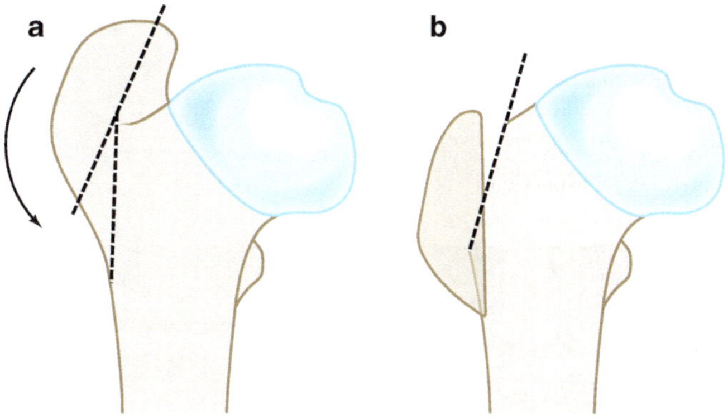

Fig. 13.7 (**a**, **b**) Further advancement of the trochanter. (**a**) **short** dotted line indicates osteotomy in line with the lateral cortex. (**b**) tip of the trochanter levels now the center of the head and the muscular lever arm is longer. The gap between GT and femur can be filled with bone chips to support the fragment from tilting

provisionally fixed with one or two K-wires. The position can be assessed with intraoperative fluoroscopy. Impingement free range of motion is checked, and if necessary the position of the trochanter is adjusted.

- Sometimes, in cases with significant distalization, the trochanter rotates posteriorly. This is caused by the pull of the gluteus minimus tendon. Lengthening the G. minimus tendon at the trochanter solves this problem and the trochanter can be distalized without rotation of the fragment. It is important to plan the osteotomy of the greater trochanter carefully to avoid excessive obliquity so as to enable proper lateralization and distalization of the trochanter without inadvertently tilting the trochanter while repositioning.
- There are two options where to place the trochanter. In hips with sufficient femoral offset, the trochanter is moved distally along the osteotomy plane (Fig. 13.6a, b). If the femoral offset is short, it may be preferable to lateralize the tip of the trochanter. In this case an oscillating saw is used to prepare a new bed more parallel to the shaft of the femur to increase the distance between femoral head and greater trochanter. A piece of bone may be interposed proximally to support the position of the trochanter (Fig. 13.7a, b). Prior to fixation of the greater trochanter it is helpful to confirm radiographically that the trochanter is positioned accurately.
- The trochanter is osteosynthesized with 2 3.5 mm screws. In some situations, 3 screws may be necessary. In sufficiently large trochanters, osteosynthesis using two 4.5 mm can be used sometimes supplementing with washers. The disadvantage of 4.5 mm screws is that they always cause irritation of the iliotibial band and have to be removed, whereas 3.5 mm screws often are asymptomatic, without need for removal,
- The distal gap between the trochanter and the femoral shaft is filled with cancellous bone.
- Some hips may need an additional intertrochanteric osteotomy. In such cases the trochanter is reduced and preliminarily fixed with K-wires. After execution of the intertrochanteric osteotomy, the osteotomy plate is fixed to the proximal femur, including the greater trochanter, before it is screwed to the distal part. The choice of the implant depends on the experience of the surgeon. Classic osteotomy plates or osteotomy plates with screws (e.g., pediatric osteotomy plates) can be used. Additional intertrochanteric osteotomy can reduce the blood supply to the fragment resulting in longer healing times. Also, the purchase in the proximal fragment may be weaker because of the shorter working length of the blade or screws in the neck. The choice of implant can influence the proximal-to-distal orientation of the trochanter and must be planned accordingly.

13.12 Postoperative Follow-Up

The postoperative regime follows the requirements of the SHD. Toe touch weight bearing for 6 weeks with gradual increase of weight bearing thereafter, depending on the applied procedures. Early range of motion exercises are important to prevent intra-articular adhesions.

Exercises for abductor strengthening and hip stabilization are started after 6 weeks, if consolidation of the trochanter is complete.

13.13 Intra-/Postoperative Complications

Avascular Necrosis (AVN) of the femoral head can occur if:

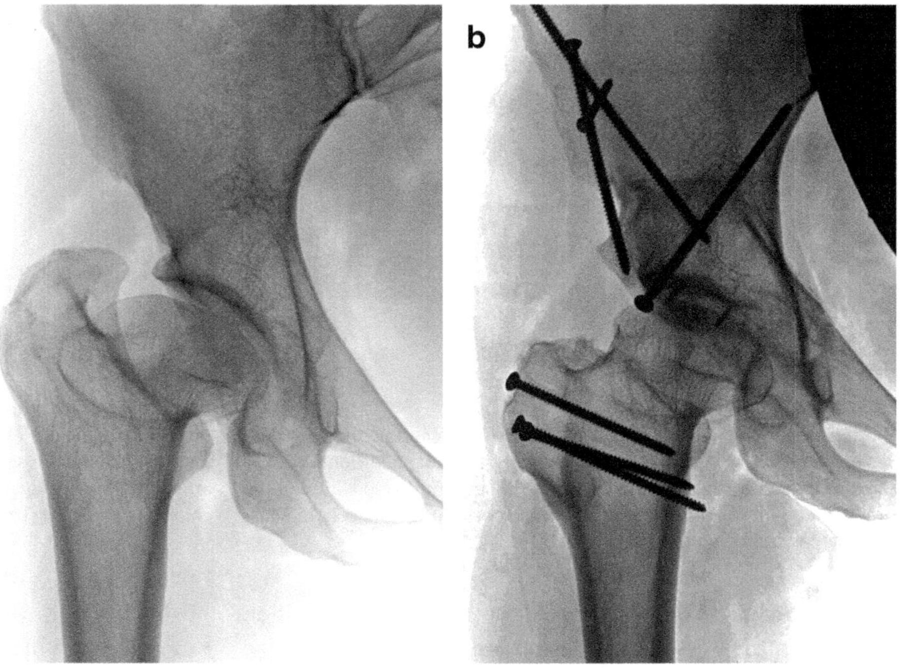

Fig. 13.8 (**a**) Preoperative radiograph of a 33 years-old patient with a post Perthes deformity and acetabular dysplasia (**b**) Postoperative radiograph 2 years after surgery

- The osteotomy of the trochanter is too medial, extending into piriformis fossa where the blood supply is endangered.
- Reducing the size of the trochanter may also risk the blood supply. Care has to be taken to a strictly subperiosteal dissection. If the trochanter compresses the retinaculum after reduction, the blood supply can be compressed.

Transverse fracture of the trochanter. This may occur if the femoral support of the trochanter is not over its length, leading to a bending leverage with a fatigue fracture during the healing period.

Nonunion or secondary dislocation of the trochanter

Implant breakage

Ectopic ossifications

Painful screwheads. Removal may be necessary

13.14 Case Studies

Case of a 33 years-old female patient with groin pain and fatigue pain over the abductor muscles after walking. On clinical examination she had a positive impingement sign but also posterior pain on external rotation. Range of motion was F/E 110-0-0°; IR/ER in 90° flexion was 30-0-15°. Abduction was limited to 15°. Radiographically, she had a post-Perthes deformity with a high-riding trochanter and a dysplastic acetabulum with a spherically congruent hip joint (Fig. 13.8a). MRI showed preserved acetabular and femoral cartilage along with a hypertrophic degeneration of the labrum. She was treated with a surgical dislocation, resizing and reattachment of the labrum, and osteochondroplasty, combined with a relative neck lengthening and PAO to correct dysplasia (Fig. 13.8b). She had a well-functioning hip with an OHS 46/48 for 11 years after surgery, time of the last follow-up. At that time, she had slight joint space narrowing.

13.15 Controversies

Advancement of the GT and intertrochanteric osteotomies alter the anatomy of the proximal femur. The implantation of the THA, as will be necessary in many of these patients, may be more difficult, and have a higher risk for intraoperative complications. Long-term survival, however, doesn't seem to be jeopardized.

13.16 Results

In general, the technique of relative neck lengthening is part of a comprehensive treatment for post-Perthes and DDH deformities suffering from intra- and extra-articular impingement. Intra-articular work may include offset correction, acetabular rim resections, treatment of labral disorders, and head reduction osteotomies, sometimes even combined with a periacetabular osteotomy. Relative neck lengthening is important to treat femoro-acetabular impingement caused by the shortened neck and to improve lever arm and muscle mechanics. The advancement of the trochanter alone does not yield good results if the intra-articular pathology remains untreated [13]. Relative femoral neck lengthening in hips with combined intra- and extra-articular impingement results in pain reduction and improved function of the hip [14, 15].

13.17 Outlook

Relative lengthening of the femoral neck with advancement of the greater trochanter often is an adjunct procedure in hips with complex deformities. It is not only used to treat intra- and extra-articular causes of FAI but also aims at improving muscle mechanics by correcting lever arm dysfunction and may be critical for a successful outcome. Therefore, this technique will be necessary for the future of hip preserving surgery. However, the technique is demanding, requiring a diverse skill-set and detailed knowledge of the vascular anatomy, and should be performed by surgeons with proper experience and the skill to do so safely and effectively.

References

1. Pozdnikin I, Baskov V, Barsukov D, Bortulev P, Krasnov K. Pediatric traumatology. Orthop Reconst Surg. 2019;7:15–24.
2. Gage JR, Cary JM. The effects of trochanteric epiphyseodesis on growth of the proximal end of the femur following necrosis of the capital femoral epiphysis. J Bone Joint Surg Am. 1980;62:785–94.
3. Langenskiöld A, Salenius P. Epiphyseodesis of the greater trochanter. Acta Orthop Scand. 1967;38:199–219.
4. Knapik DM, McCarthy C, Liu RW. Developmental patterns of the greater trochanter in skeletally immature patients. J Pediatr Orthop. 2019;39:e412–6.
5. Batailler C, Weidner J, Wyatt M, Dalmay F, Beck M. Position of the greater trochanter and functional femoral antetorsion: which factors matter in the management of femoral antetorsion disorders? Bone Joint J. 2018;100-B:712–9.
6. Beck M, Sledge JB, Gautier E, Dora CF, Ganz R. The anatomy and function of the gluteus minimus muscle. J Bone Joint Surg Br. 2000;82:358–63.
7. Gardner MJ, Robertson WJ, Boraiah S, Barker JU, Lorich DG. Anatomy of the greater trochanteric 'bald spot': a potential portal for abductor sparing femoral nailing? Clin Orthop Relat Res. 2008;466:2196–200.
8. Theivendran K, Hart WJ. Is the tip of the greater trochanter a reliable reference for the rotation centre of the femoral head in total hip arthroplasty? Acta Orthop Belg. 2009;75:472–6.
9. Beck M, Kruger A, Katthagen C, Kohl S. Osteotomy of the greater trochanter: effect on gluteus medius function. Surg Radiol Anat. 2015;37:599–607.
10. Ganz R, Huff TW, Leunig M. Extended retinacular soft-tissue flap for intra-articular hip surgery: surgical technique, indications, and results of application. Instr Course Lect. 2009;58:241–55.
11. Leunig M, Ganz R. Relative neck lengthening and intracapital osteotomy for severe Perthes and Perthes-like deformities. Bull NYU Hosp Jt Dis. 2011;69(Suppl 1):S62–7.
12. Najima H, Gagey O, Huten D, Cottias P. Vascularization of the trochanter fragment after digastric trochanterotomy in man. Morphologie. 1999;83:57–8.
13. Joo SY, Lee KS, Koh IH, Park HW, Kim HW. Trochanteric advancement in patients with Legg-Calvé-Perthes disease does not improve pain or limp. Clin Orthop Relat Res. 2008;466:927–34.
14. Anderson LA, Erickson JA, Severson EP, Peters CL. Sequelae of Perthes disease: treatment with surgical hip dislocation and relative femoral neck lengthening. J Pediatr Orthop. 2010;30:758–66.
15. Albers CE, Steppacher SD, Schwab JM, Tannast M, Siebenrock KA. Relative femoral neck lengthening improves pain and hip function in proximal femoral deformities with a high-riding trochanter. Clin Orthop Relat Res. 2015;473:1378–87.

Morscher Osteotomy

14

Etienne L. Belzile, Xia-dong Chen, and Ira Zaltz

14.1 Introduction

Legg-Calve-Perthes disease (LCPD), proximal femoral focal deficiency (PFFD), childhood septic arthritic of the hip, and sequalae of treatment of developmental dysplasia of the hip (DDH) can all lead to early subcapital physeal fusion leading to a coxa breva, coxa magna deformity, and leg length discrepancy, along with varying degrees of coxa vara. This unique deformity decreases the lever arm of the abductor mechanism causing abductor dysfunction with a Trendelenburg limp and hip pain, and leads to a loss of range of motion, intra- and extra-articular impingement, and eventually hip osteoarthritis [1].

The Morscher technique offers the possibility of diminishing pelvi-trochanteric impingement and improving the abductor's lever arm by repositioning the greater trochanter while using the power of the SHD (Chap. 7) and the surgical mobilization of the retinacular vessels (Chap. 8) to perform an oblique intertrochanteric osteotomy. Hence, upon proximal femoral fixation, femoral neck length, lateral offset, and the resulting leg length can by increased [2].

14.2 Background

Coxa breva is commonly associated with Legg-Perthes disease, the sequelae of developmental hip dysplasia, or other conditions that cause growth disturbance of the upper femur. Growth disturbances in the proximal femur due to injuries to the subcapital physis will lead to an enlarged femoral head (coxa magna), a shorter femoral neck (coxa breva, coxa vara), with most often a normally shaped greater trochanteric (GT). The resulting high-riding GT combined with a shorter femoral neck intrinsically deceases abductor lever arm and may lead to extra-articular impingement with the iliac or ischial bone, limiting hip motion. This complex association of deformities has puzzled many until Hefti and Morscher proposed a procedure addressing all items of the deformity at once [3]. The initial technical description of the procedure was prior to the contemporary understanding of the retinacular flap or the surgical dislocation procedure. The original procedure combined a reduction of the GT overhang, a distalization of the GT, along with a true neck-lengthening sliding intertrochanteric (IT) osteotomy. Recent advances using the Ganz surgical hip dislocation (Chap. 7) now allows intra-articular treatment of labral pathology, femoral head reduction procedures, or osteochondroplasty of the femoral head-neck junction [2, 4] to be performed simultaneously with the Morscher osteotomy. Even if the original proximal femoral deformity is severe, once bone remodeling occurs and abductor strength improves, patients undergoing the Morscher osteotomy via surgical hip dislocation can benefit from a true leg lengthening (1.5–3 cm), an optimized hip range of motion, better abductor muscle function (gain in offset averaging 12 mm), and minimized limping [2].

14.3 Indications

14.3.1 Indications

- Short femoral neck due to growth disturbance
- Greater trochanter overgrowth
- Leg length inequality of more than 1.5 cm

E. L. Belzile (✉)
Division of Orthopedic Surgery, CHU de Québec – Université Laval, Québec, QC, Canada
e-mail: etienne.belzile.med@ssss.gouv.qc.ca

X.-d. Chen
Department of Orthopedic Surgery, Xin-hua Hospital, Affiliated to Jiao Tong University School of Medicine, Shanghai, People's Republic of China
e-mail: chenxdmd@163.com

I. Zaltz
Pediatric Orthopedic Surgery Clinic, C.S.Mott Children's Hospital, Ann Arbor, MI, USA
e-mail: zaltz@med.umich.edu

M. Leunig et al. (eds.), *Surgical Hip Dislocation*, https://doi.org/10.1007/978-3-031-70622-6_14

14.3.2 Relative Contraindications

- Advanced osteoarthritis over Tönnis Grade II or MRI evidence of advanced chondral damage
- Inability to establish a congruent joint following reorientation of the upper femur and/or acetabulum

14.3.3 Contraindications

- Ongoing femoral head osteonecrosis.
- Lack of patient compliance and reliability to follow postoperative precautions and undergo abductor muscle strength rehabilitation.

14.4 Preoperative/Pre-Interventional Diagnostics

- Careful physical examination to evaluate the affected hip range of motion and lumbar spine flexibility.
- Anteroposterior (AP) pelvic radiograph and a 45° Dunn lateral of affected hip (Fig. 14.1).
- Standing long leg film with compensation to correct pelvic obliquity (Fig. 14.2).
- MRI of the symptomatic hip may help assessing for articular cartilage damage in chronic proximal femoral deformity or the status and maturity of the osteonecrosis in the femoral head.
- In exceptional cases, CT with special sequences for preoperative computer simulation of the oblique intertrochanteric osteotomy to optimize lengthening of neck and femur.
- Eventually, intraoperative abduction view after trochanteric osteotomy to show the new relation of head and acetabulum, and to see whether or not an additional periacetabular osteotomy (PAO) is necessary.

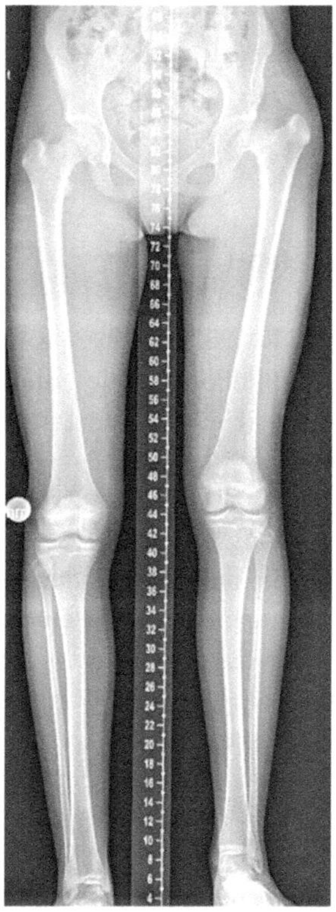

Fig. 14.2 Full-length long-leg standing radiograph with a 2 cm lift on the left side, of a 13-year-old girl presenting with a healed osteonecrosis after DDH open treatment

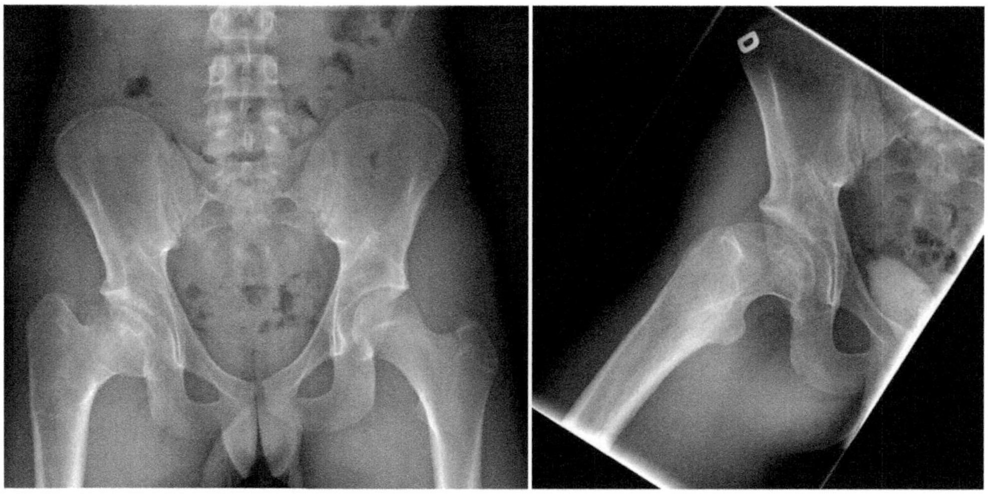

Fig. 14.1 AP pelvis radiograph and a 45° Dunn lateral view of a 15-year-old boy presenting with a Legg-Calve-Perthes hip after sustaining a varus IT osteotomy

14.5 Preoperative Planning/Computer Modeling

To date, no routine preoperative planning is performed for this procedure. However, paper (computational) planning/simulation is helpful to define the amount of lateral shift of the distal femoral fragment and the necessary extrusion over bone level of the head neck implant.

14.6 Applied Anatomy

- A prerequisite for the preparation of the retinaculum soft flap is the completely performed SHD [4] (see Chap. 7) as well as preparation of the extended soft tissue retinacular flap [5] (see Chap. 8).
- Dislocation of the femoral head is necessary to optimize joint congruence and minimize intra-articular impingement. Retinacular dissection requires special attention to optimize relative neck lengthening prior to real neck lengthening and avoid retinacular vessel entrapment when the greater trochanter is distalized.
- Subperiosteal dissection around the lesser trochanter requires protection of the deep branch of the medial femoral circumflex artery which bypasses the lesser trochanter proximally, runs posteriorly along the undersurface of the obturator externus muscle, and crosses its tendon posteriorly to finally undercrosses the tendon of the triceps coxae to reach the hip capsule (Chap. 6). The area is covered by the quadratus femurs muscle.

14.7 Specific Risks

- Impairment of the blood supply to the femoral head may result in avascular necrosis of femoral head during mobilizing retinacular flap, especially while performing the relative femoral neck lengthening.
- Excessive periosteal dissection, especially in multiple operated hips, may critically diminish the blood supply of the metaphysical bone after intertrochanteric osteotomy.
- Head collapse and subsequent advanced osteoarthritis.
- Loss of reduction or implant failure.
- Greater trochanteric nonunion.
- Abductor muscles chronic insufficiency due to incorrect trochanter positioning.
- Delayed or nonunion of osteotomy site.
- Heterotopic ossifications in soft tissues around the surgical approach (gluteal muscles, vastus lateralis, external rotators, piriformis, hip capsule).
- Contracture of the abductor apparatus with resulting in pelvic obliquity.

14.8 Type of Anesthesia

General anesthesia with or without additional regional block for pain management

14.9 Positioning

- Radiolucent operating table
- Lateral positioning with tunnel cushion and lateral bag
- Stabilization of the pelvis perpendicular to the floor along with the operated leg in the horizontal position with possibility to stabilize the femur in abduction will facilitate tensioning the abductor mechanism.
- Access to contralateral knee/ankle to monitor leg length
- Fluoroscopy and X-ray possibility

14.10 Instruments/Implants

Standard instrument set for surgical hip dislocation and extended soft tissue flap (see Chaps. 7 and 8)

- Soft tissue dissector.
- Curved soft tissue dissector
- Oscillating saw and saw blade
- Straight chisel 10 mm, 15 mm, 1 each
- Fixation device: 130° blade plate (or proximal femoral locking plate) with the blade inserted as far as possible to optimized fixation
- Alternative fixation device for small individuals: locking plates with 5.0 mm screws into the femoral neck with choice of a few angles between 110° and 140° depending on the manufacturer

14.11 Access

- Access as for a surgical hip dislocation with trochanteric osteotomy (see Chap. 6) with a skin extension distally to allow proper fixation of the fixation device (three to four-hole plate) onto the femoral shaft.
- Trochanteric osteotomy should be performed according to the orientation of the greater trochanter respecting its overhanging position. As a rule, the trochanteric osteotomy is rather horizontal and can be planned to safeguard a segment of trochanter to be used as autograft to lengthen the neck (Fig. 14.3).
- The trochanteric fragment should not be thicker than 1.5 cm. If the trochanteric osteotomy is too superficial, it will be at risk of fracture upon fixation or at risk of fragmentation. If the trochanteric osteotomy is too deep, the tendon of the piriformis muscle may adhere to the mobile

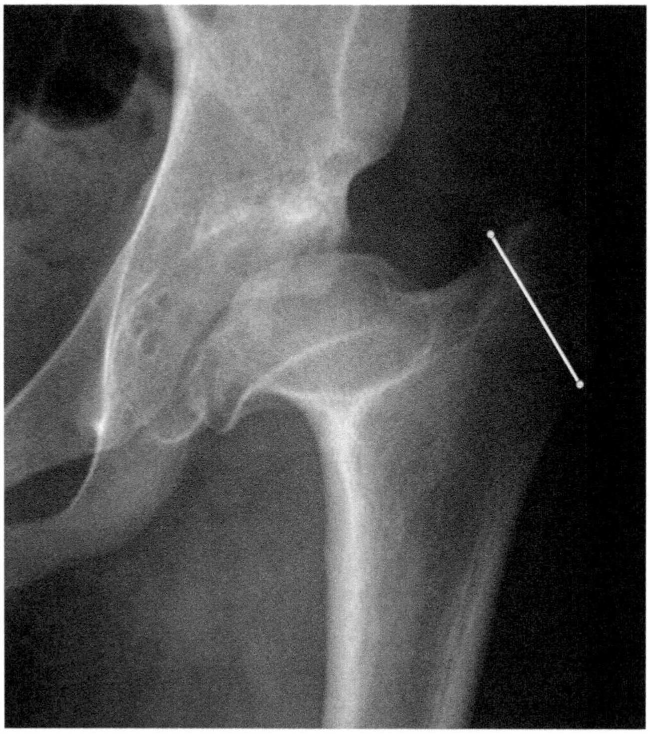

Fig. 14.3 AP of left hip radiograph of a healed hip post osteonecrosis after DDH treatment and a high-riding GT. The line drawn represents the proposed position of the GT osteotomy during de initial surgical hip dislocation procedure

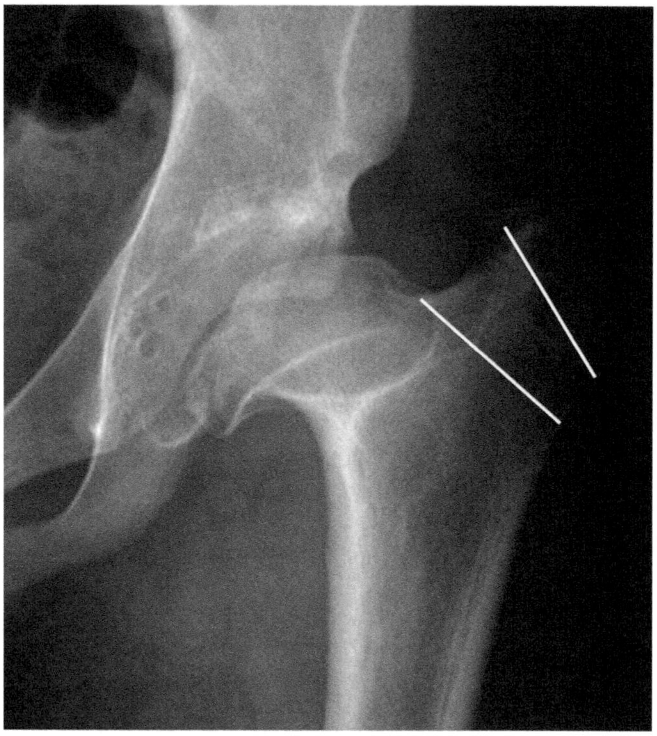

Fig. 14.4 AP of left hip radiograph of a healed hip post osteonecrosis after DDH treatment and a high-riding GT. The inferior line drawn represents the proposed position of the neck lengthening dissection and osteotomy line for the bone bridge resection that will later be used as a bone autograft to supplement the femoral neck during the true neck lengthening phase of the Morscher osteotomy

trochanteric fragment limiting its mobilization or endanger the deep branch of the medial circumflex artery with the risk of head necrosis.

- A proximal subvastus approach is developed over a segment of 10–15 cm to expose the femoral shaft subperiosteally.
- The resulting flat and trigastric trochanteric osteotomy is elevated anteriorly (with gluteus medius, gluteus minimus, and vastus lateralis attached) to expose anterior capsule. A Z-shaped capsulotomy is performed to allow for further intra-articular surgery or femoral head dislocation.

14.12 Technical Steps

- A retinacular soft-tissue flap is developed from the superior and posterior corner of the remaining base of the greater trochanter as in Chap. 8. A relative femoral neck lengthening procedure can be performed as well as a femoral head and neck junction osteoplasty can be performed as needed (Chap. 9).
- The femoral neck-lengthening bone graft is then harvested from the excess bone that represents parts of the overgrown greater trochanter from the trochanteric osteotomy level and the real neck level (Fig. 14.4). The bone graft donor segment is meticulously mobilized and peeled out of its medial and posterior periosteum, preferably in one intact piece and set aside. A block of bone of at least 1-cm-thick can usually be harvested.
- The first step toward achieving adequate fixation after the Morscher osteotomy is the optimized positioning of the cephalic fixation (blade plate or locking screws). Center-to-center pin placement into the neck may not be possible in aspherical growth arrested femoral heads. AP and lateral fluoroscopic views are taken as the pin placement advances into the neck to avoid intra-articular perforation or pin malposition. Once the optimal pin placement is obtained, the pin is measured for length adding to this value the harvested bone autograft thickness value as well as the desired lateral offset increment value planned. This step will dictate the length of the fixation holding the neck.
- When positioning the chisel (or the fixed angle aiming device), the flat portion of the blade must remain perpendicular to the long axis of the distal femur to avoid inducing extension or flexion malposition of the distal fragment upon plate reduction to the femoral shaft. Before hammering in the chisel (or drilling-in the fixed angle aiming device), enough of a bony bridge must remain between the entry point in the femoral neck and the planned position of the intertrochanteric osteotomy. At least 1.5 cm of bony bridge but as few as 1 cm has been proposed

(Fig. 14.5). In cases with narrow clearance between lesser trochanter and ischium (low offset), it is preferable that the medial end of the osteotomy is proximal to the lesser trochanter.

- Infra-blade femoral neck fracture rarely leads to catastrophic complication, but it may render completion of the up-sloping medial translation lengthening procedure more challenging.
- After the intertrochanteric bone area has been exposed circumferentially with a blunt retractor to allow positioning of soft tissue protectors (preferentially radiotransparent), the level of the intertrochanteric osteotomy is visualized via intraoperative fluoroscopy.
- As in the preoperative planning, the intertrochanteric osteotomy should be parallel to the cephalic fixation, upsloping from the lateral femoral cortex to the junction between lower femoral neck and lesser trochanter.
  - The leg length increase will depend on the up-sloping pitch of the IT osteotomy and the femoral shaft diameter at the level of the lesser trochanter.
  - The placement of K-wires may help predict the osteotomy site and orientation (Fig. 14.5). Longitudinal markings along the anterior femur can also help avoid rotational malposition.
- After the IT osteotomy is performed using an oscillating saw with continuous saline instillation, the femoral neck fragment is freed from the femoral shaft. The blade plate (or fixed angle locking plate) is inserted into the greater trochanter, the bony autograft, and then the femoral neck. The fixation device is then progressively deduced into lateral cortical apposition to the femoral shaft avoiding any malrotation.
  - Using bone reduction clamp or a femoral distractor may avoid bending the fixation device if used as a "joystick" upon final reduction maneuvers.
- Final GT fixation is completed using two 4.0 or 4.5 mm cortical screws oriented parallel to each other, on each side of the blade plate or cephalic locking screws, toward the lesser trochanter (Fig. 14.6).
  - Addition of a tension band cerclage wire may help limit GT migration.
  - Release of the long tendon of the gluteus minimus at the medial aspect of the trochanteric fragment may facilitate manipulation of the fragment.

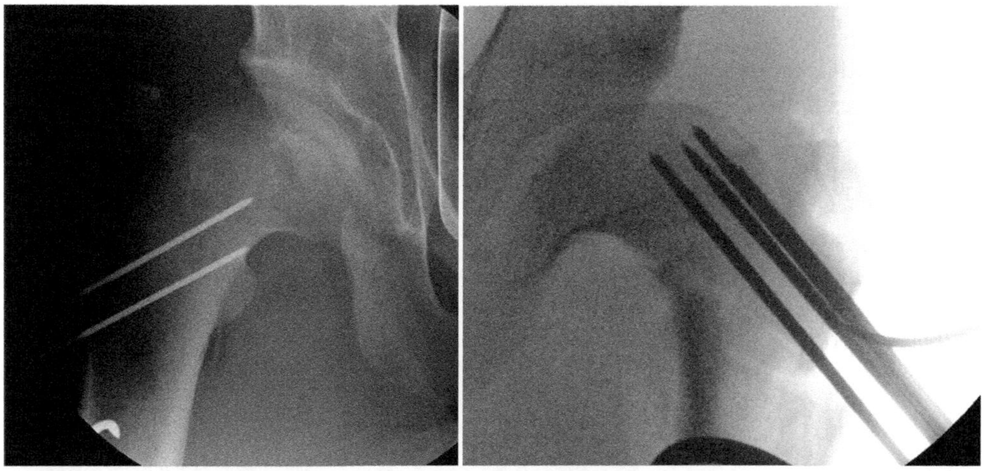

Fig. 14.5 AP of the hip radiographs of hips with proximal femoral growth disturbances. The image on the left demonstrates how K-wires can be used to plan future IT osteotomy position in reference to a blade plate position before surgical dissection. The image on the right demonstrates guide wires being positioned into the femoral neck after IT osteotomy and respecting IT osteotomy angulation for a proximal femoral locking plate positioning

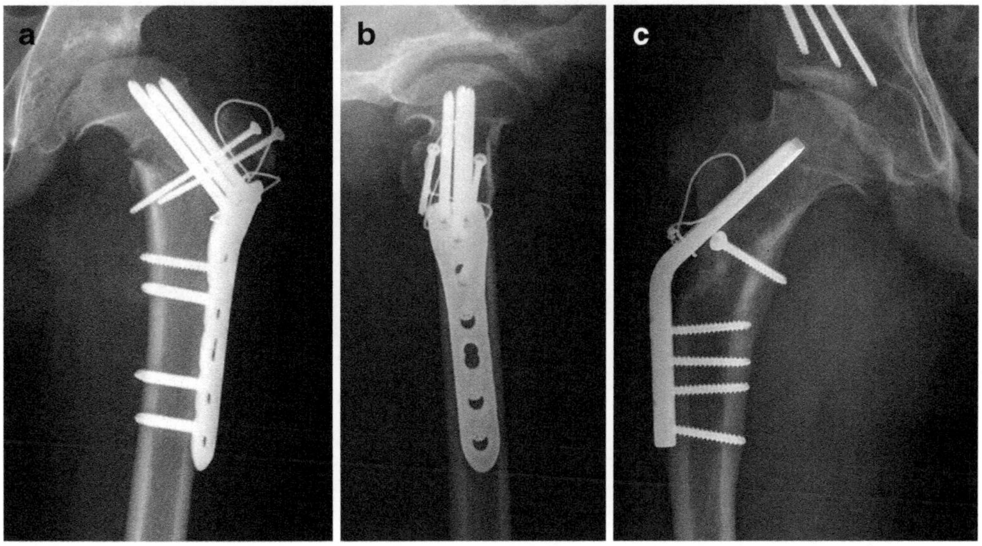

Fig. 14.6 (**a**-**b**) AP and lateral radiographs of the hip after fixation of a Morscher osteotomy using a locking plate and screw and tension band cerclage of the GT. PAO for subluxation will be staged (**c**) AP radiograph of the hip after fixation of a Morscher osteotomy using a blade plate and screws presenting at 12 months post-operative with an escaped, proximally displaced GT fragment

14.13 Postoperative Follow-Up

- Wound care is a routine with primary dressing change after 3 days and subsequent dressing change every 2 days as needed.
- Continuous passive motion is prescribed in hospital for the first 48 hrs.
- Thromboprophylaxis is prescribed in mature patients for 30 days.
- Physical therapy is initiated rapidly with partial weight bearing and avoidance of active abduction exercises for the first 6 weeks.
- Early follow-up at 6 weeks help judge GT union and would lead to full weight bearing and hip abductor exercises.

14.14 Intra-/Postoperative Complications

The Morscher procedure is an amalgamation of many different techniques within the same operation that are all performed using the surgical dislocation approach. As detailed, the steps include performing a trochanteric osteotomy, developing a retinacular flap to resect the stable trochanter, recontouring of the femoral head, and repairing or reconstructing chondral and labral defects along with a three-part geometrically complex upper femoral osteotomy. As such, complications associated with each individual step are possible and have been described in other chapters of this text so they will not be restated in this chapter.

Intraoperative and postoperative complications that are specific to the Morscher procedure largely involve problems with the osteotomy. In addition to delayed union and nonunion of either or both the trochanter or the femur, improper design and execution of the osteotomy will not allow optimal restoration of the upper femoral anatomy to as normal as possible. Since the morphology of each patient is substantially different, each osteotomy must be individually planned. Therefore, failure to understand the principles of osteotomy design frequently result in inadequate or over-correction that mechanically compromises hip function. Historically, fixation of the osteotomy using blade plates and limited availability of intraoperative fluoroscopy posed an exceptional technical challenge. Nowadays, fluoroscopy and the use of proximal femoral locking plates of varying angles have obviated the challenges of inserting a blade plate; however, the locking plate can give surgeons a false sense of confidence. The relative ease of the locking plate use does not simplify the geometric complexity of the procedure, and careful planning is still necessary to avoid inexact trochanter alignment, neck lengthening, and reestablishment of the neck-shaft angle. Thus, over- or under-correction of any part of the procedure will fail (1) to normalize abductor mechanics, (2) to correct leg length discrepancy, and (3) to restore hip motion.

14.15 Case Study

A 13-year-old female present with a history of DDH at birth, who was treated by open reduction, Salter osteotomy, and adductor tenotomy at age 2. She later presented with femoral osteonecrosis that led to a proximal femoral growth disturbance. She presents with hip pain in her school sporting activities and a limb and a leg length inequality of 2.5 cm. Preoperative AP pelvis shows a healed femoral head with coxa magna, coxa breva, coxa vara, and a GT overhang with pelvis obliquity correcting with a 2 cm lift on the affected side. She underwent a staged (6 months apart) Morscher osteotomy followed by a periacetabular osteotomy to correct all her bony anatomy. The hip healed uneventfully (Fig. 14.7).

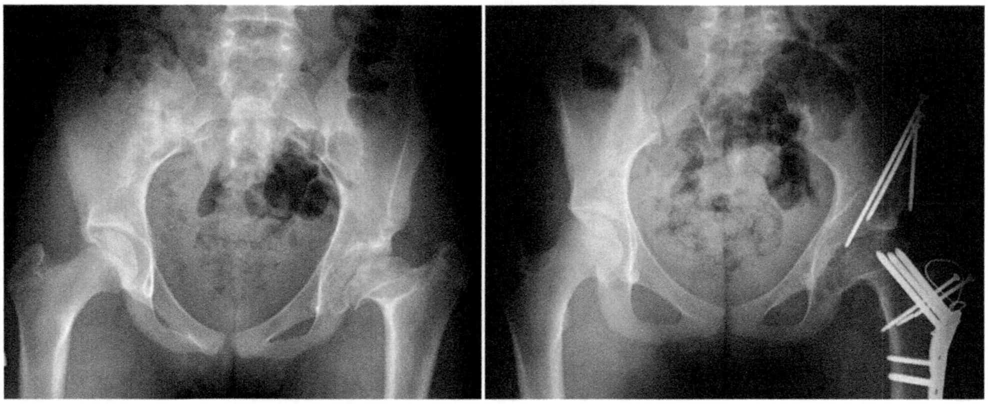

Fig. 14.7 The left image is an AP pelvis radiograph of a 13-year-old girl presenting with a hip growth disturbance after sustaining an osteonecrosis following an open reduction and Salter osteotomy for a DDH at age 2. The right image is an AP pelvis radiograph of the same patient after a Morscher osteotomy combined with a staged periacetabular osteotomy (same patient as in Fig. 14.3 and 14.6a–b)

14.16 Controversies

Since the Morscher procedure is a complex reconstruction of the upper femur that can affect subsequent hip operations, especially total hip replacement, the decision to undertake a Morscher must be weighed primarily against the expected benefit of performing a total hip replacement. There are multiple competing limitations and benefits that must be evaluated based upon the individual patient. Age of the patient, health of the articular cartilage, expected congruity of the reconstruction, and the impact of post-reconstruction geometry of the upper femur and the ability to insert a femoral component are the most critical considerations. For each factor, patients who are younger and have healthy articular cartilage and spherically or aspherically congruent hip joints are more suitable candidates for reconstruction.

The stability of the hip joint must be assessed, and performing a concomitant acetabular reorientation is a point of controversy. Some surgeons will judge the need for acetabular reorientation upon the radiographic anatomy of the acetabulum, and others will make an intraoperative decision based upon observed instability of the hip immediately following the osteotomy. The precise criterion upon which to base this decision is still discussed. Most surgeons agree that acetabular reorientation is needed if Shenton's line is disrupted, if there are preoperative signs and symptoms of instability, and if there is intraoperative clinical evidence of instability.

Last, reconstruction of the hip often necessitates a prolonged recovery that includes both extensive physical rehabilitation and a second procedure to remove hardware. Therefore, the patient must possess the psychological reserve, motivation, and commitment to fully participate in the recovery process.

14.17 Expected Outcomes

The outcome that is expected by both the surgeon and patient following full recovery following the Morscher procedure are diminished pain, improved hip mobility and stability, improved functional capacity, and preservation of the hip joint. In addition, there are specific anatomic scenarios especially when the upper femur is extensively deformed and would not otherwise easily tolerate insertion of a femoral component that an inferior clinical outcome is tolerated and expected so that the anatomy can be altered so that the patient is a more suitable candidate to insert a total hip replacement.

14.18 Future Direction

The future for complex femoral reconstructions may involve computer planning using patient-specific guides designed from three-dimensional CT data. Such guides can be anatomically applied to the patient to assist with precision surgery and plate application. They will likely greatly minimize the use of intraoperative fluoroscopy, improve the efficiency of the procedure, and minimize inexact corrections.

References

1. Larson AN, Sucato DJ, Herring JA, Adolfsen SE, Kelly DM, Martus JE, Lovejoy JF, Browne R, Delarocha A. A prospective multicenter study of Legg-Calvé-Perthes disease: functional and radiographic outcomes of nonoperative treatment at a mean follow-up of twenty years. J Bone Joint Surg Am. 2012;94:584–92.
2. Faure PA, Zaltz I, Côté K, Pelet S, Forsythe C, Beaulé PE, Belzile EL. Morscher osteotomy through surgical dislocation approach for true femoral neck lengthening with greater trochanter transposition. J Bone Joint Surg Am. 2020;102(Suppl 2):66–72.
3. Hefti F, Morscher E. The femoral neck lengthening osteotomy. Orthop Traumat. 1993;2:144–51.
4. Ganz R, Gill TJ, Gautier E, Ganz K, Krugel N, Berlemann U. Surgical dislocation of the adult hip a technique with full access to the femoral head and acetabulum without the risk of avascular necrosis. J Bone Joint Surg Br. 2001;83:1119–24.
5. Ganz R, Huff TW, Leunig M. Extended retinacular soft-tissue flap for intra-articular hip surgery: surgical technique, indications, and results of application. Instr Course Lect. 2009;58:241–55.

Inter–/Subtrochanteric Femoral Osteotomy

15

Wudbhav N. Sankar and Hannes Manner

15.1 Introduction

Intertrochanteric or subtrochanteric osteotomies may be performed as stand-alone procedures or in combination with a surgical hip dislocation (SHD) approach (see Chap. 7). Whenever a surgeon wishes to address any coexisting intra-articular pathology along with proximal femoral deformity correction, the SHD offers a clear advantage of a single surgical approach with unmatched intraoperative flexibility. Depending on the type of osteotomy to be performed, the implant choice and age of the patient (child, adolescent, or adult), the details of the surgical technique may vary substantially.

15.2 Background

Inter- and subtrochanteric femoral osteotomies have been performed for years to correct proximal femoral malalignment, optimize leg position and hip range of motion, and to improve the weight-bearing region (coverage) of the femoral head [1, 2]. Conditions that may require these osteotomies include excessive femoral version (both ante and retro), residual Legg-Calve-Perthes disease (LCPD), slipped capital femoral epiphysis (SCFE), osteonecrosis, chondral defects, and other disorders that affect hip joint congruity and stability [3].

Intertrochanteric osteotomies are more proximal and are generally performed to address varus/valgus, extension/flexion deformities and can simultaneously address torsional problems. Advantages of doing the osteotomy in this location include larger surface areas for bony healing and correction closer to the point of maximal deformity in most cases.

Subtrochanteric osteotomies are more distal and more often performed for rotational and/or shortening purposes. Advantages of this osteotomy include less secondary deformity and preservation of the lesser trochanter position and psoas insertion although rotational osteotomies may be performed in the intertrochanteric region as well. Angular corrections in the subtrochanteric region can lead to secondary deformities.

Classically both these osteotomies have been performed as stand-alone procedures either in the supine or lateral position. However, with the advent of the SHD our ability to address intra-articular pathology including cartilage lesions, cam deformities of the head-neck junction, etc. has revolutionized the approach—as many of these coexist with associated proximal femoral deformity. Performing inter–/subtrochanteric osteotomies through a SHD enables one to address both the joint and the proximal femur through a single surgical approach [2, 4, 5]. In addition, intraoperative findings within the joint may dictate the type and magnitude of proximal femoral osteotomy to be performed. Furthermore, SHD enables the surgeon to assess whether the amount of correction is sufficient to solve the intra-articular problem, whether joint rotation is well balanced and confirm that altered range of motion does not lead to new impingement problems anteriorly or posteriorly.

15.3 Indications

15.3.1 Indications

- Varus-retroversion of the proximal femur (e.g., healed deformity in slipped capital femoral epiphysis)
- Aspherical head with accompanying retroversion (residual Legg-Calve-Perthes disease) with poor congruency
- Femoro-acetabular impingement (FAI) with coexisting femoral retroversion

W. N. Sankar (✉)
Division of Orthopaedic Surgery, Children's Hospital of Philadelphia, Philadelphia, PA, USA
e-mail: SANKARW@chop.edu

H. Manner
Pediatric Service, Department of Orthopedics, Schulthess Clinic Zurich, Zurich, Switzerland
e-mail: Hannes.Manner@kws.ch

M. Leunig et al. (eds.), *Surgical Hip Dislocation*, https://doi.org/10.1007/978-3-031-70622-6_15

- Hip joint incongruity associated with growth disturbance
- Other complex proximal femoral deformities in need of combined intra-articular repair and extra-articular correction (e.g., multiple hereditary exostoses)
- Anterior hip instability with coexisting femoral anteversion
- Epiphyseal dysplasia (focal Avascular Necrosis (AVN))

15.3.2 Relative Contraindications

- Absence of intra-articular pathology requiring dynamic assessment.
- Intra-articular pathology which may be better addressed by arthroscopy rather than SHD (e.g. isolated cam deformity)
- Poor articular cartilage with guarded prognosis. In these cases, performing a sub–/intertrochanteric osteotomy may overly complicate future total joint arthroplasty without sufficiently improving the natural history.
- In cases with combined relative lengthening of the femoral neck and intertrochanteric osteotomy, the stability of the blade plate or screws may be at risk since the lateral and parts of the posterior cortex of the metaphysis are removed. In such situations a rotational correction is better performed at the subtrochanteric level.

15.4 Preoperative/Preinterventional Diagnostics

- Pelvic anteroposterior (AP) as well as Lauenstein or cross table lateral views.
- Standard or arthro-MRI of the symptomatic hip
- CT with 3D reconstructions, radial sequences, and cuts through the distal femur to allow assessment of femoral version.

15.5 Preoperative Planning/Computer Simulation

3D-printed models and computer simulation allow the surgical steps of an osteotomy to be specified more precisely and the production of cutting devices (see Chap. 5). This is particularly useful for complex multiplanar corrections such as slipped capital femoral epiphysis and severe Perthes deformity.

15.6 Applied Anatomy

- A prerequisite for the combined procedure with sub–/intertrochanteric osteotomy is the fully executed SHD (see Chap. 7).
- With external rotation of the leg, the postero-medially located Weitbrecht ligament with the medial retinaculum becomes visible. With internal rotation, the laterally located retinaculum at the femoral neck becomes visible. Both contain the vessels from the medial circumflex artery for the blood supply of the femoral head. Smallest vessel branches from the lateral circumflex artery are insignificant for the head blood supply. The same applies to the artery in the ligamentum teres, vessels in the capsule, and vascular branches in the metaphysis of the head-neck transition (see Chap. 6).

15.7 Special Risks

Disturbance of the blood supply to the femoral head with consequences such as the following:

- Loss of reduction, head collapse, resulting follow-up surgery including joint replacement
- Nonunion or delayed union of osteotomy site

Undesired side deformities with angular corrections

- Iatrogenic impingement

15.8 Type of Anesthesia

Since the procedure is performed in lateral position and usually takes more than 90 min, general anesthesia is preferable over spinal anesthesia, especially since the patients are mostly children and adolescents. Regional anesthesia via a fascia iliaca block or lumbar plexus catheter may be helpful to limit the need for postoperative narcotics.

15.9 Positioning

- Standard or radiolucent operating table
- Lateral positioning with tunnel cushion, lateral bag, or peg board
- Fluoroscopy and X-ray possibility

15.10 Instruments/Implants

Because of the transtrochanteric approach, implant choice is critical when performing combined SHD and inter–/subtrochanteric osteotomies as this effectively becomes a three-part osteotomy which can be more challenging to handle. Meticulous implant-specific technique can limit the mobility of the trochanteric fragment and greatly facilitate surgical correction.

In addition to standard instrumentation for SHD (see Chap. 7), the following implants might become necessary for the sub-/intertrochanteric osteotomy:

- 3.5–4.5 mm solid or cannulated screws (for trochanteric fixation)
- Straight 3.5 mm or 4.5 mm DCP plate (for subtrochanteric derotational osteotomies)
- Adult/adolescent/children 90–110° blade plate (preferred by some for varus/valgus and/or flexion/extension osteotomies, especially when trochanteric advancement has to be included)
- Adult/adolescent 90 proximal femoral locking plate (preferred by others for varus/valgus and/or flexion/extension osteotomies—usually intertrochanteric osteotomies)

15.11 Access

- Access as for surgical hip SHD (see Chap. 7). Incision should be extended more distal to allow full exposure to the proximal femoral shaft.

15.12 Technical Steps of Deep Dissection

- *Reduction of the joint and internal rotation*

After completion of the SHD, the lower leg is first removed from the sterile bag, and the femoral head is reduced back into the acetabulum. The joint capsule should be closed if an intertrochanteric osteotomy is planned (it can be left open at this point for subtrochanteric osteotomies which do not require that the trochanter be fixed first). If performing a significant flexion osteotomy, the inferior limb of the capsulotomy should be left open in order to prevent a postoperative hip flexion contracture.

- *Subperiosteal exposure of the proximal femoral shaft*

For *intertrochanteric osteotomies*, this sub-/epiperiosteal exposure should extend proximal to the lesser trochanter. For *subtrochanteric osteot*omies in children and adolescents, the thicker periosteum is sharply split distal to the trochanteric osteotomy bed, and the periosteum is elevated circumferentially around the proximal femur with a Cobb, Crego, or another elevator. In adults, an epiperiosteal approach is preferred using decortication at the level for the subtrochanteric osteotomy to accelerate healing.

- *Intertrochanteric (flexion, extension, varus, or valgus)*

Multiplanar osteotomies are often performed in the intertrochanteric region since it is closer to the site of deformity but also in order to facilitate osteotomy healing due to the higher vascularization and broader surface area of the cancellous bone. Blade plates and proximal femoral locking plates of various angles are typically used for these procedures. Regardless, the first step is to minimize the instability of a three-part osteotomy by obtaining provisional trochanteric fixation. The trochanter is reduced anatomically (or advanced if desired), and one or two K-wires are placed proximally in the trochanteric base to temporarily stabilize the fragment. A proximal femoral locking plate is applied to the lateral cortex of the trochanter and the proximal femur. Flexion of the proximal fragment is achieved by rotating the plate anterior to the femoral axis (with extension the opposite) (Fig. 15.1a). Coronal plane corrections (varus and valgus) are achieved by adducting or abducting the plate relative to the femur axis (Fig. 15.1b). The proximal guide pins are inserted via towers mounted on the plate into the trochanter and across the trochanteric osteotomy site prior being checked on fluoroscopy. The plate can be removed from the guide pins (which now act to hold the greater trochanter in place) and the osteotomy performed at a distance from the pins as specified by the particular implant design. The plate can be slid back over the guide wires and the wires replaced with proximal femoral locking screws. The femoral shaft can then be reduced to the plate, derotation may be added if necessary, and distal fixation can be achieved in compression to aid in osteotomy healing.

If a blade plate is preferred, the central guide wire should be placed after achieving provisional trochanteric fixation at an angle to the shaft depending on the intended coronal plane correction. Flexion or extension at the osteotomy can be achieved by rotating the chisel around the guide wire as it is inserted through the trochanteric fragment and into the stable base. The osteotomy can then be performed as above and the femur reduced to the plate followed by definitive distal fixation. Alternatively, the chisel can be inserted into the stable base to create the path for the blade plate without involving the mobile trochanteric fragment. A small hole can then be carved into the trochanteric fragment, and the blade can be inserted through this hole into the stable base before reducing the femoral shaft. Fixation of the osteotomized trochanter can be adjusted to achieve more or less abductor tension. The amount of flexion osteotomy can be increased and residual flexion contracture be minimized, when the trochanter is not part of the flexion (Fig. 15.2a–d).

To avoid further shortening, wedge resection in order to increase the contact area of the intertrochanteric osteotomy site should not be performed. Consolidation of the osteotomy is not prolonged, but leg shortening may stay in tolerable ranges.

- *Subtrochanteric (rotational) osteotomy*

Rotational osteotomies to address abnormal femoral version are either performed at the intertrochanteric or subtrochanteric level [6]. The consolidation of osteotomies through cortical bone at the subtrochanteric level takes longer compared to the cancellous bone of the intertrochanteric area. The osteotomy level should allow the placement of half of the plate length proximal to it and should not interfere with fixation of the greater trochanter. Nevertheless plate position should be as

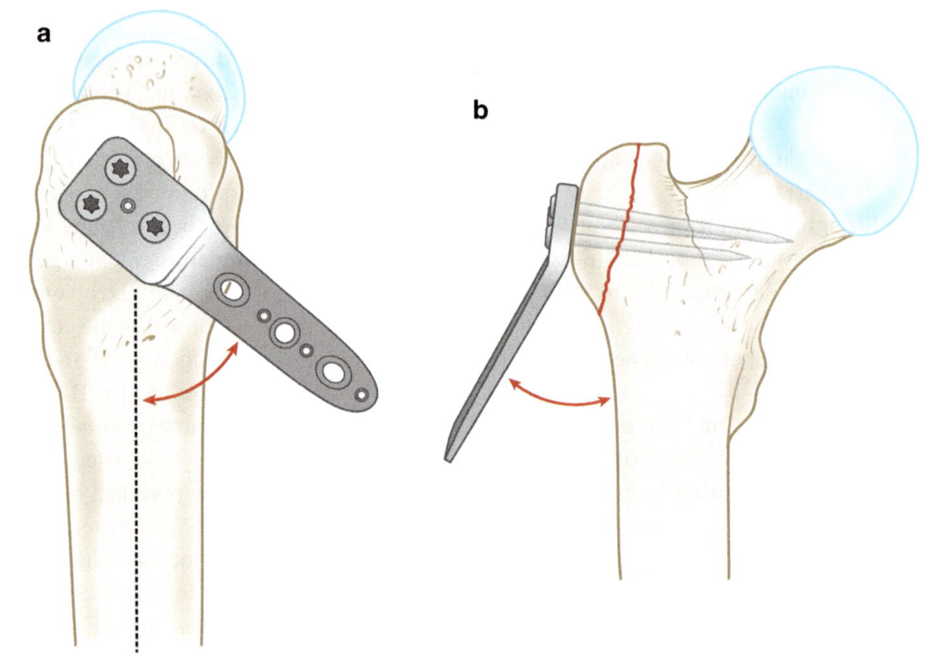

Fig. 15.1 (**a**) Line drawing demonstrating technique for adding flexion correction to an intertrochanteric osteotomy. Flexion is introduced by rotating the plate anterior to the femoral shaft. (**b**) Line drawing demonstrating technique for adding coronal plane correction to an intertrochanteric osteotomy. Coronal plane corrections (varus and valgus) are achieved by adducting or abducting the plate relative to the shaft

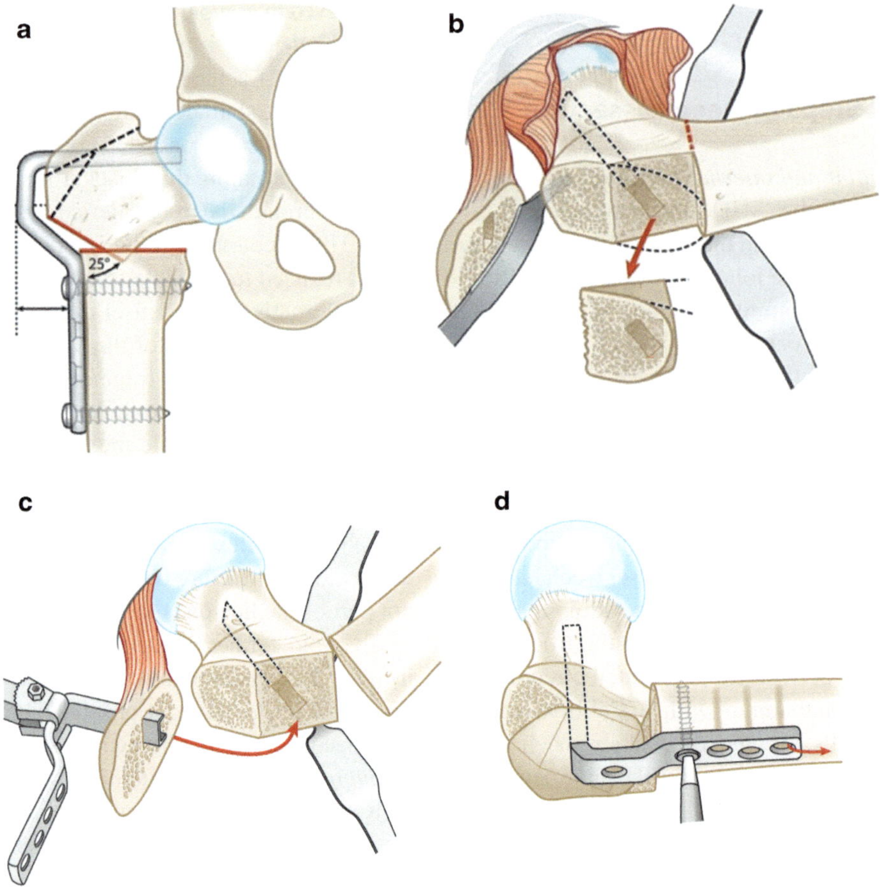

Fig. 15.2 (**a-d**) Planning and correction of multiplanar intertrochanteric deformity with a blade plate. (**a**) Planning of the correction. Intertrochanteric varus osteotomy. Advancement of the trochanteric fragment and enhancement of the muscular lever arm can be increased by a second cut (dotted lines). The plate offset comes with 10, 15, and 20 mm, allowing consideration of the mechanical axis of the leg. (**b**) In the case of a flexion osteotomy, the channel for the blade is neutral in the trochanteric fragment and turned in the head-neck fragment according to the amount of desired flexion. (**c**) Reduction of the trochanter, loaded with the blade plate can be delicate, because the channel direction in the neck is hidden when the trochanteric fragment is reduced. Intertrochanteric reduction and fixation with K-wires reduce the problem. (**d**) Final correction of a flexion-varus OT. Rotational correction is also possible. A trochanteric fragment excluded from the flexion allows higher intertrochanteric flexion with less risk of a flexion contracture. Interfragmentary compression is sufficient with the gliding hole. A compression device (red arrow) is rarely necessary

proximal as possible to avoid unnecessary exposure and a too distal osteotomy. Decortication at the osteotomy site is helpful to enhance bony healing particularly in the adult patient. Exposure is done such that a six- or seven-hole plate can be placed under full visibility especially in the distal region. A seven-hole plate leaves more space for the osteotomy but, on the other hand, reaches more distally. A steel plate with a thickness of 4.5 mm is recommended in adolescent and adult patients. A drill tower is placed in the second most distal plate hole, and the plate is placed on the lateral cortex of the femur as proximal as possible underneath the trochanteric osteotomy and may be bent according to the anatomy proximally. Over the drill sleeve, a 2.5 mm K-wire with a threaded tip is placed bicortically, which then serves as the distal derotation wire. Placing the derotation wire in this location avoids interference with the muscles and avoids the need for further distal exposure. The third most distal plate hole is then stocked with a locking screw. The site of the osteotomy is marked with a chisel. It should be at least 5 mm proximal to the inserted screw. The proximal rotation (orientation) wire is placed proximal to the plate in the desired rotational angle. To correct femoral retrotorsion, this proximal wire should be internally rotated in comparison to the distal wire and for correction of excessive antetorsion vice versa. The plate and the screw are then removed. Decortication is done over a length of 3–4 cm with a sharp chisel anterior and posterior to the osteotomy. Blunt Hohmann retractors are placed between decortication and bone. The transverse osteotomy can be performed using an oscillating saw (using saline to cool the bone) or with drill holes and an osteotome. The inserted distal derotation wire serves as orientation for the direction of the osteotomy. Finally, using a Lexer chisel or a bone spreader, the osteotomy is opened, to make sure it is complete without spikes of bone interfering with the correction. With the help of the Hohmann retractors, the fragments are held in position while correction is performed. An additional table or Mayo-stand on which to place the foot is helpful. By increasing the height of the table, internal rotation of the distal fragment is performed and vice versa. When the rotation (orientation) wires are parallel, the plate is put back in place over the distal derotation wire, and the screw is reinserted. Usually, reduction clamps are not needed. Therefore, a large subperiosteal exposure of the femur can be avoided. Then, the plate hole proximal to the osteotomy is fixed with a 4.5 screw in compression technique by prior eccentric drilling. Care is taken that the drilling is performed exactly parallel to the distal rotation wire to avoid loss of correction when compression is performed, which is one of the problems that might occur. If compression in the planned correction is clinically sufficient, additional locking screws are inserted (Fig. 15.3a–d). Drainage is not needed.

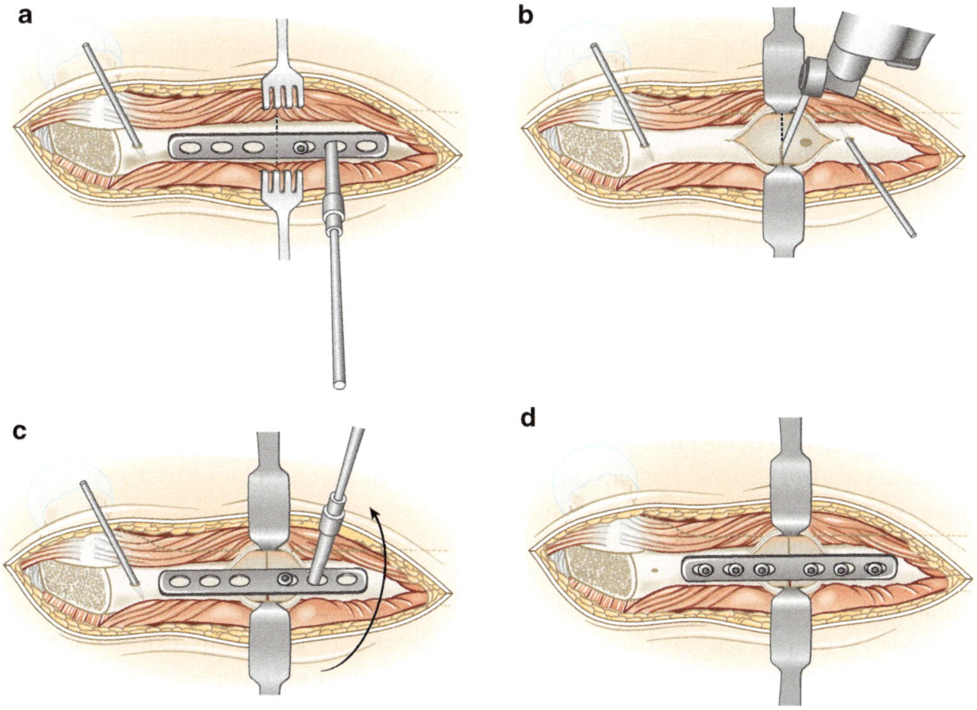

Fig. 15.3 (**a-d**) Technique for subtrochanteric osteotomy with a six-hole plate. (**a**) A locking plate is placed as proximal possible below the trochanteric osteotomy. The second most distal hole is used for placing a 2.5 mm distal derotation wire over the drill sleeve. The third most distal plate hole is stocked with a locking screw. The proximal derotation wire is rotated and placed in the desired amount of torsional correction proximal to the plate. (**b**) After marking the osteotomy, the plate is removed with its screw, leaving the distal derotation wire in place. After decortication, the osteotomy is performed with an oscillating saw. The distal derotation wire is a perfect directional guide for the osteotomy. (**c**) After repositioning the plate and reinsertion of the screw, the distal fragment is derotated to the desired position. (**d**) Proximal derotation is possible with the help of a reposition clamp under visual control of the joint relation. The distal plate fixation is accomplished, compression is performed by eccentric drilling and screw fixation proximal to the osteotomy (**d**)

In cases of additional SHD, the correction can also be performed on the proximal fragment with the help of a derotation clamp. Proximal derotation allows fine tuning of the torsional correction under visual control of the joint relation.

15.13 Postoperative Follow-Up

- *Postoperative partial weight-bearing depending on the osteotomies performed*

The period of partial weight-bearing is determined by the procedure performed. After multiplanar intertochanteric osteotomy, weight-bearing can be advanced after 6–8 weeks with signs of early callus formation on postoperative radiograph and 8–10 weeks in adults. After a transverse subtrochanteric femoral derotation osteotomy, weight-bearing can be increased after 4–6 weeks in children and 6–8 weeks in adults and activity advanced with further consolidation of the osteotomy. Athletic activities are allowed once the osteotomy has fully consolidated and abductor strength has returned (typically ~6 months).

- *Secondary procedures*

Screw heads may cause bothersome pain with direct pressure or interfere with iliotibial band gliding; these may disappear after removal of the metal. Most plates are removed after 6–12 months to avoid complicating future total hip arthroplasty.

15.14 Intra-/Postoperative Complications

Complications can be generalized to those related to the SHD (see Chap. 7) and those specific to inter–/subtrochanteric osteotomies. The primary complications related to osteotomies are implant failure and/or nonunion. Insufficient bony bridges with proximal fixation can lead to "cut out" of the proximal locking screws or the blade especially in osteopenic bone. Careful placement of the proximal implants in the central neck and intertrochanteric region can help avoid this. Nonunion can be an issue especially in multiplanar osteotomies where apposition of the bony fragments may not be perfect and with plate fixation that can be overly rigid. Optimizing osteotomy apposition through wedge resections and performing osteotomies with cooled saw blades or drill holes/osteotomes can help improve union rates. Malunion can also occur if osteotomy planning and execution is not performed meticulously. It is critical that the surgeon understand the direction that the limb must be moved intraoperatively in order to achieve the desired correction (e.g., derotation of the proximal vs. distal segment and in what direction). The oval cross section of the femur, especially in the intertrochanteric region, can lead to over- or under-correction of femoral torsion while tightening the plate screws. Other complications related to the use of plate systems in the proximal femur include peri implant fractures of the trochanter, joint penetration that may induce chondrolysis or limit movement, or complications related to excessive or inadequate correction.

15.15 Case Studies

Case study surgical dislocation with combined intertrochanteric flexion-valgus-derotation osteotomy:

An otherwise healthy 10-year-old female presented with worsening right hip pain after in situ pinning of a right slipped capital femoral epiphysis 6 months previous. She initially recovered well from her surgery but developed worsening pain over the last 2 months as well as increasing frustration with her limited motion and persistent limp. On clinical examination she walked with an extremely external knee and foot progression angle. She could flex to 90° with approximately 50° of obligate external rotation. AP (Fig. 15.4a) and frog lateral view (Fig. 15.4b) of the hip demonstrated a characteristic residual SCFE deformity. Postoperative (Fig. 15.4c) AP and (Fig. 15.4d) frog lateral view 7 months after combined surgical dislocation with flexion-valgus-internal rotation proximal femoral osteotomy. The surgical dislocation approach was chosen in order to fully resect the metaphyseal prominence and evaluate any potential intra-articular injury. This approach also allowed for more accurate assessment of the desired osteotomy correction. In situ screw was maintained due to incomplete physeal closure. Postoperatively, the child had 20° of internal rotation in flexion and 95° of flexion without pain, and her external foot progression angle was much improved.

Case study surgical dislocation with combined subtrochanteric derotation osteotomy:

An otherwise healthy 22-year-old male presented with long-term groin pain on both sides. In a clinical examination there were severe impingement symptoms in both hips as well as an internal rotation of 0°. He showed evident external rotation gait with a kneeing-out of 20°. Radiographic and MRI workup showed only some reduced anterior waisting of the head-neck junction (Fig. 15.5a, b). Torsional profile showed retroversion of 5° on both sides. Decision was made to perform a surgical hip dislocation to improve the waisting with a burr in combination with a subtrochanteric derotation osteotomy with a six-hole plate in the technique described above. The labrum showed no lesion. By the subtrochanteric osteotomy, the femoral retrotorsion was corrected by 20°. The postoperative course showed healing of the osteotomies as expected (Fig. 15.5c–e), and the patient outcome was highly satisfactory.

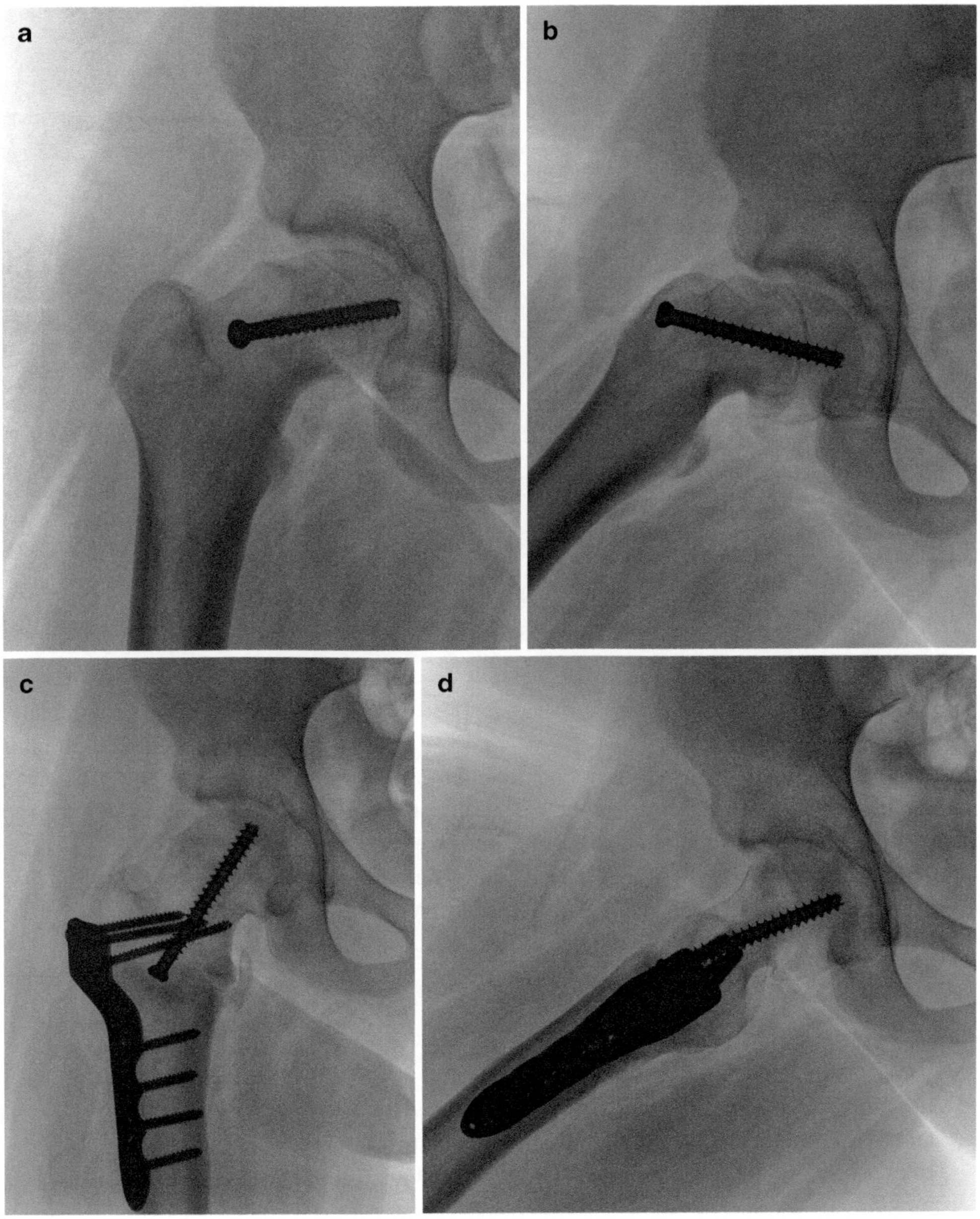

Fig. 15.4 (**a-d**) Preoperative (**a**) anteroposterior (AP) and (**b**) frog lateral view demonstrates characteristic residual SCFE deformity. Postoperative (**c**) AP and (**d**) frog lateral view 7 months after surgical dislocation for cam decompression combined with flexion-valgus-internal rotation proximal femoral osteotomy. In situ screw was maintained due to incomplete physeal closure

15.16 Controversies

- With the advent of hip arthroscopy, certain pathologies that once required a SHD to allow access and appropriate treatment are more often addressed arthroscopically. This is particularly true for most cases of femoro-acetabular impingement (FAI). For those patients that need a corrective osteotomy in addition to intra-articular treatment, it is not known when it is beneficial to perform a hip arthroscopy and concomitant extra-articular proximal femoral osteotomy vs a SHD. One advantage of the latter approach is the use of a single surgical exposure and setup to accomplish both operative goals (address intra-articular pathology and perform proximal femoral realignment) as well as the ability to accurately assess both the intra-articular and even more important the extra-articular effects of the osteotomy.
- Specifically for residual deformity from SCFE, some controversy exists over the limits of SHD with sub–/intertrochanteric femoral osteotomy and when to consider a modified Dunn procedure. The former is a safe procedure but does introduce secondary deformity since the osteotomy is performed distal to the deformity. The latter corrects the deformity at its original site but has higher risks of osteonecrosis.

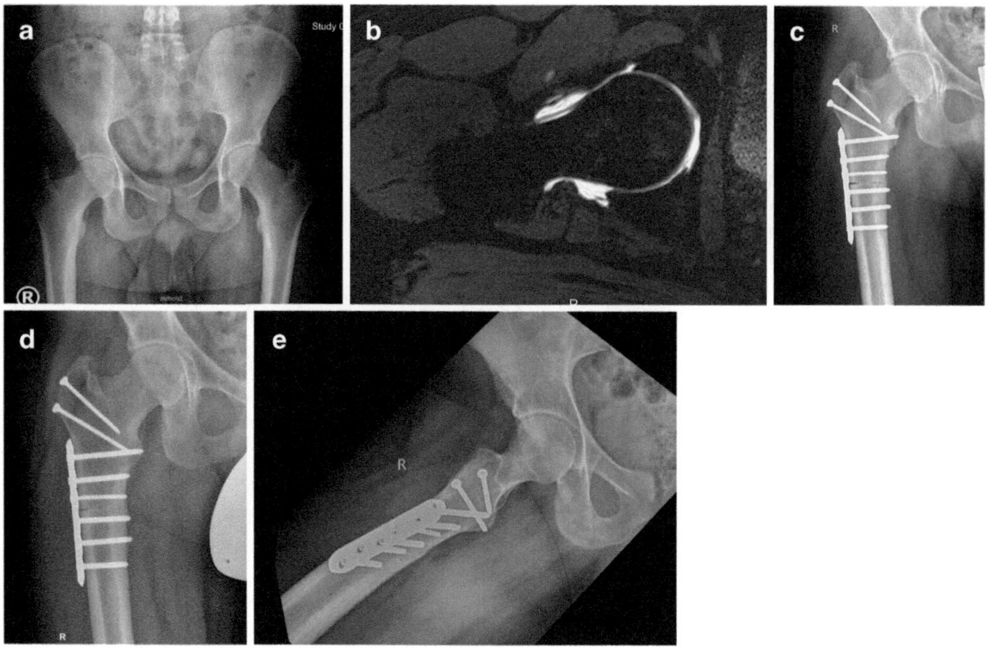

Fig 15.5 (**a**-**e**) Preoperative X-ray (**a**) MRI (**b**) demonstrates low anterior waisting of the head neck junction. In addition, there is a 5° retroversion. Postoperative X-rays after 8 (**c**) and 12 (**d**, **e**) weeks with on-time healing of the trochanteric and anteverting subtrochanteric osteotomy and a restored head-neck offset

15.17 Results

SHD with concomitant sub–/intertrochanteric femoral osteotomy can be safely performed without significant risk of avascular necrosis. Several studies suggest improved radiographic indices as well as functional outcome scores (depending on the specific pathology being addressed) with this approach. Delayed or frank nonunion can occur.

15.18 Outlook

- For complex deformities such as residual Perthes disease and SCFE deformity, the combined SHD and sub–/intertrochanteric osteotomy looks to have an important role moving forward. For mild to moderate deformities, advances in hip arthroscopy have improved treatment of intra-articular bony and chondral pathology. As such, it may be that combined arthroscopy and osteotomy procedures may supplant some of the cases currently being performed via a surgical dislocation/osteotomy approach. More recently, femoral neck osteotomies (Chap. 16) challenge the intertrochanteric osteotomy for its lesser side deformities and hardware problems.

References

1. Erickson, et al. Treatment of chronic, stable SCE via surgical hip dislocation with combined osteochondroplasty and Imhauser osteotomy. J Child Orthop. 2017;11:284–8.
2. Rebello, et al. Surgical dislocation in the management of pediatric and adolescent hip deformity. Clin Orthop Relat Res. 2009;467:724–31.
3. Dunn DM. The treatment of adolescent slipping of the upper femoral epiphysis. J Bone Joint Surg (Br). 1964;46:621–9.
4. Baraka, et al. Combined Imhauser osteotomy and osteochondroplasty in SCFE through a surgical dislocation approach. J Child Orthop. 2020;14:190–200.
5. Hellman, et al. Operative treatment of FAI: open hip preservation surgery. Curr Rev Musculoskelet Med. 2013;6(3):258–63.
6. Kamath AF, Ganz R, Zhang H, Grappiolo G, Leunig M. Subtrochanteric osteotomy for femoral mal-torsion through a surgical dislocation approach. J Hip Preserv Surg. 2015;2:65–79.

Femoral Neck Osteotomy

16

Paulo Rego, Dianzhong Luo, and Reinhold Ganz

16.1 Background

- Proximal femoral osteotomies are well-established realignment procedures performed to address hip deformities, non-union or avascular necrosis (AVN). Nevertheless, the use of more conventional osteotomies specifically intertrochanteric osteotomy (ITO) or subtrochanteric osteotomies (STO) appears to be declining in current clinical practice in the context of modern hip surgery [1].
- A broader acceptance for THA even in younger patients and some technical limitations of osteotomies could explain why proximal femoral osteotomy has been rarely considered as the first option in the surgical management of a painful hip.
- In the case of the classic ITO, the approach is always extra-articular, and there is no direct access to intra-articular pathology. The correction is also performed distant from the main anatomic anomaly, creating a secondary deformity and eventually a long-term loss of abductor strength in the case of a varus osteotomy [2]. The femoral shaft is either medialized, lateralized, or shifted anteriorly or posteriorly dependent on the inclination of the proximal fragment. As such it alters the mechanical axis of the lower limb [3]. Varus ITO also has the potential to create extra and intra-articular impingement. THA following ITO is also technically more demanding and can be associated with higher complication rates.
- With the development of the extended vascular retinacular flap (Chap. 8), a technique that allows mobilization of the femoral neck periosteum containing the retinacular branches of the deep branch of the medial branch of the medial circumflex artery (MFCA) [3–5], it was possible to consider a more proximal level for the osteotomy cut(s). By performing the correction closer to the deformity, at the femoral neck, it is possible to obtain a larger correction and improve the joint congruency with less angular displacement of the proximal fragment and less shortening or lengthening of the limb (Fig. 16.1). Understanding and having experience with the SHD (Chap. 7) is a prerequisite to performing a retinacular flap and neck osteotomy safely. With the dislocation, the hip can be inspected for femoro-acetabular impingement before and after the osteotomy; it is possible to treat labral and chondral pathologies and, if needed, to perform a head-neck junction osteochondroplasty proximal to the osteotomy line (Chap. 9). In dysplastic hips with a high fovea capitis and a negative delta angle (angle between two lines extending from medial edge of sourcil and superior edge of fovea capitis to centre of femoral head (Fig. 16.2)), a varus neck osteotomy can significantly normalize the load distribution without changing the relation between the femoral head and greater trochanter.
- With the dissection of the lateral retinacular flap towards the lesser trochanter, the technique of relative neck lengthening is almost completed (Chaps. 8 and 13).
- With meticulous dissection of the flap, the risk of avascular necrosis (AVN) is very low, and ongoing perfusion of the femoral head can be controlled with laser-Doppler flowmetry or 2 mm drill holes in the head.

P. Rego (✉)
Orthopaedic Department, Hospital da Luz, Lisbon, Portugal

D. Luo
Joint Department of Orthopaedic Centre of PLAGH, Beijing, China

R. Ganz
Emeritus, Faculty of Medicine, University of Berne, Berne, Switzerland

M. Leunig et al. (eds.), *Surgical Hip Dislocation*, https://doi.org/10.1007/978-3-031-70622-6_16

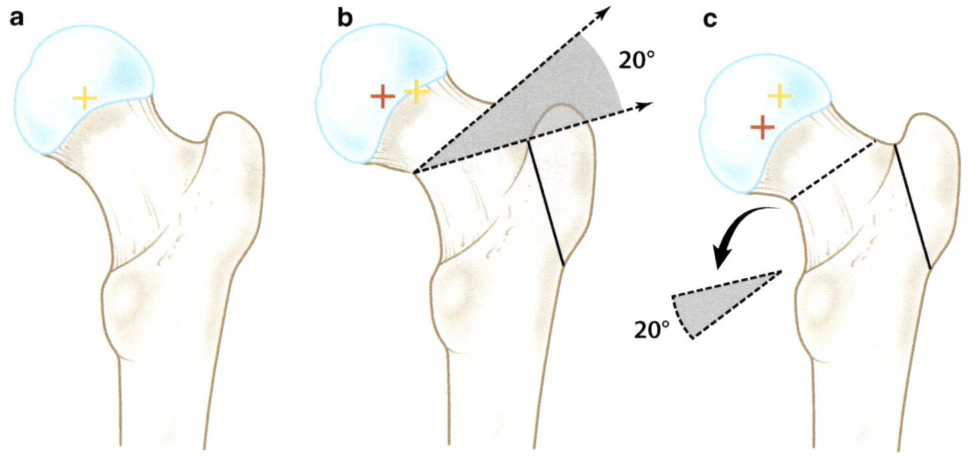

Fig. 16.1 Displacement of the femoral head centre in different varus femoral neck osteotomies: (**a**) normal proximal femur; (**b**) femoral neck open wedge varus osteotomy (20°) causes negligible shortening but some relative lateral displacement of the diaphysis; (**c**) closing wedge varus osteotomy (20° medial fragment removed) causes some more shortening but less lateral displacement of the diaphysis (yellow vs red cross sign)

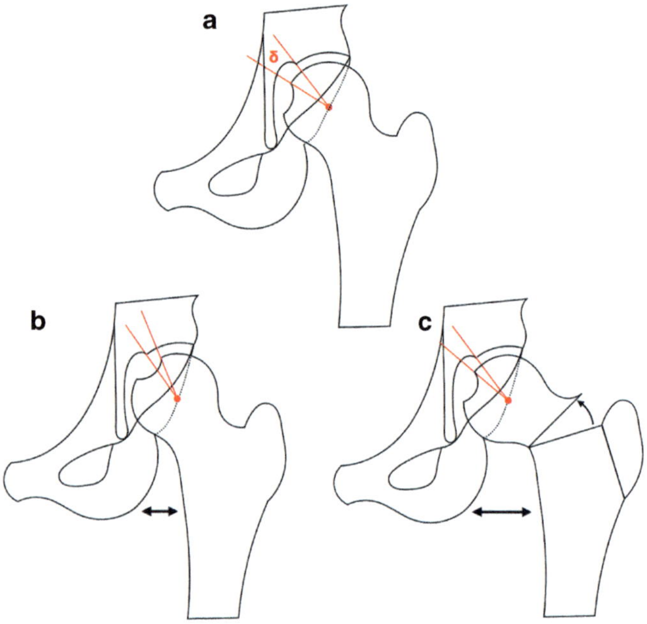

Fig. 16.2 (**a**) Normal position of the fovea capitis. The delta angle (δ) is measured between the lateral margin of the fovea capitis and the medial margin of the acetabular weight bearing area (red lines); (**b**) a high position of the fovea capitis has a negative delta angle; (**c**) varus femoral neck osteotomy restores the lower position of the fovea. Leg shortening is minimal. Femoral shaft is slightly lateralized (double arrows)

16.2 Indications

16.2.1 Indications

Best indication is in the age group between 15 and 30 years, when the periosteum and the retinacular tissues are still thick enough to allow easy circumferential detachment and mobilization from the femoral neck with a low risk of tearing. The bone quality is also usually sufficient to allow significant corrections with stable fixation:

- Severe valgus deformities.
- Deformities resulting from slipped capital femur epiphysis (SCFE) after growth plate closure.
- Post-traumatic deformities.
- Epiphyseal dysplasia.

16.2.2 Relative Indications

- Osteonecrosis of the femoral head. The correction must be able to unload the necrotic sector. In post-traumatic necrosis, the retinacular area may be altered by scaring and the number of open retinacular vessels may be critical.
- Osteochondral lesions as long as healthy cartilage surface can take the main load.
- Open epiphyseal growth plate in children 10 years old or older.

16.2.3 Contraindications

- Younger children with open femoral epiphysis growth plate.
- Extensive avascular necrosis.
- Presence of substantial degenerative changes.
- Inability to correct the deformity using a femoral neck osteotomy (e.g. rotational deformity).

16.3 Preoperative/Preinterventional Diagnostics

- Supine pelvis anteroposterior (AP) radiograph.
- Hip cross-table view and Lauenstein radiographs.
- Abduction or adduction standing AP pelvic dynamic views.
- Magnetic resonance imaging (MRI) including radial sequences and determination of femoral neck and acetabular version.
- Full-length AP lower limbs radiograph to access limb length discrepancies (optional).
- Enhanced (angio) MRI for evaluation of the vessel shape along the lateral retinaculum (in a case with previous trauma to the neck region). Further point to be added: CT with 3D reformat.

16.4 Preoperative Planning/Computer Simulation

- The AP pelvis standing view obtained before surgery can be used to simulate the position of the femoral head after correction and check for the position of the fovea capitis and for joint congruency.
- In the case of varus or valgus osteotomies, digital or manual templating of the proximal fragment can also be used to calculate the amount of angular correction needed to obtain the desired congruency of the joint and the final position of the greater trochanter (Fig. 16.3).

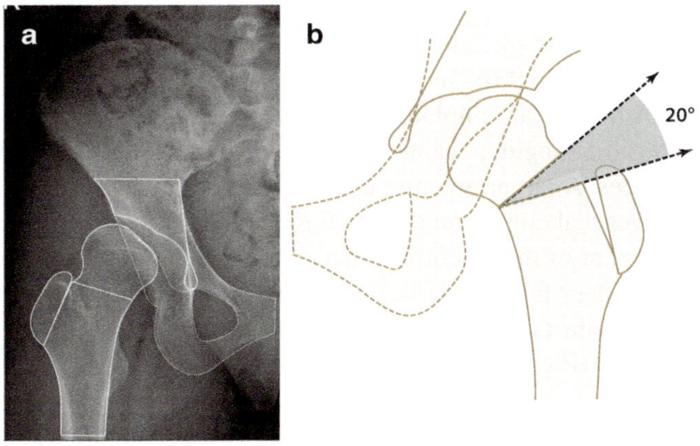

Fig. 16.3 Preoperative planning of varus neck osteotomy and PAO. Anteroposterior radiography of the left hip presenting with mild acetabular dysplasia, coxa valga and a high position of the fovea capitis. (**a**) The contours of proximal femur and acetabulum and desired level of osteotomy are drawn. (**b**) Using the same contours, the amount of angular correction necessary to achieve the best possible corrections can be measured

- Changes in limb length and femoral diaphysis axis can also be predicted using digital templating. The influence of a varus open wedge osteotomy on the total limb length is negligible. Limb length will be decreased minimally by performing a varus closing wedge osteotomy (Fig. 16.1).

16.5 Applied Anatomy

- To approach the femoral neck and prepare it to perform a safe osteotomy, the periosteum containing both retinacula needs to be detached circumferentially from the cortical bone down to the lesser trochanter (see Chap. 8). The deep branch of the MFCA runs from anterior to posteriorly between pectineus muscle medially and psoas muscle laterally, exiting posterior 5–10 mm proximal to the lesser trochanter.
- In cases where the neck is very short as after severe posterior epiphyseal slip, extreme care should be taken during positioning of the posterior Hohmann retractor, to avoid overstretching of the already shortened soft tissue flap. Additional relative neck lengthening will help to overcome such problems (Chap. 13).
- When performing closing wedge osteotomies (varus or valgus) or posterior rotation of the femoral head, the soft tissue flap becomes redundant and may risk being entrapped in the osteotomy site. Therefore, it should be constantly monitored to ensure that the flap is unfolded. In open wedge varus osteotomies or anterior rotation osteotomies, a certain risk for the perfusion of the femoral head comes from overstretching the postero-superior retinaculum. The tension of the flap and femoral head perfusion should be constantly monitored during the correction. If necessary, slight neck shortening or distal mobilization of the retinacular flap can relieve excessive tension.

16.6 Special Risks

- Compromise of the integrity of the soft tissue flap with interruption in the femoral head perfusion and development of AVN of the femoral head.
- Mechanic instability of the osteotomy due to poor bone quality, lack of adequate cortical bone contact, or inadequate hardware fixation. This can result in loss of reduction and retinacular flap tearing.
- Delayed union has been observed in cases with open wedge neck osteotomy.

16.7 Type of Anaesthesia

General anaesthesia is preferred as the surgery may take more than 120 minutes and the position is lateral decubitus or lateral followed by supine decubitus (in case a PAO is added).

16.8 Positioning

- Standard operating table.
- Lateral positioning with tunnel cushion and lateral bag.
- Supine positioning if PAO is added.
- Fluoroscopy and X-ray possibility.

16.9 Instruments/Implants

Standard instrumentation for surgical hip dislocation (see Chap. 7). In addition, the following instruments ensure an optimal surgical procedure:

- 2 rounded Hohmann retractors, 22 mm.
- 1 Dockhorn retractor 55/14 mm.
- Curved periosteal elevators, 6 mm, and 14 mm, 1 each.
- Straight chisel type Lexer, 5 mm, 10 mm, 15 mm, 1 each.
- Straight chisel type Lambotte 5 mm, 10 mm, 15 mm, 1 each.
- 1 metal hammer 300gr.
- Bone hooks small and medium, curved, 1 each.
- 1 capsule pliers.
- 1 curved haemostasis clamp.
- Small laminar spreader.
- Low-vibration oscillating saw.
- Sawblade thickness 0.60 mm, length 49 mm, width 27 mm.
- Sawblade thickness 0.60 mm, length 49 mm, width 14 mm.
- Triangular positioning template 90°/50°/40°.
- Triangular positioning template 80°/70°/30°.
- Triangular positioning template 100°/60°/20°.
- Threaded tip Kirschner (K) wires 1, 2, and 3 mm diameter and 15 mm length.
- Laser-Doppler flowmetry (optional).

16.10 Access

Access as for SHD with trochanteric osteotomy and extended retinacular vascular flap (see Chaps. 7 and 8). If a periacetabular osteotomy (PAO) is planed, the lateral access can be used for the ischial cut and later, an anterior modified Smith Petersen approach should be used for the remaining cuts of the PAO (see Chap. 19).

16.11 Technical Steps of Deep Dissection

- *Preparation and exposure of the neck*

After development of the extended reticular flap (see Chap. 8), both operative gaps resulting from anterior and posterior periosteal detachment from the neck need to be connected posteriorly. This can be done with the hip reduced using the 6 mm curved periosteal elevator to increase the gap so that two rounded 22 mm Hohmann retractors, one from anterior and the other from posterior, can be inserted in order to protect the flap from the oscillations of the saw blade while performing the osteotomy [5, 6] (Fig. 16.4). Constant care should be taken not to put tension on the flap with the retractors in place.

Before the development of the extended retinacular flap (Chap. 8) or before the osteotomy is performed, the joint should be inspected for the presence of femoro-acetabular impingement, cartilage, or labral damage. All lesions should be treated at this time.

- *Open wedge varus osteotomy*

With the hip reduced, under fluoroscopic control a 1 mm K-wire should be used to define the direction of the osteotomy cut. The tip of a K-wire should run perpendicular to the shaft and perforate the calcar levelling the undersurface of the head (Fig. 16.4). The osteotomy should follow the K-wire to achieve the best possible mechanical stability. Care should be taken to leave the medial border of the osseous calcar intact, allowing a gradual opening of the gap with a small bone spreader. Doing so prevents medial migration of the proximal fragment during correction.

A triangular template should be used at this time to confirm the angular value that should not exceed 30–35 degrees. A larger opening angle of the osteotomy increases the vertical component of the force exerted on the proximal fragment of the osteotomy, decreases medial bone contact, and is less favourable to bone healing. The gap should be filled with bone from the piece-meal resection of the trochanter (Fig. 16.4). Correction is provisionally stabilized with two K-wires (2 mm) under fluoroscopic control. Definitive fixation is achieved with two or three parallel cortical 4.5 mm fully threaded screws to avoid compression and loss of correction. Neutralization of the fixation can also be performed in certain cases by inserting a proximal femoral locking plate with the locking screws in the inferior femoral neck. Constant visual control of the soft tissue flap is advised during the entire procedure. Visual and palpatory control is also used to prevent overhanging of the bone graft.

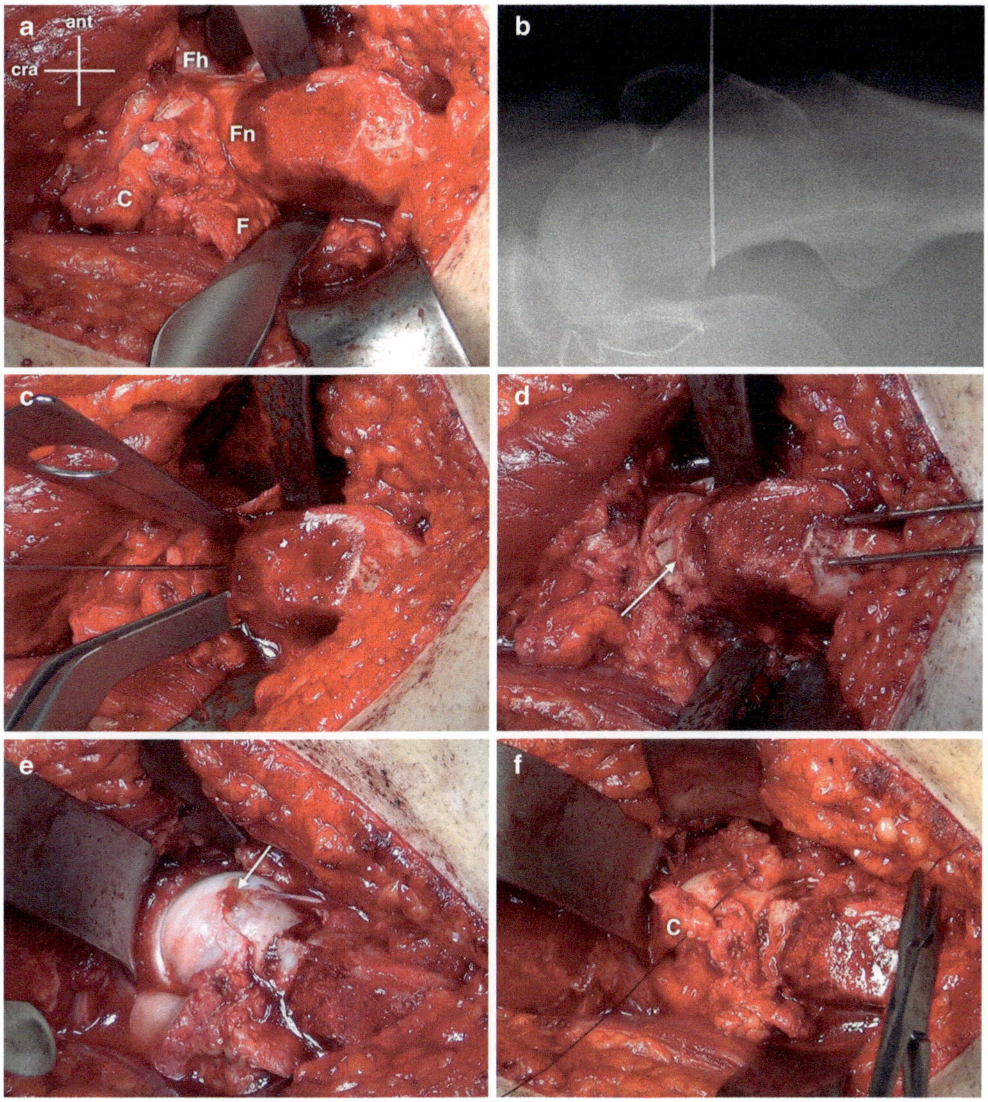

Fig. 16.4 Intraoperative pictures of an open wedge varus osteotomy of the right hip. (**a**) Circumferential exposure of the femoral neck with the rounded tip retractors in place around the calcar area. (**b**) Guide wire position controlled by fluoroscopy. (**c**) Opening of the osteotomy gap with a bone spreader until the desired angle of correction is achieved. (**d**) After provisional fixation of the osteotomy with two K-wires, the gap is filled with bone graft (arrow). (**e**) After definitive fixation of the osteotomy, the perfusion of the femoral head is checked by exit of blood at a drill hole on the antero-lateral area of the femoral head. (**f**) Capsular closure should be performed with loose sutures avoiding compression of the soft tissue flap containing the reticular vessels. Fn, femoral neck; Fh, femoral head; C, capsule; F, soft tissue flap; cran, cranial; ant, anterior

- *Close wedge varus osteotomy*

In a closing varus osteotomy, the cuts are easier to perform with the hip dislocated. The head can be prevented from relocation with several small wet sponges placed into the acetabulum. Again, K-wires and a triangular template should be used to control the osteotomy cuts, which should result in an approximately horizontal course of the resulting contact line.

The medially based wedge fragment should be removed, and the proximal fragment should be manually adapted to the distal fragment and secured with two K-wires. A half-diameter wedge will lead to even less shortening; the lateral gap can be filled with the wedge.

It is essential to keep anterior and medial cortical contact. Again, provisional fixation is performed using two K-wires. After that the hip is reduced, and a fluoroscopic control image should be obtained. The screws for final fixation are inserted in a lag fashion to allow interfragmentary compression. Proper screw length should be controlled with fluoroscopy and redislocation. During closing the gap and during final relocation of the head, caution is advised to prevent entrapment of the flap.

- *Close wedge valgus osteotomy*

For this osteotomy, the head can remain reduced. Again K-wires are used to control the amount of correction. After removal of the lateral-based bone fragment, the osteotomy gap should be closed and secured with a reduction clamp. Again, the screws for definitive fixation are inserted to create compression across the osteotomy. With this type of osteotomy, the retinacular flap becomes redundant and must be carefully adapted to avoid kinking with a potential stop of perfusion. Normally the outer cortex is strong enough to insert the screws without supplemental washers.

- *Neck osteotomy in slipped capital femur epiphysis (SCFE) with close physis*

In this case, deformity is usually more complex due to the posterior tilt of the epiphysis. The dissection of the posterior neck is particularly difficult when the tilt is so severe that the posterior border of the epiphysis lies close to the posterior neck cortex (Fig. 16.5). When the physis is already closed, the realignment of the epiphysis can only be achieved by performing a femoral neck osteotomy. Usually in cases of severe tilt, there is also shortening of the postero-superior retinaculum. The flap in cases like this needs to be developed more distal than usual to avoid over-stretching the vessels caused by the retractor positioning and manipulation of the epiphysis after the osteotomy. The osteotomy line should start in the area where the soft tissue flap cannot be further dissected from the posterior neck due to the posterior tilt of the epiphysis. We advocate the use of manual osteotomes to perform the osteotomy since the vibration of the oscillating saw can cause damage to the vascular supply of the femoral head. After separation from the neck, the proximal fragment should be carefully repositioned usually in a flexion and valgus position, avoiding stretching the soft tissues. However, rarely it is necessary to shorten the neck.

- *Femoral neck rotation osteotomy*

The described technique to unload an osteonecrotic area of the femoral head and to re-establish a healthy lateral pillar of the femoral head is a modification of the Sugioka technique [7], which lost consideration due to the difficulty mobilizing the deep branch of the MFCA and for the difficulty unloading necrotic sectors that are located in the centre of the head,

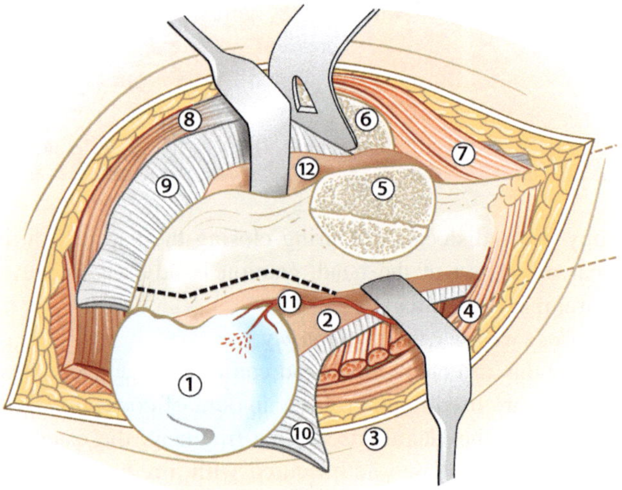

Fig. 16.5 Drawing showing a SCFE deformity after development of the soft tissue flap. Double pointed arrow shows the usual distal extension of separation of the flap from the bone. Dotted arrow shows the distal extension of the flap sometimes necessary in severe deformities. The blue line shows the osteotomy line started in the posterior neck cortical bone as near as possible to the posterior border of the tilted epiphysis and progressed parallel to the scar of the physis. 1- femoral head, 2- soft tissue flap, 3- external rotators, 4-lesser trochanter, 5-trochanter bed after bone trimming of the posterior trochanter, 6-trochanter free fragment, 7-vastus lateralis muscle, 8-gluteus medius muscle, 9-anterior capsule flap, 10-posterior capsule flap, 11-terminal branches of the MCFA, 12-anterior periosteal flap

where rotation does not turn sufficiently a healthy sector into the weight-bearing zone. By dissecting the retinacular flaps (Chaps. 7 and 8), the blood supply to the head is better protected, and the amplitude of rotation is slightly higher compared to the classic technique. The optimal indication is necrotic sectors located more in the periphery of the head. Theoretically, varus tilt of the head fragment could be included in the rotation with an osteotomy direction oblique to the rectangular line of the neck axis. The necessary amount of inclination is dependent on the amount of rotation needed to unload the necrotic segment. The required rotation can be calculated or simulated preoperatively. Though this technique is discussed between experienced surgeons, to date, such an extension of the rotational osteotomy has not been published.

The technical execution starts with the head reduced. A 3 mm K-wire is inserted under fluoroscopic control along the geometric axis of the femoral neck. Two other parallel 3.0 mm K-wires are inserted perpendicular to the first, one medial and the other lateral, to the osteotomy line in the basicervical area (Fig. 16.6). Using the oscillating saw and straight 5 mm and 10 mm manual osteotomes, the osteotomy is executed perpendicular to femoral neck axis. Rotation of the femoral neck around the first axial K-wire can be than performed. The medial perpendicular to the neck K-wire is used to rotate the medial fragment and confirm the angular value of the rotation with respect to the lateral K-wire.

The direction of rotation can be anterior or posterior according to the desired effect of unloading the necrotic area of the femoral head. Posterior rotation, opposite to anterior rotation, has much less potential to develop tension over the vascular flap allowing a larger amount of correction without endangering arterial perfusion to the femoral head [8]. The osteotomy can then be fixed using half-threaded cannulated screws inserted parallel to the axial K-wire. However, due to the reduced cortical contact area, the stability of the assembly is not as high as with a standard neck osteotomy and may need more strict postoperative unloading of the hip.

- *Relocation of the flap and refixation of the trochanteric fragment*

After definitive stabilization of the osteotomy, the perfusion of the femoral head should be checked by drilling the epiphysis near the anterior (around 2 o'clock) head-neck junction area (Fig. 16.4) or through the fovea capitis. After the neck osteotomy is performed, the only possible blood supply to the proximal osteotomy fragment (femoral head and part of the proximal femoral neck) comes from both retinacular flaps. If a constant blood flow is observed, this is sufficient evidence that there is an intact perfusion. However, not infrequently the blood flow is slow due to vascular spasms following the manipulations.

The anterior borders of the retinacular flaps should be reapproximated without any tension, and contact of the flaps should not be achieved (Fig. 16.4). Similarly, the capsular closure, especially following SCFE reconstruction, is performed using few sutures without putting the capsule under tension. The trochanteric fragment should be fixed against the remaining trochanteric bed without compressing the retinacular tissue. Maintaining the abductor lever arm should be controlled with fluoroscopy; excessive advancement and high positioning should be avoided. For definitive fixation two 3.5 or 4.5 mm screws are sufficient depending upon the trochanter size (Chap. 7). Tightening of the screws may compress the underlying retinaculum and may reduce the lever arm distance. Interposition of a bone fragment can avoid such adverse effects.

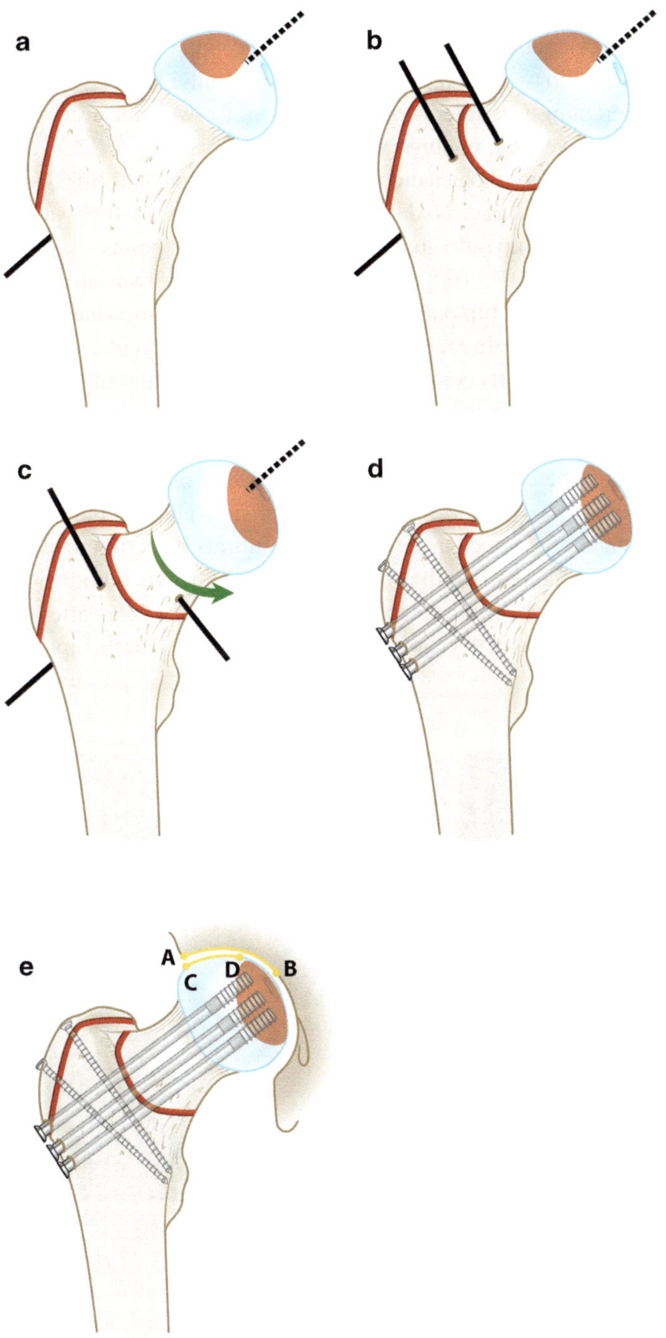

Fig. 16.6 Schematic drawing of the femoral neck rotational osteotomy. (**a**) One 3.0 mm K-wire is inserted into the axis of the femoral neck, avoiding to perforate the femoral head; (**b**) two 3.0 mm parallel K-wires are inserted perpendicular to the femoral neck, proximal and lateral to the planed osteotomy line; (**c**) anterior (or posterior) rotation of the medial osteotomy fragment until the desired angle of correction is achieved; (**d**) fixation of the osteotomy using half-threaded cannulated screws; (**e**) schematic drawing of lateral pillar intact ratio (LPIR), LPIR = CD/AB. It is claimed that if the LPIR>34%, the femoral head would not collapse in long-term follow-up in AVN hips

- *Additional periacetabular osteotomy (PAO) during the same anaesthesia*

  In some cases, an additional PAO may be needed to improve joint congruency and femoral coverage. An added benefit of the lateral approach is that the first and incomplete ischial osteotomy can be executed through this approach using the interval between the *inferior gemellus* and *quadratus femoris*/obturator externus muscles. It allows direct visualization and protection of the sciatic nerve with a soft tissue retractor. For the remaining PAO cuts, the patient should be turned to supine decubitus position [3], and the remaining cuts are performed from anterior as in the conventional technique (Chap. 19).

16.12 Postoperative Follow-Up

- The period of reduced weight bearing after a FNO should not be less than 10–12 weeks. Adding a PAO does not increase this period.
- Abductor strengthening program can be started at about 4 weeks. In open wedge varus osteotomy, the period of reduced weight bearing is prolonged, and the end is defined by complete radiological healing of the bone graft filling the lateral osteotomy gap.
- After radiological consolidation, the patient is encouraged to start walking using just one crutch for another 3–4 weeks. At 4 months full weight bearing is allowed. Impact activities should be postponed for 6 to 9 months after surgery. Deep venous thromboembolism prophylaxis should be carried for at least 6 weeks after surgery.

16.13 Intra-/Postoperative Complications

- The most severe intraoperative complication is the interruption of blood supply to the femoral epiphysis. This complication is rare. It can occur with poor technical preparation of the retinacular tissue flaps.
- Excessive tension on the posterior flap resulting from pressure of the retractors can potentially lead to a laceration of the retinaculum at the base of the femoral head.
- After the osteotomy manipulation of the proximal osteotomy fragment should also be done very carefully to avoid overstretching of the vessels.

- The flap should never be interposed in the osteotomy during fragment reduction and fixation or during interposition of a bone graft.
- Entrapment with resulting compression of the flap can also occur when refixing the trochanteric fragment without sufficient clearance from the neck. To avoid this last complication, the distal 3.5 mm screw should be put in place first (see also Chap. 8).
- Postoperative complications can include non-union of the osteotomy or hardware failure. In this case a revision surgery with bone graft and refixation might be necessary.

16.14 Case Studies

We present five illustrative cases of the femoral neck osteotomy technique. In two an additional PAO was performed to correct acetabular dysplasia:

Case 1 (Fig. 16.7): A 27-year-old female suffered from pain which was related to a combination of coxa valga, caput valgum, and high fovea capitis on the right side. The opposite side with a similar deformity was pain-free, probably because the fovea was corresponding with the fossa acetabuli and not with the acetabular cartilage, a configuration which potentially would never become symptomatic. Therefore, the femoral neck was determined as level of the unilateral osteotomy, leading to much less leg shortening when compared with an osteotomy at the intertrochanteric level. The MRI of the right side confirmed the large fovea and parts of the round ligament corresponding with the acetabular cartilage. The varus correction of about 20° was fixed with two screws and healed uneventfully. The minimal leg shortening was tolerated, and a shoe raise was not necessary. Fifteen years after surgery, the patient remained pain-free, and control radiographies did not show signs of osteoarthritis. Non-arthritic hip score (NAHS) reached 92.5 points, mHHS was 91 points, and hip outcome score (HOS) was 0.98 points.

Case 2 (Fig. 16.8): An 18-year-old female was suffering from bilateral hip pain. The symptoms were somewhat dominant on the right side. There was bilateral acetabular dysplasia (right > left) combined with caput valgum and high fovea capitis. The abduction view showed that on the right side, a PAO alone would be sufficient, while on the left side, PAO should be combined with a femoral varus osteotomy to normalize the joint relation. This decision also included the choice of the neck as level for the femoral correction to avoid substantial leg length difference. Interval between both sides was 1 year beginning with the right side. Eight years after the right side and 9 years after the left surgery, both hips are

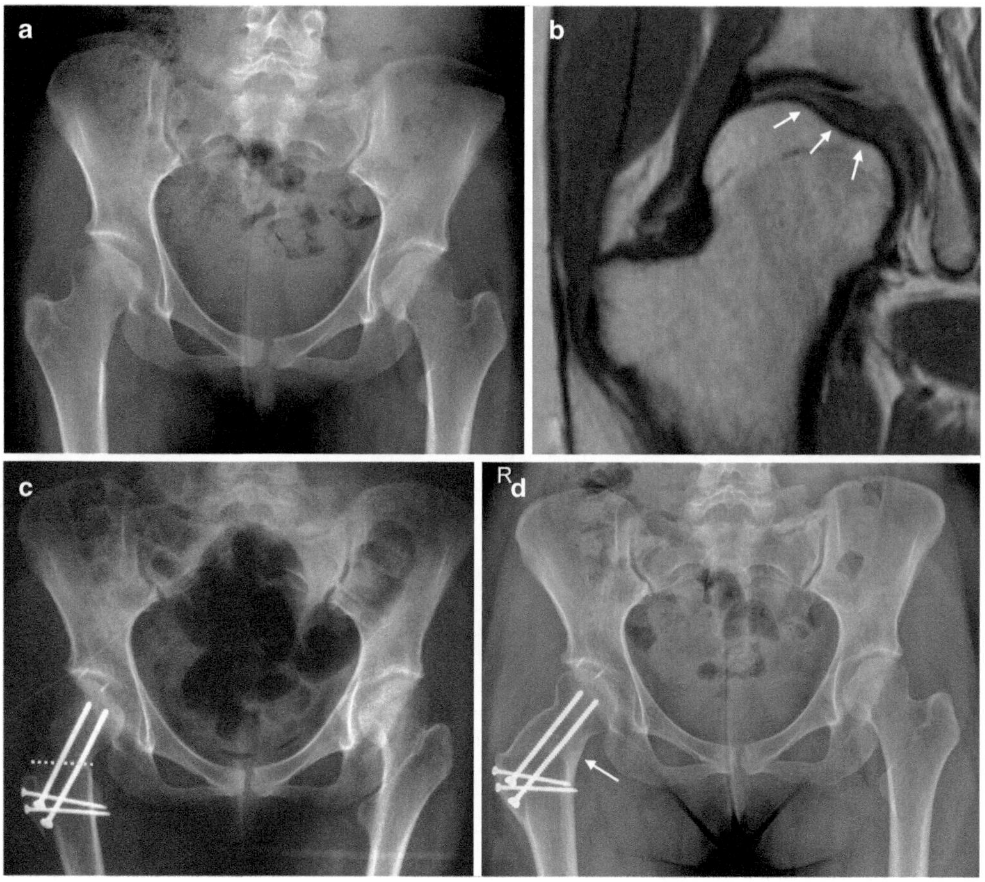

Fig. 16.7 (**a**) Coxa valga, caput valgum, and high fovea capitis on the right side of a 27-year-old female patient. (**b**) The MRI shows the large fovea and *ligamentum teres* under the acetabular cartilage (arrows). (**c**) Postoperative radiograph after a close wedge varus femoral neck osteotomy (dotted line). (**d**) Result at 15-year follow-up without signs of osteoarthritis, no pain, a non-arthritic hip score (NAHS) of 92.5 points, a modified Harris hip score (mHHS) of 91 points, and a hip outcome score (HOS) of 0.98 points. Note the extensive remodelling of the calcar area as a response to the varization (arrow)

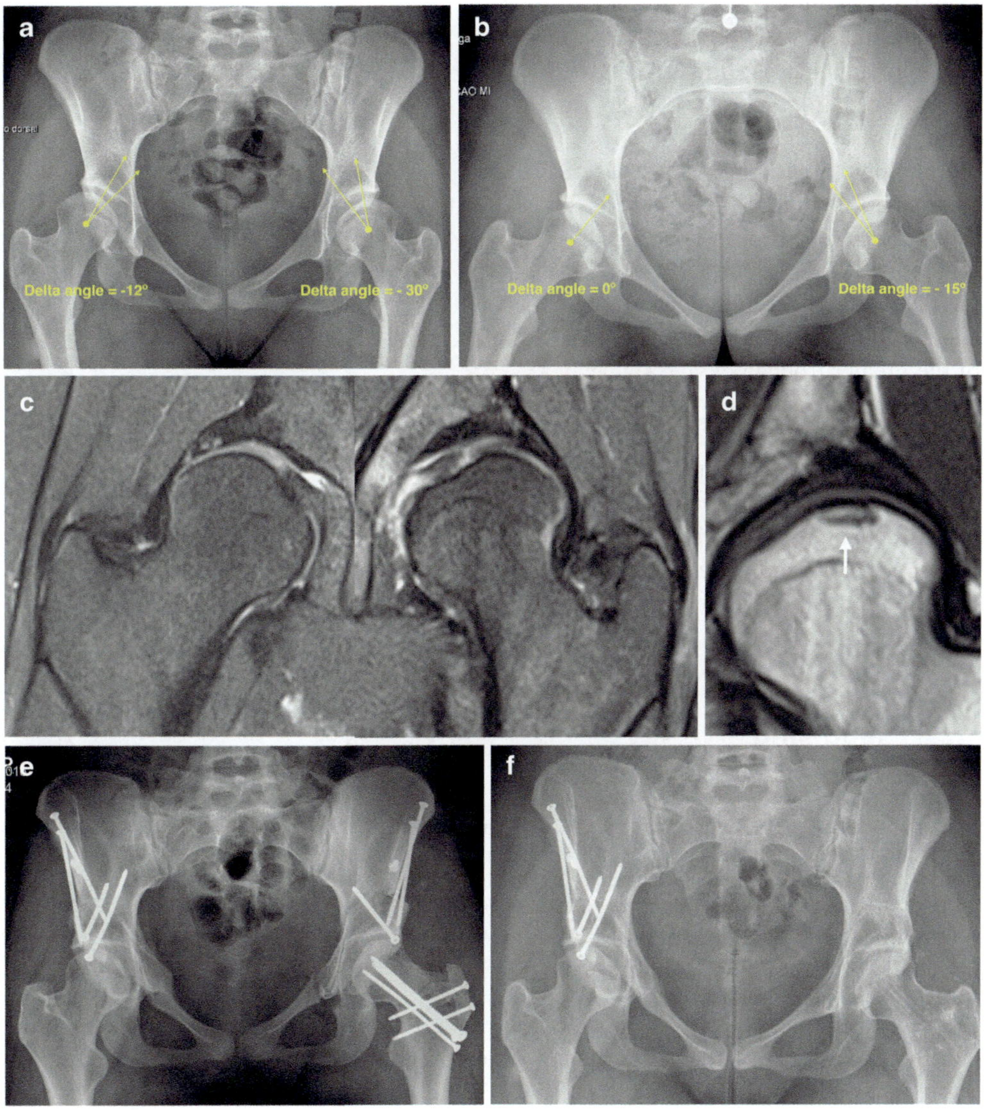

Fig. 16.8 (**a**) Bilateral acetabular dysplasia combined with caput valgum and high fovea capitis with bilateral negative delta angle in an 18-year-old female patient. (**b**) In the abduction view, on the left side, the negative angle persists. (**c**) MRI of the left and right hips (pd-tse with fat suppression). On the left hip, the fovea presents with a higher position, and the load sharing area is shorter. (**d**) MRI sequence without fat suppression showing on the left side an area of sequestration of 8 mm related to increased stress on the articular surface. (**e**) Postoperative radiograph showing 1 year result after PAO on the right side and immediate result after FNO and PAO on the left side (the decision to add a varus osteotomy on the left side was to avoid overcorrection of the PAO with a resulting negative roof angle). (**f**) 7- and 8-year results on the right and left hips. The patient presented no pain, a NAHS of 95 points, a mHHS of 84 points, and a HOS of 97%. On the left side, screws were removed due to hardware intolerance

pain-free. On the left side, the metal was removed successfully for intolerance. NAHS reached 95 points, mHHS was of 84 points, and HOS was 0.97 points.

Case 3 (Fig. 16.9): An 18-year-old female with severe unilateral acetabular dysplasia of the right side, coxa valga, high-positioned fovea capitis, significant subluxation, and an intraosseous cyst in the lateral edge of the acetabulum. Instability will lead to rapid further degeneration, reason why surgery is urgent despite relative moderate pain. A radiography in abduction alluded to a femoral varus osteotomy in addition to a PAO. Pre-existing leg shortening of 1 cm fostered the decision for an open wedge type osteotomy at the level of the neck; healing time was prolonged up to 16 weeks until sufficient consolidation. The result 5 years after surgery was excellent with normalization of the joint parameters and painless function. NAHS and mHHS reached 100 points and HOS 100%.

Case 4 (Fig. 16.10): A 17-year-old female deplored pain and limitation of ROM from chronic SCFE deformity of the right hip. Radiographies showed a severe slip with step formation in varus and retrotilt, the growth plate was consolidated. MRI revealed a vital epiphysis. It was obvious that a distant osteotomy could not sufficiently correct the complex pathomorphology, on the other hand dissection of the retinacular flaps to access the deformed neck area was expected to be delicate and laborious; MRI sequences helped to better understand details of the area of deformation. During dissection the integrity of the retinacular flaps was visually controlled. The osteotomy immediately distal to the retinacular origin at the head-neck junction had to be executed with straight and curved osteotomes. Raising of the freed epiphysis had to be made under constant control of the retinacular tension; final position was possible only by some bone resection. Joint

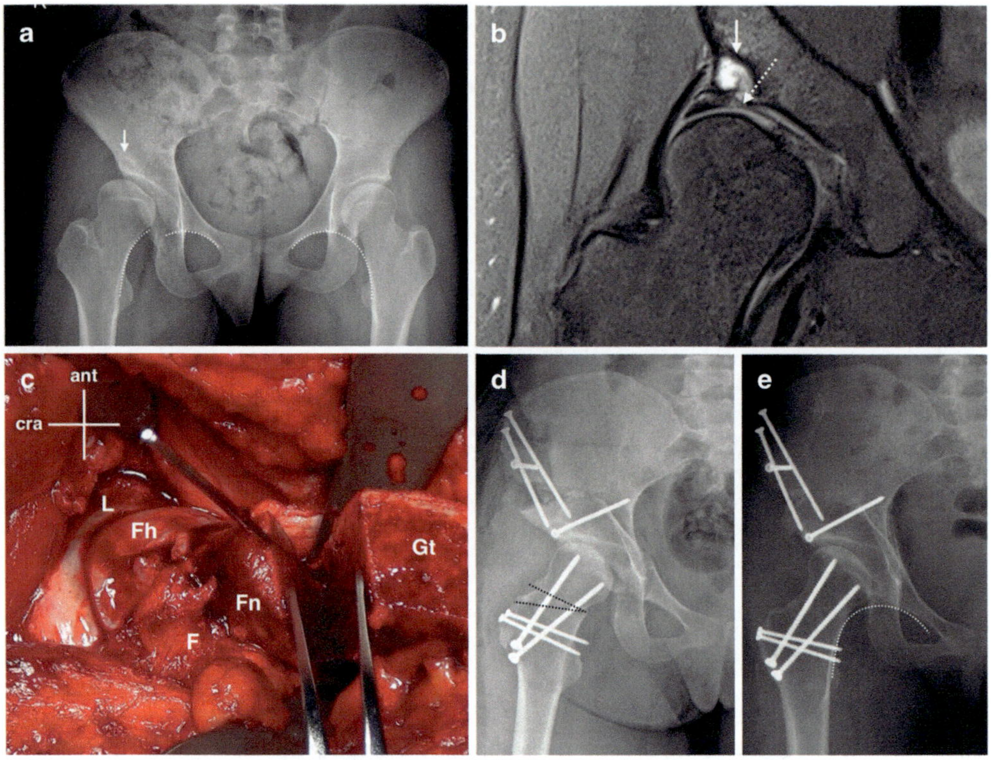

Fig. 16.9 (**a**) Severe acetabular dysplasia, coxa valga, high-positioned fovea capitis, and significant lateral migration of the femoral head (Shenton's line interruption) in an 18-year-old female patient. A degenerative cyst is already seen on the superolateral acetabular area (withe arrow). (**b**) The MRI shows the cyst more striking and a complex inside out avulsion of cartilage and labrum (dotted arrow). (**c, d**) Intraoperative picture showing the lateral opening (25°) with the spreader still in place. (**d**) Postoperative radiograph of the open wedge osteotomy (solid lines) plus PAO. (**e**) Result at 5-year follow-up with significant improvement in joint congruency, re-establishment of the Shenton's line continuity, healing of the cyst a NAHS of 100 points, a mHHS of 100 points, and a HOS of 100%. L, labrum; Fn, femoral neck; Fh, femoral head; F, soft tissue flap; Gt, greater trochanter; cran, cranial; ant, anterior

stability of the best epiphyseal position was secured with subtrochanteric rotational osteotomy. Osteotomy gaps were filled with resected bone from the resection. Five years after surgery, the head-neck junction is smoothly remodelled. ROM and leg length are nearly normal. NAHS reached 95 points and mHHS 91 points. HOS was 91.7%.

Case 5 (Fig. 16.11): A 14-year-old male patient presented with AVN of the right femoral head after neck fracture and internal fixation. The preoperative evaluation with standard radiographies and computer tomography gave the necessary understanding of localization and extension of the necrosis, necessary for the indication of a rotational neck osteotomy. The definitive amount of anterior rotation was controlled by fluoroscopy. The achieved position was primarily fixed with K-wires and finally secured with three screws. The osteotomies of neck and greater trochanter healed uneventfully. A radiographic control 3 years after surgery showed a healthy head contour corresponding with the acetabulum; nHHS reached 97 points.

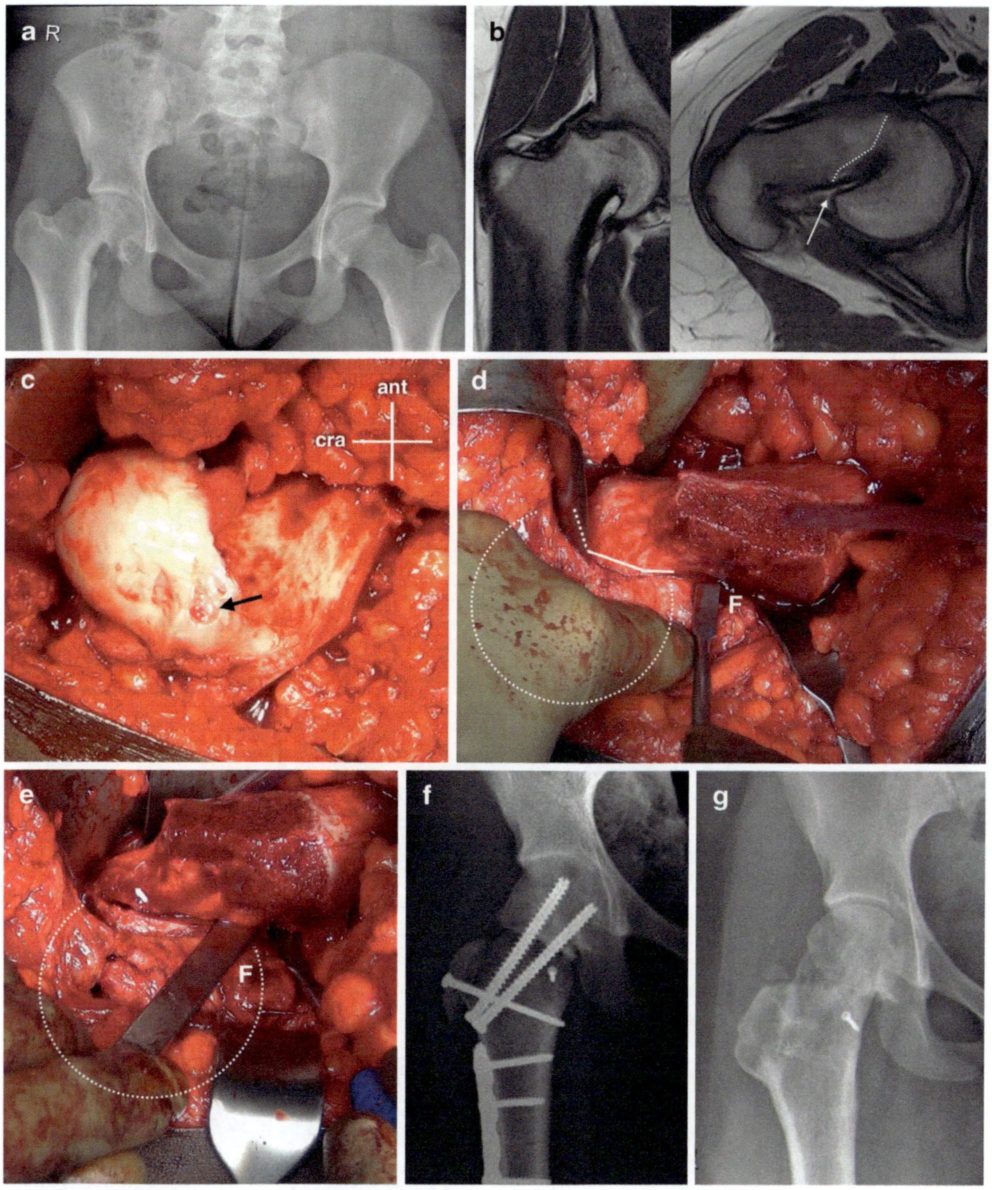

Fig. 16.10 (**a**) SCFE deformity of the right hip in a 17-year-old female patient. (**b**) Coronal and axial MRI sequences showing the severe inferior and posterior tilt of the epiphysis. Arrow points to the posterior border of the tilted epiphysis overlapping the bone penetration area of the retinacular vessels. Doted white line represents the path of the planed FNO. (**c**) Intraoperative picture showing the deformity with a protruding antero-superior metaphysis (arrow). (**d**) The flap (**f**) was separated from the posterior femoral neck up to the posterior border of the tilted epiphysis. Shortening of the soft tissues increases the difficulty of the circumferential approach to the neck. The white circle represents the position of the femoral head and the white line the planed osteotomy path. (**e**) The osteotomy was performed under visual control using straight and curved osteotomes. (**f**) Postoperative radiograph showing the reduced epiphysis. A sub-trochanteric osteotomy was added to increase the anteversion of the femoral neck. (**g**) Result at 5-year follow-up with complete healing of the osteotomies, remodelling of the head-neck junction, a NAHS of 95 points, a mHHS of 91 points, and a HOS of 91.7%

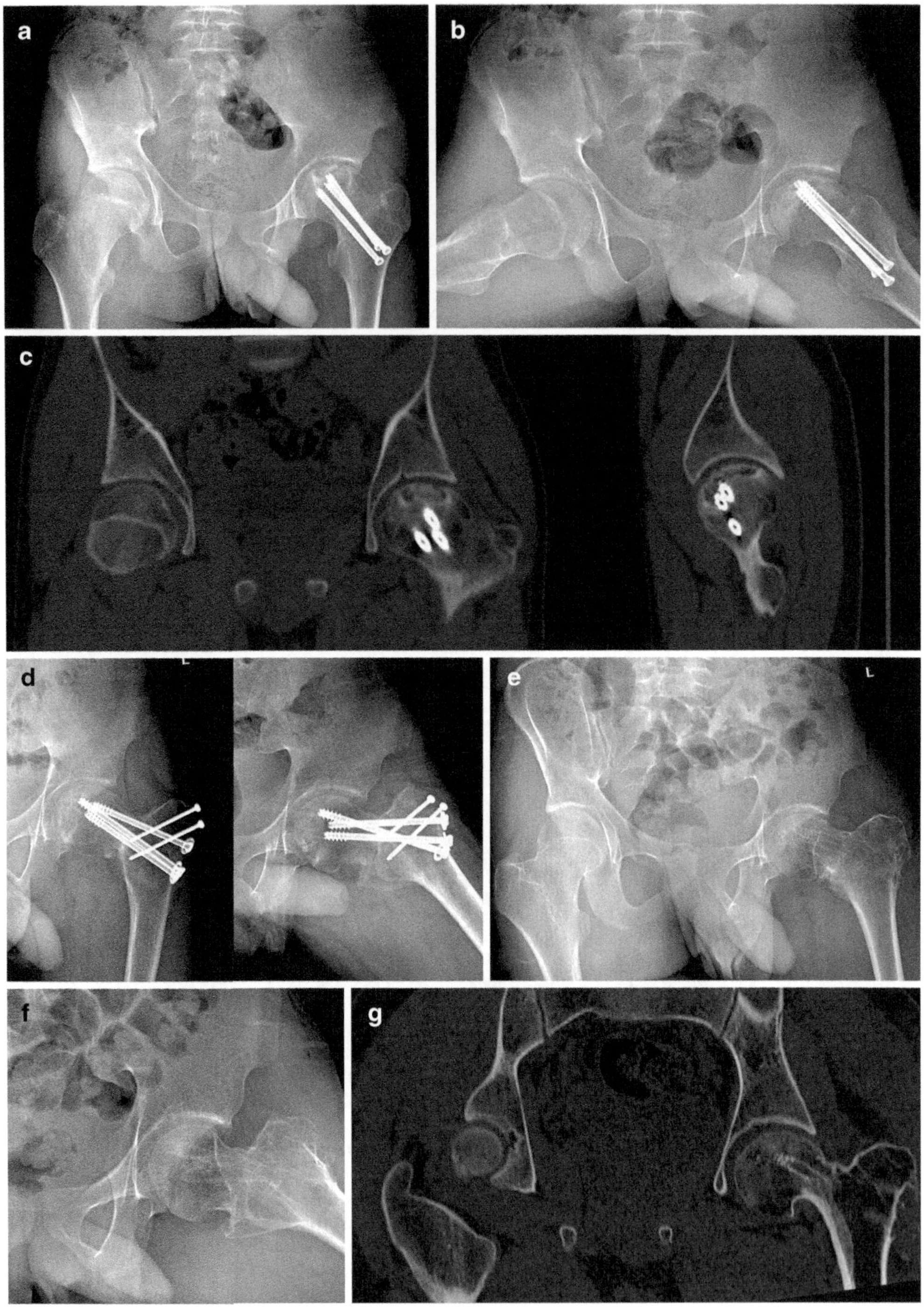

Fig. 16.11 (**a**) A 14-year-old male patient presenting with extensive AVN after left femoral neck fracture and internal fixation. (**b**) Frog lateral view confirms the extensive collapse of the femoral head. (**c**) CT scan coronal and sagittal reconstructions show collapse in the anterior and superior area of the left femoral head. (**d**) Six months after femoral neck rotational osteotomy, the AP and frog lateral view radiographs show a congruent joint with no visible collapse in the weight-bearing area of the femoral head. (**e**) Radiographic result at 3-year follow-up after hardware removal. (**f**) In the frog lateral view, it is visible a normal contour of the anterior head-neck area. (**g**) CT coronal reconstruction shows accomplished remoulding of the necrotic area of the femoral head without collapse. The mHHS was 97 points

16.15 Controversies

- The ideal location for a proximal femoral osteotomy depends on hip morphology and surgeon experience. FNO has several advantages over more distal procedures but is a demanding procedure. Performing this procedure in a safe way requires a long learning curve.
- In contrast to ITO, FNO does not influence the torsional profile of the femur. If it is needed, one may add a subtrochanteric rotational osteotomy or perform an ITO instead of a FNO.
- The question of whether to do an open or closed wedge varus osteotomy is controversial. The open wedge osteotomy creates nearly no shortening. However, healing time is longer and non-union is a risk factor. Closing wedge osteotomy is technically more demanding, and shortening can be up to 1 cm, but healing time is shorter, and the risk of non-union is very low.

- Lower and upper age limits remain controversial. We have good experience with a lower limit around 10 years. FNO should probably not be performed over the age of 30 years. Bone quality and adequate psychological profile of the patient (long healing time) are also important when recommending this osteotomy level.
- The technique should be learned in centres with an adequate case load. Sufficient expertise may need about 25 personal cases per year.
- Risk of avascular necrosis and the demanding execution of the osteotomy may discourage, especially when the expected case load is low.

16.16 Results

- There are few published studies [3, 8–10] reporting the results of femoral neck osteotomy based on the surgical technique of the extended retinacular flap. The midterm outcome of 103 hips (103 patients) was analysed regarding short-term surgical complications, presence of avascular necrosis, and conversion to total hip replacement (THR). The indications for FNO were varus/valgus deformities, SCFE malunion (closed physis), post-traumatic deformities, and avascular necrosis.
- The osteotomies performed were: 45 cases of varus close wedge, 30 varus open wedge, 6 valgus close wedge, 18 flexion-valgus osteotomies (to correct SCFE malunion), and 4 anterior rotation osteotomies for AVN.
- Reported complications varied from 6 to 25%. The most frequent complications were delayed union (five cases) and AVN (five cases, after previous surgery, scar-adhesions between neck and the epiphysis in SCFE). Two cases of hardware failure, one case of trochanteric non-union, and a postoperative infection were also reported. In three patients the hip function did not improve after anterior rotation FNO for AVN. Five hips had to be converted to THR due to AVN.
- According to Ganz et al. [9, [3], further possible risk for development of AVN could come from excessively tight closure of the capsule, tamponade secondary to a hematoma, and a retinacular fold under the refixed trochanter leading to compression of the retinacular vessels. Hips with previous surgery at the level of proximal femur can also be at risk due to unpredictable abnormalities in the circulation to the head. Anderson et al. [10] also point to the existence of adhesions between posterior vasculature and the epiphyseal scar in malunited SCFE as a risk factor to AVN.

16.17 Outlook

- Precise indications and detailed outcomes of FNO are still not fully established. Concentrating such surgery in centres, interaction of centres, and publishing the results with detailed analysis of complications, especially AVN, could help to further reduce failure rates.

References

1. Haverkamp D, Eijer H, Besselaar PP, Marti RK. Awareness and use of intertrochanteric osteotomies in current clinical practice. An international survey. Int Orthop. 2008;32(1):19–25. https://doi.org/10.1007/s00264-006-0270-0.
2. Leunig M, Puloski S, Beck M, Siebenrock K-A, Ganz R. Proximal femoral osteotomy: current indications and techniques. Semin Arthroplast. 2005;16(1):53–62. https://doi.org/10.1053/j.sart.2004.12.006.
3. Ganz R, Horowitz K, Leunig M. Algorithm for femoral and periacetabular osteotomies in complex hip deformities. Clin Orthop Relat Res. 2010;468(12):3168–80. https://doi.org/10.1007/s11999-010-1489-z.
4. Gautier E, Ganz K, Krügel N, Gill T, Ganz R. Anatomy of the medial femoral circumflex artery and its surgical implications. J Bone Joint Surg Br. 2000;82(5):679–83. https://doi.org/10.1302/0301-620x.82b5.10426.
5. Kalhor M, Beck M, Huff TW, Ganz R. Capsular and pericapsular contributions to acetabular and femoral head perfusion. J Bone Joint Surg Am. 2009;91(2):409–18. https://doi.org/10.2106/JBJS.G.01679.
6. Kalhor M, Horowitz K, Gharehdaghi J, Beck M, Ganz R. Anatomic variations in femoral head circulation. Hip Int. 2012;22(3):307–12. https://doi.org/10.5301/HIP.2012.9242.
7. Xiao K, Luo D, Cheng H, Zhang Z, Zhang H. Rotational osteotomy on the base of femoral neck in treating osteonecrosis of the femoral head. Chinese J Orthop. 2018;38:425–32. https://doi.org/10.3760/CMA.J. ISSN. 0253-2352.2018.07.007
8. Rego P, Mascarenhas V, Mafra I, Oliveira F, Pinto P, Ganz R. Femoral neck osteotomy in skeletally mature patients: surgical technique and midterm results. Int Orthop (SICOT). 2020; https://doi.org/10.1007/s00264-020-04822-4.
9. Ganz R, Huff TW, Leunig M. Extended retinacular soft-tissue flap for intra-articular hip surgery: surgical technique, indications, and results of application. Instr Course Lect. 2009;58:241–55.
10. Anderson LA, Gililland JM, Pelt CE, Peters CL. Subcapital correction osteotomy for malunited slipped capital femoral epiphysis. J Pediatr Orthop. 2013;33(4):345–52. https://doi.org/10.1097/BPO.0b013e31827d7e06.

Subcapital Osteotomy

17

Eduardo Novais and Michael Leunig

17.1 Introduction

Correction of a deformity at the center of rotation of angulation is the most anatomical correction possible with the slightest secondary deformity. However, for correction of a SCFE deformity, the vascular supply to the femoral head [1] (Chap. 6) must be left intact. With the combination of surgical hip dislocation (Chap. 7) and a soft tissue flap developed subperiosteally from the retinaculum and external rotators (Chap. 8), the vascular supply to the femoral head through the medial circumflex femoral artery can be preserved [2]. This soft tissue flap allows release of the epiphysis and complete callus resection from the femoral neck without tensioning the retinacular flap supplying the blood flow to the femoral head.

17.2 Background

Theoretically, the best long-term results of surgical treatment for slipped capital epiphysis (SCFE) would be expected from techniques that allow anatomic reduction of the slipped epiphysis while preserving blood flow. However, such techniques were rarely used until a few years ago because of the risk of femoral head necrosis and associated with surgical techniques that were considered very technically demanding especially when infrequently applied. These concerns have helped the much less complex "pinning in situ" to gain popularity over many years. Historical studies with medium to long-term results seemed to justify the popularity of in situ fixation [3, 4]. However, more recent work has shown that long-term results are not as good as historically presented, mainly because of the frequent secondary hip impingement even following minor slippage. Indirect corrective osteotomies, such as those proposed at the base of the femoral neck or the intertrochanteric level for more severe deformity, are also unable to sufficiently eliminate the "cam-like impingement" localized at the head and neck junction and the retroversion deformity in moderate and severe SCFE. Even after mild SCFE, the residual cam deformity that persists after the remodeling associated with in situ pinning is an anatomic risk factor that can lead to anterosuperior acetabular cartilage damage through the inclusion of the bump.

Dunn was the first to reduce the risk of head necrosis by local mobilization of the lateral retinaculum before directly correcting the deformity of the SCFE [5]. Although his technique was sufficiently safe for minor corrections, the risk of overstretching the retinacular flap increases with the extent of correction required mainly due to deformity of the femoral neck and significant amounts of posterior femoral neck subperiosteal new bone formation. Furthermore, if surgical dislocation of the head is not used, as was described in the original Dunn's technique [5], the manipulation of the femoral neck is more complex and complicated.

Like the rest of the periosteum, the retinaculum flap containing the nutrient vessels to the femoral head is significantly thicker in children than in adults. Following the osteotomy of the greater trochanter, an additional resection of the remaining portion of the greater trochanter to the level of the femoral neck with the capsulotomy, the lateral retinaculum can be detached from the bone down to the level of the lesser trochanter under visual control. If the trimming of the base of the trochanter is omitted, the dorsal and distal parts cannot be seen, which significantly complicates safe visualization and increases the tension of the retinaculum containing the vessels.

E. Novais (✉)
Department of Orthopedics, Boston Children's Hospital, Harvard Medical School, Boston, MA, USA
e-mail: eduardo.novais@childrens.harvard.edu

M. Leunig
Hip Service, Department of Orthopedics, Schulthess Clinic, Zurich, Switzerland
e-mail: Michael.leunig@kws.ch

M. Leunig et al. (eds.), *Surgical Hip Dislocation*, https://doi.org/10.1007/978-3-031-70622-6_17

17.3 Indications

17.3.1 Indications

- Acute, unstable displaced SCFE
- Moderate and severe stable chronic or acute on chronic SCFE with an open growth plate with an epiphyseal diaphyseal angle (Southwick angle) [6] greater than 30°.

17.3.2 Relative Indications

- Residual deformity after moderate or severe stable SCFE (after growth plate closure) if cam resection to improve the impingement-free flexion and internal rotation would require to remove more than one-third of the femoral neck diameter. The surgery is technically performed in this setting as a femoral neck osteotomy [7].

17.3.3 Contraindications

- Advanced osteoarthritis
- Lack of patient compliance and reliability to follow post-operative precautions risking hip stability and fixation integrity
- Closed growth plate (femoral neck osteotomy)

17.4 Preoperative/Preinterventional Diagnostics

- Hormonal status including vitamin D
- Anteroposterior (AP) pelvic radiograph and a lateral (Lauenstein or cross table lateral) (Fig. 17.1).
- MRI of the symptomatic hip may help assessing for articular cartilage damage in chronic SCFE deformity.
- In exceptional cases, CT with special sequences for preoperative computer simulation of a subcapital osteotomy.

17.5 Preoperative Planning/Computer Simulation

To date, no routine preoperative planning is performed for this procedure.

17.6 Applied Anatomy

- A prerequisite for the preparation of the retinaculum soft flap is the completely performed surgical dislocation of the joint [8] (see Chap. 7) as well as preparation of the extended soft flap [2] (see Chap. 8).
- Dislocation of the femoral head is used for manual securing during curettage of the growth plate and finally for anatomical reduction under visual control of the retinaculum. With the head dislocated, undesired manipulation of the leg is less likely to compromise the integrity of the retinaculum than would be the case with the head remaining in the socket.

17.7 Special Risks

Circulatory disturbance of the femoral head with consequences such as

- Damage to the femoral head blood supply due to rough intraoperative manipulation
- Loss of reduction
- Avascular necrosis of the femoral head with head collapse and advanced osteoarthritis
- Instability of the hip with subluxation or complete dislocation
- Ossifications in the area of the surgical approach (external rotators, piriformis, trochanter)

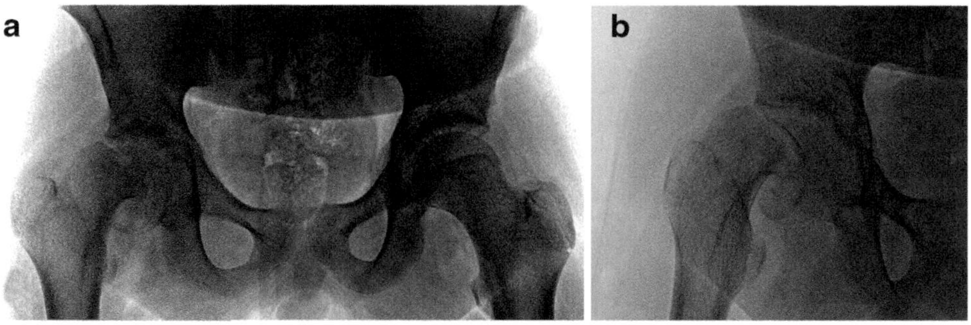

Fig. 17.1 (**a**) Preoperative anteroposterior pelvic radiograph showing a completely displaced slipped capital femoral epiphysis of the right hip. (**b**) A lateral radiograph was limited to hip pain but showed a complete displacement of the femoral epiphysis

17.8 Type of Anesthesia

General anesthesia with or without additional regional block for pain management.

17.9 Positioning

- Radiolucent operating table
- Lateral positioning with tunnel cushion and lateral bag
- Fluoroscopy and X-ray possibility

17.10 Instruments/Implants

Standard instrument set for surgical hip dislocation and extended soft tissue flap (see Chaps. 7 and 8).

For fixation of the epiphysis, 3.0 mm fully threaded wires (Hausmann Spitalbedarf, Hubstrasse 104, 9501 Wil, Switzerland). Alternatively, fixation can be performed with two 6.5 mm cannulated screws (DePuy Synthes West Chester PA, USA).

17.11 Access

- Access as for a surgical hip dislocation with trochanteric osteotomy (see Chap. 7). In the not infrequently overweight children, the skin incision should be sufficiently long (up to 30 cm).
- Trochanteric osteotomy in SCFE is particularly challenging due to the increased external rotation malposition and the thicker subcutaneous adipose tissue. In extreme cases, performing the osteotomy with straight and curved chisels from the dorsal-distal direction may be advantageous than using a saw.
- As a rule, the trochanteric fragment should not be thicker than 1.5 cm. If the trochanteric osteotomy is too superficial, there may be fixation problems and risk of fracture of the trochanteric fragment. If the trochanteric osteotomy is too deep, the tendon of the piriformis muscle adheres to the mobile trochanteric fragment in toto. This may result in insufficient mobilization of the trochanteric fragment as well as endangerment of the deep branch of the medial circumflex artery with the risk of head necrosis.
- With abduction and additional external rotation, the tendon of the piriformis muscle is relaxed, facilitating visualization of the gap to the inferior border of the gluteus minimus muscle. By gradually detaching the gluteus minimus muscle from the capsule dorsally, cranially as well as ventrally, the capsule is exposed to above the acetabular rim. All external rotators remain attached to the stable trochanter for the time being.
- A z-shaped capsulotomy follows, starting with its axial component parallel to femoral neck and close to the anterosuperior corner of the stable trochanter. To avoid injury to the retinaculum, cartilage, or labrum, it is proximally performed from the inside out. This is followed by the ventral limb of the capsulotomy, which aims toward the anteroinferior acetabular rim, and the dorsal capsulotomy along the acetabular rim.
- An 8-mm Hohmann retractor is driven into the supra-acetabular bone below the capsular rim but above the labrum and retains the soft tissues. A Langenbeck retractor may also suffice for this purpose. Now it becomes apparent how far the head has displaced dorsally, whether synovitis is present, and whether the epiphysis is still stably connected to the femoral neck and whether the retinaculum has been ruptured at the junction of the femoral neck and epiphysis.
- If the epiphysis is unstable it should be immediately fixed with two to three 2-mm threaded Kirschner wires. During a reduction maneuver, no attention is paid to completeness; the visible retinaculum must not come under tension under any circumstances (Fig. 17.2).
- Now an initial check of the epiphyseal blood supply is performed, either with a 2-mm drill hole, from which there should be active (and even pulsatile) bleeding. If none of the measures gives a clear indication of perfusion of the epiphysis, the operation should still be accomplished as planned.
- This should be followed by dislocation of the femoral head, for which the leg should be placed in flexion, adduction, and external rotation and the lower leg placed in the sterile bag. During this maneuver, the suction seal of the joint is broken, and the femoral head is subluxated out of the acetabulum; a bone hook around the medial neck (calcar) can be used to help. If the verification of the slippage shows that a reduction of the ventrally protruding metaphysis is sufficient and that the femoral neck would not become too thin after an osteochondroplasty, then a full dislocation can be avoided. The intervention then consists of offset correction, immediately followed by screw stabilization of the epiphysis.
- If, on the other hand, dislocation is necessary, the round ligament (ligamentum teres) is cut with scissors. With manipulations of the leg by the assistant and by special levers on the anterior edge of the acetabulum and in the incisura acetabuli, 360° of the acetabulum can be viewed. When the knee is lowered, the femoral head can be elevated from the incision, which with rotations makes approximately three-quarters of the head circumference

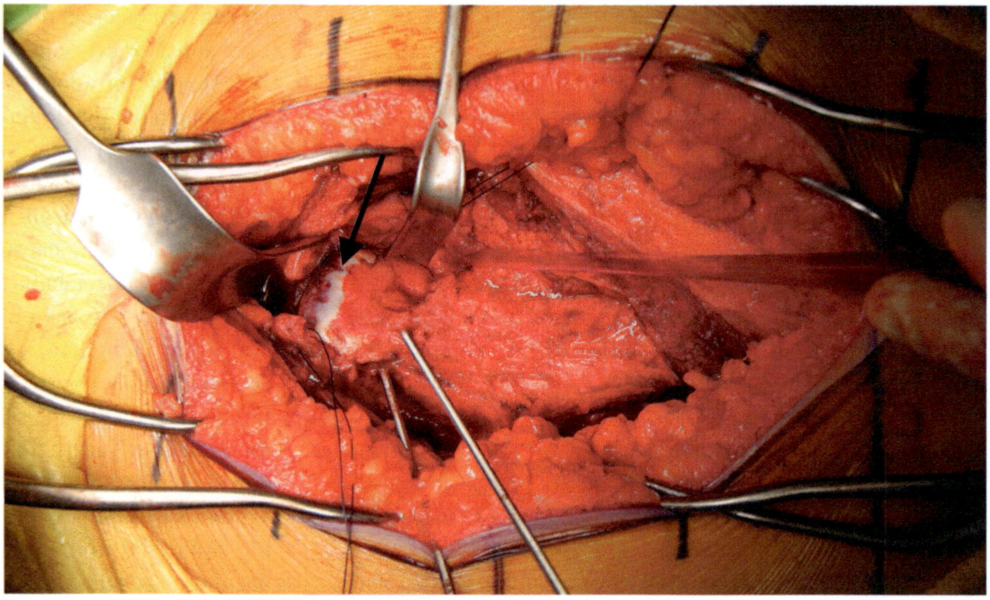

Fig. 17.2 The intraoperative picture shows the provisional fixation of an unstable SCFE, performed immediately after the capsulotomy. The black arrow points to the anterior aspect of the femoral metaphysis, which is severely displaced from the epiphysis. Note that the fixation of the epiphysis is performed without any attempt to reduce or manipulate it

visible. Once exposed, the cartilage should be protected from desiccation by constant sprinkling with physiologic saline. Cartilage and labral damage to the acetabulum is documented and treated as necessary.

17.12 Technical Steps of Deep Dissection

- Preparation of the soft tissue flap, which contains the feeding blood vessels to the epiphysis, is started with the femoral head reduced in the acetabulum [2, 9]. Therefore, after completion of the surgical dislocation approach, the lower leg is first removed from the sterile bag, and the femoral head is reduced back into the acetabulum. For an optimal view of the osteotomy surface of the stable trochanter, especially its posterior corner, the operating table is tilted slightly to the side facing away from the surgeon, and the hip is rotated inward. Full extension of the hip and as little flexion of the knee as possible improve relaxation of the posterior soft tissue structures.
- Development of the soft tissue flap consisting of the retinaculum and external rotators, which contains the ascending branch of the Medial Femoral Circumflex Artery (MFCA) and epiphyseal nourishing blood vessels, is started with the femoral head reduced. The piriformis muscle is covered by the capsular flap. The area of the stable trochanter proximal to the visible growth plate is carefully mobilized with a chisel and then peeled out of its periosteum, preferably piece by piece, from the inside to the outside.
  - Special tip or consideration: the periosteal dissection may begin at the level of the trochanteric apophysis before its resection and move distally and posteriorly. This portion of the periosteal dissection is typically easy and serves as a guide to the proximal dissection that follows (Fig. 17.3).
- Starting at the anterosuperior corner of the stable trochanteric apophysis, the periosteum of the femoral neck is incised femoral neck—axially in the direction of the head (see dashed line in Fig. 17.4). Then, the stable portion of the greater trochanter is resected.
  - A major pitfall in performing the modified Dunn occurs when performing the release of the stable portion of the greater trochanter and freeing the periosteal flap posteriorly. Careful dissection should be performed especially around the piriformis fossa. Although the trochanter can be resected in one piece, when the periosteum is thick, it is probably safer to use a piece-meal technique.
- The retinaculum is then gradually detached from the femoral neck with the aid of a knife and raspatory without tearing the head-neck junction. Uncontrolled internal rotation is dangerous, especially if a retractor is inserted between the soft tissue flap and the bone. Finally, after resection of the stable portion of the greater trochanter, the entire dorsal aspect of the femoral neck becomes visible up to the level of the lesser trochanter (Fig. 17.5).
- A similar procedure is performed with the anteromedial periosteum, although this step is more easily performed with the head dislocated. Similarly, care is taken to ensure that the periosteal flap does not tear from the neck. Now the perfusion of the femoral head can be checked again, preferably with the head still reduced, using the techniques listed above. The head is then dislocated out of the acetabulum again.
- After the bone of the femoral neck has been exposed circumferentially and visualized with a blunt retractor,

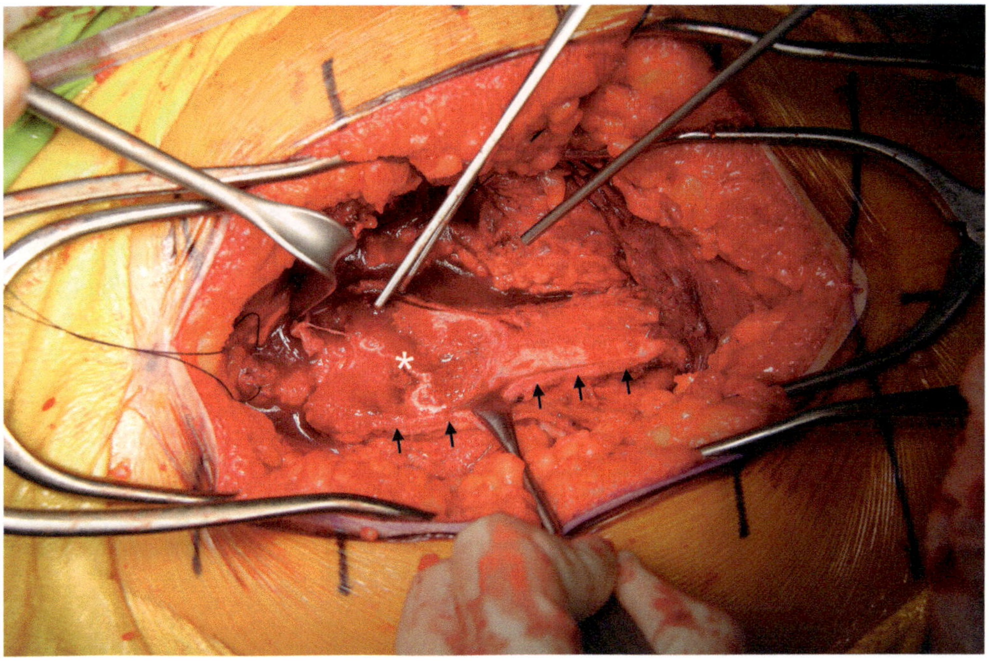

Fig. 17.3 The intraoperative picture shows the periosteal dissection from the lateral surface of the femur and the greater trochanter toward the posterior aspect. The black arrows mark the periosteum that is dissected with a mini Cobb. The asterisk (*) marks the trochanteric apophysis, which is the reference for the stable trochanter resection following the initial periosteal dissection

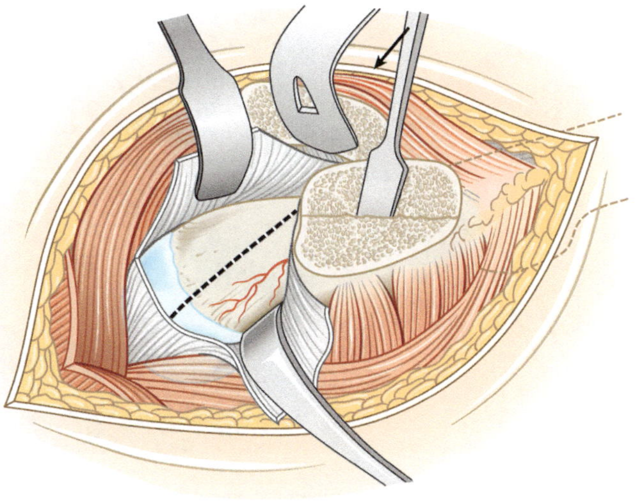

Fig. 17.4 Development of the soft-tissue flap consisting of retinaculum and external rotators, which contain the nutrient blood vessels to the epiphysis commence at the reduced femoral head. The piriformis muscle is hidden behind the capsular flap. The region of the stable trochanter proximal to the visible growth the plate is carefully mobilized with a chisel and then gradually eased out of its periosteum

while not applying tension to the retinaculum, the head is gradually disconnected from the femoral neck with a 10-mm-wide curved osteotome (Fig. 17.6). Note that the growth plate is running concavely within the epiphysis. Removal of a wedge at the metaphysis for better visualization is usually not necessary and should be avoided to not shorten the neck. Simultaneous careful pushing with the curved osteotome and controlled external rotation of the leg further tilts the head and rotates the femoral neck stump out of the periosteal tube. Removal of a medial portion of the dorsal callus spur (not visible), most easily in external rotation, facilitates release of the epiphysis. The epiphysis remains dorsomedial, but it should not be reduced back into the socket, because now its redislocation would be difficult due to suction in the joint even with a Kirschner wire drilled in. Inserting several small sponges in the acetabulum helps prevent this from happening. First, at the femoral neck stump, the regular dorsal callus bulge is resected down to the visible or palpable femoral neck level with a straight chisel. Then the surface of the end of the stump is rounded slightly, taking care to align it perpendicular to the femoral neck axis (Fig. 17.7).

- By controlled movements of the leg, the femoral neck stump can be rotated to such an extent that one hand of the surgeon can grasp the head with two fingers (Fig. 17.8), while the other hand removes the residual tissue of the growth plate with periosteal elevator and curette, if possible under visual control. Usually, spontaneous blood leakage from the exposed epiphyseal bone can be detected afterward. Caution is advised when the curette approaches the rim of the epiphysis at the junction with the retinaculum.
- Once all callus and tissue fragments are removed, the epiphysis is reduced back onto the neck of the femur with visual inspection of the retinaculum, facilitated by internal rotation of the leg. If tension of the retinaculum develops during reduction, the maneuver must be discontinued and the cause identified. Occasionally, part of the dorsal soft tissue flap is trapped and must be freed. Very rarely, the height of the femoral neck must be reduced slightly (neck shortening).

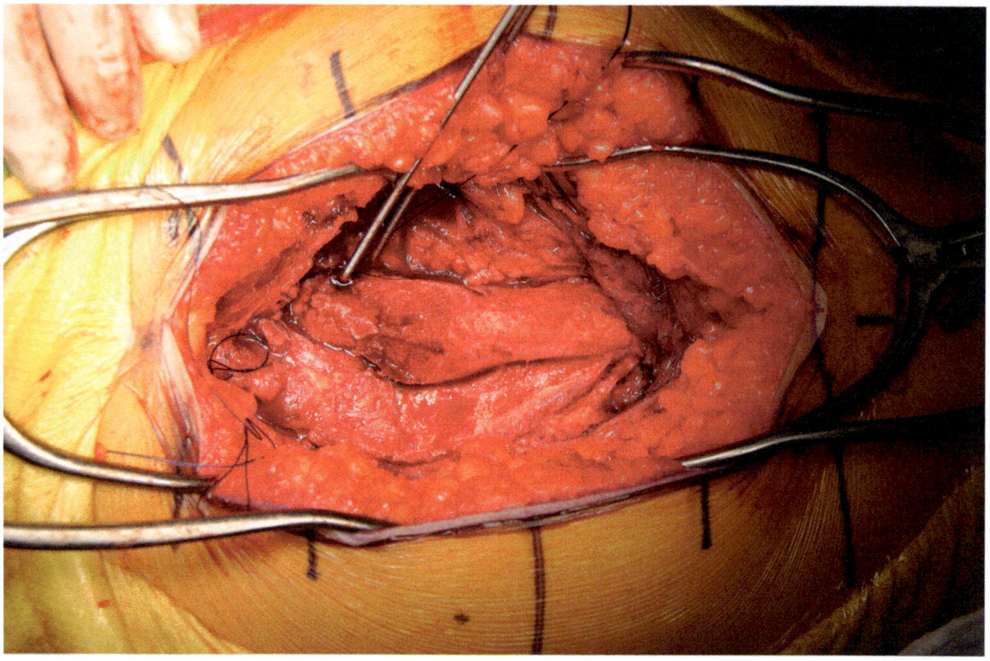

Fig. 17.5 The intraoperative picture shows that the retinaculum is ultimately released after the resection of the greater trochanter's stable portion at the apophysis level. Subsequently, the entire posterior femoral neck is visible to the lesser trochanter level. Here, attention is also paid to ensuring that the periosteal flap does not tear off the head. Optimally, with the head still reduced, perfusion of the head can be re-evaluated using the techniques mentioned earlier. The head will then be dislocated to release the anterior periosteum from the neck

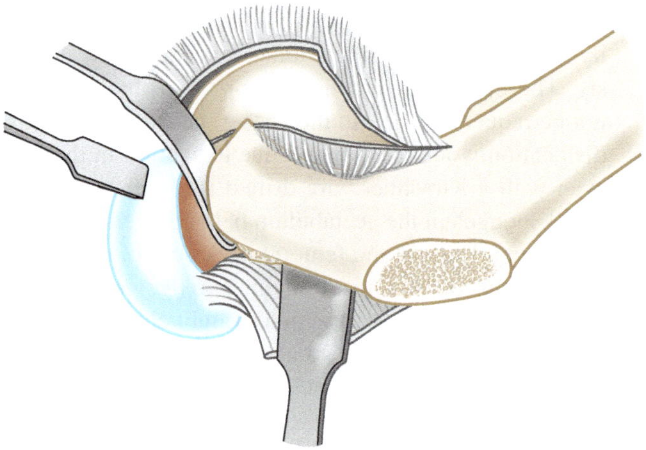

Fig. 17.6 After the bone of the femoral neck is exposed with a blunt retractor so that no tension is applied to the retinaculum, a 10-mm-wide, bent chisel is used to gradually separate the growth plate from the head (not shown here). Excision of a wedge at the metaphysis to improve vision is usually not necessary. By careful levering with a retractor and controlled external rotation of the leg, the head can be tilted further, and the femoral neck stump can be worked out of the periosteal sheath. Removal of a medial part of the posterior callus bridge (not visible), which is most accessible in external rotation, facilitates separation of the head. The head remains posteromedial but should not slip back into the acetabulum since a dislocation at this stage will be tricky, even with an in situ Kirschner wire due to suction in the joint. A sponge placed in the acetabulum helps to prevent this from happening

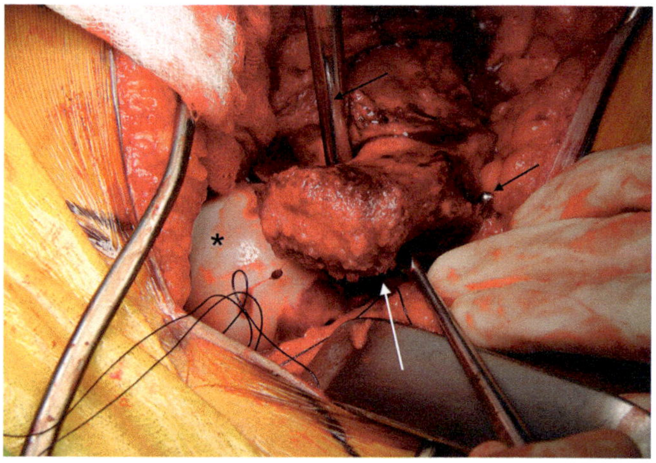

Fig. 17.7 The intraoperative picture shows the resection of the constant posterior callus spur on the femoral neck stump. The stump is rounded off slightly and aligned perpendicular to the axis of the femoral neck. A black asterisk (*) marks the femoral epiphysis. A bone hook (black arrows) is used to slightly lift the femoral neck and facilitate access to the posterior aspect of the neck

- Tip: Shortening of the neck is not recommended, but if inadvertently performed, then the greater trochanter should be fixed with slight advancement. Shortening of the femoral neck may reduce the lever arm of the abductor musculature and lead to hip instability after surgery. An additional 1–2 mm of shortening is reasonable, however, if there is excessive tension in the retinaculum after reduction of the epiphysis. In these cases, the trochanter should be fixed with slight advancement.

- If the position of the epiphysis is anatomic, a fully threaded wire is first inserted retrograde through the fovea capitis, and the position is assessed (Fig. 17.9).
- Subsequently, two additional fully threaded wires are usually inserted antegrade to secure the position of the head. Care must be taken to avoid distraction when screwing the wire tips into the hard cancellous bone of the

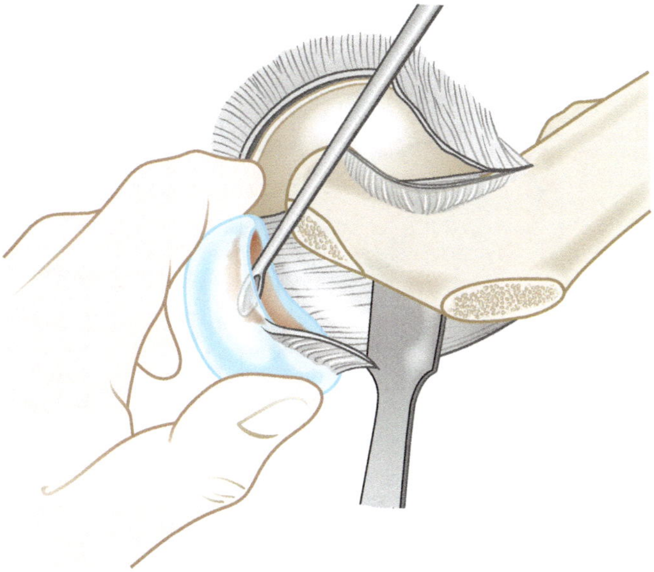

Fig. 17.8 The femoral neck stump can be turned by controlled leg movements so that the surgeon can grip the head with two fingers of one hand while the other removes the residual tissue of the growth plate with a curette under direct vision. As a rule, spontaneous bleeding from the exposed epiphyseal bone is seen. Meticulous preparation is required as the curette approaches the margin of the head at the junction of the retinaculum

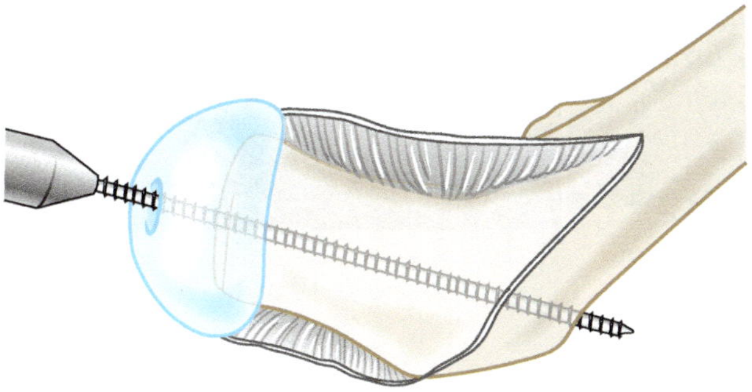

Fig. 17.9 The precise spatial alignment of the head is essential. There should be the same-size step-off around its border to the femoral neck at the anterior, posterior, medial, and lateral aspects, which can initially be verified visually or by palpation with a freer. Correct head rotation can be estimated based on the relative position of the retinaculum to the femoral neck and the position of the fovea for the ligament of the head. It is hardest to adjust the varus-valgus position correctly; intraoperative fluoroscopy is recommended for this control. First, a 3.0-mm fully threaded wire is drilled through the fovea for the head ligament in the retrograde technique so that it exits the lateral cortex slightly below the trochanter. The wire is further introduced from that position until it disappears into the fovea. Next, the head can be carefully repositioned in the acetabulum. This is followed by an evaluation of head position with the image intensifier and a repeat perfusion assessment

epiphysis. Fully threaded Kirschner wires are usually easier to remove later compared to 3.5-mm screws, where it is not uncommon for the hex to give way or for the screw to break, leaving part of the thread in the bone. The correct length of the wires can be checked with re-

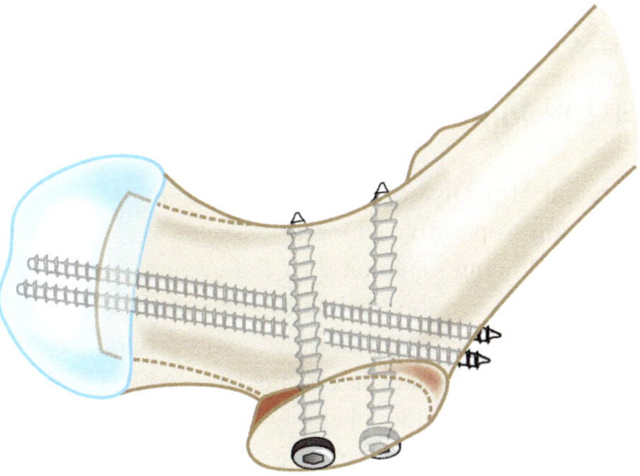

Fig. 17.10 The final aspect of the subcapital osteotomy and the greater trochanter fixation. If the head is in the anatomic position, one or two more fully threaded wires are inserted in an antegrade technique to secure the position of the head. It is vital to ensure that distraction does not occur when inserting the wire tips into the hard cancellous bone of the head. The correct length of wire can be checked by repeated dislocation or with fluoroscopy. The wires should be uniformly distributed in the head

dislocation and/or image intensifier control. They should be evenly distributed in the head. If the caliber gap between the head and femoral neck is filled with bone crumbs, there is a risk of losing the desired offset between the head and neck; thus it is not recommended. Spontaneous bony bridging occurs within a few weeks and months and results in a harmonious waist.

- The periosteum-retinaculum tube is restored with a few sutures, which must be free of tension. The capsular suture must also not be made under tension; otherwise the retinaculum can be compressed and could endanger the supply to the femoral head. If the piriformis muscle subsequently exerts traction on the capsule, its tendon can be slightly released. Trochanteric refixation is performed with two to three 3.5 mm screws, and distalization can be adjusted as needed (Fig. 17.10).
  - Special tip or consideration: Alternatively, the guide wires to the 6.5-mm fully threaded screw (DePuy Synthes West Chester PA, USA) are inserted in a retrograde fashion to stabilize the epiphysis (Fig. 17.11). Fixation with a fully threaded screw is preferred in obese adolescents (Fig. 17.12).
- We close the bursal tissue layer over the trochanter with continuous sutures and make sure to do a tight and stable fascial suture for a correct suspension of the dorsal subcutaneous adipose tissue layer. Suturing of the adipose tissue is performed in multiple layers, with only the septa being grasped. With careful, layered reconstruction of the soft tissue layers, a drain is usually unnecessary.
- As a dressing, we apply a light compressing spica bandage for 2 days. The leg is placed in neutral rotation in a

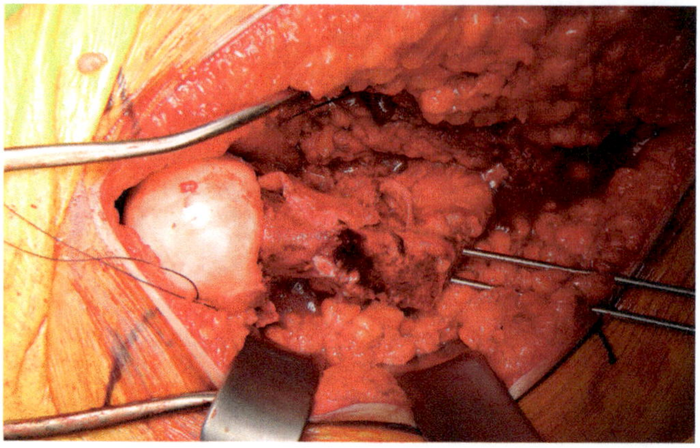

Fig. 17.11 The intraoperative picture shows the provisional fixation of the epiphysis with the two guide wires for the 6.5-mm cannulated screw system (DePuy Synthes West Chester PA, USA). The wires are inserted in an anterograde fashion

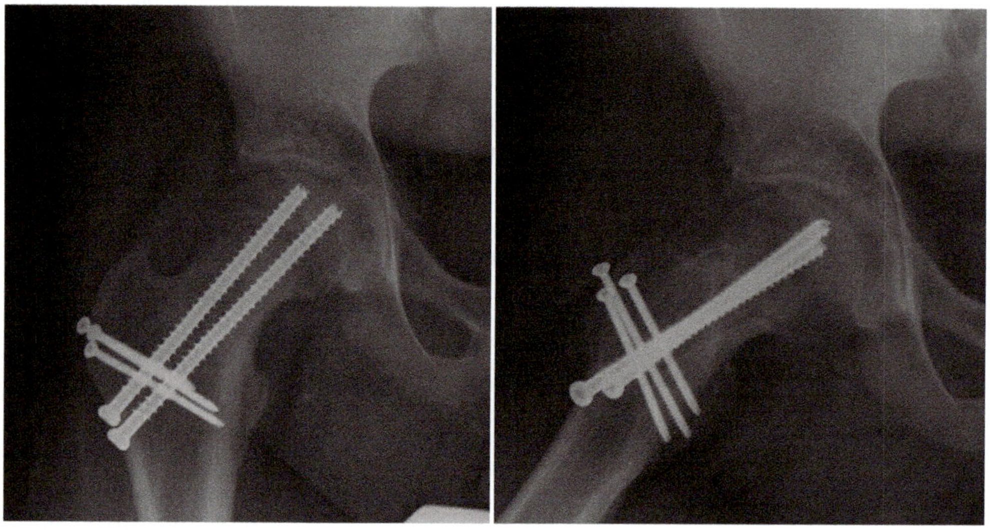

Fig. 17.12 The final radiographic aspect of the subcapital osteotomy performed on the patient presented previously (Fig. 17.1) shows complete restoration of the proximal femoral anatomy with the realignment of the epiphysis at 1-year postoperative without any signs of osteonecrosis of the femoral head

foam splint. If prophylactic pinning of the contralateral side is planned, it can be performed under the same anesthesia after appropriate repositioning.

17.13 Postoperative Follow-Up

- The dressing is removed after 2 days and replaced by a simple wound dressing for another 2–3 days. The absorbable and colorless material of the intracutaneous suture does not need to be removed. We prescribe a motorized motion device during the inpatient stay. The physical therapist instructs the patient how to lift the operated leg out of bed with the support of the opposite leg without its active muscle tension. Instruction also includes how to roll the foot on two sticks when touching the floor and how to sit down and stand up. Chairs should be as high as possible and have arm rests. Instruction includes climbing and descending stairs.
- Thromboprophylaxis is not routinely given in these young patients.
- After 8 weeks, radiographs will show the progress of consolidation and will help determine if weight-bearing should already be increased or, if in doubt, postponed for another 3–4 weeks.

17.13.1 Secondary Interventions

- Screw or wire removal should be performed no sooner than 1 year after surgery but may be performed later depending on circumstances. However, if the implants are left in place for too long, it may be difficult to remove the metal during a secondary procedure, since the wire and especially the 3.5-mm screws are often firmly integrated. The implants of the prophylactically screwed opposing hip should be left in place until the growth plate has ossified.

17.14 Intra-/Postoperative Complications

- The most common "mistake" is the lack of detail in performing the procedure. The course of the medial circumflex femoral artery, the most important blood supply to the epiphysis, must be known in relation to the external rotators along the posterior edge of the greater trochanter (Chap. 6), and meticulous knowledge in developing and manipulating the retinacular flap is a prerequisite.
- Access proximally too short, therefore poor overview, damage to musculature, difficult dislocation: widen access proximally.
- Tearing of the retinaculum at the head-neck junction during subperiosteal dissection with risk of head necrosis: subperiosteal mobilization of the retinaculum with care and caution when using the sharp periosteal elevator, which must not slip off. Use caution with internal rotation of the leg when a lever is inserted subperiosteally at the femoral neck.
- Tearing of the retinaculum during manipulations for callus removal from the femoral neck and reduction. If the epiphysis detached from the femoral neck is also dislocated from the socket, the retinaculum is much less at risk from involuntary movements, such as on the leg, or from manipulations by the instruments because the free head can escape. During curettage of the growth plate cartilage, the dislocated epiphysis can be manually stabilized, a procedure that must take place in a much more uncontrolled manner when the epiphysis is reduced in the acetabulum. Finally, the dislocated epiphysis can be reduced by hand in a well-dosed and spatially perfect manner under visual control of the retinaculum, which is much less dangerous for the retinaculum compared to reduction of the femoral neck onto the epiphysis located in the acetabulum. Insufficient callus removal dorsal to the femoral neck or incomplete removal of loosened callus pieces, resulting in circumscribed tension in the retinaculum, blood flow stoppage, and danger of head necrosis.
- Perforation of the threaded wires into the joint with risk of damage to the acetabular cartilage: the wires must be withdrawn immediately.
- Mechanically insufficient screw placement during trochanteric fixation: in case of trochanteric pseudarthrosis, renewed stable osteosynthesis (screw osteosynthesis, rarely cerclage or plates).
- Bending or breakage of the threaded wires or screws due to overload, mispositioning of the epiphysis: depending on the extent, revision surgery, and renewed fixation.

17.15 Case Study

An 11-year-old female with bilateral hip pain, limp, and severe limited flexion with obligatory external rotation in flexion. Preoperative AP and frog-leg radiographs revealed a severe stable SCFE (Fig. 17.13). The patient was treated with staged (3 weeks apart) subcapital realignment osteotomy. Intraoperatively the slip was confirmed to be stable with a severe retroversion deformity of the head in relation to the metaphysis (Fig. 17.14). The hips healed uneventfully without any signs of osteonecrosis of the femoral head after 2 years (Fig. 17.15).

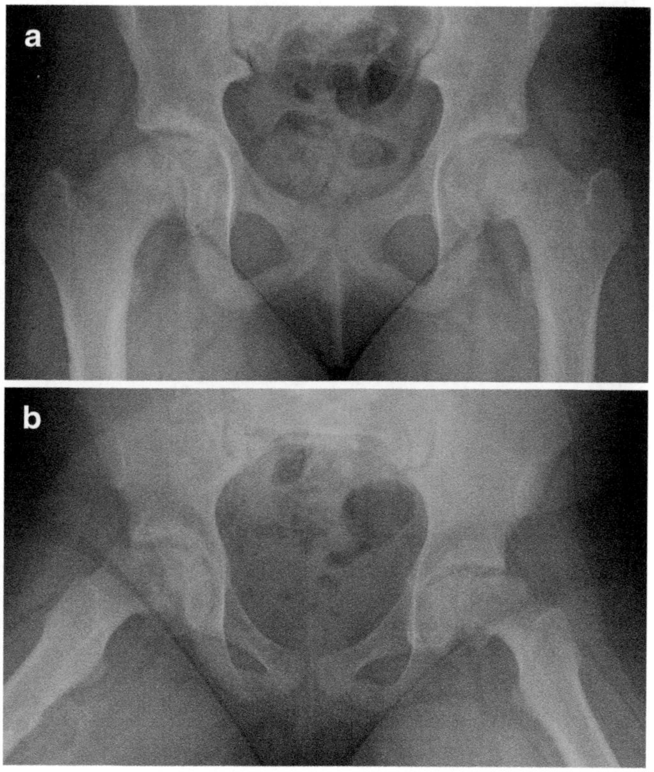

Fig. 17.13 Preoperative radiographs of an 11-year-old girl who presented to clinic with a long history of bilateral hip pain, limp, and severe restricted motion. (**a**) Anteroposterior pelvic radiograph. (**b**) Bilateral frog leg radiograph

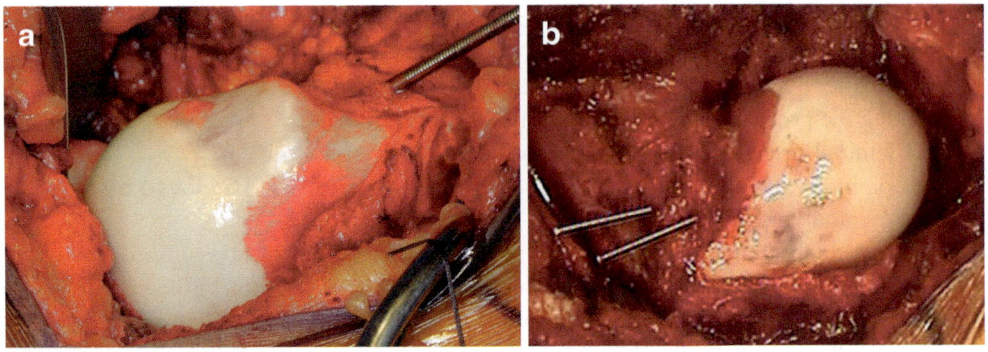

Fig. 17.14 Intraoperative pictures ((**a**) right hip and (**b**) left hip) obtained at the time of the subcapital osteotomy performed at the level of the open growth plates. Note the severe retroversion deformity of the femoral epiphysis in relation to the metaphysis

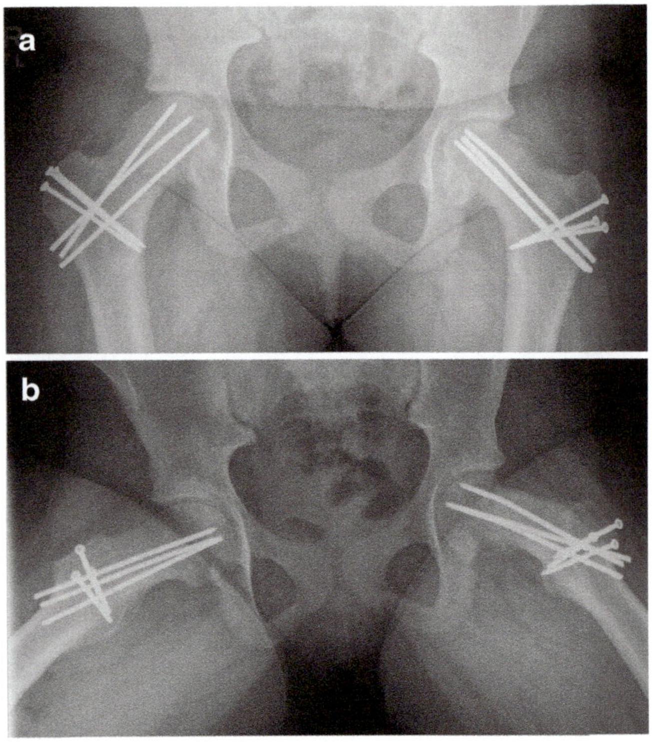

Fig. 17.15 Postoperative radiographs obtained at 2-year follow-up visit. The patient has remained asymptomatic with full hip range of motion without any limitation of activities. The only complication noted was one of the pins broke at the left hip

17.16 Controversies

- The most frequently mentioned counter-arguments to the method presented here are related to the treatment of SCFE and refer to reports from the 1980s about good results with the surgically much less complex "pinning in situ" [3, 4]. This technique convinced many pediatric orthopedic surgeons because of its ease of performance and its almost certain avoidance of head necrosis. However, recent reports of in situ pinning showed persistent mild pain was common in one-third of patient treated with in situ pinning [10] and the association of poorer clinical and radiological long term in hips with persistent deformity and impingement [11, 12].
- One response to this has been screw fixation following a "gentle manual reduction." There is little literature on results of this method; the head necroses seen repeatedly are presented as isolated cases. It is difficult to define how far a surgeon is willing to go with a "gentle" reduction if his goal is to achieve a better to ideal head-neck relationship. On the other hand, it is known today that even in the case of the so-called acute slipped neck, a callus can already exist dorsally on the neck, which imposes a detour on the retinaculum, which can lead to overstretching of the vessels running through it.
- Because of this problem, Fish [13] recommended circumscribed detachment of the retinaculum with removal of the dorsal new bone formation (callus), thereby achieving substantial risk reduction of head necrosis. The extension of retinaculum detachment described here has largely eliminated the risk when used correctly. Our own results show that necrosis that can nevertheless be observed is more correctly explained by nonsurgical factors, such as traumatic retinaculum avulsion or too long of a perfusion stop [14–18].
- Especially established pediatric orthopedists object that the technique of extended retinaculum flap is too complex and difficult to learn. Small numbers of cases also make it difficult to gain sufficient experience. The safest alternative is to bundle the cases in centers where the necessary expertise can be developed.

17.17 Results

Several studies have showed that the modified Dunn technique is safe, reliable, reproducible, and achieve good short- and midterm results for hips with stable SCFE [19]. In a comparative study, Novais et al. [20] reported that the subcapital realignment with the modified Dunn procedure resulted in better anatomic features of the femur, a higher rate of good and excellent clinical outcome scores, a lower reoperation rate, and similar occurrence of complications when compared with in situ pinning for treatment of severe stable SCFE. Similarly, Galleta et al. [21] also reported that the modified Dunn provided best deformity correction and highest functional scores at long-term follow-up and similar rates of osteonecrosis compared to in situ fixation. In an intermediate-term study, Ziebarth et al. [22] reported that the cumulative survivorship was 93% at 10 years with few hips showing secondary impingement deformity. Lerch et al. [23] performed gait analysis of 22 patients treated with modified Dunn for severe SCFE and reported that patients with severe SCFE treated with modified Dunn procedure had mostly symmetrical foot progression angle and good hip scores at midterm follow-up.

However, the results for the modified Dunn for unstable SCFE have been controversial with some studies reporting low rate of osteonecrosis [14, 18, 24] and others reporting a proportion as high as a quarter of patients developing osteonecrosis [25–27]. Novais et al. [28] reported that compared to inadvertent reduction and percutaneous pinning, the modified Dunn procedure provided better clinical and radiographic outcomes with similar proportion of osteonecrosis and unplanned reoperations following an unstable SCFE.

17.18 Outlook

The modified Dunn subcapital realignment osteotomy is a safe and reliable surgical technique to restore the anatomy of the proximal femur in moderate and severe SCFE. The details of the surgical technique describe herein will help the orthopedic surgeon navigate this laborious procedure.

References

1. Gautier E, Ganz K, Krugel N, Gill T, Ganz R. Anatomy of the medial femoral circumflex artery and its surgical implications. J Bone Joint Surg Br. 2000;82:679–83.
2. Ganz R, Huff TW, Leunig M. Extended retinacular soft-tissue flap for intra-articular hip surgery: surgical technique, indications, and results of application. Instr Course Lect. 2009;58:241–55.
3. Boyer DW, Mickelson MR, Ponseti IV. Slipped capital femoral epiphysis. Long-term follow-up study of one hundred and twenty-one patients. J Bone Joint Surg Am. 1981;63:85–95.
4. Carney BT, Weinstein SL, Noble J. Long-term follow-up of slipped capital femoral epiphysis. J Bone Joint Surg. 1991;73:667–74.
5. Dunn DM. The treatment of adolescent slipping of the upper femoral epiphysis. Journal of bone and joint surgery. 1964;46:621–9.
6. Southwick WO. Osteotomy through the lesser trochanter for slipped capital femoral epiphysis. J Bone Joint Surg Am. 1967;49:807–35.
7. Rego P, Mascarenhas V, Mafra I, Oliveira F, Pinto P, Ganz R. Femoral neck osteotomy in skeletally mature patients: surgical technique and midterm results. Int Orthop. 2021;45:83–94.
8. Ganz R, Gill TJ, Gautier E, Ganz K, Krugel N, Berlemann U. Surgical dislocation of the adult hip a technique with full access to the femoral head and acetabulum without the risk of avascular necrosis. J Bone Joint Surg Br. 2001;83:1119–24.
9. Leunig M, Slongo T, Kleinschmidt M, Ganz R. Subcapital correction osteotomy in slipped capital femoral epiphysis by means of surgical hip dislocation. Oper Orthop Traumatol. 2007;19:389–410.
10. Larson AN, Sierra RJ, Yu EM, Trousdale RT, Stans AA. Outcomes of slipped capital femoral epiphysis treated with in situ pinning. J Pediatr Orthop. 2012;32:125–30.
11. Wensaas A, Gunderson RB, Svenningsen S, Terjesen T. Femoroacetabular impingement after slipped upper femoral epiphysis: the radiological diagnosis and clinical outcome at long-term follow-up. J Bone Joint Surg Br. 2012;94:1487–93.
12. Wensaas A, Svenningsen S, Terjesen T. Long-term outcome of slipped capital femoral epiphysis: a 38-year follow-up of 66 patients. J Child Orthop. 2011;5:75–82.
13. Fish JB. Cuneiform osteotomy of the femoral neck in the treatment of slipped capital femoral epiphysis. J Bone Joint Surg. 1984;66:1153–68.
14. Lerch TD, Vuilleumier S, Schmaranzer F, Ziebarth K, Steppacher SD, Tannast M, Siebenrock KA. Patients with severe slipped capital femoral epiphysis treated by the modified Dunn procedure have low rates of avascular necrosis, good outcomes, and little osteoarthritis at long-term follow-up. Bone Joint J. 2019;101-B:403–14.
15. Novais EN, Sink EL, Kestel LA, Carry PM, Abdo JC, Heare TC. Is assessment of femoral head perfusion during modified Dunn for unstable slipped capital femoral epiphysis an accurate indicator of osteonecrosis? Clin Orthop Relat Res. 2016;474:1837–44.
16. Tannast M, Jost LM, Lerch TD, Schmaranzer F, Ziebarth K, Siebenrock KA. The modified Dunn procedure for slipped capital femoral epiphysis: the Bernese experience. J Child Orthop. 2017;11:138–46.
17. Ziebarth K, Leunig M, Slongo T, Kim YJ, Ganz R. Slipped capital femoral epiphysis: relevant pathophysiological findings with open surgery. Clin Orthop Relat Res. 2013;471:2156–62.
18. Ziebarth K, Zilkens C, Spencer S, Leunig M, Ganz R, Kim YJ. Capital realignment for moderate and severe SCFE using a modified Dunn procedure. Clin Orthop Relat Res. 2009;467:704–16.
19. Leunig M, Manner HM, Turchetto L, Ganz R. Femoral and acetabular re-alignment in slipped capital femoral epiphysis. J Child Orthop. 2017;11:131–7.
20. Novais EN, Hill MK, Carry PM, Heare TC, Sink EL. Modified Dunn procedure is superior to in situ pinning for short-term clinical and radiographic improvement in severe stable SCFE. Clin Orthop Relat Res. 2015;473:2108–17.
21. Galletta C, Aprato A, Giachino M, Marre' Brunenghi G, Boero S, Turchetto L, Masse A. Modified Dunn procedure versus percutaneous pinning in moderate/severe stable slipped capital femoral epiphyses. Hip Int. 2021;11207000211004862.
22. Ziebarth K, Milosevic M, Lerch TD, Steppacher SD, Slongo T, Siebenrock KA. High survivorship and little osteoarthritis at 10-year Followup in SCFE patients treated with a modified Dunn procedure. Clin Orthop Relat Res. 2017;475:1212–28.
23. Lerch TD, Boschung A, Leibold C, Kalla R, Kerkeni H, Baur H, Eichelberger P, Steppacher SD, Liechti EF, Siebenrock KA, Tannast M, Ziebarth K. Minimal out-toeing and good hip scores of severe SCFE patients treated with modified Dunn procedure and contralateral prophylactic pinning at minimal 5-year follow up. J Pediatr Orthop. 2022;42:e421–6.
24. Slongo T, Kakaty D, Krause F, Ziebarth K. Treatment of slipped capital femoral epiphysis with a modified Dunn procedure. J Bone Joint Surg. 2010;92:2898–908.
25. Davis RL 2nd, Samora WP 3rd, Persinger F, Klingele KE. Treatment of unstable versus stable slipped capital femoral epiphysis using the modified Dunn procedure, vol. 38. J Pediatr Orthop; 2017. p. 3.
26. Sankar WN, Vanderhave KL, Matheney T, Herrera-Soto JA, Karlen JW. The modified Dunn procedure for unstable slipped capital femoral epiphysis: a multicenter perspective. J Bone Joint Surg. 2013;95:585–91.
27. Upasani VV, Birke O, Klingele KE, Millis MB, International, S. S. G. Iatrogenic hip instability is a devastating complication after the modified Dunn procedure for severe slipped capital femoral epiphysis. Clin Orthop Relat Res. 2017;475:1229–35.
28. Novais EN, Maranho DA, Heare T, Sink E, Carry PM, O'Donnel C. The modified Dunn procedure provides superior short-term outcomes in the treatment of the unstable slipped capital femoral epiphysis as compared to the inadvertent closed reduction and percutaneous pinning: a comparative clinical study. Int Orthop. 2018;43:669.

Intra-Capital Osteotomy

18

Daniel J. Sucato, Diego Collado Gastalver, and Reinhold Ganz

18.1 Background

More than 120 years ago, Mickulicz published a method to resect a prominence of the head neck junction [1].

Today, a surgical step at the periphery of the head is popular as osteo-chondro-plasty in the treatment of the femoro-acetabular impingent (Chap. 9).

Surgery of the center of the head is occasionally performed as curettage for intra-capital tumors, cyst, and, in the treatment of femoral head necrosis, osteochondritis dissecans and Pipkin fractures.

Segmental resection of the middle of the head became possible with more detailed understanding of the blood circulation within the head [2–4] (Chap. 6) (Fig. 18.1).

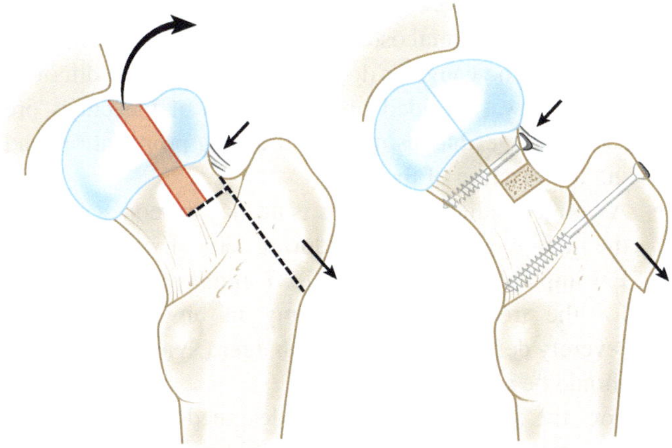

Fig. 18.1 Drawing of the intra-capital osteotomy. The stable medial head-neck segment will remain perfused by the medial branch of the MFCA. The lateral mobile segment is pedicled on the lateral retinacular flap and perfused by the retinacular branches of the deep branch of the MFCA (short arrows). Often relative lengthening of the neck and distal advancement of the greater trochanter are necessary (long arrows)

18.2 Indications

- Ideal indications are a hinge abduction of a Perthes head with coxa magna extruded and/or subluxated, a camel saddle-like upper contour, or a central necrosis and a healthy and rounded lateral pillar of reasonable size.
- Best age range is between 10 and 20 years.
- Open growth plate is not a contraindication at the age of 8 and older.
- Mushroom-type contour of a coxa magna, as well as an acetabular radius smaller than the radius of the head may be an indication, often together with an acetabular reorientation.
- In posttraumatic necrosis, careful preoperative evaluation of the integrity of the lateral retinaculum is mandatory with enhanced MRI.
- Lack of a healthy lateral pillar may still be an indication before closure of the growth plate.
- After growth plate closure, substantial cartilage damage of the lateral pillar may be a contraindication.
- Reduction of the head size may become necessary during Codivilla/Colonna capsular arthroplasty (Chap. 20).

18.3 Preoperative Diagnostics

- Classic anteroposterior (AP) radiography of the pelvis (including the entire opposite hip) and lateral radiography of the diseased hip.
- To distinguish between hips which qualify for a periacetabular osteotomy (PAO) only and an intra-capital osteotomy, an AP radiography of the diseased hip with maximum

D. J. Sucato
Department of Orthopaedic Surgery, University of Texas Southwestern Medical Center, Dallas, TX, USA
e-mail: dan.sucato@tsrh.org

D. Collado Gastalver
University Hospital Vall d'Hebron, Barcelona, Spain
e-mail: collado@institutocot.es

R. Ganz (✉)
Emeritus, Faculty of Medicine, University of Berne, Bern, Switzerland

M. Leunig et al. (eds.), *Surgical Hip Dislocation*, https://doi.org/10.1007/978-3-031-70622-6_18

abduction in neutral rotation is necessary; it should show hinged abduction produced by the deformed head and not by the greater trochanter. If it is caused by the greater trochanter, the radiography may be repeated intraoperatively after trochanteric osteotomy. If hinged abduction cannot be documented, isolated PAO may be discussed.
- MRI with radial sequences can help to differentiate between necrotic and vital tissue of the epiphysis.
- Today's standard before executing the intra-capital osteotomy is computer simulation of the osteotomy [5]. It helps for the decision-making of cut directions while looking for best approximate sphericity and size of the final head. For this purpose, a computer tomography following a special program is necessary. It allows one to produce cutting guides to precisely execute the osteotomy cuts (Chap. 5).

18.4 Preoperative Planning/Computer Modeling

- The cuts must be placed to respect the lateral retinaculum and minimum 15 mm thickness of the stable medial segment.
- For computer modeling see Chap. 3.

18.5 Applied Anatomy

- Detailed knowledge of the vascular anatomy of the femoral head [3, 4] is of outmost Importance.
- Knowledge of the topography of the retinacula is also needed (Chap. 2).
- Practical experience with the techniques of surgical dislocation and dissection of the retinacular flaps is mandatory (Chaps. 7 and 8).

18.6 Specific Risks

- Necrosis of the entire mobile segment has not yet been observed. In one case of posttraumatic necrosis, the vitality of the neck part of the mobile fragment was questionable. In another case a small necrosis like, subchondral sector of the mobile segment appeared after 1 year of good function. Necrosis of the stable segment has not been observed.
- Fracture of the stable medial segment is possible when the residual neck diameter (thickness of the stable segment) is 10 mm or smaller. It can become a problem in patients with spasticity.
- Residual joint instability can persist when additional PAO is not performed. Therefore, stability testing after completion of the head reduction is recommended.

18.7 Type of Anesthesia

- General anesthesia is preferred because there is a potential need for changing the position from lateral to supine during the case to allow one to perform a combined PAO.
- Cell saver should be used, and the possible need for blood transfusion should be taken into consideration.

18.8 Positioning

- The patient is completely draped for femoral osteotomy and PAO.
- The procedure starts out in the lateral decubitus to execute the intra-capital osteotomy and eventually the ischial cut of the PAO.
- Before suture of the skin, the patient is turned supine for the PAO.

18.9 Instruments/Implants

- For the femoral side, the same instruments are needed as for surgical dislocation (Chap. 7) and extended retinacular flap (Chap. 8).
- For the intra-capital osteotomy, a saw blade must be available with the gauge as decided when the slot width of the template was decided upon; a length of 6.5 cm is preferred; longer blades may bend during propagation leading to deviation of the cut.
- A pointed reduction forceps is needed to reduce and hold the mobile lateral segment during screw fixation.
- For implants the 3.5 mm and 2.7 mm screw sets, 4.5 mm for the trochanteric osteotomy in bigger patients or severely deformed greater trochanter (Synthes catalogue) should be available.
- For the PAO a specially designed instrument set (Accuratus AG, Berne, CH) should be available.
- As implants for the PAO 3.5 mm screws between 60- and 130-mm length are needed.
- If available cutting templates.
- If available equipment for measuring perfusion (probe for measuring intracranial.
- pressure).

18.10 Access

- First step for the intra-capital osteotomy is the SHD approach (Chap. 7).
- It may include the execution of the ischial cut of the PAO to be executed between gemellus inferior and obturator

externus muscles (Chap. 19). Optimal overview on this muscle group and best differentiation of the different muscles are given immediately after the trochanteric osteotomy. Be aware that the anatomy of the external rotators can be altered by the proximal femur deformities.

- The sciatic nerve is identified and mobilized in order to protect it mechanically and optically during the cut.
- The risk of injury to the deep branch of the MFCA is minimized when developing of the gap is started in close contact with the palpable ischial bone.
- By gently increasing the gap, one reaches the axilla between ischium and postero-inferior acetabular rim, the place where the incomplete ischial cut will be performed. The osteotomy is executed with straight and curved osteotomes, the direction being controlled using a sterile plastic model of the pelvis held in the same spatial orientation during the cutting process.
- Fluoroscopic control may help to increase precision of the cut. The osteotome should penetrate the inner cortex, but not advance posteriorly more than 2–2.5 cm in order to keep the continuity of the posterior ilio-ischiatic column [6].

18.11 Technical Steps

- The surgical dislocation is completed as described in Chap. 7.
- Final confirmation of the indication is provided with careful inspection of acetabular cartilage and labrum as well as of the femoral head cartilage.
- First step is the working out of the lateral retinaculum as described in Chap. 8.
- **The medial retinaculum is not dissected for this procedure**!
- For the intra-capital cutting process, the head is dislocated, and the leg is placed for best visualization of the anterior head-neck junction.
- When a cutting template is used, the periosteum at the anterior neck area must be removed in order to permit optimal and stable placement of the device.
- Before the template is definitively fixed with K-wires, the position should be controlled with the ideal position on a sterilized, identical plastic model.
- Before starting the cutting process, a final check confirms that the more lateral cut does not perforate the bone posteriorly within the zone of the 2-cm-wide lateral retinaculum and that the medial cut will preserve a minimum15 mm or larger bridge of the neck bone along the calcar area; these aspects have been already respected during the simulation process (Chap. 5) (Fig. 18.2).
- Using an oscillating saw, the cutting through both slots is advanced slowly under constant cooling (Figs. 18.3 and 18.4). Do not bend the saw blade while advancing!
- At first, the blade should penetrate deep in the bone but not perforate the posterior border of head and neck.
- During the second cut, stability of the cutting template may be increased with a blade left in the first cut during the cut through the second slot.
- Caudad propagation of the cuts should include at least 1 cm of the neck (Fig. 18.5).

	X	Y	Z
Scaling	100.000 %	100.000 %	100.000 %
Rotation	-16.035°	2.837°	-36.892°
Translation	2.340 mm	-6.670 mm	-19.093 mm

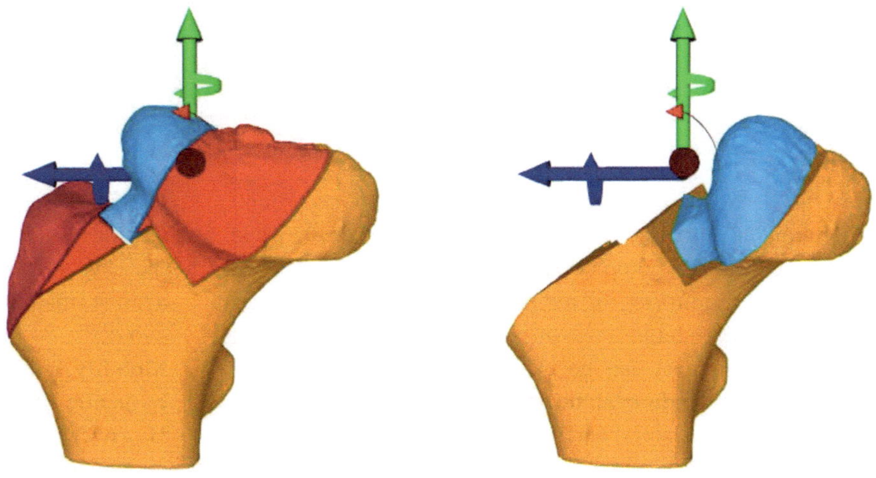

Fig. 18.2 Computer simulation with the segment to be resected (red), matched contour (blue against yellow), and definitive head size. While doing so, the topography of the retinacula, the width of the stable neck portion, and the length of the neck remaining on the mobile segment are respected

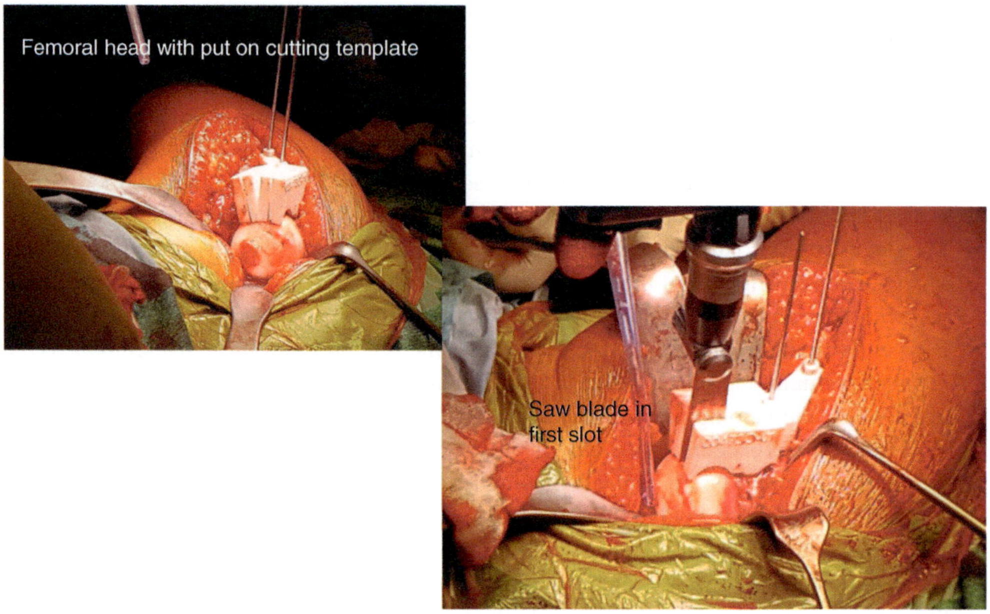

Fig. 18.3 Intraoperative view on the head with the cutting template, fixed with two K-wires and a saw-plate held in one of the cutting slots

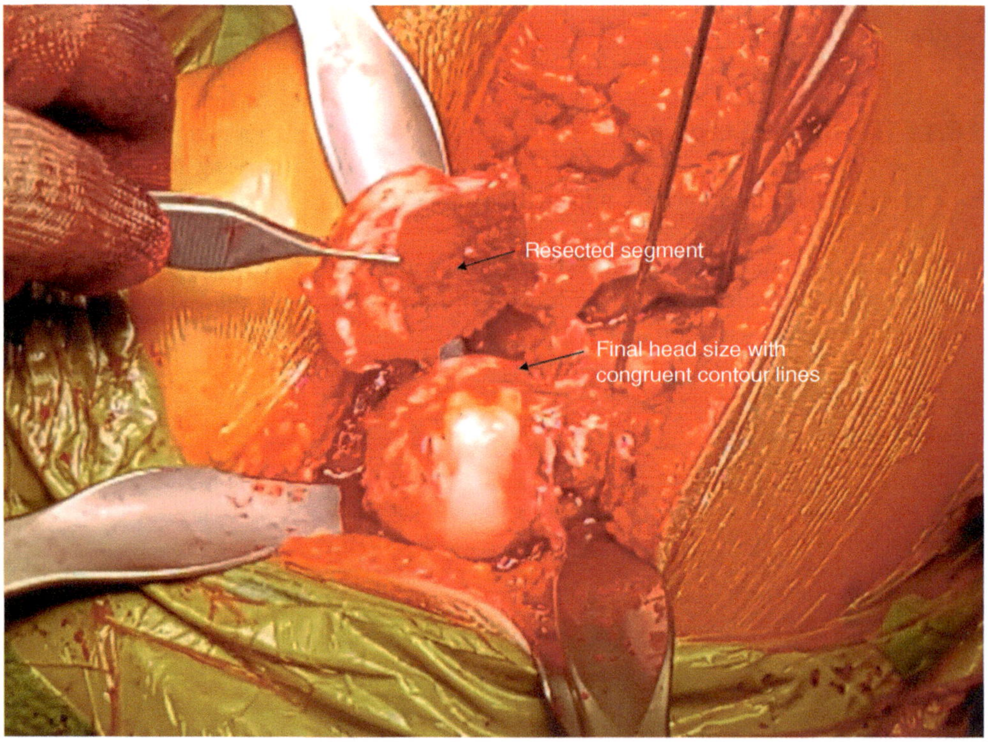

Fig. 18.4 Resected segment held in front of the "new" head showing stepless contour of the cartilage surface

- After the second cut, the template is removed, and round Hohmann retractors are placed to protect the soft tissue during posterior completion of the cut.
- Optional monitoring of the perfusion (technically rather easy for the stable segment and more difficult for the mobile segment) can be executed with Laser Doppler flowmetry or indo-cyanine green (ICG) angiography.
- Thereafter, the lateral and intermediate segments are freed with a transverse cut keeping the abovementioned neck distance connected with the two resulting segments.
- Freeing the segments is rather delicate and should be advanced slowly with back-and-forth maneuvers, using the saw and thin osteotomes. Levering out movements against the stable medial segment should be always avoided.
- Mobility of the lateral segment can be somewhat increased by gentle further dissection of the posterior periosteum. However, extension of this dissection into the retinacular attachment at the head should strictly be avoided.

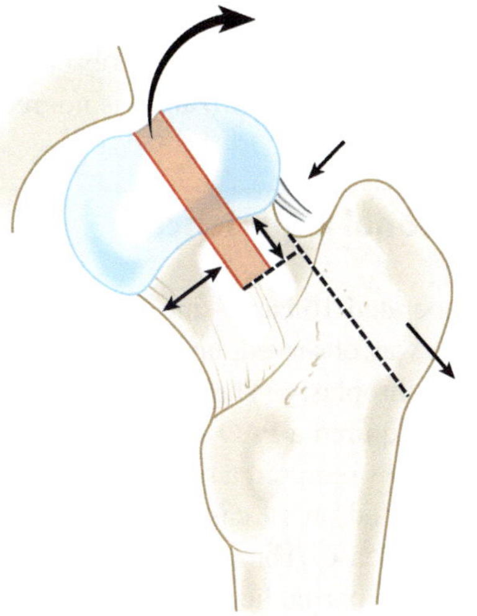

Fig. 18.5 Drawing with a minimum width of 15 mm of the calcar pillar and a neck portion left on the mobile segment, long enough to allow placement of a more anterior and a more posterior screw

- Similar dissection of attached posterior periosteal tissue may be necessary for removal of the intermediate segment.
- Both remaining segments should have a flat cutting surface. With some patience, bleeding of the surfaces can be demonstrated.
- Adjustment of the mobile segment is achieved manually and should result in a cartilage surface without a step-off or mayor gap.
- Provisional fixation is achieved with a pointed reduction forceps. It should be placed in a way to allow best screw placement in the neck extension. After relative neck lengthening, the neck extension may have lost its cortical cover. Screw tightening should be executed with special care, or even placed through the near cartilage; in such a case, the screw head should be countersunk clearly below the cartilage surface.
- Screws are placed at the neck portion of the mobile fragment and directed to the opposite stable neck cortex. Two screws are sufficient. Optimal length of the two 3.5 mm screws can be palpated at the opposite cortex. The screw heads and tips should not project.
- Before repositioning of the head into the socket, care must be taken that the retinaculum is unfolded, and without any tension, be aware of Hohmann retractor placement and leg mobility during all the procedure.
- • Careful movements of the head may show that the head can be shifted within the widened socket. It may be used as confirmation for additional periacetabular osteotomy (PAO). It could have been foreseen already with computer simulation.
- It is important that readaptation of the retinacular flap is executed without any tension. One or two knots are sufficient. The same applies for closure of the capsule.
- Refixation of the greater trochanter (Chap. 7) should not create pressure on the retinaculum. Some distal advancement may be necessary; excessive advancement should be avoided. Optimal position may be controlled with fluoroscopy.
- Soft tissue closure is executed layer by layer; skin suture is postponed and happens together with the wound closure of the PAO.
- Consideration for performing a concomitant PAO will allow for proper draping and easy turning into the supine position.
- For the execution of the PAO, see Chap. 19. It takes less time compared with an isolated PAO, because the first ischial cut is already done [6–9].

18.12 Postoperative Follow-Up

- The operated leg is placed in full extension, neutral rotation, and ab–/adduction using a foam rubber splint until the patient can actively control the leg position.
- On postoperative day 1, gentle passive flexion and rotation is started, and, depending on pain tolerance, toe-touch loading can begin.
- As soon as possible, active movements are initiated and completed by passive flexion-extension on a motorized frame.
- At 4 weeks loading can be increased to 15 kg, and abductor training can be started.
- A radiographic control is recommended at 8 weeks.
- Walking with one crutch in the opposite hand can be started at 10–12 weeks.
- Walking without external support can be started when the abductor force has reached M4–5 and a new radiography has shown sufficient consolidation of femoral and acetabular osteotomies.
- Sportive activities should be postponed at least for 6 months.

18.13 Intra-/Postoperative Complications

18.13.1 Intraoperative

- Wrong cut into the head. When only superficial, it may be corrected without vital consequences. When already propagated deeper into the head bone, it may be accepted, hoping that it does not exit posteriorly within the retinacular attachment on the head.
- Wrong cuts when using a cutting template is caused by incorrect placement of the template.
- Injury to the retinaculum with the oscillating saw. There is no correction possible. The only alternative is prevention

with careful observation and protection of the retinaculum during the process of cutting.

- The primary cause of intraoperative fracture through the neck area of the stable medial segment is leverage against it during mobilization of the intermediate segment. It can be stabilized immediately with a screw inserted from the lateral cortex into the medial head segment. If a fracture is impending because the residual neck diameter is very small, prophylactic screw reinforcement is recommended.
- While bleeding of the stable segment can be observed immediately on the cutting surface, it may take a while to be seen on the mobile segment due to spasms of the capillaries. Unfolding of the retinaculum is sometimes helpful. ICG angiography may be repeated.
- A mismatch of the articular contour can happen as gap or step. A gap can be treated with recutting of an uneven surface. Localized and superficial gaps may be left alone or filled with osteochondral material from the resected segment.
- Projection of one segment may be treated with re-reduction of the mobile segment. Localized anterior or posterior projection may be resected. Trimming of good cartilage of the stable segment should be avoided.
- When sufficient cephalad displacement of the mobile segment is not possible, careful further dissection of the posterior periosteum may be attempted.
- If the purchase of the two screws is not sufficient, cancellous screws or a third screw may be used. If the neck portion is very small, one screw may be inserted into the epiphyseal bone; the head of such a screw must be countersunk clearly below the cartilage level.
- If the resulting head is still too large, recutting should be performed. A resulting head which is too small can only be compensated with increased acetabular correction.
- The majority of cutting mistakes can be minimized with computer simulation and cutting templates.

18.13.2 Postoperative

- Postoperative fracture through the neck of the stable segment does normally not result in definitive stop of its perfusion. Nevertheless, immediate stabilization is necessary, using the technique as described above.
- Recurrent subluxation or even dislocation is possible when the additional PAO has not been executed or the correction of the PAO was not sufficient.
- Postoperative necrosis of the mobile fragment has not been observed so far by these authors. In one hip of traumatic necrosis, a partial necrosis of the neck portion was seen.
- Severe joint stiffness after a correctly executed intra-capital osteotomy has not been observed. In any case, closed manual joint mobilization is not recommended.

18.14 Personal Experience

- DC has operated 16 cases since 2008. So far, no necrosis or fracture was observed, and no case was converted to a total hip arthroplasty. Three hips with sole intra-capital osteotomy required a PAO shortly after due to joint instability. Two hips required a secondary osteochondroplasty.
- **DS** has operated on 14 cases with 11 having a diagnosis of Perthes disease. The other diagnoses were a postop-SCFE hip with partial head avascular necrosis (AVN) and associated large femoral head, one hip with coxa magna following treatment for developmental dysplasia of the hip and one hip with posttraumatic AVN. There are no cases of avascular necrosis or neck fracture postoperatively. The optimal results are seen with healthy medial and lateral columns and associated limited hip abduction. There was a surprisingly good "remodeling" that seems to occur following surgery and improved concentricity between the femoral head and acetabulum. One patient required revision surgery after the procedure for Perthes disease, who had residual adduction contracture (better than preop.)_despite improved range of motion. He had a proximal femoral valgus osteotomy to position the leg to improve his gait. Another patient may require future revision surgery, who had subluxation following the intra-capital reduction and subsequently underwent a PAO but may have continued symptoms. Patient selection is critically important to achieve good results, and only one patient has had a concomitant PAO although some patients may have been better having both.
- RG follows more than 50, mainly elsewhere operated cases. The majority of hips were treated with additional PAO. So far total necrosis of the medial or the lateral segment has not been observed. One hip, treated for a deformity after traumatic avascular necrosis, developed a necrosis of the neck extension of the lateral segment which did not have consequences for the contour of the head. One case had localized subchondral sequestration within the healed lateral segment and required THR 1 year after surgery. In two patients with neurological disorders and reduced mechanical bone quality, a fracture of the neck of the stable medial segment occurred shortly after surgery; open screw fixation led to uneventful consolidation. One Perthes hip with total head involvement healed with partial joint stiffness.

- The first cases operated in Berne showed surprisingly good 10-year results [10]. Good early results were also reported from other institutions [11, 12].

18.14.1 Exemplary Cases

1. A 13-year-old boy suffered from bilateral Perthes disease and received nonsurgical treatment so far. While problems on the right side were minimal, the left side became increasingly symptomatic with pain, limping, and reduced ROM. Conventional radiographies of the right hip showed a mild mushroom-like deformity of the head corresponding with a slightly dysplastic acetabulum. The joint space was wide and congruent. In contrast, the left proximal femur was severely deformed, and the partially necrotic head was subluxated. The acetabulum showed a substantial secondary dysplasia. Surgery took place before computer simulation was available. It was planned to perform relative lengthening of the femoral neck, distal advancement of the greater trochanter, femoral head reduction osteotomy, and PAO in one anesthesia. The femur was approached first in lateral decubitus, and surgery was completed with the PAO in supine position. Healing of the osteotomies was uneventful. Sixteen years later the hip is pain-free during ADL and has a reasonable ROM, and the walking pattern is normal (Fig. 18.6).
2. A 9-year-old boy suffering from Perthes disease with nearly total head involvevent. Pain and limping continued after valgus intertrochanteric osteotomy for adduction contracture. Subluxation persisted. Size reduction osteotomy of the head stabilized the joint, reason why an additional PAO seemed to be unnecessary. He remained pain-free and fully active during 15 years, when he noticed recurrency of pain after playing soccer. New radiographies in abduction showed better congruency and containment of the head. The possibility of a PAO was discussed, but the patient is hesitating, because he is pain-free when refraining from soccer (Fig. 18.7).

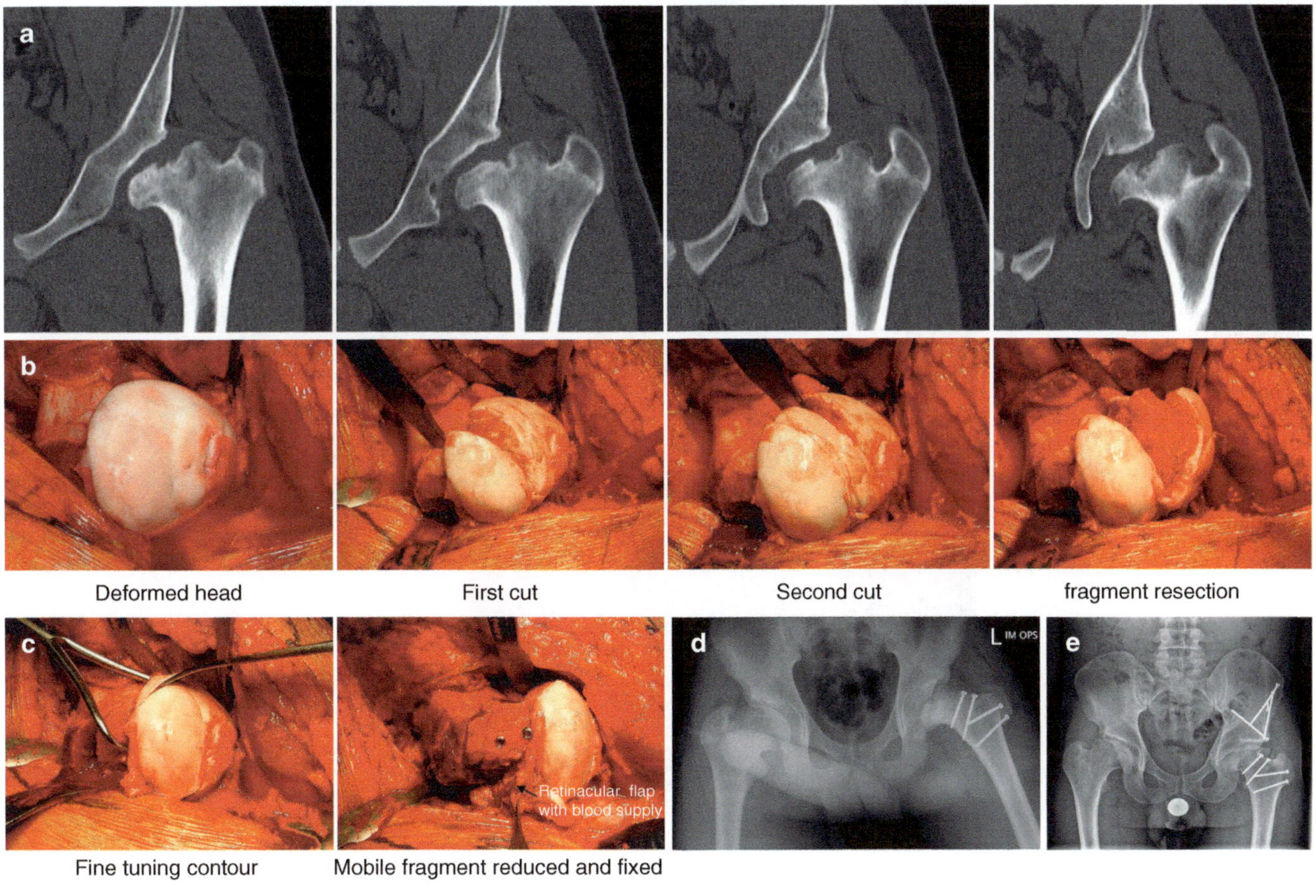

Fig. 18.6 A 13-year-old male with Perthes disease left>right. (**a**) Tomographic series of the left hip showing severe deformity of the proximal femur with central necrosis of the subluxated head, short neck, and high-riding greater trochanter; the acetabulum is dysplastic accordingly. (**b**) Sequence of the intra-capital osteotomies. (**c**) Sequence of segment reduction and fixation. (**d**) Intraoperative abduction view to understand the necessary amount of PAO correction. (**e**) 16-year-result. The patient is pain-free, walks normal, and has a good ROM

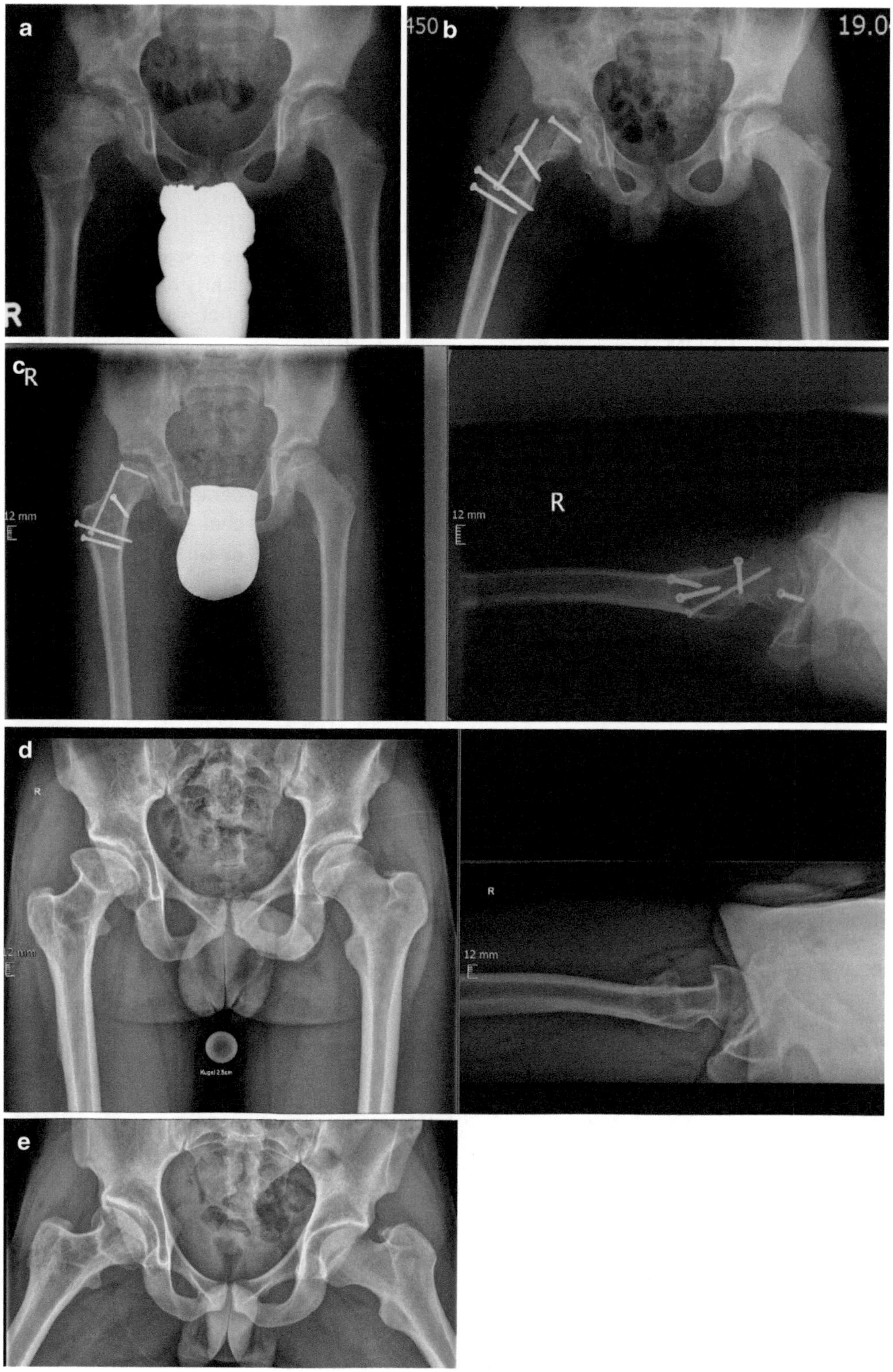

Fig. 18.7 A 9-year-old male patient with nearly total epiphyseal necrosis. (**a**) Subluxation after valgus osteotomy for severe adduction contracture. Rather little reactive acetabular adaptation; ongoing pain and limping. (**b**) Radiography after head reduction osteotomy; the coaxial neck screw was necessary to protect the thin neck of the stable segment. PAO was planned but was waived because of good intrasoperative joint stability. (**c**) 1-year-result with visible remodeling of the epiphyseal contour. (**d**) Control radiography 17 years after surgery for recent pain recurrency after playing soccer. (**e**) Better congruency in abduction; however, patient is not ready for PAO

18.15 Controversies

So far, the procedure is only practiced in centers with experience with intracapsular surgery.

- Others regard the technical execution of the procedure as too demanding and risky when considering the rather infrequent indication. Furthermore, it may be difficult to get access to computer simulation and cutting templates.
- Routine additional PAO is not executed in all centers. Follow-up studies are needed to clarify this important aspect.
- When performing an additional PAO, it can be executed the classical way or as described here.
- Routine use of perfusion monitoring during surgery may not always be available.

18.16 Expected Outcomes

Considering the severe deformity and the rather modest results of other treatments, previous publications with the described technique have already shown surprisingly good results. Routine application of computer simulation and the routine use of corresponding cutting templates will increase the accuracy of correction and further reduce intraoperative complications.

18.17 Future Directions

In view of the rather infrequent indication, the procedure should be concentrated in institutions with considerable case load. Computer assistance and template production should be simplified to an extent that no outside technical assistance is necessary. Intraoperative ICG angiography may become routine.

References

1. Mickulicz-Radecki J. in Vulpius Handbuch der Orthopädische Chirurgie. Stuttgart: Enke Verlag; 1913. p. 382.
2. Ganz R, Huff TW, Leunig M. Extended retinacular soft tissue flap for intraarticular hip surgery: surgical technique, indications, and results of its application. Instr Course Lect. 2009;58:241–55.
3. Sewitt S, Thompson RG. The distribution and anastomosis of the arteries supplying the head and neck of the femur. J Bone Joint Surg Br. 1965;47:560–73.
4. Kalhor M, Horowitz K, Gharehdaghi J, Beck M, Ganz R. Anatomic variations in femoral head circulation. Hip Int. 2012;22:307–12.
5. Fürnstahl P, Casari FA, Ackermann J, Marcon M, Leunig M, Ganz R. Computer-Assisted femoral head reduction osteotomies: An approach for anatomic reconstruction of severely deformed Legg-Calvé-Perthes hips. A pilot study of six patients. BMC Musculoskelet Disord. 2020;21:759. https://doi.org/10.1186/s12891-020-03789-y.
6. Ganz R, Horowitz K, Leunig M. Algorithm for femoral and periacetabular osteotomies in complex hip deformities. Clin Orthop Relat Res. 2010;468:3168–80.
7. Ganz R, Klaue K, Vinh TS, Mast JW. A new periacetabular osteotomy for the treatment of hip dysplasias, technique and preliminary results. Clin Orthop Relat Res. 1988;232:26–36.
8. Leunig M, Siebenrock KA, Mahomed MN, Ganz R. Bernese periacetabular osteotomy: technical aspects and clinical results. Hip Int. 1999;9:119–26.
9. Kalhor M, Collado D, Leunig M, Rego P, Ganz R. Recommendations to reduce risk of nerve injury during Bernese periaceabular osteotomy (PAO). JBJS Essential Surgical Techniques. 2017;7(4):e34. https://doi.org/10.2106/JBJS.ST.17.00017. Subspecialty Procedures
10. Siebenrock KA, Anwander H, Zurmühle CA, Tannast M, Slongo T, Steppacher SD. Head reduction osteotomy with additional containment surgery improves sphericity and containment and reduced pain in Legg-Calvé-Perthes disease. Clin Orthop Relat Res. 2015;473:1274–83.
11. Paley D. The treatment of femoral head deformity and coxa magna by the Ganz femoral head reduction osteotomy. Orthop Clin North Am. 2011;42:389.
12. Clohisy JC, Pascual-Garrido C, Duncan S, Pashos G, Schoenecker PL. Concurrent femoral head reduction and periacetabular osteotomies for the treatment of severe femoral head deformities. Bone Joint J. 2018;100-B:1551–8.

Surgical Hip Dislocation Combined with Periacetabular Osteotomy

19

John C. Clohisy, Xiadong Chen, and Michael Leunig

19.1 Introduction

The surgical hip dislocation and periacetabular osteotomy (SHD/PAO) is a combination of procedures used to manage complex deformities involving both the proximal femur and acetabulum. The most common indication for this surgical strategy is to treat residual, symptomatic Legg-Calve-Perthes deformities (Perthes deformities) or "Perthes-like" deformities resultant from other developmental disorders. These hips commonly have an aspheric femoral head, intra-articular abnormalities (labrum, articular cartilage, and ligamentum teres), intra-articular impingement, extra-articular impingement, and instability from secondary acetabular dysplasia. The SHD/PAO procedure allows comprehensive correction of all aspects of the disease and is the optimal strategy for many patients with these challenging deformities. Hips with epiphyseal dysplasia, e.g., Morquio disease with similar complex deformities can also present an indication.

19.2 Background

Patients may present in adolescence or young adulthood with hip pain and functional limitations. Symptomatology and progressive joint degeneration are common, and many patients present later in life with more severe joint degeneration. Femoral deformities variably include a large aspheric femoral head (coxa plana), a short, wide femoral neck (coxa breva), coxa vara, and relative overgrowth of the greater trochanter [1] and torsional abnormalities of the femur. These femoral abnormalities can result in complex intra- and extra-articular femoroacetabular impingement (FAI) and instability. On the acetabular side, secondary dysplasia is common and characterized by insufficient femoral head coverage and variable acetabular version with retroversion being common. Intra-articular abnormalities are also common and include osteochondral lesions of the femoral head, acetabular labral tears, acetabular and femoral chondromalacia and chondral flaps, and ligamentum teres tears. This combination of structural and intra-articular abnormalities presents a major treatment challenge. In cases with both acetabular dysplasia (instability) and FAI, treatment of both sides of the joint may be necessary for comprehensive correction. Surgical treatment requires access to the intra-articular disease elements, wide exposure for reconstruction of the proximal femur, and adequate exposure for acetabular reconstruction. A combined surgical hip dislocation and periacetabular osteotomy (SHD/PAO) is our preferred method for managing these complex hip abnormalities [2, 3].

The safe surgical hip dislocation approach [4] and the Bernese periacetabular osteotomy [5] were both described by Ganz and colleagues (see Chap. 7). The SHD is performed through a lateral transtrochanteric approach with anterior dislocation and is characterized by wide exposure of the proximal femur and acetabulum with preservation of femoral head vascularity via the terminal branches of the deep branch of medial femoral circumflex artery. This exposure of the hip allows treatment of lesions in the central compartment, reshaping of the femoral head (peripheral or central head reduction), relative neck lengthening with trochanteric advancement, and proximal femoral osteotomy in selected cases. Historically, the PAO is performed through a modified Smith-Petersen approach and includes a series of periacetabular osteotomies, acetabular mobilization, and multiplanar deformity correction. With improved understanding of Perthes deformities and the associated complex pathomechanics, the combined SHD/PAO procedure has been adopted for comprehensive surgical treatment of these challenging deformities.

J. C. Clohisy (✉)
Department of Orthopaedic Surgery, Washington University Medical School, St. Louis, MO, USA
e-mail: jclohisy@wustl.edu

X. Chen
Department of Orthopaedic Surgery, Shanghai Jiaotong University School of Medicine, Shanghai, China

M. Leunig
Hip Service, Department of Orthopaedic Surgery, Schulthess Clinic, Zurich, Switzerland
e-mail: michael.leunig@kws.ch

M. Leunig et al. (eds.), *Surgical Hip Dislocation*, https://doi.org/10.1007/978-3-031-70622-6_19

19.3 Indications

- Older children and relatively young patient (<30 years).
- Well-conditioned patient with body mass index (BMI) ≤ 30.
- Adequate radiographic congruency (aspherical congruency).
- Combined FAI and instability (confirmed during the surgical procedure).
- Radiographically healthy hip without significant (≥50%) joint space narrowing.
- Adequate hip range of motion (flexion ≥80°, abduction ≥10°).

19.3.1 Relative Contraindications

- Age > 30 years.
- BMI > 30.
- If joint is determined to be stable after SHD, then PAO may not be indicated even in the setting of mild acetabular dysplasia.

19.3.2 Contraindications

- Minimally symptomatic hip not affecting daily activity or quality of life (relative).
- Major restriction of hip motion (< 85° hip flexion, < 10° hip abduction).
- Radiographic evidence of secondary osteoarthritis (OA) with joint space loss (≥ 50%).
- Major joint incongruity that is not surgically correctable by peripheral or central femoral head reduction osteotomy (aspherical incongruency).

19.4 Preoperative/Preinterventional Diagnostics

- Plain radiographs include a standing and/or supine anteroposterior (AP) pelvis, frog lateral, cross table, 45° Dunn, and a false profile view of the involved hip (see also Chap. 2).
- Selective functional radiographic views to assess congruency and suitability of osteotomy correction.
- MR arthrogram of the involved hip to assess articular cartilage integrity, acetabular labrum, and femoral head lesions (see also Chap. 3).
- Low radiation dose 3D CT scan with transverse images through the knee to assess hip structural anatomy and femoral version.

19.4.1 Preoperative Planning/Computer Simulation

- Preoperative planning is fundamental to a successful reconstruction. The transtrochanteric osteotomy should be planned, and the amount of advancement (distalization) determined. We usually aim to align the proximal tip of the greater trochanter with the vertical position of the femoral head center. The specific techniques to be used via the SHD should also be planned and may include intra-articular repair (labrum, acetabular articular cartilage, femoral head osteochondral lesions), peripheral or central femoral head reduction, relative femoral neck lengthening, and occasionally concomitant proximal femoral osteotomy. Acetabular morphology should be examined in detail to plan the PAO. Lateral center edge angle, acetabular inclination, horizontal hip center position, anterior coverage, and acetabular version (anterior and posterior walls) should be considered when planning the PAO reorientation goals.
- Computer simulation holds promise in providing more precise surgical planning and creation of custom cutting guides or templates as discussed in Chap. 5. Recently, a new technique was developed that combines computer simulation for preoperative planning and additive manufacturing for surgical navigation with patient-specific instruments, with the goal to perform head reduction osteotomies in a more controlled manner [6] (Chap. 5).

19.5 Applied Anatomy

Preservation of the vascular supply to the femoral head is fundamental to the SHD approach. Of paramount importance is the protection of the deep branch of the medial femoral circumflex artery as described in Chaps. 6 and 7.

The PAO procedure enables remarkable mobility of the acetabulum with preservation of the vascularity to the acetabulum. Most importantly, the supra-acetabular and acetabular branches of the superior gluteal, obturator, and inferior gluteal arteries provide acetabular vascularity despite the remarkable mobility of the acetabulum [7]. The location and proximity of the sciatic and femoral nerves must also be appreciated. Most importantly, excessive medial soft tissue retraction for the superior pubic ramus osteotomy can result in femoral nerve injury. Retraction during this part of the procedure should not be excessive and should be as brief as possible. Flexion and adduction of the hip relaxes the medial soft tissue envelope. The sciatic nerve is at risk for injury during the lateral ischial and distal lateral posterior column cuts. Knee flexion, abduction, and external rotation will relax the nerve during these cuts [8]. Care must also be taken to not impact the osteotome beyond the lateral cortex in these areas.

19.6 Special Risks

Retinacular dissection must be executed with special care to avoid avascular necrosis (AVN) of the femoral head during head reduction or neck osteotomy. The peripheral head reduction (common) and central head reduction osteotomy (uncommon) can be complicated by over resection and/or joint instability due to the resultant excessively small femoral head. We routinely combine a PAO with the central head reduction osteotomy [9] as previous reports have emphasized the risk of femoral head subluxation (after central femoral head reduction osteotomy) and the potential need for a subsequent surgery to correct residual instability [10]. Inadequate decompression of all components of FAI can also compromise the reconstruction. Dynamic range of motion exam should be used to confirm adequate decompression of the femoral head, low femoral neck, intertrochanteric ridge, and anterior superior greater trochanter. The intraoperative decision to perform a PAO after the SHD can be challenging and but is fundamental to optimizing the clinical outcome. If the hip is deemed stable after the SHD, we do not perform the PAO as this may create secondary FAI. Alternatively, if the hip is judged to be unstable after the SHD, we continue with the PAO to stabilize the hip. Prior to capsular closure the stability of the hip is assessed. The presence of instability is determined by direct observation of femoral head subluxation during the dynamic examination. Subluxation observed in any of three positions (10° extension and 15° external rotation; 45° flexion, 20° adduction, and 30° internal rotation; 90° flexion and neutral rotation) is considered to indicate instability and the need for PAO. A PAO is performed for radiographic evidence of acetabular dysplasia and documented dynamic instability. In the setting of severe radiographic dysplasia, intraoperative instability is uniformly present. In the setting of mild or moderate radiographic dysplasia without intraoperative instability, no PAO is performed. Adequate hip range of motion (90° of flexion and 20° of abduction) and excellent or good congruity as assessed by intraoperative fluoroscopy are additional criteria to indicate the PAO. The acetabular reduction is assessed by intraoperative radiography and range-of-motion examination. Care was taken to preserve at least 90° of hip flexion after the PAO to prevent secondary FAI. The PAO reduction is distinct in that even after surgical reconstruction of the proximal femur, there remains the risk of both intra-articular and extra-articular FAI. In these hips our acetabular reduction is less aggressive than in "classic dysplasia" as there is a higher risk for secondary FAI.

19.7 Type of Anesthesia

We use general endotracheal anesthesia for the combined SD/PAO because the procedure is relatively lengthy (3.5–5 hours depending upon complexity) and the patient is repositioned between the two procedures.

19.8 Positioning

The SHD procedure is performed in the lateral decubitus position, and the patient is repositioned supine for the PAO. A radiolucent table is used and the patient stabilized for the SHD with a peg board, bean bag or tunnel pillow, and lateral bag. All bony prominences and peripheral nerves are padded, and the ipsilateral arm is placed on a padded Mayo stand. After completion of the SHD approach, the patient is repositioned and re-prepped and draped for the PAO. Alternatively, a floppy lateral position can be used where the patient is turned on the back after SHD without new re-prepping and re-draping for the PAO.

19.9 Instruments/Implants

The basic instruments and implants for the SD approach have been presented in Chaps. 7 and 8. For Perthes-like hips, it is important to have suture anchors for labral refixation and the needed implants/systems for managing femoral osteochondral lesions. Articular cartilage repair of the femoral head may include a variety of techniques including microfracture, mesenchymal stem cell/matrix repair, osteochondral autograft, osteochondral allograft, and/or osteochondral fragment fixation (see Chap. 11). After preoperative planning the surgeon should have the appropriate implant systems to facilitate the selected cartilage repair techniques. Stainless steel screws that are 3.5 or 4.5 mm should be available for trochanteric fixation.

The PAO procedure requires specific instruments and retractors that may vary between surgeons (Fig. 19.1).

- 2 Hibbs retractors
- 3 Sofield (narrow, deep) retractors
- 1 long Mayo surgical scissors
- 1 hip skid
- 1 curved (or angled) ½ inch, handled ischial osteotome
- 1 metal mallet
- 1 Cobb elevator
- 1 small/long periosteal elevator (300 mm length/6 mm width)

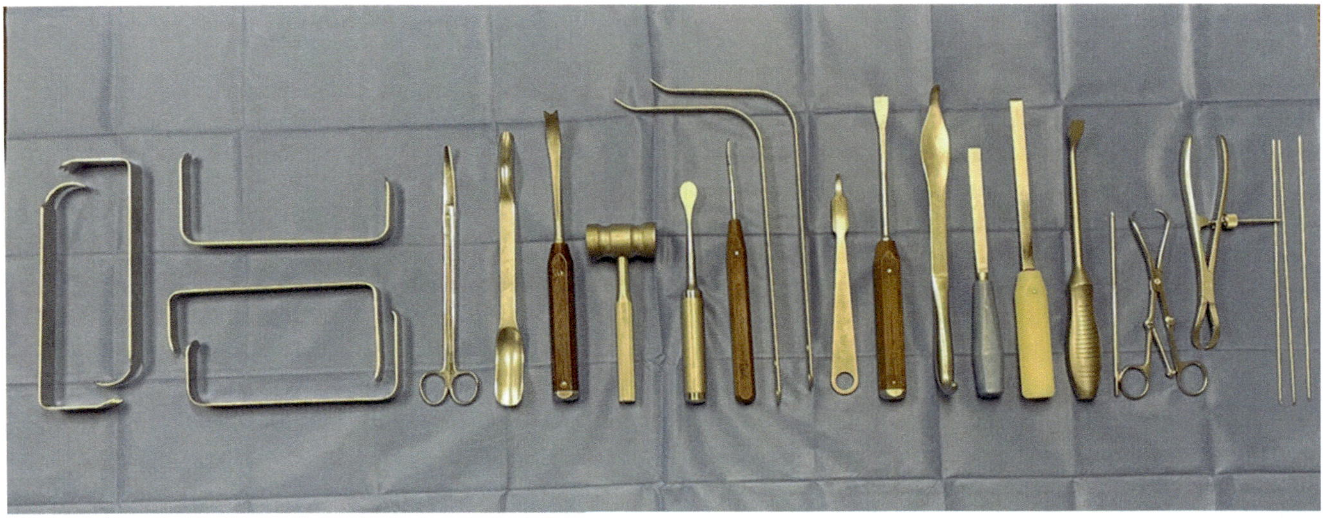

Fig. 19.1 Set of instruments used by Dr. Clohisy as described above

- 2 thin and long 90° blunt-tipped retractors (for ramus exposure) (320 mm handle length/150 mm right angle/10 mm/2 mm at tip/)
- 1 long pointed Homan retractor (245 mm/18 mm/3 mm at tip)
- 1 ½ inch, long, straight, handled superior pubic ramus osteotome (325 mm/15 and 20 mm)
- 1 straight cobra retractor for quadrilateral plate exposure
- 1 ½ inch saw blade for iliac osteotomy (12.5 mm/0.68 mm/73.8 mm)
- 1 ½ inch long, slightly curved, handled osteotome (posterior column cut) (295 mm)
- 1 ½ inch long, straight, handled osteotome (posterior column cut) (312 mm)
- 1 angled ½ inch handled osteotome (270 mm/15 mm/20 degree angle)
- 1 Schanz pin (5.0 x 200 mm) and T handle
- 1 Weber pointed bone reduction clamp (240 mm)
- 1 large serrated reduction clamp (Synthes reduction forceps with serrated jaw/240 mm)
- 3 2.5 mm K-wires (285 mm trocar point) and wire driver
- 3.5 or 4.5 stainless steel bone screw system.

19.10 Access

- Access for the SHD approach and the extended retinacular flap is covered in Chaps. 7 and 8. Trochanteric osteotomy, preservation of the terminal branches of the deep medial femoral circumflex artery, z-type capsulotomy, and anterior dislocation of the femoral head are fundamental.
- The access for the PAO is classically through the modified Smith-Petersen interval via a longitudinal or anterior ilioinguinal incision. The lateral femoral cutaneous nerve is protected by incising the fascia over the tensor fascia muscle belly and reflecting the fascia medially. Proximally in the wound, the external oblique and iliacus muscles are reflected medially providing access to the inner table of the ilium. Distally the interval between the tensor and sartorius muscles is developed. The anterior superior iliac spine is osteotomized and reflected medially.

19.11 Technical Steps of Deep Dissection

- ***SHD deep dissection.***
- Deep access for the SHD approach is summarized in detail in Chaps. 7 and 8. The same dissection steps are used with Perthes deformities although these hips can be more difficult to expose due to the proximal femoral morphology and restricted range of motion. The anterior arm of the z-type capsulotomy can be extended inferiorly to the level of the anterior acetabular labrum to provide additional mobility of the femur. Proximal femoral exposure is usually not complicated, but access along the medial and posterior femoral head can be more restricted. To access the medial head, the assistant should flex, externally rotate, and push the femur posteriorly. This maneuver also assists with acetabular exposure which can be more challenging in these hips. Exposure of the posterior femoral head can be further improved by placement of a small hip skid under the posterior neck to elevate the femoral head away from the acetabulum. Some surgeons prefer to perform the ischial cut for the PAO under direct visualization during the SD procedure. This is done by developing the interval between the inferior gemellus and

obturator externus. The sciatic nerve is palpated and protected during this maneuver.

- ***PAO deep dissection.***
- The PAO deep dissection is first carried distal along the medial edge of the direct head of the rectus (without rectus takedown) with elevation of iliacus and iliocapsularis muscle fibers to expose the anterior hip capsule. The hip is flexed, and the interval between the psoas tendon and hip capsule is developed with a large Mayo scissors, and a small hip skid is placed in this interval to guide insertion of the osteotome for the ischial osteotomy. After positioning of the osteotome at the infracotyloid groove, the hip is brought into less flexion, while knee flexion is maintained to relax the sciatic nerve. The superior pubic ramus is then exposed with a small periosteal elevator. This subperiosteal dissection is initiated along the anterior pelvic brim and extended medially under the superior aspect of the superior pubic ramus and into the obturator foramen. The dissection is then advanced medially approximately 1 cm along the anterior aspect of the ramus and then carried inferiorly around the inferior aspect of the ramus. Long blunt-tipped retractors are then placed around the superior and inferior aspects of the ramus. A pointed Homan retractor is impacted into the anterior ramus approximately 15 mm medial to the iliopectineal eminence to provide access for the ramus osteotomy. Retraction with the Homan should not be excessive and should be brief to prevent injury to the femoral nerve during the ramus osteotomy. The subperiosteal dissection is then extended posteriorly along the inner wall of the ilium and over the pelvic brim to expose the quadrilateral plate. A straight cobra retractor is used to palpate and localize the sciatic notch and then positioned on the ischial spine to facilitate access for the ilium and posterior column cuts. A small tunnel is then developed along the lateral side of the ilium and a thin retractor placed to protect the lateral soft tissues during iliac osteotomy. Once the periacetabular cuts are complete the mobility of the acetabulum is assessed, the same deep dissection steps can be repeated (if needed) to revisit any area(s) of incomplete osteotomy.

19.12 Postoperative Follow-Up

- ***Postoperative rehabilitation and activity resumption.***

The majority of these procedures require a trochanteric advancement which is usually the limiting factor for weight bearing. We maintain 10 to 15 kg foot flat weight bearing for the first 6 weeks and then advance to 50% for 4 additional weeks and full weight bearing at 10 weeks. A continuous passive motion machine is used for the first 4 weeks (4–8 hours per day), and hip flexion motion is limited to 90° during this time. Active hip strengthening exercises start at 6 weeks with resistance added at 10 weeks. Four months is the target for release to full activity including the initiation of sport, although some patients require 6 months for complete recovery and return to athletics. Patients are seen in clinic with radiographs (to assess bone healing) at 6 weeks, 4 months, and 1 year postoperatively.

- ***Secondary procedures.***

We routinely recommend hardware removal primarily for trochanteric screws that may cause lateral hip pain/trochanteric bursitis and may complicate (screw breakage) future total hip arthroplasty (THA). This is performed 6 to 12 months postoperatively, and unrestricted activity is allowed 6 weeks after screw removal. Trochanteric screw size can affect ease of removal with 4.5 mm having a lower risk of breakage than 3.5 mm screws.

19.12.1 Intra-/Postoperative Complications

Potential complications of the SHD/PAO reconstruction are important to consider. The SHD approach has the risk of compromising blood supply to the femoral head which can uncommonly result in head osteonecrosis, collapse, and joint failure. Reported complications of the SHD/PAO procedure suggest that there is an approximate 13% risk of any complication [11] with the majority being minor (9%) including asymptomatic heterotopic ossification, asymptomatic superior pubis ramus nonunion, and superficial wound dehiscence not requiring surgery. Major complications can also occur (4%) and may include persistent symptomatic intra-articular disorders requiring surgery and deep infection. Additional potential risks include thromboembolic disease, neurovascular injury, and symptomatic nonunion.

19.13 Case Studies

19.13.1 Case 1

See Fig. 19.2.

19.13.2 Case 2

See Fig. 19.3

19.13.3 Case 3

See Fig. 19.4

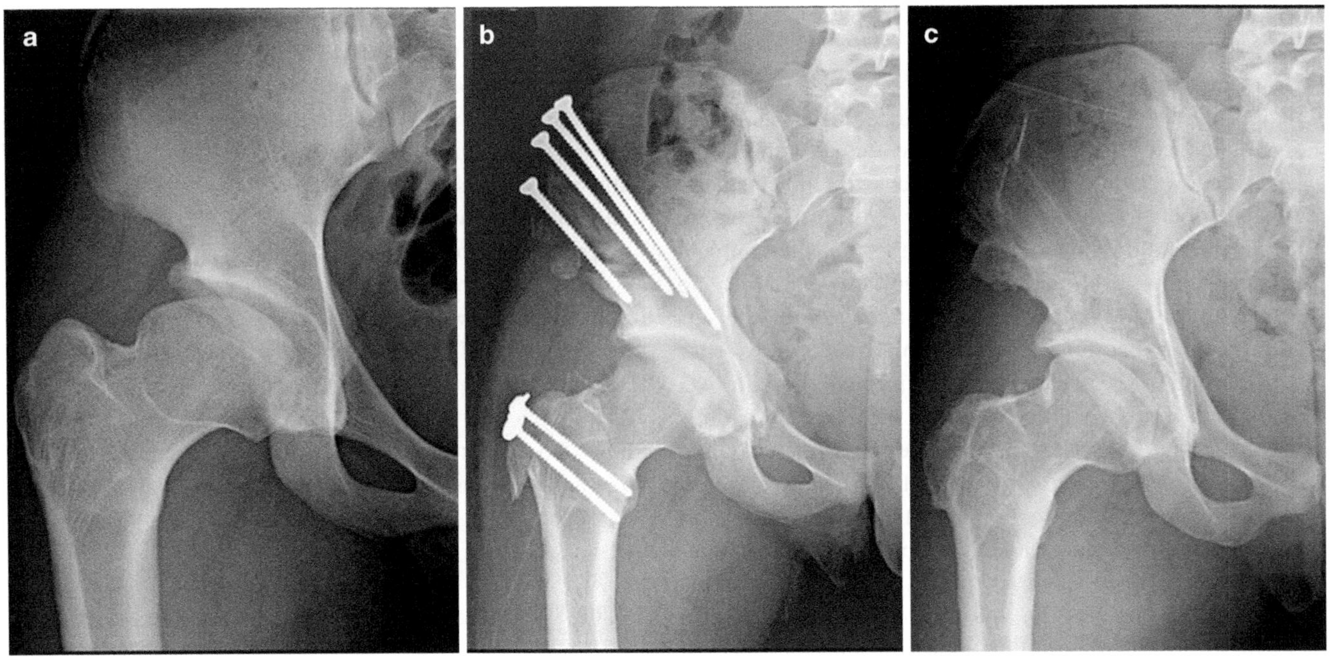

Fig. 19.2 (a–c) Radiographs of a 16-year-old girl treated with SHD including osteochondroplasty, relative femoral neck lengthening, and trochanteric advancement. A PAO was then performed to stabilize the hip. (Fig. 19.2a) Preoperative anteroposterior pelvic radiograph (cropped from AP pelvis) showing an aspheric femoral head, coxa breva, coxa vara, and relative trochanteric overgrowth on the femoral side. The acetabulum is noteworthy for secondary dysplasia with retroversion. The hip demonstrates aspheric congruency and was unstable after the SHD. (Fig. 19.2b) Initial postoperative anteroposterior pelvic radiograph demonstrating improved head sphericity, relative neck lengthening with trochanteric advancement, improved acetabular coverage, and version correction. (Fig. 19.2c) A 10-year postoperative radiograph associated with an excellent clinical result. (Reproduced from [3])

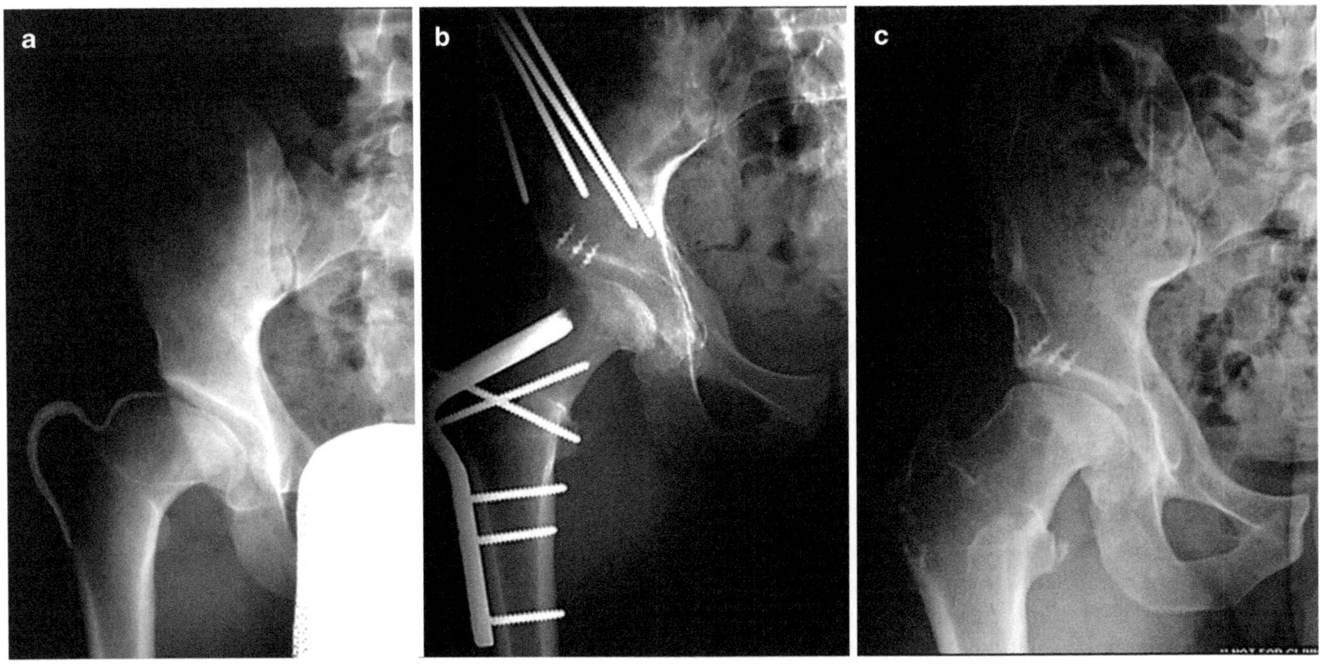

Fig. 19.3 (a–c) Radiographs of a 17-year-old boy with symptomatic, complex, residual Perthes deformity. (Fig. 19.3a) Preoperative anteroposterior pelvic radiograph (cropped image from AP pelvis). The patient was treated with combined SHD/PAO including peripheral head reduction, labral repair, relative neck lengthening with trochanteric advancement, proximal femoral valgus osteotomy (to improve congruency, range of motion and length) followed by the PAO. (Fig. 19.3b) One-year postoperative radiograph showing healed osteotomies, improved head sphericity, containment, and joint congruency. (Fig. 19.3c) Nine-year postoperative radiograph showing a well-maintained joint space and congruency associated with an excellent clinical result. (Reproduced from [3])

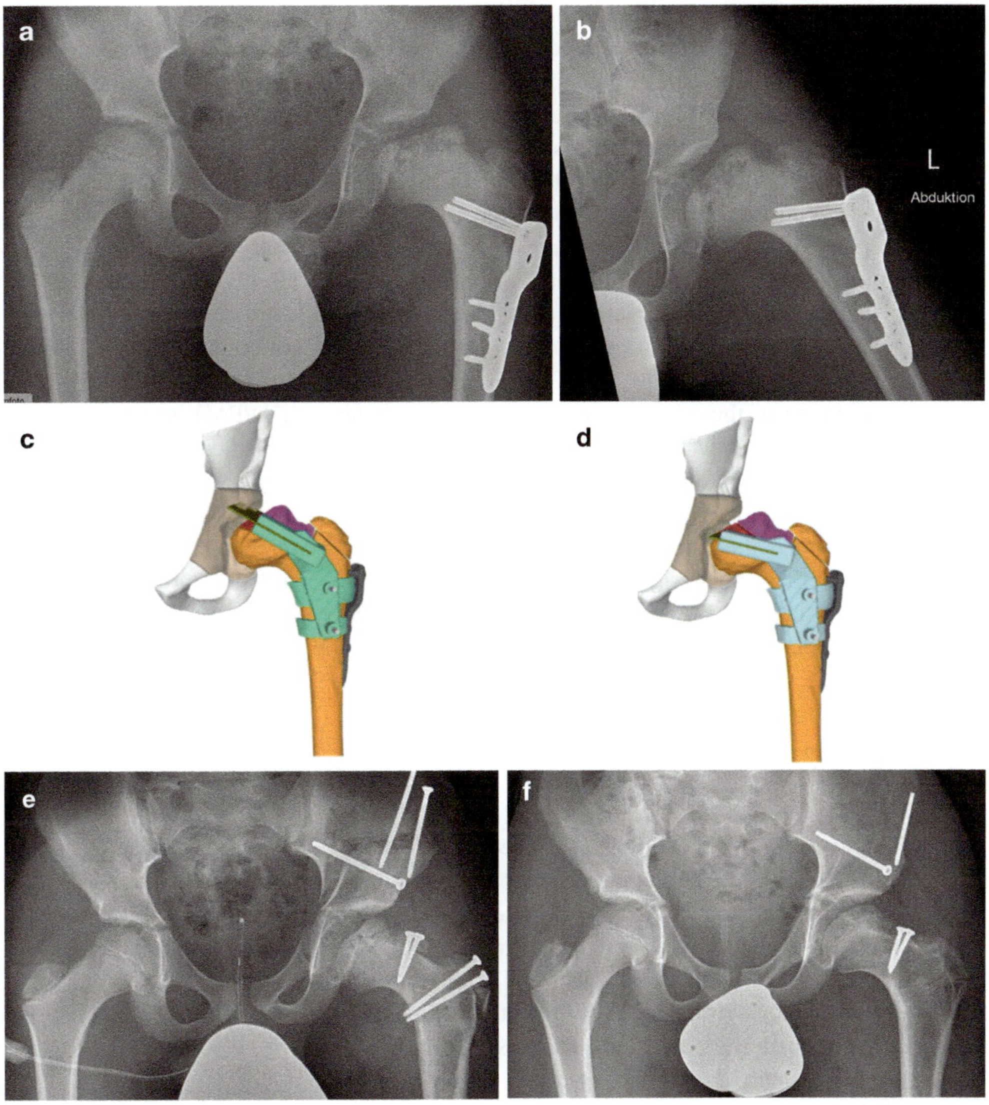

Fig. 19.4 (a–f) A 10-year-old boy from Italy who started to limb 2–3 years earlier diagnosed early Legg-Calve-Perthes disease (LCPD) underwent intertrochanteric varization intertrochanteric osteotomy (ITO) (Fig. 19.4a). Persistent pain, limited abduction, short extremity, abduction of only 10° in internal rotation of the left extremity (Fig. 19.4b). Radiographically hinged abduction with coxa magna. Femoral head too big to fit socket. Therefore, patient specific instrument (PSI)-based head reductions (first step) followed by PAO (second step) as described in Chap. 5 (Fig. 19.4c, d). Postoperatively well-centered femoral head after PAO and head reduction osteotomies (Fig. 19.4e). Excellent 2-year result after partial hardware removal with a well-centered healthy-appearing femoral head and normal joint space (Fig. 19.4f)

19.14 Controversies

- A common challenge in treating Perthes-like deformities is determining the optimal timing of surgical intervention. While early intervention is optimal before substantial intra-articular damage occurs, it is important to note that many of these hips will function well through adulthood. We do not recommend SHD/PAO reconstruction in asymptomatic hips and only indicate patients who are symptomatic, have failed nonoperative treatment, and have hip dysfunction that limits activity and/or quality of life. Worsening hip symptoms over time is a strong indicator for surgical intervention.
- Indicating patients for surgery is also controversial due to the multiple factors that may impact the clinical outcome. These include patient age, BMI and physical conditioning, articular cartilage health, joint congruency, femoral head osteochondral lesions, and preoperative range of motion. We have relatively strict criteria that generally include age < 30 years, BMI < 30 and adequate physical condition, at least fair joint congruency, a well-preserved joint space, treatable femoral head lesions, and preoperative range of motion of at least 85° flexion and 15° abduction.
- Head reduction osteotomies to lessen the size of the head to fit the acetabulum is best indicated in younger patients (children or adolescents) with classic Perthes disease. Older patients (> 16 years) and patients with posttraumatic AVN as seen in dancers have shown poor mixed results after head reduction osteotomies [12]. Neck osteotomies show remarkable good results [13] (Chap. 16).
- A major source of controversy includes the use of other surgical techniques to treat these deformities. Some surgeons have favored arthroscopic treatment, while others feel that total hip replacement may be a better option in some patients. The role of hip arthroscopy remains

unclear as much of the structural deformity is not corrected and mid- to long-term outcomes are not known. We prefer open treatment for these complex deformities as it allows comprehensive surgical correction of all aspects of the disease. Total hip arthroplasty is an excellent option when secondary osteoarthritis is established (50% joint space narrowing) and there is severe incongruency (that is not correctable) and/or limited hip range of motion. In a young person with a healthy joint and correctable deformity, we prefer hip preservation with the SHD/PAO procedure.

- Determining the need for concurrent PAO is another controversy. Many of these hips have features of acetabular dysplasia, but this doesn't necessarily translate to joint instability. Perthes-like hips are unique in that the very large femoral head and hypertrophic labrum may lend the hip stable even in the setting of some dysplastic characteristics on the acetabular side. The intraoperative assessment of hip stability, radiographic congruency, and range of motion is important in determining the need for concurrent PAO.

19.15 Results

The clinical results of the SHD/PAO procedure are documented in the literature, yet it is important to note that these are relatively uncommon procedures and large case series are not available. In general, the reported clinical outcomes endorse major improvements in pain relief, function, and deformity correction. Promising early results of the procedure are maintained at the mid-term for most patients. One recent study summarized the mid-term (average 8.4 years) results of 27 hips treated with the SD/PAO for symptomatic Perthes-like deformities. Deformity correction was consistent, and 85% of the hips remained preserved (no conversion to THA). The survivorship estimates at 5 and 10 years were 93% and 85%, respectively. Clinically significant improvements were noted with the modified Harris hip score (improved from 64 to 92 points) and the WOMAC pain score (improved from 60 to 86 points). Average UCLA activity improved and average one grade. Fifteen percent of the hips underwent conversion to THA. Two factors were associated with failure, including a greater preoperative center-trochanter distance with hips that failed measuring −47 mm compared with −23 mm in surviving hips. This difference is substantial and may be an indicator of deformity severity at baseline, which may limit the clinical outcome. Additionally, lower postoperative ACEA was present in hips undergoing THA, suggesting less postoperative anterior coverage. This finding suggests that adequate anterior coverage may play a role in optimizing clinical outcomes and is a potential target as a modifiable variable [2]. Regarding head reduction osteotomies in severe coxa magna with hinged abduction, the 10-year results of our first hips in children and adolescents with classic Perthes deformities are favorable [10], while Perthes like AVN in young gymnasts was associated with mixed outcomes in three cases [12]. Neck osteotomies have so far excellent results after 2 years [13].

19.16 Outlook

The treatment decision-making and surgical management of Perthes-like deformities are challenging. In selected hips the SHD/PAO seems to be the optimal treatment strategy. Published clinical results indicate that the combined procedure is safe and effective for most patients at mid-term follow-up. Improved indications for treatment, computational modeling, and/or articular cartilage repair techniques may further improve the clinical outcomes and survivorship of these reconstructions.

References

1. Stulberg SD, Cooperman DR, Wallensten R. The natural history of Legg-calve-Perthes disease. J Bone Joint Surg Am. 1981;63(7):1095–108.
2. Ganz R, Horowitz K, Leunig M. Algorithm for femoral and periacetabular osteotomies in complex hip deformities. Clin Orthop Relat Res. 2010;468(12):3168–80.
3. Nepple JJ, Freiman S, Pashos G, Thornton T, Schoenecker PL, Clohisy JC. Combined surgical dislocation and Periacetabular osteotomy for complex residual Legg-calve-Perthes deformities: intermediate-term outcomes. J Bone Joint Surg Am. 2022;104(9):780–9.
4. Ganz R, Gill TJ, Gautier E, Ganz K, Krugel N, Berlemann U. Surgical dislocation of the adult hip a technique with full access to the femoral head and acetabulum without the risk of avascular necrosis. J Bone Joint Surg Br. 2001;83(8):1119–24.
5. Ganz R, Klaue K, Vinh TS, Mast JW. A new periacetabular osteotomy for the treatment of hip dysplasias. Technique and preliminary results. Clin Orthop Relat Res. 1988;(232):26–36.
6. Fürnstahl P, Lanfranco S, Leunig M, Ganz R. Computer simulation and jig cutting of femoral head osteotomy in severe Perthes' deformities. Abstract Orthop Proceedings. 2018:100-B, SU. https://doi.org/10.1302/1358-992X.2018.1.061.
7. Beck M, Leunig M, Ellis T, Sledge JB, Ganz R. The acetabular blood supply: implications for periacetabular osteotomies. Surg Radiol Anat. 2003;25(5–6):361–7.
8. Kalhor M, Collado D, Leunig M, Rego P, Ganz R. Recommendations to reduce risk of nerve injury during Bernese Periacetabular osteotomy (PAO). JBJS Essent Surg Tech. 2017;7:e34.
9. Clohisy JC, Pascual-Garrido C, Duncan S, Pashos G, Schoenecker PL. Concurrent femoral head reduction and periacetabular osteotomies for the treatment of severe femoral head deformities. Bone Joint J. 2018;100-B(12):1551–8.
10. Siebenrock KA, Anwander H, Zurmuhle CA, Tannast M, Slongo T, Steppacher SD. Head reduction osteotomy with additional containment surgery improves sphericity and containment and reduces pain in Legg-calve-Perthes disease. Clin Orthop Relat Res. 2015;473(4):1274–83.

11. Edelstein AI, Duncan ST, Akers S, Pashos G, Schoenecker PL, Clohisy JC. Complications associated with combined surgical hip dislocation and periacetabular osteotomy for complex hip deformities. J Hip Preserv Surg. 2019;6(2):117–23.
12. Blümel S, Leunig M, Manner H, Tannast M, Stetzelberger V, Ganz R. Perthes-like necrosis in young female gymnasts—a pursuit of etiology and therapy. Bone JtOpen. 2022;3–9:666–73.
13. Rego P, Mafra I, Viegas R, Oliveira F, Pinto P, Ganz R. Femoral head reduction osteotomy approach for severe proximal femur deformities: surgical technique and minimum 2-year results. Unpublished results.

20 Capsular Arthroplasty (Modified Codivilla-Colonna)

Ira Zaltz, Hong Zhang, and Reinhold Ganz

20.1 Background

The idea of wrapping the capsule of a congenitally dislocated femoral head goes back to Codivilla, who published a drawing in 1901, but neither described the technique in detail nor reported results [1]. Based in Bologna, Italy, he travelled frequently to the leading hospitals of that time. His conference in Berlin at the Charité Hospital is published in detail and includes the mentioned drawing [1]. His presentation in New York at the Hospital for the Ruptured and the Crippled (today HSS) only exists as an abstract [2]. However, it is interesting that it is the same hospital where 30 years later Colonna described his two-stage technique which experienced some popularity during the subsequent decades [3]. Even before Colonna, Hey Groves published a similar operation, which did not find wide acceptance due to its technical difficulty [4]. The last paper on Colonna's capsular arthroplasty was published in 1999, and the authors stated that "they do not support revival of this now obscure procedure." [5]

Analysis of the available literature, especially comparison of excellent results and failures brought us to the conclusion that the operation should be reconsidered, especially for the unilateral congenital dislocation, which is a major handicap and cannot be properly treated with other joint preserving procedures. With simultaneous femoral shortening (Chap. 15) and newer surgical techniques (Chaps. 7 and 8), complications such as head necrosis, joint stiffness, and secondary subluxation should be greatly diminished.

I. Zaltz (✉)
Department of Orthopaedic Surgery, C.S. Mott Children's Hospital, University of Michigan, Ann Arbor, MI, USA
e-mail: zaltz@med.umich.edu

H. Zhang
Department of Joint Surgery, The Orthopedic Institute of C.P.L.A., The First Affiliated Hospital of PLA General Hospital (Beijing 304 Hospital), Beijing, People's Republic of China

R. Ganz
Emeritus, Faculty of Medicine, University of Berne, Berne, Switzerland

20.2 Indications

20.2.1 Indications

1. The classical indication is a unilateral congenital dislocation between the age of 10 and 25 years [6]. The femoral head should be reasonably round. MRI should confirm healthy femoral articular cartilage and substantial integrity of the gluteus medius muscle. The procedure is also useful for younger children with unilateral and bilateral dislocated hips and severe acetabular hypoplasia that are unsuitable for open reduction.

20.2.2 Relative Indications

1. Bilateral, symmetric hip dislocations are usually well tolerated with less disability; therefore, the need for a capsular arthroplasty, especially in the absence of symptoms, is questionable; however, if surgery on one side is indicated, it is obligatory to perform surgery on the second side.
2. Subluxated hips with pseudo-acetabula have significantly less available capsular tissue that is sufficient for a complete wrapping. Dissection of the lateral retinacular flap may help to mobilize the capsule to some extent. In extreme situations, fascia lata material may be required for closure of a residual medial deficiency or to supplement a very thin capsular layer.
3. Prior hip surgery can induce substantial scarring and stiffness that prevents adequate mobilization of the head and the availability of healthy, pliable capsular tissue for wrapping and interposition.
4. Insufficient acetabular coverage following reaming can be anticipated. Superior bony deficits of coverage can be treated with a shelf-type augmentation, while anterior or posterior deficits can be prevented by a head reduction (see Chap. 18).

M. Leunig et al. (eds.), *Surgical Hip Dislocation*, https://doi.org/10.1007/978-3-031-70622-6_20

5. Very small femoral head size accompanying high dislocation such as in a congenital short femur can be difficult to stabilize.
6. Strict, intensive, and regularly controlled strengthening of the gluteus medius is crucial to the success of the procedure with the goal to achieve normal strength. Hips with reduced strength of the muscle function poorly and probably are less durable. Inability to follow the strengthening regime may be a relative contraindication for the procedure.
7. Use of the procedure in Down's syndrome, cerebral palsy, and myelodysplasia can substantially help to restore stability and pain-free range of motion despite the low likelihood of achieving normal muscle strength.
8. The large majority of patients are female.

20.2.3 Contraindications

1. Absent or degenerated femoral head cartilage.
2. Severely aspherical femoral head.
3. Congenital short femur with absent abductors.
4. Multiple previous surgical procedures.
5. Lack of patient compliance (abductor reinforcement).

20.3 Preoperative/Pre-Interventional Diagnostics

1. History and result of earlier interventions as well as the skin scars give information about extent and localization of eventual internal scaring.
2. Mobility of the hip, especially adduction in full extension (leg held under the other leg) gives an idea about the stretchability of the gluteal musculature and allows to speculate about the extent of distal advancement of the greater trochanter and head. Reduced hip extension may indicate the need for an anterior tendon release.
3. Standard radiology of hip and pelvis including orthoradiography gives basic information.
4. MRI permits assessment and extent of pericapsular scaring, size of gluteus medius, and quality of femoral hyaline cartilage.
5. Computer tomography with three-dimensional reconstruction enables calculation of femoral and acetabular version, sphericity of the femoral head, and geometry of the acetabulum. Understanding the maximal anteroposterior diameter of head and acetabulum enables an estimation of endpoints of reaming in order to avoid loss of anterior or posterior acetabular wall.
6. Computer modeling may give even more precise information but has not yet been introduced into practice.

20.4 Preoperative Planning/Computer Simulation

To date, no routine preoperative planning is performed for this procedure.

20.5 Applied Anatomy

1. *Muscles* attached to the hip area, originating cephalad to the level of the paleo-acetabulum, are shortened to some extent, while muscles originating at the same level or even caudad did undergo some lengthening depending on the amount of dislocation; this applies especially for muscles with tendinous attachment. Although the topographic anatomy is basically unchanged, muscle trajectory and, thus, surgical orientation may be altered by the dislocation. If muscle release is necessary at all, it would be rectus femoris, psoas, gluteus maximus, piriformis, and/or long head of gluteus minimus.
2. In high dislocations *the joint capsule* is elongated to a kind of tube, furnishing ample material for wrapping the femoral head. The densest area of the capsule is the part that is covering the head, and flaps should be designed to place this part on the top of the head in the weight-bearing zone. Low dislocations, generally, have sufficient capsular material; however, the dissection must be executed as close as possible to the pelvic bone and orifice of the native acetabulum. High subluxations may not have sufficient capsular tissue for easy wrapping of the head. Dissection of the lateral retinacular flap may solve the problem, in rare conditions fascia lata can be used to fill a medial gap but is not appropriate to cover the superior curvature of the head.
3. *Sciatic, femoral, and obturator nerves* are also short to some extent; with simultaneous flexion of hip and knee, all three are substantially relaxed. To avoid stretch-related neurapraxia, femoral shortening is recommended.
4. *The blood supply* to the proximal femur area comes from medial and lateral femoral circumflex artery [7, 8]; the obturator artery admittedly has some anastomoses with the medial circumflex artery but provides mainly part of the acetabular perfusion. Both medial and lateral arteries are elongated with a dislocated head, and reduction of the head into the newly reamed acetabulum should be well tolerated. Only the medial artery is supplying the femoral head, while the lateral artery gives blood to capsule and muscles. In practice, perfusion of the head is not reduced if the lengthening does not exceed the tensioning tolerance of the sciatic nerve. Preservation of the ascending division of the transverse branch of the lateral femoral circumflex artery may keep at least the anterior capsule vital.

20.6 Special Risks

1. The capsular arthroplasty procedure requires intimate knowledge of developmental hip dislocation. Specific attention to surgical detail is of paramount importance for a successful result and inexperience with open reduction of developmental dislocations and the capsular arthroplasty, specifically, is a significant risk. We suggest mentorship for those with limited experience.
2. *Femoral head necrosis*, the most frequent and severe complication with the classic Colonna procedure can only be prevented by strict observation of the topography of the vascular supply of the hip (Chap. 2) especially when releasing the capsule from the inferior aspect of the acetabulum. Inadequate femoral shortening may be another reason.
3. *Stiffness* after surgery may be the result of insufficient suture strength to maintain the capsular flaps, rapid deterioration of the capsule due to inferior quality tissue, and/or substantial damage of the head cartilage. Finally, excessively long-lasting postoperative immobilization can lead to stiffness.
4. *Recurrent subluxation* can occur due to insufficient acetabular coverage, due to inability to ream deeply or due to eccentric reaming. Alternatively, overcoverage of the femoral head after excessive reaming may lead to impingement that can lever the head out of the acetabulum. Finally, insufficient correction of femoral anteversion or excessive femoral shortening can lead to redislocation.
5. *Nerve paralysis, especially involving the sciatic nerve,* is primarily the result of insufficient shortening of the femur.
6. *Persistence of abductor muscle weakness is* a major functional limitation and can occur after excessive trochanteric distalization or inadequate physical rehabilitation. Bilaterally operated hips may exhibit more problems with abductor reinforcement.
7. *Leg length inequality* can lead to persistent limping and can be managed by epiphysiodesis at the appropriate age or contralateral limb shortening.

20.7 Type of Anesthesia

Since the procedure is performed in lateral positioning and usually takes more than 90 min, general anesthesia is the recommendation of choice, especially since the patients are mostly children and adolescents.

20.8 Positioning

- Standard operating table
- Lateral positioning with tunnel cushion and lateral bag
- Intraoperative fluoroscopy and X-ray

20.9 Instruments/Implants

- Besides the instruments and implants for SHD (Chap. 7), Total Hip Replacement (THR)-reamers, including small-size reamers (36–50 mm), are needed for enlarging the new socket. (Beware! 36 mm reamer may not be included in a standard set.)
- For the subtrochanteric derotation/shortening osteotomy, a 10 mm curved periosteal elevator is helpful. Decortication before osteotomy is best done with a 15 mm osteotome. Two-millimeter K-wires help to control the desired amount of derotation. A straight six-hole plate for 3.5 or 4.5 mm screws is needed for fixation. For the rare indication to perform the osteotomy at the intertrochanteric level, angled blade plate osteotomy systems according to preop planning are to be provided.

20.10 Access

Straight lateral incision as for the SHD (Chap. 7). Cephalad extension makes the presentation of the high dislocated head easier. Distal extension for the subtrochanteric osteotomy using a subvastus approach (Chap. 15). If necessary, relative neck lengthening (Chap. 13) or head reduction osteotomy (Chap. 18) can easily executed with the extended retinacular flap (Chap. 8).

1. **Technical Steps of Deep Dissection**
    1. The SHD approach (Chap. 7) with some proximal extension allows circumferential dissection of the capsule from the overlying muscles and permits exposure of the acetabular cavity. It is quite important during this technique that the capsule is not incised before it is freed from the attached muscles up to the pelvic insertion. The topographic relation of the muscles may be somewhat different from normal. Sharp dissection is necessary for the superior and anterior isolation of the capsule from the surrounding muscles, while blunt dissection may be preferred for the posteroinferior dissection. Accurate dissection is greatly facilitated by proper limb positioning during exposure.

2. Be mindful of the perforating nutrient vessels of the head near the capsular insertion on the lateral neck!
3. The capsular incision itself is clearly different from the one for the classic approach.
4. Prior to the capsular incision, an overview is facilitated by manual traction on the leg. The anterior incision is straight and runs from the anterosuperior edge of the trochanteric osteotomy to the most cephalad point of the native acetabular rim. From there the dissection continues in a caudad direction in an outside to inside fashion, staying as close to the anterior bony rim as possible (Fig. 20.1a).
5. For the posterior capsular incision, the leg is placed in a sterile bag on the opposite side of the table (surgeon is standing on the posterior side of the patient), the elongated ligamentum teres is resected when still present, and the head is dislocated and held apart with a 10 mm curved Hohmann retractor which is hooked against the posteroinferior rim. The incision starts at the superior edge, first outside in, then inside out, but always close to the acetabular rim (Fig. 20.1b).
6. Detachment of the capsule at the acetabular notch is best performed from inside after it has been tensioned with a blunt Hohmann retractor around the notch. Use special care when incising the inferior capsule due to the proximity of the underlying vascular plexus between medial femoral circumflex artery (MFCA) and obturator artery! This area is surrounded by fatty tissue and is readily identifiable. When all capsular connections with the pelvic bone are detached, the head can be lifted easily away from the pelvis with a bone hook around the neck, a test to confirm that the necessary mobility has been established in order to permit reduction into the newly reamed acetabulum.
7. Provisional reduction at this stage can show whether relative lengthening of the neck is necessary to avoid impingement at the acetabular rim. It also gives an idea about the necessary femoral derotation.
8. Provisional wrapping of the capsule will demonstrate if sufficient capsular material is available, or whether additional technical steps are needed (see above). The width of the head with the capsule wrapped can be measured using calipers to assist in estimating the ultimate size required for acetabular reaming.
9. The widening process of the paleo-acetabulum can be best visually controlled with spiked Hohmann retractors surrounding the acetabular rim and with the femur flexed, externally rotated and the foot in the leg bag. Palpation of the rim circumferentially gives an idea about the reaming tolerance. Reaming starts with the smallest reamer head at the original fossa but should preserve the bone at the bottom. Identification of the acetabular notch greatly facilitates identifying the center of the native acetabulum where reaming should commence. Continue the reaming until the transverse head diameter plus twice the thickness of the wrapped capsule would fit into the cavity. Reaming should repeatedly be interrupted to control the result. Normally, most of the bone can be reamed from the posterior wall. In rare cases when reaming at the extreme is still not sufficient, the procedure can only be continued with a reduction of the femoral head size or the addition of a shelf arthroplasty (Chap. 18).
10. After reaming of the new socket is completed, the capsular flaps are sutured together. First sutures approximate the posterior capsular margins which is facilitated with the head pulled up with a hook around the neck (Fig. 20.2a).
11. It is followed by the anterior suturing. Closure of the capsule over the head must be firmly without tissue overlapping (Fig. 20.2b).
12. Nonabsorbable sutures are used taking care to avoid passing suture material adjacent to the articular cartilage of the femoral head to prevent abrasive wear.
13. In subluxed hips with insufficient capsular tissue for coverage, dissection of the lateral retinacular flap will permit shifting the capsule more proximally; however, excessive tension in the flap should be avoided.
14. During provisional reduction of the wrapped head, the tension of the sciatic nerve should be tested manually, thereby, providing some information about the necessary shortening, which is normally executed at the subtrochanteric level. Overstretching the sciatic nerve during provisional reduction can be avoided by performing the femoral osteotomy first.
15. The area of shortening is freed from periosteum in children, while for adults a decortication is preferred. Sufficient distal femoral exposure is required to facilitate room for attachment of the femoral plate. The plate is provisionally attached to the proximal femur just distal to the vastus tubercle. Proximally, space should be reserved for refixation of the greater trochanter prior to selecting the location of the plate. The plate is then removed from the femur.
16. The wrapped head is reduced into the acetabulum, and then a transverse femoral osteotomy is performed. Sufficient diaphysis is removed so that there is no tension on the reduction or the sciatic nerve. The plate is then reattached to the proximal femur, and then the distal femur is reduced to the plate while properly correcting the femoral anteversion. Kirschner wires inserted proximal and distal can be used as guides to correct rotation. As a guide for adequate correction of femoral anteversion, with

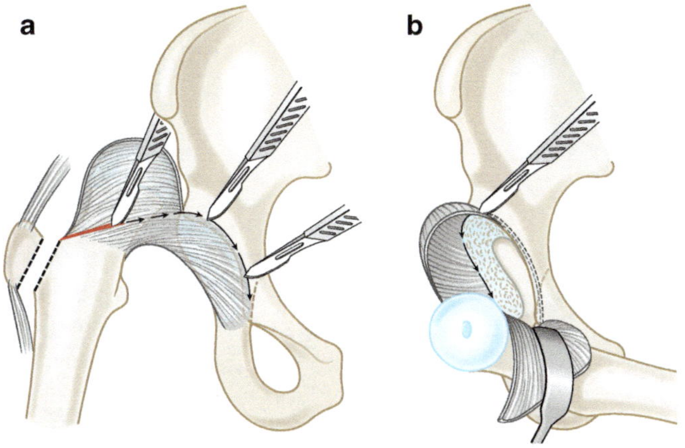

Fig. 20.1 (a) Anterior capsular incision and (b) posterior capsular separation from the periacetabular bone

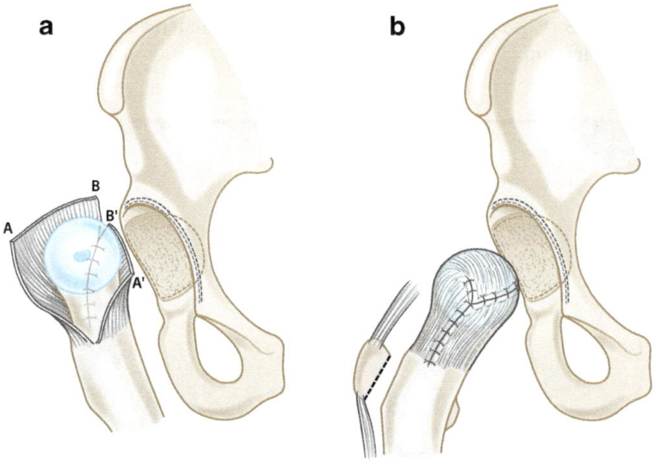

Fig. 20.2 (a) Deepening of the original acetabulum and (b) posterior suturing of the capsule over the femoral head

the patient in a true lateral decubitus position, the patella should face directly anteriorly, and there should be equal internal and external femoral rotation.

17. The resected femoral segment is reserved if shelf augmentation of the acetabulum is necessary. When the graft is used for augmentation of the bony roof, it can be shaped and best fixed with two to three small screws.
18. Finally, examining the range of motion of the reduced hip is important in order to ascertain the amount of flexion that is possible without visible tugging of the capsule that could endanger the suture line. This information is needed to guide physical therapy when the patient begins passive motion exercises of the hip.
19. The final step is refixation of the trochanteric fragment. If necessary, release of the long head of the gluteus minimus at the trochanter will facilitate distal advancement. It is crucial not to over distalize the greater trochanter which can overlengthen and permanently weaken the gluteus medius.
20. Final radiographs can be obtained to document the reduction of the femoral head and position of the trochanter. Beware, in younger children eccentric ossification of the epiphysis may make the reduction appear incomplete. Suction drainage is usually not needed.

20.11 Postoperative Management

1. Adequate time and protection are required to allow the capsule to heal to the reamed acetabulum; however, the hip should be mobilized to prevent stiffness.
2. For children a spica with slight abduction and neutral rotation, including the thigh of the opposite side, is applied and bivalved immediately. Beginning on the first postop day, assisted flexion maneuvers to the intraoperatively tested level are started. For adults the leg position may be secured with pads. Passive flexion maneuvers are repeated several times/days. Range of flexion may become increased gradually after 2–3 weeks which provided adequate time for capsular adhesion. Mobilization out of bed with toe touch loading can be started after postop day 2 with restricted flexion and neutral position of the leg. Plaster or external padding can be removed as soon as the patient is able to actively maintain control the position of the extremity.
3. Starting 4 weeks after surgery, the trochanter should be solid enough to start passive and active ab–/adduction as well as rotation, while continuing toe-touch weight bearing (approximately 15 kg). Repeat X-rays are taken between 4 and 6 weeks after surgery to assess healing; however, restricted loading of the hip should be maintained until 8 weeks after surgery or until the femoral osteotomy is sufficiently consolidated. Thereafter, rigorous abductor exercises should be started under the supervision of a physical therapist with the goal of regaining full muscle strength.

20.12 Intra-/Postoperative Complications

1. Using the new basic approach, the major complications associated with the classic Colonna procedure, like femoral head necrosis, recurrent subluxation, and stiffness, have been dramatically reduced, although, some patients still have persistent stiffness and muscle weakness.
2. Compared to a normal hip, the anatomy of the proximal femur can be considerably different including trochanteric hypoplasia and decreased neck length. Therefore, caution should be exercised when performing the trochanteric osteotomy to avoid inadvertently cutting into the neck and risking osteonecrosis.

3. In order to protect the blood supply, when dissecting the pericapsular muscles, it is important to avoid dissecting close to the femoral insertion where the deep branch of the medial femoral circumflex artery (MFCA), feeding the femoral head, [7] as well as the ascending branch of the lateral femoral circumflex artery (LFCA), perfusing the anterior capsule, [8] can be damaged.
4. Eccentric or over-reaming of the acetabulum can create a central perforation or ablation of the anterior or posterior wall leading to hip instability or protrusion. In cases of severe acetabular hypoplasia, in addition to very judicious reaming, shelf augmentation or acetabular reorientation should be considered.
5. Postoperative stiffness may be caused by complications related to the capsular tissue, femoral cartilage degeneration, or significant aspherical femoral head. When the capsule is insufficient or insecurely sutured, the joint space may appear narrow on plain X-ray, or there may be no interposed tissue between the femoral head and the acetabulum on MRI. Poor postoperative management, especially excessive motion of the hip early in the postoperative phase may also lead to rupture of the capsular suture and stiffness.
6. For possible complications of the rarely executed additional techniques of extended retinacular flap or reduction of the femoral head size, see Chap. 7.
7. For complications of the femoral osteotomy, see Chap. 15.
8. Provided abductor muscles are normally developed, persistent abductor weakness can occur if the trochanter is not repaired anatomically, if the length of the femoral neck is short or if patients do not rehabilitate properly.

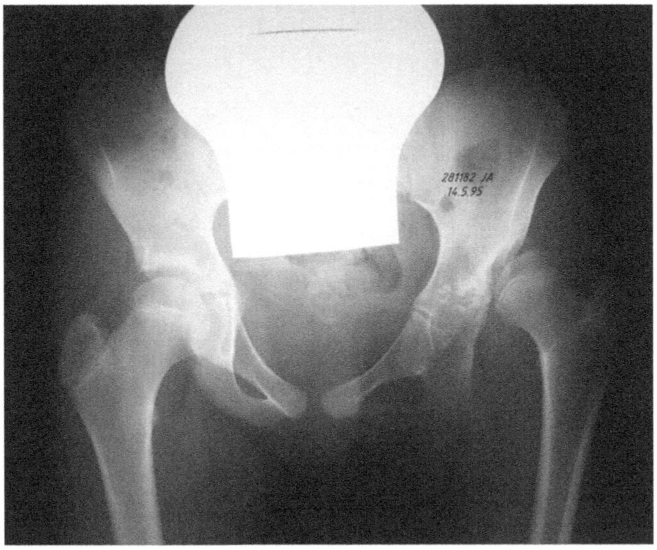

Fig. 20.3 Case 1: A 13-year-old female with unilateral low dislocation of the left hip

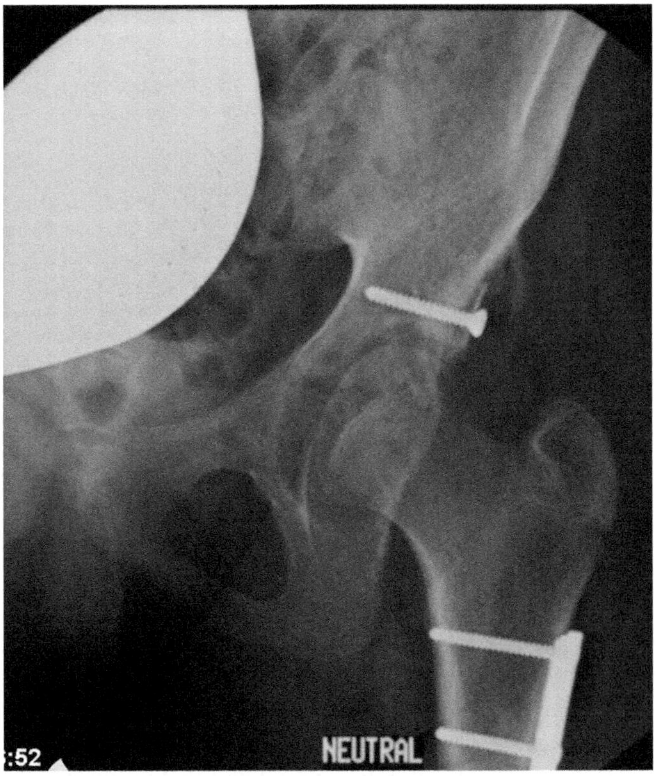

Fig. 20.4 Case 1: Postoperative control showing a well-reduced head after capsular arthroplasty, shelf augmentation, and plate fixation of a subtrochanteric shortening and derotation osteotomy

20.13 Case Studies

(Case 1) A 13-year-old girl with unilateral low dislocation. No previous surgery. She had occasional pain, limping was moderate, Range of motion (ROM) was excellent, and abductor force M4 and leg length difference was 3 cm. MRI confirmed a spherical head with a good cartilage cover—all together a good indication for capsular arthroplasty (Fig. 20.3). Preparation of the capsule from the surrounding musculature was easy. Care was taken to preserve the vessels near the femoral insertion during the dissection. Complete presentation of the original acetabular socket was possible after transsection of the inferior capsule next to the notch. During deepening of the original acetabulum using reamers from the THR set, care was taken to preserve the anterior and posterior wall as well as the acetabular floor. Reaming was interrupted several times for inspection. Trial reduction revealed that soft tissue was stretched especially during motion and that femoral torsion was high, reasons to perform a subtrochanteric derotation, including 1 cm shortening. Trial reduction also confirmed the need for augmentation of the acetabular cover. After these additional steps, joint stability was high and soft tissue tension was acceptable. The shelf bone was taken from the femoral shortening; fixation of the femoral osteotomy was achieved with a straight plate.

Figure 20.4 shows the early postop radiographs with good containment of the femoral head. Figure 20.5 shows the 28-year follow-up radiography with a good joint space width and minor only osteophytic reaction. Patient is pain-free even after jogging three times/week and thinks that her hips are identical. Leg shortening is about 1.5 cm. ROM is nearly normal (Fig. 20.6). Gluteus medius is M5 (Gait Video).

(Case 2) A 21-year-old female with arthrogryposis. Left hip with low dislocation; right hip with slightly abnormal shape (Fig. 20.7). Considerable pain and limitation of motion on the left side. Tedious walking using one crutch. The dissection was laborious due to the reduced tissue elasticity. The femoral head turned out as too big even after reaming the acetabulum to the extremes. Continuation of the surgery was only possible by choosing between THR and femoral head size reduction with an intra-capital osteotomy (see Chap. 18). To do the latter, dissection of the lateral retinacu-

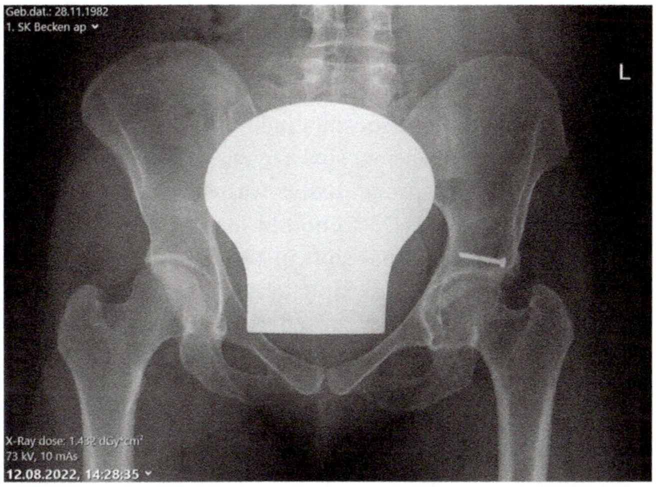

Fig. 20.5 Case 1: 28-year result with large and congruent joint lines. Minimal osteophytic reactions. Femur plate is removed

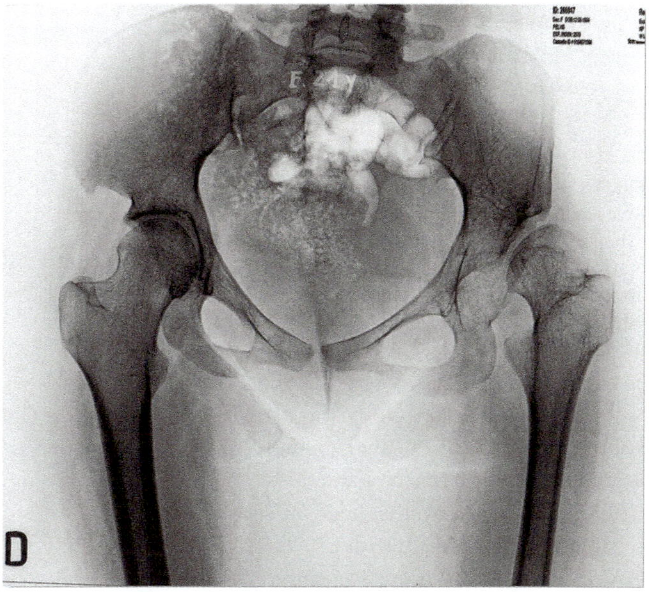

Fig. 20.7 Case 2: A 21-year-old female with arthrogryposis. Low dislocation of the left hip, slight coxa profunda of the right hip. Substantial limitation of ROM on both sides. Considerable pain on the left side

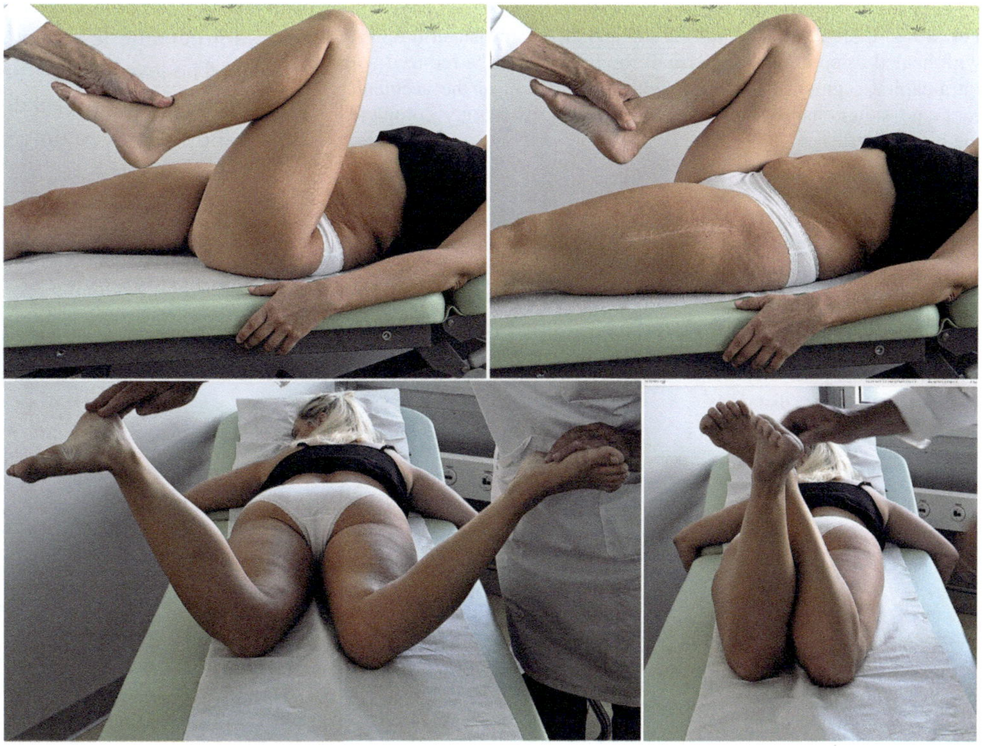

Fig. 20.6 Case 1: Good ROM with slightly reduced external rotation in full extension

lum was necessary, a step which also facilitated the closure of the capsule over the head. For best alignment of the proximal femur and best possible hip motion, a subtrochanteric derotation and shortening osteotomy had to be added on. For best containment of the head, the acetabulum had to be augmented with bone from the shortening. Healing of the osteotomies was uneventful (Fig. 20.8). The patient became pain-free and could walk without external support. Mobility increased to some extent and was slightly better than the right hip. Three years after surgery, femoral plate and trochanteric screws were removed for discomfort. The patient enjoyed an unchanged function of the hip at 17 years after surgery, although osteophytic reactions increased over time (Fig. 20.9).

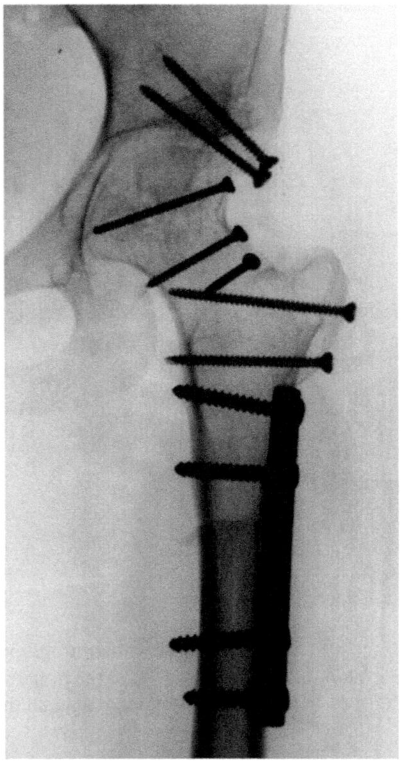

Fig. 20.8 Case 2: Radiography 6 months after capsular arthroplasty with healed osteotomies. The size of the head had to be reduced with intra-capital segment resection. Shelf augmentation of the acetabular roof and subtrochanteric derotation/shortening osteotomy completed the procedure

(Case 3) A 24-year-old male with high subluxation of the right hip. During adolescents he had a subtrochanteric derotation osteotomy (Fig. 20.10). Pain forced him to give up his work, which included regular handling of heavy items. With good quality of the femoral head cartilage on MRI, the decision was to do a capsular arthroplasty. With normal femoral anteversion, a subtrochanteric osteotomy was unlikely to be necessary; in addition, repositioning of the head did not create excessive tissue tension. However, as anticipated for subluxated hips, the capsular tissue was short for complete wrapping of the head. Dissection of the lateral retinaculum resulted in some proximal shift of the femoral insertion of the capsule allowing its complete anterior closure. A bone graft from the iliac crest was used as shelf for a minor deficiency of the lateral acetabular roof. The patient returned to his former job 5 months after surgery and works there without restrictions since 10 years (Fig. 20.11).

(Case 4) A 20-year-old female with high dislocation of the right hip articulating with the iliac bone (Fig. 20.12). Chronic trochanteric pain with distal irradiation. Difficulty in walking and increasing lumbar pain. No earlier surgery. Dissection of the capsule and elaboration of the paleo-acetabulum became easier after trochanteric flip osteotomy and subtrochanteric osteotomy allowing the bone ends to overlap. The level of the transverse osteotomy was chosen to allow screw fixation of the grater trochanter and plate fixation of the shaft osteotomy without interference. Tenotomies

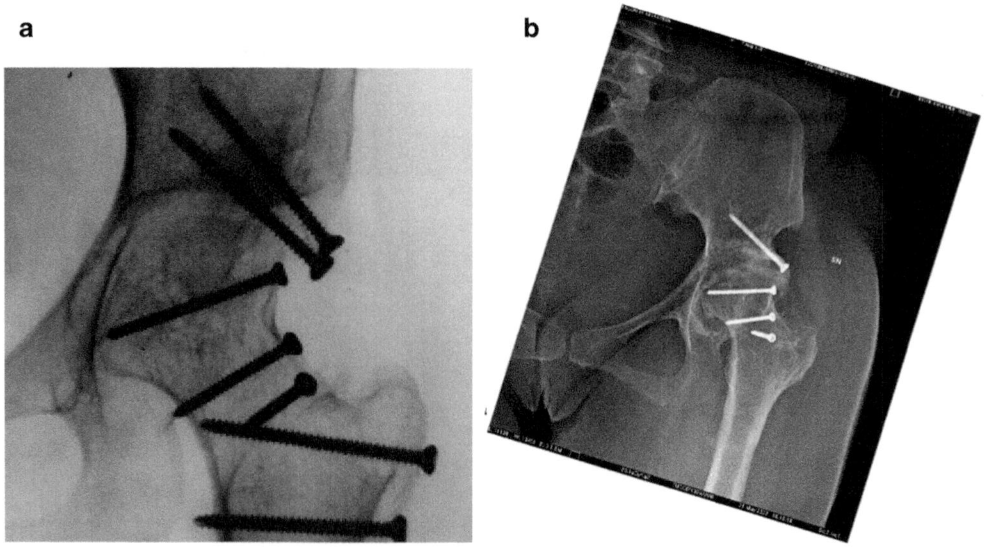

Fig. 20.9 Case 2: Three- (**a**) and 17-year (**b**) results. Joint space remains maintained over time. Motion is still reduced but better than on the other side. No external support needed. Pain only after walking longer distances

Fig. 20.10 Case 3: A 24-year-old male with high subluxation of the right hip. Subtrochanteric derotation osteotomy during adolescence. Unable to work for increasing pain

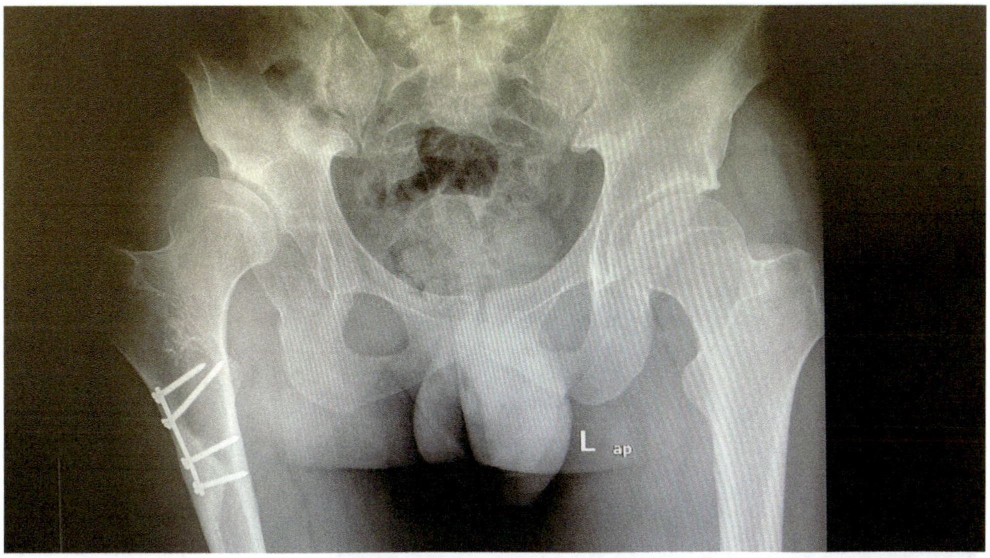

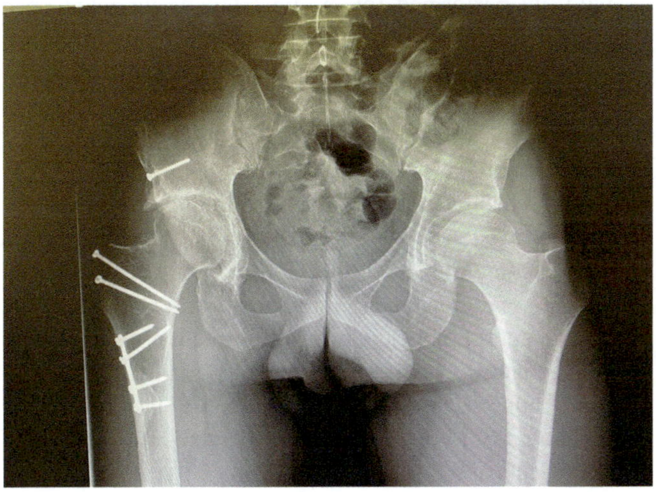

Fig. 20.11 Case 3: Ten-year result after capsular arthroplasty combined with acetabular shelf augmentation. Patient pain-free and back to work

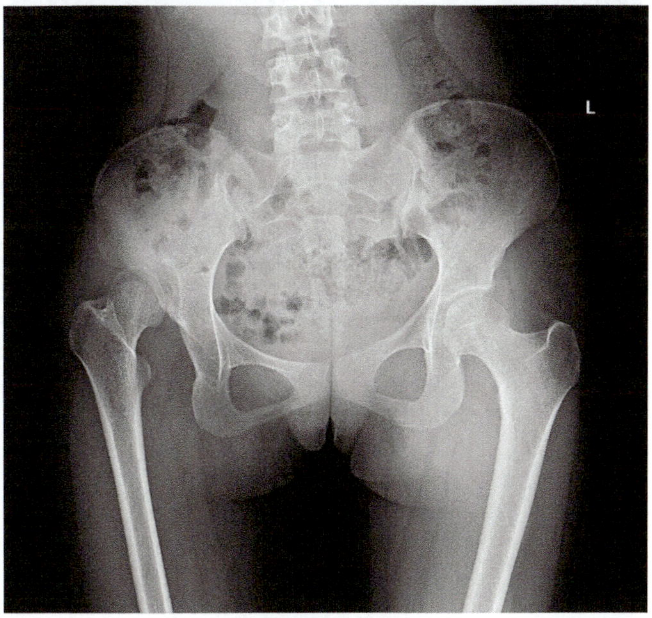

Fig. 20.12 Case 4: A 20-year-old female with high dislocation. Neoarticulation with the ilium. Chronic trochanteric and lumar pain, severe limping

were not necessary. There was ample capsular tissue for wrapping the head. Trial and definitive repositions were easy and did not create a risk for the sciatic nerve. With the wrapped head reduced into the socket, the amount of necessary femoral shortening became visible on the bony overlap. Observation of the best relation between head and acetabulum allowed to define the amount of rotation. A straight six-hole plate was sufficient for fixation. MRI was made 6 months after surgery for residual pain. The capsular growth on the acetabular bone does not seem to be completed (Fig. 20.13). The radiological result 6 years after surgery shows a reasonable joint space with some posteroinferior rim osteophyte. The patient has some pain after walking long distances and complains about some residual limping. However, all in all she is very satisfied with the result (Fig. 20.14).

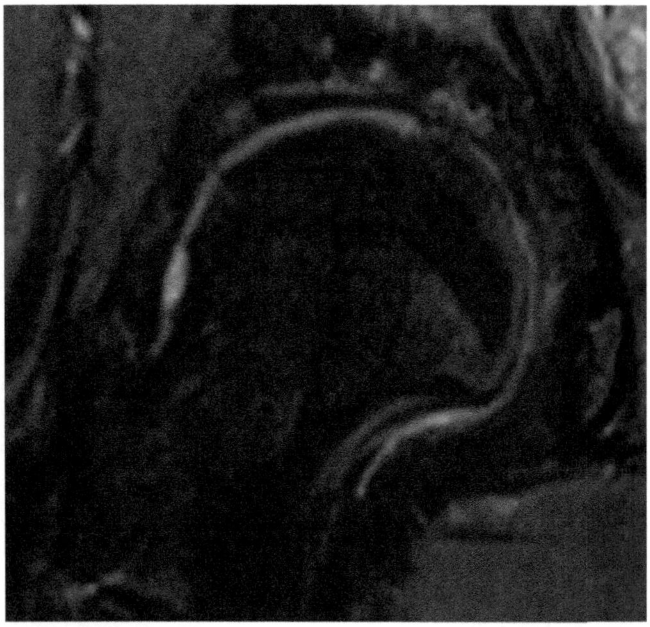

Fig. 20.13 Case 4: MRI 6 months after capsular arthroplasty for unexplained pain. Inconsistent healing of the capsule against acetabular bone

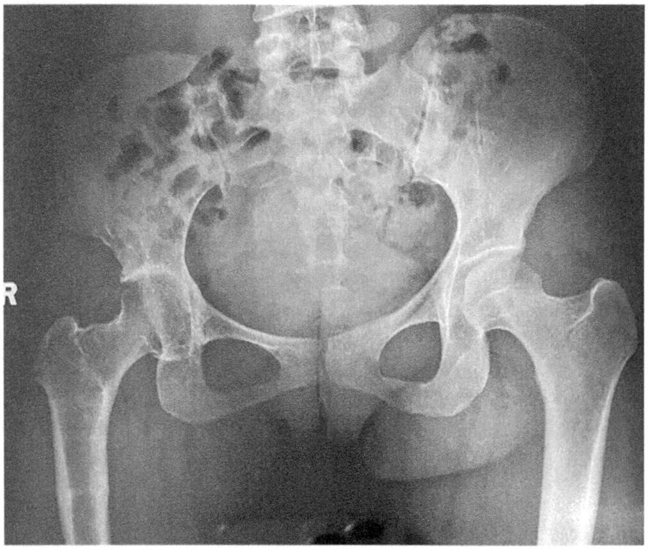

Fig. 20.14 Case 4: Six-year result with maintained joint space. Some osteophytic bone at the posteroinferior rim. Metal removed. Patient happy with the result despite occasional pain and some residual limping

20.14 Controversies

1. Essential background of controversies is the complexity of the procedure considering the decreasing case load. Both aspects speak for a concentration in few centers.
2. There are cases where the decision is not easy between PAO plus femoral reconstruction and capsular arthroplasty. Personal experience may be decisive.
3. The upper age limit for open reduction and the lower age limit for capsular arthroplasty are controversial. Some surgeons use a SHD approach in older children in order to make an intraoperative decision based upon the quality of the acetabular cartilage, the size of the acetabulum, and the contour of the femoral head.

20.15 Result

1. The US experience includes 14 hips in 13 female children between the ages of 5 and 15 years (Figs. 20.15, 20.16, 20.17 and 20.18) once developmental dysplasia of the hip (DDH) patient was operated bilaterally. Average follow-up is 5 years (range is 3–9 years). 7 patients had DDH, with 2/7 performed for multiple failed attempted open reduction. Six unilateral neuromuscular painful hips included two children with myelodysplasia and four children with Cerebral palsy (CP). One hip in a CP patient is radiographically arthritic 2 years following the Colonna, and this patient had a low dislocation with thin capsular tissue. All other patients are functioning well and have had no revision surgery to date. Formal Patient reported outcome measures (PROMs) have not been collected because of patient age. Four patients with DDH have had contralateral epiphysiodesis for correction of leg length discrepancy.
2. The Chinese experience is based on the largest group including 88 unilateral hips, operated at the age of 8–26 years and followed for a mean of 3 years. Harris hip score (HHS) improved to mean 83.7 (range: 31–97). Best results were seen when the joint capsule was thick, and the head was big. A total of 12 patients (13%) suffered from joint stiffness, two patients needed reoperation with PAO for joint subluxation, and one hip got THR. [9]
3. The Swiss experience includes 14 unilateral hips, operated at an age of 13–25 years: 9 cases have been published. [6] In this group six had low dislocations; only one case had a high dislocation. Two patients had spina bifida and one had arthrogryposis. At a mean follow-up of 7.5 years, HHS improved to mean 84 (78–94). There was one complication in a spina bifida patient, who sustained a fracture of the neck shortly after surgery; it healed uneventfully after screw fixation. In the group of the five patients operated later, in one patient with Down's syndrome and uncontrollable motor activity, radiography showed disappearance of the capsular interposition within 6 months.

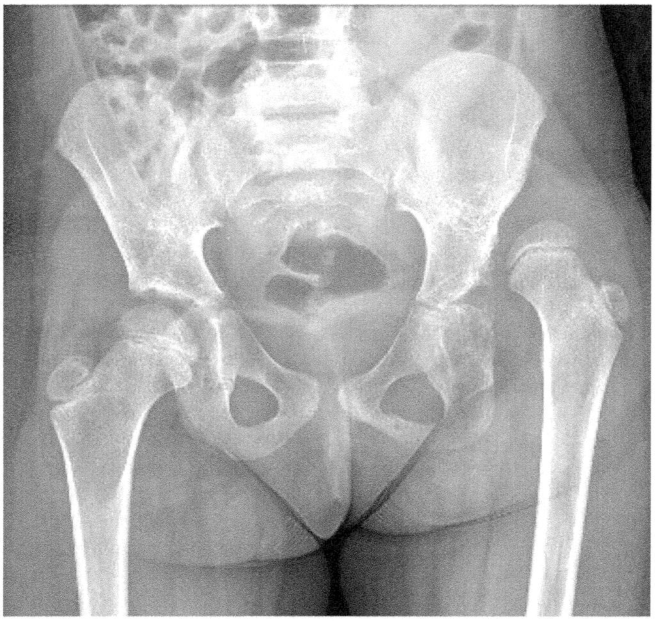

Fig. 20.15 Case 5: A 6-year-old female with high dislocation of the left side. Severe limping. Two prior attempts of open reduction

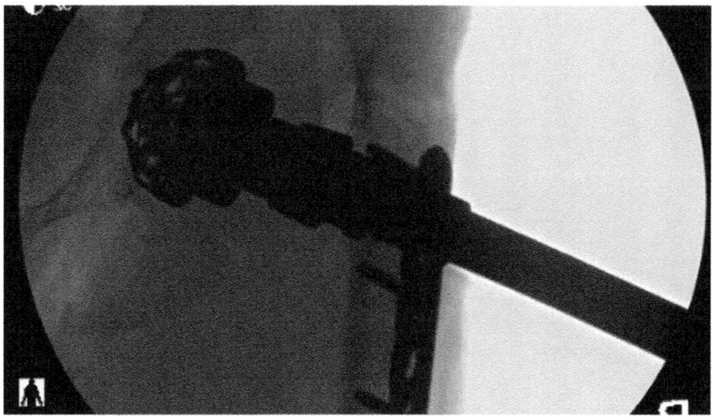

Fig. 20.16 Case 5: Fluoroscopy of the paleo-acetabulum with extra small THR-reamer to check level and depth of the enlargement

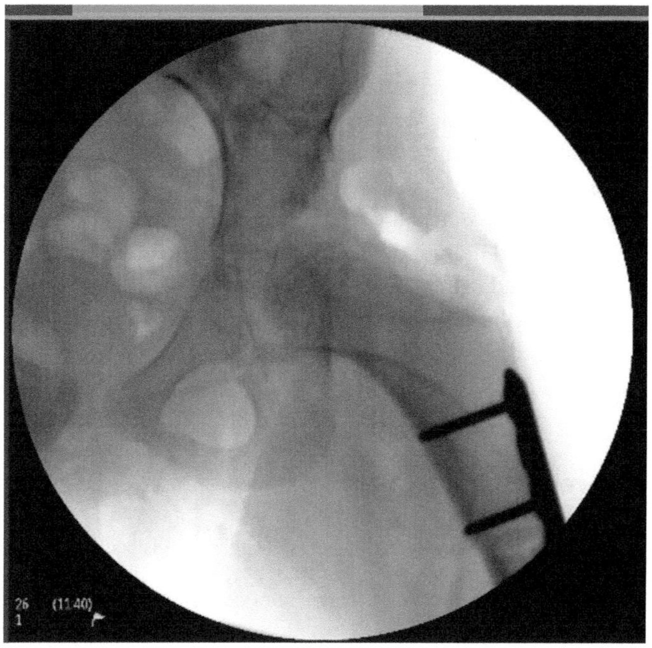

Fig. 20.17 Case 5: Fluoroscopy after reduction of the head wrapped with capsule to check the need for shelf augmentation of the acetabulum

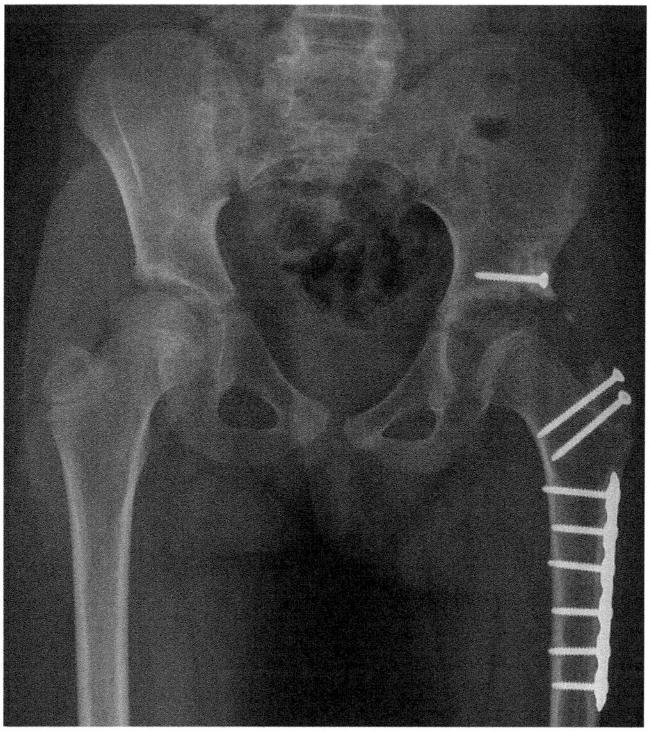

Fig. 20.18 Case 5: Two-year result after capsular arthroplasty plus subtrochanteric shortening/derotation osteotomy plus shelf with cortical bone from the shortening. The reminder of the triradiate cartilage is still open

20.16 Outlook

1. Like computer simulation for femoral head reduction osteotomy (chap. 18) simulation of the widening of the paleo-acetabulum (where to mill, maximal possible widening, extent of space requirement for the head + wrapping) could make the planning of the procedure more precise and help to avoid intraoperative mistakes.
2. Established exchange of experience between centers who practice the procedure could optimize the individual experience more rapidly.

References

1. Codivilla A. Operative treatment of congenital dislocation of the hip] [in German]. Z Orthop Chir. 1901;9:124–37.
2. Codivilla A. The operative treatment of congenital dislocations. N Y Med J. 1902;73:741.
3. Colonna PC. Congenital dislocation of the hip in older subjects: based on a study of sixty-six open operations. J Bone Joint Surg. 1932;14:277–98.
4. Hey Groves EW. Some contributions to the reconstructive surgery of the hip. Br J Surg 1926–27;14: 486–513.
5. Boardman DL, Moseley CF. Finding patients after 40 years: a very long-term follow-up study of the Colonna arthroplasty. J Pediatr Orthop. 1999;19:169–76.
6. Ganz R, Slongo T, Siebenrock KA, Turchetto L, Leunig M. The capsular arthroplasty. A useful but abandoned procedure for young patients with developmental dysplasia of the hip. Clin Orthop Relat Res. 2012;470:2957–67.
7. Gautier E, Ganz K, Krügel N, Gill T, Ganz R. Anatomy of the medial femoral circumflex artery and its surgical implications. J Bone Joint Surg (Br). 2000;82-B:679–83.
8. Kalhor M, Gharehdaghi J, Leunig GR. Lateral femoral circumflex artery (LFCA) contribution to the articular and peri-articular hip circulation. Relevance to the anterior hip approach. A cadaveric study. Eur J Orthop Surg Traumatol. 2022;33:1547. https://doi.org/10.1007/s00590-022-03310-2.
9. Zhang Z, Luo D, Cheng H, Zhang H, Ganz R, Zhang J. Modified capsular arthroplasty. Experience and results with 92 hips. J Hip Preser Surg. 2023;10:149–57. https://doi.org/10.1093/jhps/hnad017.

Part 5

Trauma

Femoral Head Fractures

21

Alessandro Massè and Michael D. Stover

21.1 Introduction

Surgical hip dislocation (SHD) reported excellent results in nontraumatic patients, providing full and safe exposure to the femoral head and the acetabulum. This technique can be a powerful tool in selected trauma cases, allowing unparalleled visualization for reduction and fixation of femoral head fractures and access to associated femoral neck and acetabular injuries. These fractures were historically approached using anterior or standard posterior approaches; however, limited exposure of the articular surface did compromise anatomical reduction and fixation. With the traditional Kocher Langenbech (KL), the femoral head blood supply may be at increased risk. Encouraging results support the advantages of SHD in specific femoral head fracture patterns with a comparable risk of avascular necrosis (AVN) to the anterior approach. The purpose of this chapter is to provide a detailed and comprehensive analysis of this technique in traumatic femoral head injuries.

21.2 Background

Often described as Pipkin fractures, articular fractures of the femoral head are rare injuries. Most often they are due to high-energy trauma resulting from motor vehicle accidents or falls from height and occur in 5–15% of posterior hip dislocations. Involved patients are usually middle-aged males [1].

Depending on the vector of the force applied on the hip, different fracture patterns can occur. Initially described by Birkett in 1869 after performing a postmortem dissection, femoral head fractures were classified as Grade IV fracture dislocations of the hip by Steward and Milford in 1954. Three years later, Pipkin further subclassified Steward and Milford Grade IV dislocations into four categories based on fracture morphology and associated injuries to better describe the outcome and sequelae of these injuries. According to Pipkin, type 1 is defined as a femoral head fracture of the inferior head below the fovea capitis, type 2 when extending cephalad to the fovea capitis and therefore involving the weight-bearing area, type 3 when a femoral neck fracture is associated with either type 1 or 2 fracture, and type 4 if associated with a fracture of the acetabulum [2]. Although not as frequently used in clinical practice, other classification systems were described. Brumback included anterior dislocations with impaction fractures as opposed to the shear injuries described by Pipkin. The AO/OTA (31C) describes infrafoveal fragments, the possible association with a femoral neck fracture and also included subchondral impaction. Yoon differentiated the fragments depending on their size relative to the femoral head; however, it does not include associated femoral neck or acetabular associated injuries. Chiron combined fragments' size relative to the femoral head, presence of free osteochondral fragments or femoral head impaction, and associated femoral neck or acetabular fractures.

Initial evaluation of the patient should include Advanced Trauma Life Support (ATLS) protocols followed by evaluation of the pelvis and extremities. Since most femoral head fractures are associated with a posterior dislocation, injured limbs may appear shortened, adducted, and internally rotated. In cases involving an associated acetabular fracture, leg position may be less reliable. If the leg is shortened, slightly flexed without obvious rotation, a locked dislocation should be suspected [3]. Neurologic status should be documented as injury to the sciatic nerve can occur.

Urgent closed reduction (CR) of the hip is indicated in the dislocated hip to limit the risk of avascular necrosis (AVN), compression damage to the sciatic nerve, and occurrence of

A. Massè
Department of Orthopedics, School of Medicine, University of Turin, Turin, Italy
e-mail: alessandro.masse@unito.it

M. D. Stover (✉)
Northwestern Center for Comprehensive Orthopaedic and Spine Care, Feinberg School of Medicine, Northwestern University, Chicago, IL, USA
e-mail: Michael.Stover@nm.org

M. Leunig et al. (eds.), *Surgical Hip Dislocation*, https://doi.org/10.1007/978-3-031-70622-6_21

heterotopic ossification. If following sedation, the hip does not feel mobile—along with the physical findings as noted above—there should be a concern for a locked dislocation, and consideration should be made for an open reduction. CR should be performed with sedation for muscle relaxation and under fluoroscopic guidance. Care should be taken to avoid an iatrogenic displaced femoral neck fracture. If one is not able to reduce easily, proceeding with open reduction as soon as possible is indicated after pelvis computed tomography (CT) scan is performed [4].

21.3 Indications

21.3.1 Surgical Indications

1. Irreducible hip dislocation or locked dislocation. This is a surgical emergency, and open reduction should be performed within 6 hours of injury, if possible.
2. Noncongruence of the joint following reduction, urgent due to likely incarcerated fragment or gross joint instability. May be secondary to displacement of associated acetabulum fracture. Traction to the extremity is indicated in this circumstance.
3. Residual displacement (>2 mm) following fracture or closed reduction.
4. Joint debris and joint irritability in the setting of a congruent reduction.
5. Congruently reduced Pipkin types 3 and 4 fractures as they may displace or re-dislocate with joint motion.

Treatment can range from non-surgical (following CR of dislocation if present), to excision, open reduction and internal fixation, or total hip arthroplasty depending on the fracture fragment morphology, associated injuries, patient age, and bone quality. Since the Pipkin article, the trend has been toward anatomic reduction of the fractures followed by internal fixation. This is especially true in the younger patient population in whom there is an interest in hip preservation.

There still is a role for nonoperative treatment of femoral head fractures. This is typically reserved for type 1 infrafoveal fractures and occasionally type 2 fractures that are anatomically reduced following CR without the presence of intra-articular debris. Secondary displacement during joint motion can happen when round ligament or part of it remains attached to the fragment. Computed tomography (CT) may be helpful for decision-making in these cases. Wait and see-nonoperative treatment may also be considered in the less active or medically compromised patients in whom a reconstruction procedure can be performed later, if necessary, following recovery from injury.

21.3.2 Operative Treatment

Different fracture patterns require specific *considerations:*

1. Pipkin types 1 and 2: Displaced fractures *can* be anatomically reduced and stabilized using the SHD, especially in the case of associated impaction or suspected cartilage lesions that should be addressed (see case example).
2. Pipkin type 3: These fractures should be approached cautiously. Femoral neck stabilization should be performed prior to head dislocation and addressing the femoral head fracture. Unique to the SHD, femoral head blood supply can be directly evaluated and determination of definitive treatment of either open reduction with internal fixation (ORIF) or total hip arthroplasty (THA) can be made following neck stabilization [5].
3. Pipkin type 4 fractures: Indications for SHD include associated fractures of the posterior wall, T-shaped, and posterior column or transverse fractures with/or without posterior wall moieties. If following approach, evaluation of the intra-articular environment (cartilage damage) precludes a satisfactory outcome, prosthetic replacement following acetabular ORIF can proceed through the SHD.

21.3.3 Relative Indications/Contraindications

1. Pipkin type 1 fractures with a non-synthesizable displaced fragment (<2 cm) or free osteochondral fragments can be excised arthroscopically or through a mini-open approach. Minimally to moderately displaced fractures may be reduced arthroscopically and synthesized percutaneously [6]. However, if anatomical reduction cannot be achieved, open reduction and internal fixation should be performed.
2. Pipkin 2 or 3 fractures that remain displaced without significant associated intra-articular pathology. The neck fracture can be stabilized percutaneously or approached by direct anterior approach for reduction. A secondary incision can be performed for neck fixation and then the head fragments exposed, reduced, and stabilized if indicated.
3. Pipkin type 3 fracture. In elderly osteoporotic patients, total hip replacement (THR) could be a more suitable option, allowing earlier weight bearing and a lower complications rate.
4. Pipkin 4 fracture in elderly osteoporotic patients or severe injuries with anteriorly based fractures (anterior column,

anterior wall, anterior column and posterior hemitransverse, associated both column) can be approached anteriorly with acetabular fixation and THR as a definitive surgical option. A posterior-based approach without trochanteric osteotomy may be indicated for acetabular reconstruction and primary THA with acetabular fractures commonly reconstructed through a posterior approach.

21.4 Preoperative/Preinterventional Diagnostics

1. The clinical examination of the patient might suggest a posterior hip dislocation with a shortened, flexed, adducted, and internally rotated limb. However, associated femoral neck or acetabular fractures might not present with this classical limb position.
2. In conscious patients, the neurological status of the affected limb should be assessed as sciatic nerve injuries are common [1].
3. Anteroposterior (AP) and cross-table pelvic X-ray is mandatory for prompt detection of hip dislocation, which will demonstrate disruption of the cervico-obturator (Shenton) line. If the hip is not dislocated or was spontaneously reduced, the radiograph should be examined for an asymmetrical joint space, fractures of the femoral neck, and associated acetabular fractures; CT of the abdomen and pelvis can be an integral part of the initial trauma evaluation in some areas and may occur prior to relocation. This can be evaluated for fractures of the femoral head, neck, acetabulum, and pelvis and for fragments remaining in the joint.
4. Full radiographic evaluation historically includes postreduction AP pelvis and Judet views (45° obliques). The obturator oblique will help to identify injuries to the posterior wall and many times allow for a better definition of the femoral head fracture morphology. These images have in many locations been replaced or supplemented by fine-cut CT scans with 2D and 3D (surfaced rendered and digitally reconstructed radiographs, DRR) images (Fig. 21.1).
5. After emergency reduction of the femoral head in case of hip dislocation, a CT scan is performed. Size, position, and congruence of femoral head fragments are determined as well as free osteochondral fragments, femoral neck, or acetabular fracture lines. CT scan is mandatory for planning future definitive treatment.
6. Optionally, MRI examination can further determine the extent of cartilage lesions, acetabular labrum, and muscle injuries. In particular, obturator externus muscle injuries may affect the femoral head's blood supply due to its close relationship with the medial circumflex femoral artery. Finally, MRI examination could provide important prognostic information.

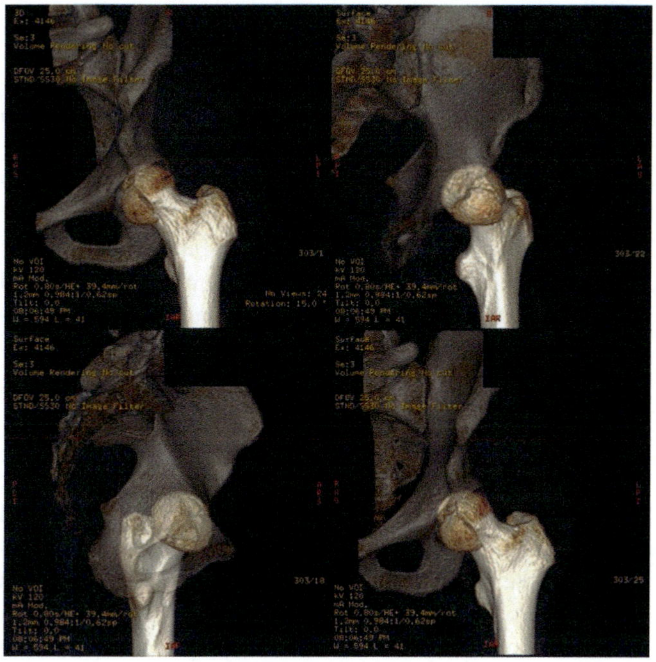

Fig. 21.1 3D reconstruction of Pipkin type 1 fracture

21.5 Preoperative Planning/Computer Simulation

Though SHD has shown promising results, it bears a steep learning curve. Given these conditions, a thorough preoperative preparation of the surgeon is mandatory to achieve satisfactory results.

The accurate analysis of preoperative CT scan allows precise understanding of femoral head's fracture patterns, associated injuries, and/or free osteochondral fragments. In recent years, the application of 3D printing in orthopedics has become more and more common in complex surgical cases. The aid of 3D-printed models could help operating surgeons define every detail in advance, i.e., the correct placement and choice of instruments/implants and visualization of reduction maneuvers. Although not compulsory, the application of this new technology could help reduce operating time, intraoperative blood loss, and implant-related complications.

21.6 Applied Anatomy

1. Either the Gibson or the Kocher-Langenbeck superficial exposure can be used. The former allows preservation of the gluteus maximus, while the latter offers a better visualization of retroacetabular surface, caudal posterior wall (Pipkin Type 4), and easier access to quadrilateral surface

for fracture evaluation and placement of reduction clamps for acetabular fracture reduction.

1. In hip dislocations, the femoral attachment of the piriformis is spared and allows for reliable identification of the cranial interval of the dissection.
2. Tenotomy of the external rotators 1.5–2 cm from trochanteric attachment can improve retroacetabular access. The obturator externus and quadratus femoris should be preserved in all circumstances to avoid damage to the deep branch of the medial femoral circumflex artery.
3. The transtrochanteric osteotomy is performed with or without a step cut as described in Chaps. 7 and 12.
4. Gluteus minimus and piriformis injuries are very common in acetabular fractures and hip dislocations. Debridement of the devitalized tissue is performed during anterior dislocation of the osteotomized trochanteric fragment or prior to closure. A standard anterosuperior Z-shaped capsulotomy is performed in case of intact capsule. In case of capsular rupture, the partial capsulotomy is completed avoiding iatrogenic injury to the lateral retinaculum.
5. In most Pipkin 1 and 2 fractures, Weitbrecht's ligament including the medial retinaculum with the medial branch of the medial femoral circumflex artery (MFCA) remains attached to the fragment providing blood supply to the fragment. The blood supply from the round ligament in Pipkin 2 fractures can be neglected.

21.7 Specific Risks

1. Sciatic nerve injury is reported in 4% of all femoral head fractures with posterior hip dislocation. In polytrauma patients unconscious upon arrival, the sciatic nerve should be inspected and eventual injuries assessed and reported [1].
2. Open reduction and fixation of associated acetabular and neck fractures present specific risks of damaging neurovascular structures. See Chap. 22 for further details on intraoperative and/or postoperative complications.
3. Integrity or amount of damage of lateral and medial retinaculum should be reported.

21.8 Type of Anesthesia

Since the procedure is performed in the lateral position and usually takes more than 90 min, general anesthesia is the recommendation of choice. Furthermore, muscle relaxation can improve joint exposure while reducing risk of iatrogenic muscle trauma. The role of postoperative adjunct local or regional anesthetic has not been examined in this population.

21.9 Positioning

1. Standard radiolucent operating table.
2. Lateral positioning with tunnel cushion, beanbag and axillary roll, arms placed comfortably on arm boards.
3. Fluoroscopy and monitor placed in front of the patient

21.10 Instruments/Implants

Standard instrumentation for SHD (see Chap. 7). In addition, the following instruments are required for proper treatment of all different patterns of femoral head fractures:

1. Cannulated headless compression screws from 2.7 mm to 4.5 mm depending on patient's body constitution and fracture characteristics.
2. Mini fragment screws (2.0–2.4 mm) with flat heads can be used.
3. Large reduction forceps with points (Weber) 130 mm and 200 mm.
4. Dental picks.

   For associated femoral neck fracture osteosynthesis (Pipkin type 3):
5. Cannulated screws from 6.5 mm to 8 mm, 16 mm, and 32 mm partially threaded, depending on patient's body constitution and fracture's characteristics.

For associated acetabular fracture osteosynthesis, we advise a dedicated pelvic instrumentation set. In particular, the following instruments/implants are useful:

1. Jungbluth large (330 mm) and small (250 mm) forceps for 3.5 mm screws, 1 each.
2. Straight ball spike with pointed ball tip and round disk.
3. Sciatic nerve Hohmann retractor, small and large.
4. 3 mm and 6 mm Schanz screws.
5. Universal chuck.
6. 3.5 mm fully threaded screws.
7. 3.5 mm reconstruction plate
8. Bending instruments to better adapt the plate to patient's anatomy.
9. Colinear clamp.
10. Angled jaw clamps.

For osteosynthesis of trochanteric osteotomy, we advise the use of 2–3 3.5 mm or two 4.5 mm fully threaded screws.

All cutting instruments should be checked for optimal sharpness prior to surgery.

21.11 Access

1. Access as for transtrochanteric SHD (see Chap. 7).

21.12 Technical Steps

A step cut osteotomy is preferred for reduction and subsequent stabilization. During the capsulotomy, care should be taken to maintain the labral attachments of any peripheral rim acetabular fragments. In case of posttraumatic capsular lesion, capsulotomy should be modified according to the existing rupture. Caution should be made not to jeopardize the already traumatized epiphyseal blood supply. Prior to dislocation and immediately following, assessment of femoral head blood supply can be done with direct visualization of the retinaculum and drilling of the femoral head or with a Doppler for decision-making regarding the potential for joint salvage. Subluxation of the femoral head can allow for manipulation and reduction of head fragments, although the fragment must be of sufficient size to allow for fixation. This fixation will not generate compression and may not be perpendicular to the fracture plane, although may allow for maintenance of soft tissue attachments to the detached fragment. In most circumstances, the reduction is not as straightforward, as it is very common to have comminution of the detached femoral head fragment and areas of intact femoral head deformed by impaction on the intact ilium. In this circumstance, full dislocation of the femoral head is necessary to achieve an adequate reduction. The ligamentum attachment may need to be released from the head or fracture fragment to perform reduction. This does not appear to affect head viability or fracture healing. The femoral head fragment might still have some continuity with the medial retinaculum and/or the ligamentum teres. Great care should be taken during dislocation and ligament release to preserve the ligament of Weitbrecht and maintain viability to the fragment. Reduction of the head fragment is typically achieved by direct manipulation of the fragment into position, maintaining this and providing compression with the use of a pointed reduction clamp. Smaller fragments may need to be held in position with small, spiked instruments and/or thin 1.25 mm wires until fragment-specific fixation is completed. Reduction is rarely anatomic due to impaction, cartilage injury, or fragmentation at the periphery of the articular injury (Fig. 21.8). Compression using mini fragment lag screws (2.0 mm, 2.4 mm) or mini fragment headless screws is the fixation of choice. These screws are easy to countersink under the cartilage as they have flat heads that can allow for compression of even very thin cortical fragments. The hip is constrained so this small fragment fixation does not see shear forces that would put the fixation at risk for failure. The screws should be inserted through the articular side avoiding, if possible, the weight-bearing area. The head of the screws should be placed deeper than the cartilage surface.

In Pipkin type 3 fractures, the femoral neck should be reduced and stabilized prior to hip dislocation. Femoral neck reduction can be facilitated by a lateral to medial Schanz pin in the femur and K-wire joysticks in the femoral head. Optimal neck fixation should be prioritized. Intact retinacula and/or active bleeding from drill holes in the head indicate preserved head perfusion.

In Pipkin type 4 fractures, a unique feature of the SHD is the reduction of the articular surface that can be performed under direct visual control. For specifics regarding acetabular fracture reduction, please refer to Chap. 22.

Following definitive fixation, closure of the capsule with absorbable monofilament should reapproximate the synovial layer to limit intra-articular adhesions and be tied with the hip in extension to avoid any tension onto the capsule. Devitalized short rotators and gluteus minimus should be debrided. Trochanteric repositioning is facilitated by the step cut, and refixation is performed with 4.5 mm or 3.5 mm cortical lag screws.

21.13 Postoperative Follow-Up

Patients are instructed to avoid active hip abduction and passive hip adduction for 30 days after surgery. Afterward strengthening of hip abductors is encouraged.

Weight-bearing is restricted for 90 days after surgery. Motion is encouraged as tolerated, and isometric strengthening is begun immediately post-op with active resistive strengthening begin when weight bearing is advanced.

Hydrotherapy can begin with wound healing. Prophylaxis against Deep venous thrombosis (DVT) and heterotopic ossification is instituted following surgery if not contraindicated. Postoperative follow-up includes clinical examination with anteroposterior view of the pelvis and cross-table lateral view of the hip at 30, 60, and 90 days.

21.14 Intra-/Postoperative Complications

Surgical exposure through SHD is excellent, giving a complete view of the femoral head and acetabulum. However, this technique has some limitations which may jeopardize the patient's outcome.

21.14.1 Intraoperative Complications

Firstly, the operating surgeon should pay attention not to compromise the vascularization of the inferior fragment of Pipkin types 1 and 2 fractures by damaging the ligament of Weitbrecht. As previously mentioned, great care should be placed in liberating the inferior fragment when sectioning the ligamentum teres.

AVN is a known outcome of femoral head fractures and may be associated with the injury as well as the approach. AVN risk does not appear to be associated with the SHD as the incidence is similar to the anterior approach. Use of the traditional KL approach has a likelihood of increasing AVN rates. Significant blood loss is uncommon when using the surgical hip dislocation for simple fractures of the femoral head (Pipkin 1, 2) and is more common with associated injuries. Secondly, associated transverse fractures (Pipkin type 4) may be more difficult to reduce in lateral decubitus: a higher rate of residual displacement has been found with respect to prone position. Thirdly, the exposure and reductions maneuvers of the anterior column can be quite challenging. With either the Gibson or the Kocher-Langenbeck approach in lateral decubitus, the inferior extra-articular portion of the anterior column is difficult to visualize. When the fracture line is medial to the iliopubic eminence, the placement of the anterior reduction clamp or Schanz screw can be demanding. Finally, the anterior column fixation is limited to the placement of one or two cortical screws.

21.14.2 Postoperative Complications

Adverse events following femoral head fractures may include heterotopic ossification, nerve dysfunction, avascular necrosis, and hip arthrosis even following nonoperative treatment.

Femoral head's AVN is reported between 0 and 24%, and it may be caused by the impairment of the blood supply at the time of injury, or it may be iatrogenic [1]. Older publications [7] suggested approaching the hip from posterior through Kocher-Langenbeck approach, as the posterior capsule or wall is often injured. However, further anatomical studies highlighted the importance of the mandatory preservation of the medical femoral circumflex artery and in particular its deep branch [8]. As a matter of fact, the posterior approach has presented a twofold higher risk of AVN with respect to the anterior approach or SHD [1]. In a recent meta-analysis, the pooled estimate of AVN incidence was 12% [9].

The reported incidence of posttraumatic osteoarthritis (OA) was 16% [9]. In comparison, anterior and posterior approaches reported a 20 to 30 times higher incidence with respect to the SHD [1]. On the other hand, SHD is associated to higher rates of heterotopic ossification (HO) with respect to the posterior approach [1], with a pooled estimate of 25% [9]. Therefore, appropriate anti-HO prophylaxis is suggested whenever possible. SHD may lead to nonunion and trochanteric bursitis which are specific complications of this surgical approach, with a reported incidence of 3.4% and 3.8% respectively [9]. Finally, one of the most common early complications is infection with a reported rate of 2.1% [9]. Adequate perioperative antibiotic prophylaxis should administered according to local guidelines.

21.15 Case Studies

Case 1: A 28-year-old man was transferred to a level-III trauma center 2 hours after being involved in a car accident with Glasgow Coma Sale of 15 at arrival. Physical examination revealed a contusion in the left hemithorax, a stable pelvic ring with flexion, adduction, and internal rotation of his right lower limb. The neurovascular status was intact with palpable pulses and no neurological dysfunction.

Figures 21.2, 21.3 and 21.4: Pelvis X-rays showed a posterior hip dislocation with a displaced femoral head fracture. No additional systemic injuries were recorded. The following day the patient was transferred to our level-I trauma center where a closed reduction attempt was unsuccessful

Figure 21.5 and 21.6: Pelvis CT where a multifragmentary displaced Pipkin type 1 fracture was detected. The patient was taken to the operatory room for open reduction and internal fixation in the lateral decubitus position. A Gibson interval was used and the femoral head was found dislocated posteriorly. Reduction of femoral head was performed followed by formal exposure

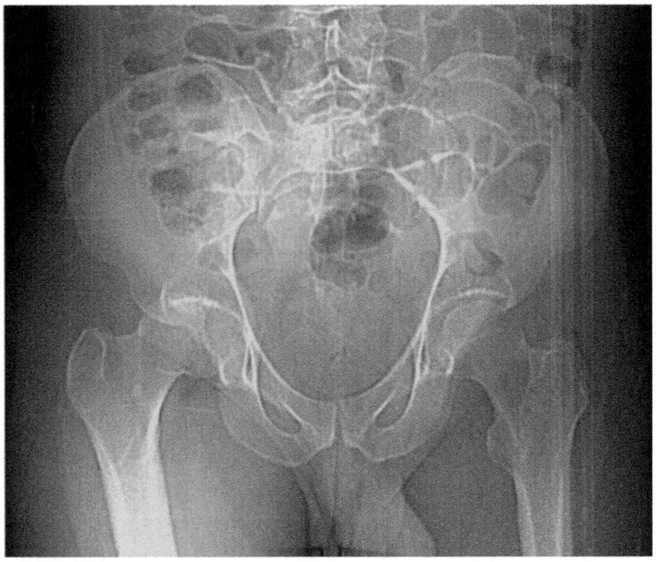

Fig. 21.2 Anteroposterior pelvis radiograph at arrival in the emergency department

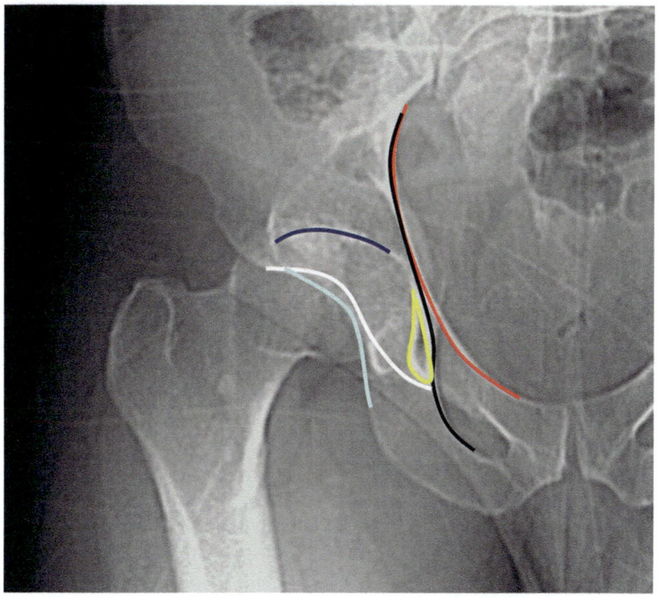

Fig. 21.3 Acetabular reference lines on anteroposterior pelvis radiograph

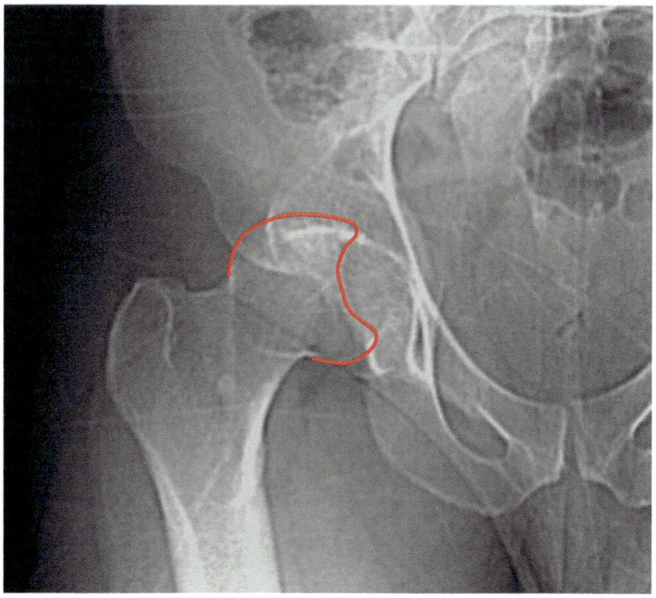

Fig. 21.4 Femoral reference lines on anteroposterior pelvis radiograph

Figure 21.7: The hip was safely dislocated through a transtrochanteric osteotomy and z-shaped capsulotomy

Figure 21.8: The femoral head's fragments were gently manipulated and then reduced with a Weber clamp and temporarily fixed with Kirschner wires. Definitive fixation was achieved through cannulated compression screws

Figure 21.9: The inferior retinaculum (white arrow) was intact and attached to the biggest femoral head fragment.

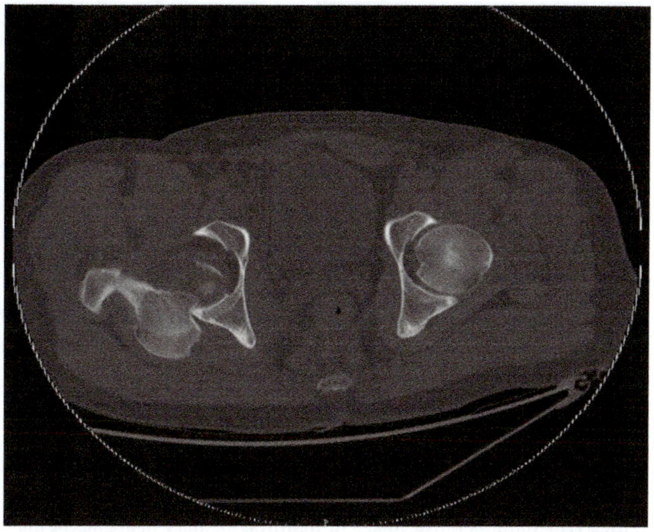

Fig. 21.5 Axial view of posterior hip dislocation and femoral head fracture

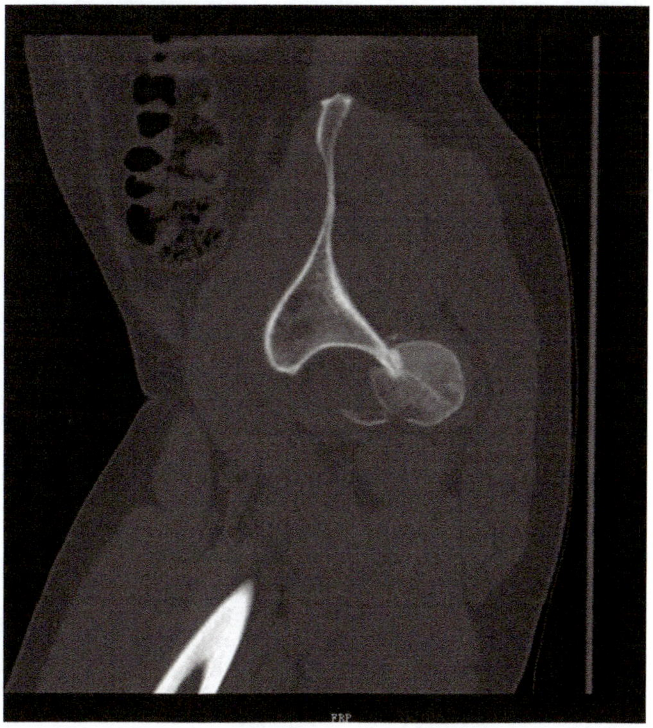

Fig. 21.6 Sagittal view of posterior hip dislocation and femoral head fracture

Confirmation of femoral head perfusion (black arrow) was performed with a 2 mm drill

Figure 21.10: The posterior detachment of acetabular labrum was repaired with two suture anchors. The femoral head was carefully reduced and closure performed according to technique

Figure 21.11: Postoperative X-rays

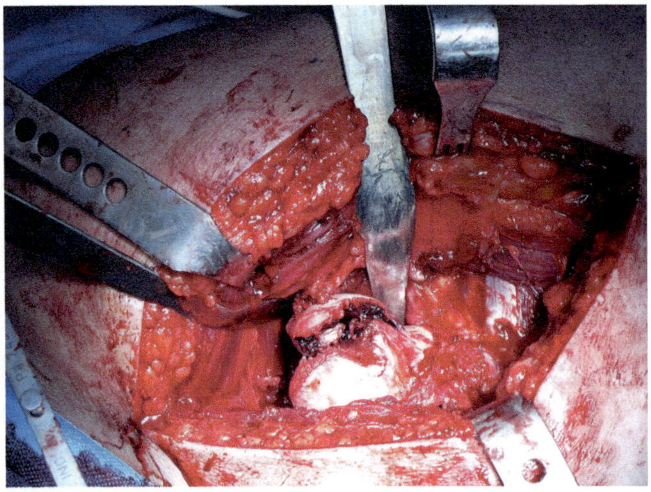

Fig. 21.7 Intraoperative image of multifragmentary dislocated Pipkin I fracture

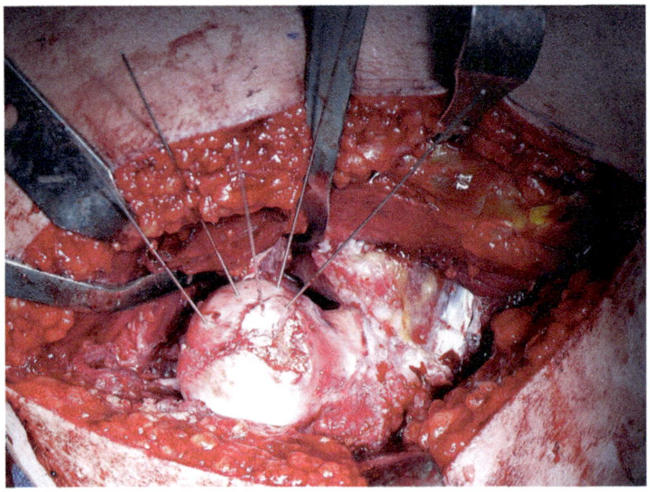

Fig. 21.8 Intraoperative image of reduction and temporary fixation of femoral head fracture

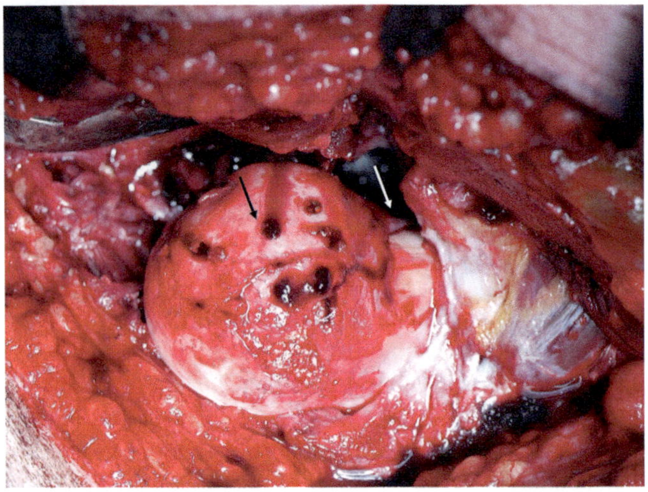

Fig. 21.9 Intraoperative image of final reduction and fixation of femoral head fracture. The black arrow shows valid vascularization of the femoral head. The white arrow points to the intact medial retinaculum

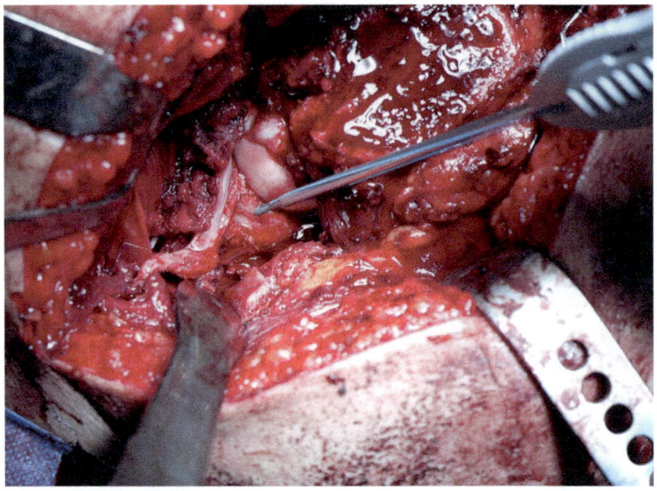

Fig. 21.10 Intraoperative image of labrum fixation with suture anchors

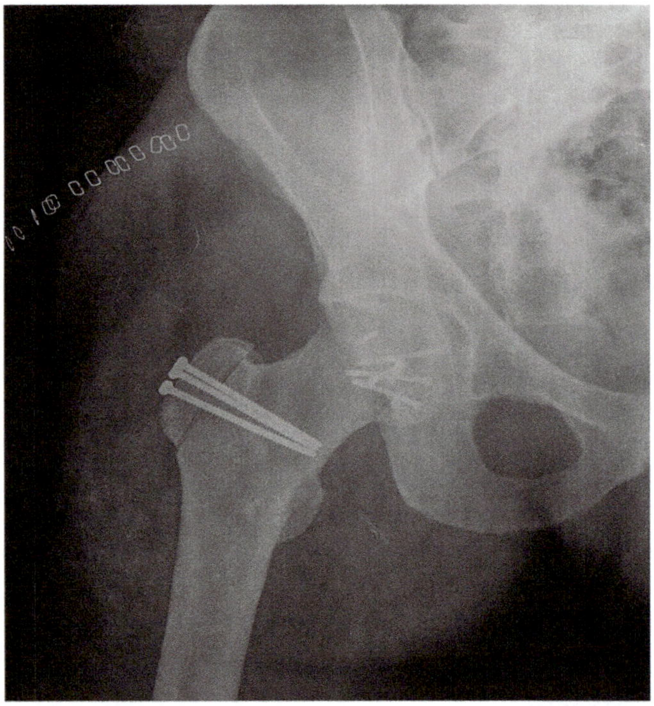

Fig. 21.11 Postoperative anteroposterior pelvis radiograph

Figures 21.12 and 21.13: Three-year follow-up with no signs of AVN and Brooker 1 heterotopic ossification. The patient remained asymptomatic with full and unrestricted range of motion of the hip

Case 2: A 20 y/o man 1 week out from an accident while out of the country. Evaluated at urgent facility. Radiographs without fracture. No history of hip dislocation. Evaluated by local physician. Hip and groin pain and difficulty walking, presented as referral to office.

Figure 21.14: Low contrast radiographs with suggested subluxation of the right femoral head

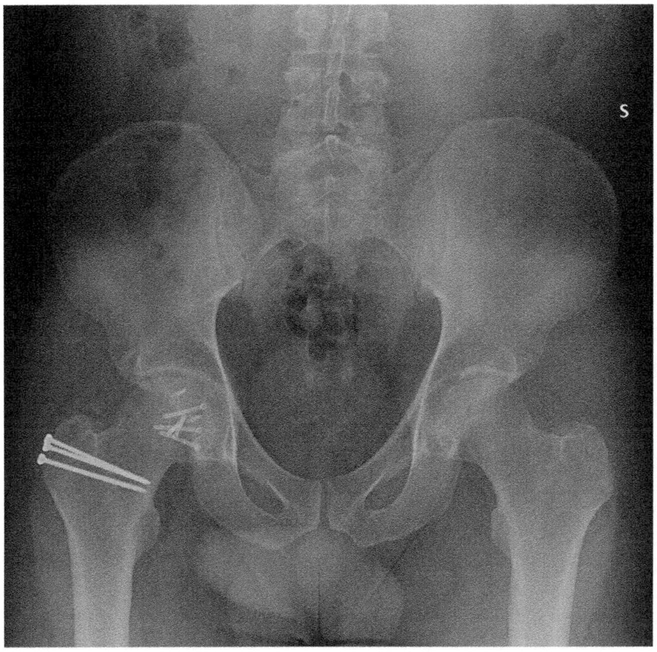

Fig. 21.12 Anteroposterior pelvis radiograph at 3-year follow-up

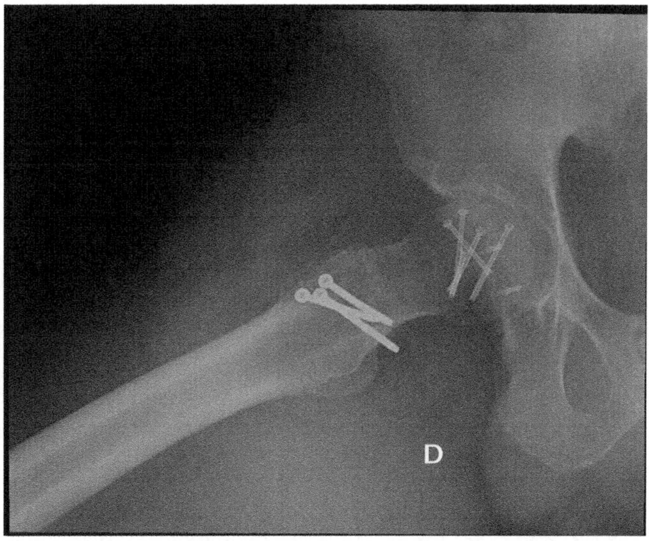

Fig. 21.13 Axial view of right hip at 3-year follow-up

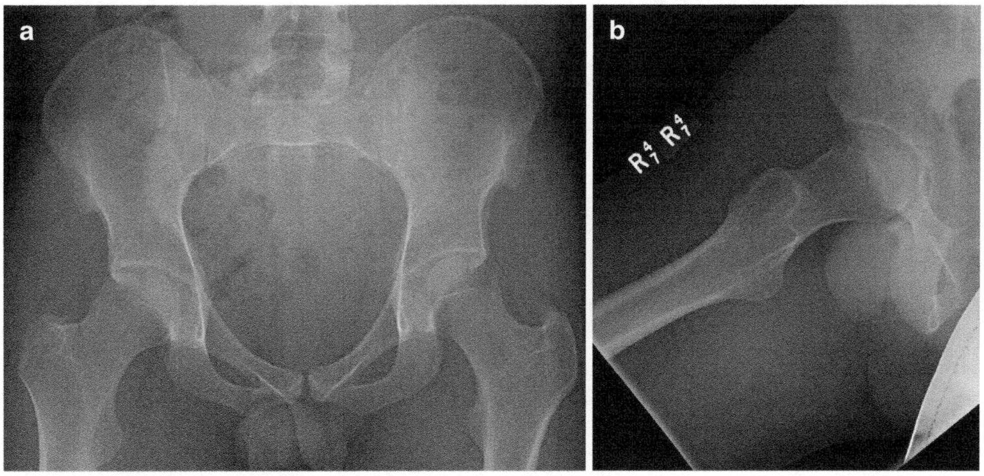

Fig. 21.14 (a) Injury AP pelvis (b) frog lateral

Figure 21.15a-c: CT scan provided visualization of femoral head fracture. SHD using the Gibson interval was performed and a thin osteochondral fragment was identified.

Figure 21.16: Large osteochondral fragment was found

Figure 21.17: Fragment was reduced and held with 2.0 mm screws, fibrin glue at periphery

Figure 21.18: Trochanteric refixation completed with 3.5 mm screws. Foot flat weight bearing for 2 months

Figure 21.19: Plain Radiographs at 6 months demonstrated fracture healing and maintained joint space, concern for prominent screws

Figure 21.20: Screws were removed with second-look SHD performed at >1 year

Figure 21.21: Plain radiographs at 6 years without evidence of AVN or significant joint space narrowing. Patient reported full function, no pain, and some limitation of motion

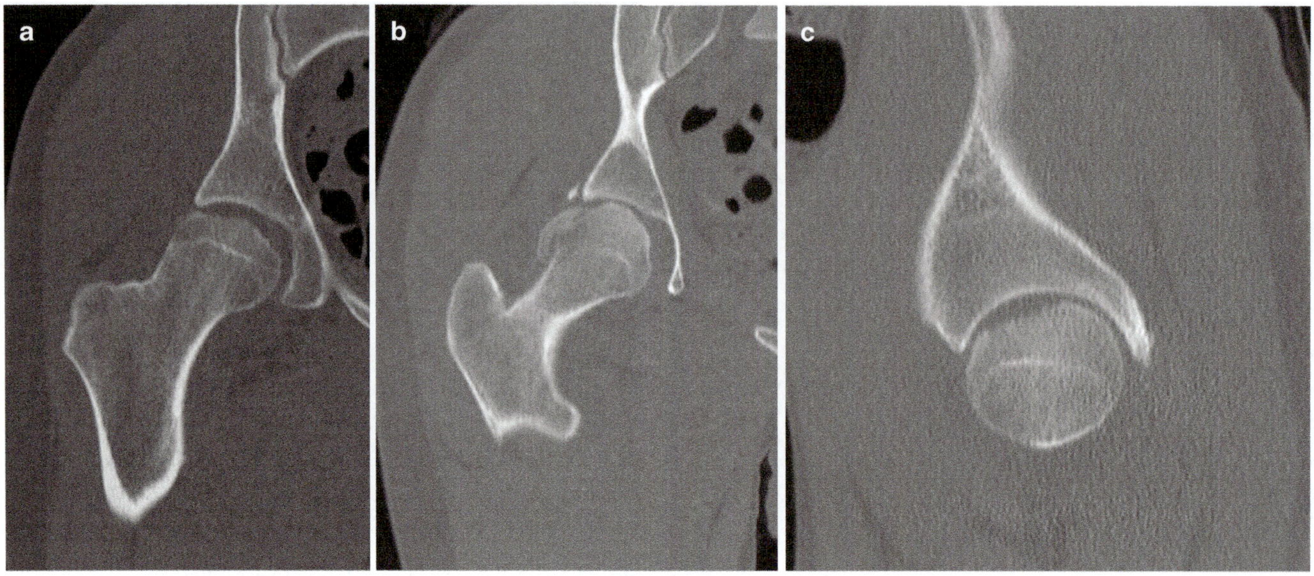

Fig. 21.15 (**a**) Anterior coronal (**b**) posterior coronal image demonstrating osteochondral fragment and posterior wall fragment (**c**) mid-sagittal reconstruction demonstrating anterior superior osteochondral defect

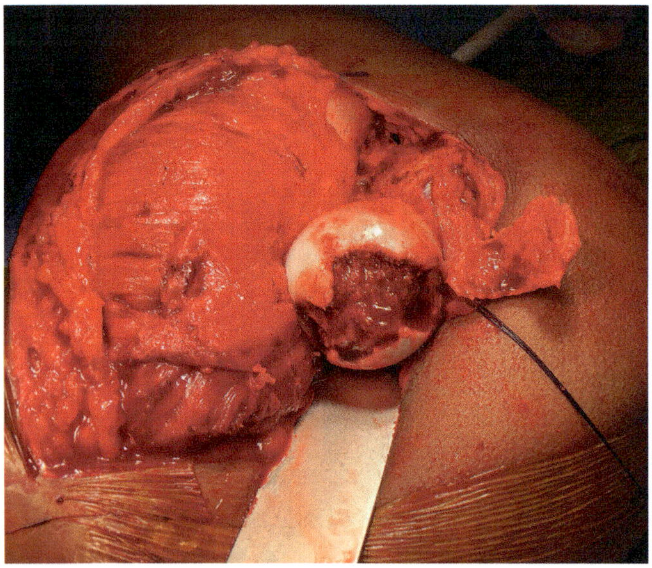

Fig. 21.16 Cranial osteochondral fragment rotated on thin cartilage attachment

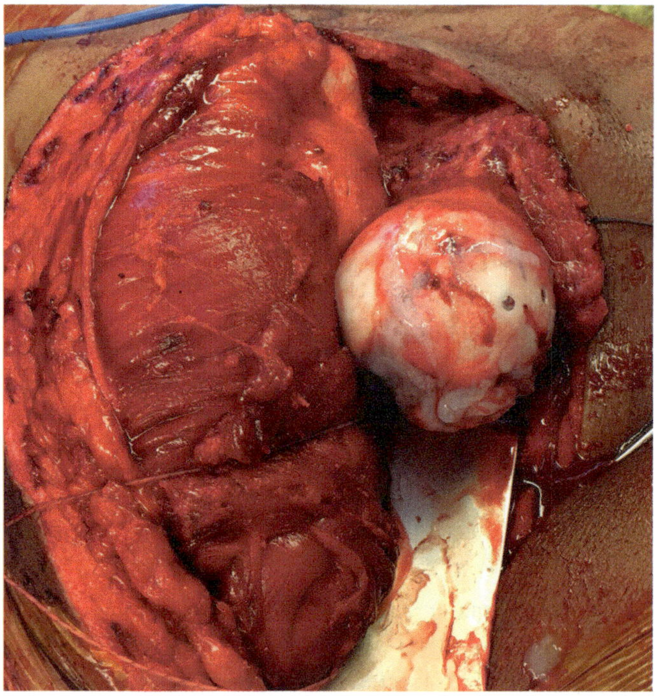

Fig. 21.17 Osteochondral fragment following fixation. Fibrin glue applied peripherally at cartilage interface, areas of cartilage defects

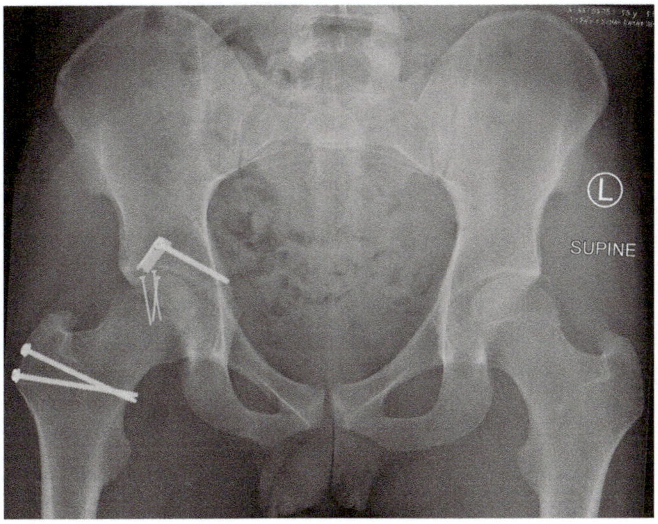

Fig. 21.18 Immediate postoperative X-ray with additional spring plate on posterior wall

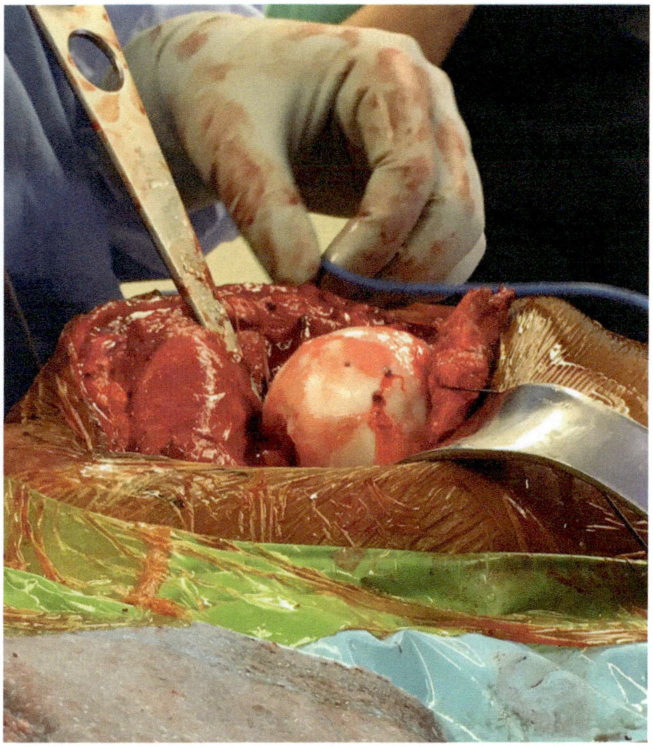

Fig. 21.20 Cartilage surface at hardware removal

Fig. 21.19 (**a**) 6 months post op AP pelvis (**b**) sagittal CT cuts demonstrating fracture healing and screw fixation at the subchondral bone

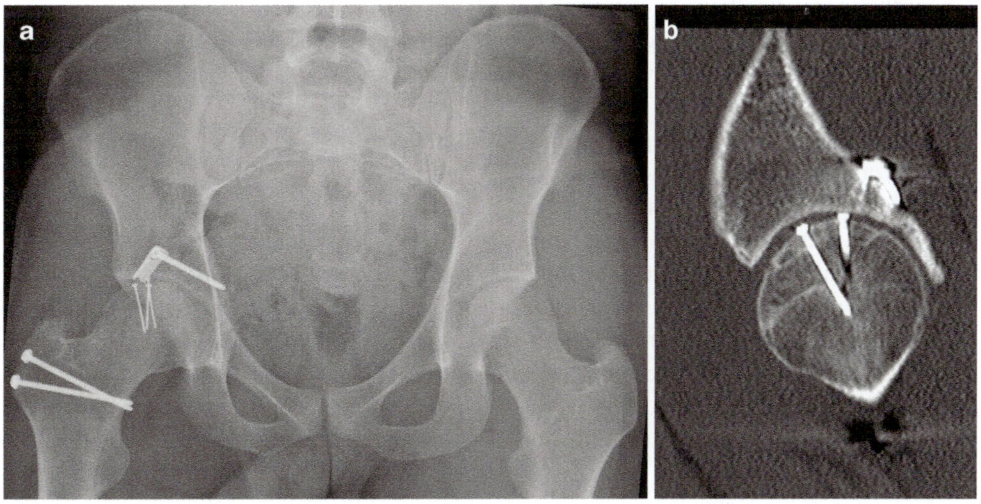

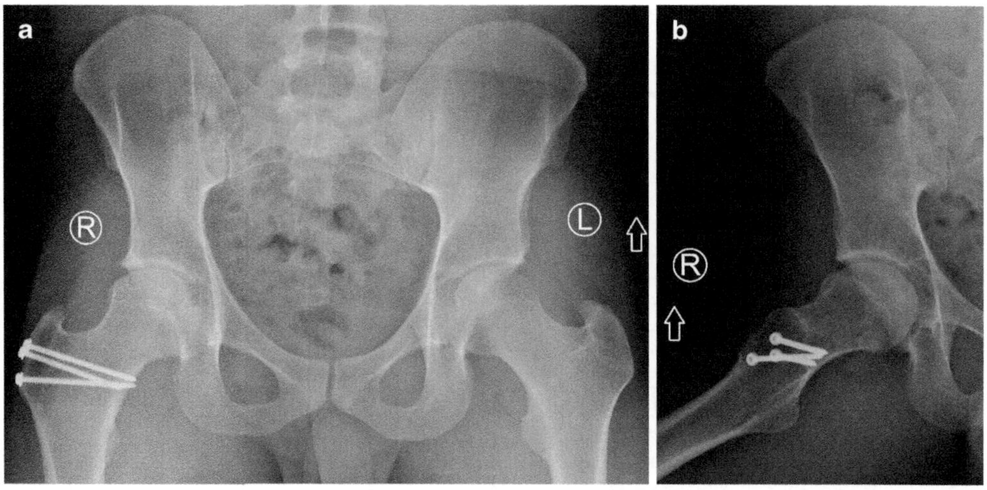

Fig. 21.21 (**a**) AP pelvis demonstrates maintained joint space, mild sclerosis. (**b**) Frog lateral reveals bone formation at the head neck junction

21.16 Controversies

1. Surgical hip dislocation of the hip allows satisfying results in the treatment of displaced Pipkin types 1 and 2 fractures. However, postoperative complications such as heterotopic ossification are common [1]. Evidence is emerging about the possibility of arthroscopic reduction and subsequent percutaneous fixation, which could allow less soft tissue damage and faster rehabilitation [6]. Furthermore, it allows excision and washout of small fragments [10]. Despite encouraging results, there is very little evidence to support arthroscopy over open reduction and internal fixation.
2. Pipkin type 3 fractures represent the 8.6% and are the least common of femoral head fractures. Therefore, there is scarce evidence on which operative treatment could provide better outcomes and fewer complications. Giannoudis et al. [1] reported fair and poor results in 50% of cases and no excellent outcomes. Further case series also reported unsatisfactory results after surgical treatment. Tonetti et al. reported four patients with a Pipkin type 3 fracture: one was treated with acute total hip replacement (THR), while the other three were converted at a later stage. Scolaro et al. treated 13 type 3 fractures with open reduction and internal fixation, and none of the native hips could be preserved during follow-up. Given the poor outcomes associated with ORIF of Pipkin type 3 fractures, acute THR has been suggested as definitive treatment [4, 11]. Acute arthroplasty in active elderly patients with femoral neck fractures has gained popularity, thanks to good clinical outcomes and few complications. Furthermore, THR as a salvage procedure after failed internal fixation presents higher rates of infection, periprosthetic fracture, and dislocation.

However, THR should not be the primary surgical option in young active patients without signs of hip arthritis. Tannast et al. [5] proposed an algorithm for the management of hip dislocations associated with a femoral neck fracture. It is suggested that intraoperative assessment of the integrity of the medial femoral circumflex artery should guide the surgeon between osteosynthesis vs arthroplasty. This approach could help the surgeon during complex cases without the need for an a priori decision but based on intraoperative evidence.

21.17 Expected Outcomes

Table 21.1 shows published studies reporting on outcomes and complications of femoral head fractures approached with SHD. Even though a recent meta-analysis was not yet able to compare different surgical approaches [19], the papers presented in Table 21.1 showed satisfying clinical scores with acceptable complication rates. The results presented in these studies are relatively similar, which may suggest that similar outcomes should be expected after 3 years of follow-up.

In a previous systematic review by Giannoudis et al. [1], according to Thompson and Epstein criteria, better clinical outcomes were found in patients treated through lateral approaches. Just 11% reported fair or poor results as compared to 35% for the anterior approach and 51% for the posterior approach. However, results are difficult to compare because the lateral approach group included both patients with and without SHD.

A recent systematic review and meta-analysis by Khalifa et al. [9], on the other hand, highlighted how SHD was used three times more often by trauma surgeons in the last 10 years. Average operative time was 123.7 minutes but was strongly affected by associated injuries: acetabular fractures (37.4%), labral tears (41.3%), and femoral head impaction (23.5%). The reported average blood loss was 491.9 ml.

Table 21.1 Comparison of published clinical results of femoral head fractures treated through the surgical hip dislocation

Study	Number of patients	Type of fracture (Pipkin)	Follow-up (months)	Outcome (Merle d'Aubigne and Postel	Outcome (Thompson and Epstein)	Outcome (modified Harris hip score)	HO	AVN
Henle et al. [1]	12	1 type 1 3 type 2 8 type 4	31	10 good or excellent 2 poor	10 good or excellent 2 poor	–	5	2
Solberg et al. [12]	12	12 type 4	47	10 good or excellent 1 fair 1 poor	10 good or excellent 1 fair 1 poor	–	4	1
Mostafa et al. [13]	12	12 type 2	31	10 good or excellent 1 fair 1 poor	10 good or excellent 1 fair 1 poor	–	2	4
Massè et al. [2]	13	5 type 1 2 type 2 6 type 4	75	–	–	11 good or excellent 1 fair 1 poor	2	1
De Mauro et al. [14]	5	4 Pipkin II 1 Pipkin IV	24	3 good or excellent 1 fair	4 good or excellent 1 fair	4 good or excellent 1 fair	1	0
Wang et al. [15]	12	4 type 1 3 type 2 5 type 4	35	10 good or excellent 2 poor	–	–	4	1
Gavaskar et al. [16]	28	6 type 1 22 type 2	36	24 good or excellent 2 fair	–	–	5	3
Engel et al. [17]	7	6 type 4	30	–	–	–	1	2
Khalifa et al. [18]	27	6 type 1 13 type 2 0 type 3 8 type 4	48	24 good or excellent 2 fair 1 poor	–	–	5	2

Functional outcomes were reported using different assessment scales. However, 85% of patients were defined as good or excellent by the Harris hip score or Merle d'Aubigne-Postel and 83.3% according to the Thompson-Epstein score. Functional results were better than what patients treated by K-L or S-P approach reported and are in line with previous data by Giannoudis et al. [1].

Anatomical reduction was reported in 74% of patients. The direct and complete visualization of the femoral head and acetabulum's articular surface is a unique feature of the SHD. Difficulties to achieve anatomical reduction could be due to osteochondral impaction and fragment comminution.

Taking in consideration complication rates mentioned in paragraph 14, preservation of the native hip was possible in 80% of treated patients.

21.18 Outlook

SHD is a reliable approach for femoral head fractures requiring open reduction and internal fixation. It also offers a 360° view of the acetabulum, which enables to address associated intra-articular injuries and acetabular fractures. Surgeons working in trauma centers treating high volumes of complex hip fractures should add this technique to their repertoire.

Better outcomes are also dependent on the quality of reduction. The visualization achieved through the SHD should allow better reduction and fixation than other approaches.

However, larger multicenter studies are required to compare outcomes and complications between different approaches. More evidence is needed to understand if SHD should be used routinely for displaced femoral head fractures or limited only to complex cases.

References

1. Giannoudis PV, Kontakis G, Christoforakis Z, Akula M, Tosounidis T, Koutras C. Management, complications and clinical results of femoral head fractures. Injury. 2009;40:1245–51.
2. Pipkin G. Treatment of grade IV fracture dislocation of the hip. J Bone Joint Surg Am. 1957;39:1027–42.
3. Roeder LF Jr, DeLee JC. Femoral head fractures associated with posterior hip dislocation. Clin Orthop Relat Res. 1980;147:121–30.
4. Tonetti J, Ruatti S, Lafontan V, Loubignac F, Chiron P, Sari-Ali H, et al. Is femoral head fracture-dislocation management improvable: a retrospective study in 110 cases. Orthop Traumatol Surg Res. 2010;96:623–31.
5. Tannast M, Mack PW, Klaeser B, Siebenrock KA. Hip dislocation and femoral neck fracture: decision-making for head preservation. Injury. 2009;40(10):1118–24.
6. Wang J, Cai L, Xie L, et al. 3D printing-based Ganz approach for treatment of femoral head fractures: a prospective analysis. J Orthop Surg Res. 2019a;14:338.
7. Epstein HC, Wiss DA, Cozen L. Posterior fracture dislocation of the hip with fractures of the femoral head. Clin Orthop Relat Res. 1985b;201:9–17.

8. Gautier E, Ganz K, Krugel N, et al. Anatomy of the medial femoral circumflex artery and its surgical implications. J Bone Joint Surg (Br). 2000;82(5):679–83.
9. Droll KP, Broekhuyse H, O'Brien P. Fracture of the femoral head. J Am Acad Orthop Surg. 2007;15:716–27.
10. Yamamoto Y, Ide T, Ono T, Hamada Y. Usefulness of arthroscopic surgery in hip trauma cases. Arthros J Arthros Relat Surg. 2003;19(3):269–73.
11. Tosounidis T, Aderinto J, Giannoudis PV. Pipkin type-III fractures of the femoral head: fix it or replace it? Injury. 2017;48(11): 2375–8.
12. Hougaard K, Thomsen PB. Traumatic posterior fracture dislocation of the hip with fracture of the femoral head or neck, or both. J Bone Joint Surg Am. 1988;70:233–9.
13. Birkett J. Description of a dislocation of the head of the femur, complicated with its fracture; with remarks by John Birkett (1815–1904). 1869. Clin Orthop Relat Res. 2000;377:4–6.
14. Muller ME. Classification and international AO-documentation of femur fractures. Unfallheilkunde. 1980;83:251–9.
15. Yoon PW, Jeong HS, Yoo JJ, Koo KH, Yoon KS, Kim HJ. Femoral head fracture without dislocation by low-energy trauma in a young adult. Clin Orthop Surg. 2011;3:336–41.
16. Chiron P, Lafontan V, Reina N. Fracture-dislocations of the femoral head. Orthopaed Traumatol Surg Res. 2013;99(1 Supplement):S53–66.
17. Wang S, Li B, Zhang Z, Yu X, Li Q, Liu L. Early versus delayed hip reduction in the surgical treatment of femoral head fracture combined with posterior hip dislocation: a comparative study. BMC Musculoskelet Disord. 2021;22:1057.
18. Ganz R, Gill TJ, Gautier E, Ganz K, Krügel N, Berlemann U. Surgical dislocation of the adult hip a technique with full access to the femoral head and acetabulum without the risk of avascular necrosis. J Bone Joint Surg (Br). 2001;83:1119–24.
19. Epstein HC, Wiss DA, Cozen L. Posterior fracture-dislocation of the hip with fractures of the femoral head. Clin Orthop Relat Res. 1985a;201:9–17.

Further Reading

Aprato A, Buzzone M, Di Benedetto P, Massè A. Surgical hip dislocation vs arthroscopy for fixation of subfoveal femoral head fractures: a new technique for Pipkin type 1 fractures. Acta Biomed. 2021;92(S3):e2021016. https://doi.org/10.23750/abm.v92iS3.11724. PMID: 34313665; PMCID: PMC8420819.

Bartels S, Gjertsen JE, Frihagen F, Rogmark C, Utvåg SE. High failure rate after internal fixation and beneficial outcome after arthroplasty in treatment of displaced femoral neck fractures in patients between 55 and 70 years. Acta Orthop. 2018;89(1):53–8.

Bettinelli G, Placella G, Moharamzadeh D, Belluati A, Salini V. Articular femoral head fracture management: a meta-analysis of literature. Indian J Orthop. 2021;55(Suppl 2):304–13.

Brumback RJ, Kenzora JE, Levitt LE, Burgess AR, Poka A. Fractures of the femoral head. Hip. 1987:181–206.

Chen C, Cai L, Zheng W, et al. The efficacy of using 3D printing models in the treatment of fractures: a randomised clinical trial. BMC Musculoskelet Disord. 2019;20(1):65–73.

Collinge C, Archdeacon M, Sagi HC. Quality of radiographic reduction and perioperative complications for transverse acetabular fractures treated by the Kocher-Langenbeck approach: prone versus lateral position. J Orthop Trauma. 2011;25:538–42.

De Mauro D, Rovere G, Smakaj A, Marino S, Ciolli G, Perna A, Battiato C, El Ezzo O, Liuzza F. Gibson approach and surgical hip dislocation according to Ganz in the treatment of femoral head fractures. BMC Musculoskelet Disord. 2021;22(Suppl 2):961.

Engel JL, Johnsen P, Patel NK, Satpathy J, Mounasamy V. Pipkin type IV femoral head fractures: a case series and review of literature. Eur J Orthop Surg Traumatol. 2021;31(4):791–5. https://doi.org/10.1007/s00590-020-02838-5. Epub 2020 Nov 19

Epstein HC. Posterior fracture-dislocations of the hip: comparison of open and closed methods of treatment in certain types. J Bone Joint Surg Am. 1961;43:1079–98.

Epstein HC. Traumatic dislocations of the hip. Clin Orthop Relat Res. 1973;92:116–42.

Gavaskar AS, Tummala NC. Ganz surgical dislocation of the hip is a safe technique for operative treatment of Pipkin fractures. Results of a prospective trial. J Orthop Trauma. 2015;29(12):544–8. https://doi.org/10.1097/BOT.0000000000000399.

Henle P, Kloen P, Siebenrock KA. Femoral head injuries: which treatment strategy can be recommended? Injury Int J Care Injured. 2007;38:478–88.

Khalifa AA, Haridy MA, Fergany A. Safety and efficacy of surgical hip dislocation in managing femoral head fractures: a systematic review and meta-analysis. World J Orthop. 2021b;12(8):604–19. https://doi.org/10.5312/wjo.v12.i8.604. PMID: 34485106; PMCID: PMC8384609

Khalifa AA, Refai O, Farouk O, Abdelnasser MK. Management of femoral head fractures through surgical hip dislocation (SHD): a demanding but safe technique. Arch Orthop Trauma Surg. 2021a;141(10):1701–10. https://doi.org/10.1007/s00402-020-03666-2. Epub 2020 Oct 28

Mahmoud SS, Pearse EO, Smith TO, Hing CB. Outcomes of total hip arthroplasty, as a salvage procedure, following failed internal fixation of intracapsular fractures of the femoral neck: a systematic review and meta-analysis. Bone Joint J. 2016;98-B(4):452–60.

Massè A, Aprato A, Rollero L, Bersano A, Ganz R. Surgical dislocation technique for the treatment of acetabular fractures. Clin Orthop Relat Res. 2013;471:4056–64.

Matsuda DK. A rare fracture, an even rarer treatment: the arthroscopic reduction and internal fixation of an isolated femoral head fracture. Arthroscopy. 2009;25(4):408–12.

Mehta S, Routt ML Jr. Irreducible fracture-dislocations of the femoral head without posterior wall acetabular fractures. J Orthop Trauma. 2008;22(10):686–92. https://doi.org/10.1097/BOT.0b013e31818e2a86.

Mostafa MF, El-Adl W, El-Sayed MA. Operative treatment of displaced Pipkin type I and II femoral head fractures. Arch Orthop Trauma Surg. 2014;134:637–44.

Park MS, Her IS, Cho HM, Chung YY. Internal fixation of femoral head fractures (Pipkin I) using hip arthroscopy. Knee Surg Sports Traumatol Arthrosc. 2014a;22(4):898–901.

Park MS, Yoon SJ, Choi SM. Arthroscopic reduction and internal fixation of femoral head fractures. J Orthop Trauma. 2014b;28(7):e164–8.

Scolaro JA, Marecek G, Firoozabadi R, Krieg JC, Routt ML. Management and radiographic outcomes of femoral head fractures. J Orthop Traumatol. 2017;18:235.

Solberg BD, Moon CN, Franco DP. Use of a trochanteric flip osteotomy improves outcomes in Pipkin IV fractures. Clin Orthop Relat Res. 2009;467:929–33.

Wang J, Cai L, Xie L, et al. 3D printing-based Ganz approach for treatment of femoral head fractures: a prospective analysis. J Orthop Surg Res. 2019b;14:338.

Surgical Hip Dislocation in the Treatment of Acetabular Fractures

22

Michael D. Stover and Klaus A. Siebenrock

22.1 Introduction

Surgical hip dislocation (see Chap. 7) allows the full exposure of the femoral head and acetabulum to achieve anatomic restoration of the acetabular joint surface while ensuring extra-articular fixation in the treatment of select transverse, T shaped, or posterior column acetabular fractures with or without involvement of the posterior wall.

22.2 Background

The "Kocher-Langenbeck" (KL) approach still represents the standard approach for fractures of the posterior column, posterior wall, T-type fractures, and certain transverse fracture patterns. However, access to the supracetabular and superior retroacetabular surfaces remains one of the limitations of this approach. Increasing retraction of the abductor muscles is one technique to gain access to these areas. Alternatively, an extended approach (as described by Letournel and Judet) where the gluteus medius muscle insertion on the greater trochanter is released also allows additional access. Unfortunately, these techniques are associated with muscle damage, prolonged postoperative gait dysfunction, and increased risk of heterotopic ossification.

As an alternative, the transtrochanteric osteotomy combined with the surgical hip dislocation (SHD) was introduced in acetabular surgery by the Bernese hip group. The trochanteric flip osteotomy was initially described by Mercati et al. in 1972 and was mainly used in difficult total hip replacement and revision surgery. As a muscle-preserving procedure, the vastus lateralis and gluteus medius muscle are left attached to the osteotomized trochanteric fragment. In addition, this approach can utilize the Gibson interval first described in 1959, which reduces the morbidity of the procedure by eliminating the need to split the gluteus maximus muscle. The interval between the gluteus maximus and the tensor fascia lata/gluteus medius is used, protecting the neurovascular supply of the anterior portion of the gluteus maximus. In rare cases where improved visual evaluation of the posterior column and digital and instrument access to the quadrilateral surface is needed, the classic Kocher Langenbeck (KL) incision along with split of the gluteus maximus may be preferred. After flipping the greater trochanter anteriorly together with the three muscles with vastus lateralis, gluteus minimus, and gluteus medius, the posterolateral hip capsule including the supraacetabular area up to the anterior inferior iliac spine can be exposed. This technique therefore provides advantages in addressing a transverse or T-type fracture with a posterior wall extending into the supraacetabular area.

Multiple large series following surgical treatment of acetabular fractures has shown that the risk factors for an unsatisfactory outcome are the quality of fracture reduction, fracture pattern, comminution, presence of intra-articular fragments, associated fractures of the femoral head, and fractures extending into the acetabular dome. Specifically, posterior wall fractures that are comminuted or combined with transverse, T-type or posterior column fractures show worse outcomes. There is universal agreement that anatomic fracture reduction is critical to offer the best possible outcome for any acetabular fracture.

The surgical hip dislocation approach has several inherent advantages. First, a full 360-degree view of the acetabular surface as well as a full 360-degree view of the femoral head is possible. This direct and complete visualization of both sides of the joint allows for direct fracture reduction and offers limited access to the anterior column. Second, both intra-articular fragments and marginal impaction can be anatomically reduced under direct visualization. Third,

M. D. Stover (✉)
Northwestern Center for Comprehensive Orthopaedic and Spine Care, Feinberg School of Medicine, Northwestern University, Chicago, IL, USA
e-mail: Michael.Stover@nm.org

K. A. Siebenrock
Emeritus, Department for Orthopaedics and Traumatology, Inselspital, University of Berne, Berne, Switzerland
e-mail: Klaus.Siebenrock@insel.ch

M. Leunig et al. (eds.), *Surgical Hip Dislocation*, https://doi.org/10.1007/978-3-031-70622-6_22

the surgeon can directly visualize the joint surface after fixation placement to either definitively verify that no hardware has penetrated the joint surface or correct the placement of any hardware that is visible in the joint. Furthermore, femoral head fractures, injuries to the femoral head cartilage of other injuries such as labral tears can be addressed using the same exposure. Finally, in elderly patients with preexisting degenerative osteoarthritis, an intraoperative decision can be made, without changing the surgical approach, to proceed with total hip arthroplasty if this is deemed most appropriate.

22.3 Indications

22.3.1 Indications

In the authors' experience, acetabular fractures are treated using the surgical hip dislocation approach in the following cases:

- Comminuted posterior wall and/or posterior column fractures.
- Posterior wall fractures with supraacetabular extension or dome impaction.
- Most transverse and T-shaped fractures.
- Pipkin type IV fractures.
- Fractures including intra-articular fragments and/or large osteochondral defects of the femoral head or acetabulum.

22.3.2 Contraindications

- Anterior-based fractures such as ABC, AW, AC, ACPHT.

22.4 Preoperative/Preinterventional Diagnostics

- AP, Judet, and inlet/outlet views of the pelvis.
- CT pelvis to further classify understand fracture morphology, marginal impaction, presence of intra-articular fragments.
- Additional imaging for concomitant injuries (e.g., femoral neck/head fracture) as needed.
- *Note*: MRI imaging is *not* routinely performed when performing a surgical hip dislocation for fracture since the presence of additional intra-articular anomalies such as a cam deformity, labral tear, cartilage lesions, etc. will be apparent at the time of surgery.

22.5 Preoperative Planning

Preoperative planning is the same as in acetabular fracture surgery performed through any other approach. Based on preoperative radiographs and computed tomography, the surgeon can determine preferred fracture reduction techniques, implants, implant placement, the need for bone grafting or void fillers, and additional equipment needed to address potential findings during surgery based on surgeon comfort and experience.

22.6 Applied Anatomy

- Crucial to the performance of any procedure through a SHD is an intimate understanding of the location and course of the medial femoral circumflex artery.
- A prerequisite for the treatment of acetabular fractures via surgical dislocation of the hip is an excellent understanding of the standard SHD technique (see Chap. 7).
- Lastly a thorough understanding of the Judet-Letournel classification of elementary and associated acetabular fractures (Fig. 22.1) is critical to making sure both that the appropriate approach is used and that appropriate reduction maneuvers/techniques are understood by the surgeon.
- Surface anatomy of the pelvic bone, acetabulum, and surrounding structures in order to safely perform reduction and subsequent fixation of the fracture.

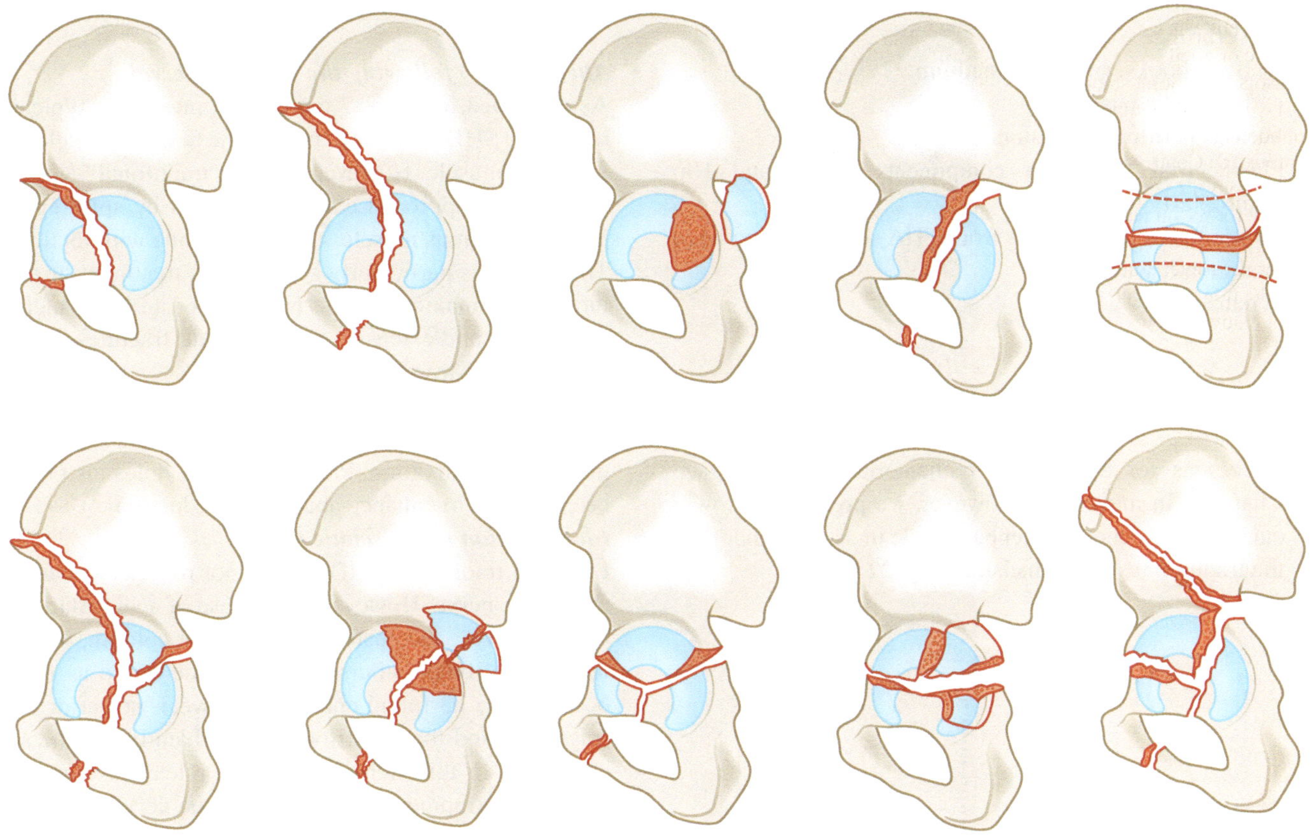

Fig. 22.1 Judet-Letournel classification of acetabulum fractures

22.7 Special Risks

- Disturbance of the femoral head blood supply resulting in:
  - Avascular necrosis.
  - Head collapse.
  - Potential loss of reduction.
  - Secondary joint degeneration (osteoarthritis).
- See also Sect. 22.14.
- Traction injury to the sciatic nerve.
- Injury to the superior gluteal Neurovascular structures (NV) as they exit the greater sciatic notch.

22.8 Type of Anesthesia

General anesthesia with or without adjunct regional anesthesia for both intraoperative and postoperative pain control is recommended.

22.9 Positioning

- Standard operating table.
- Lateral positioning with tunnel cushion and lateral bag.
- Fluoroscopy and X-ray available if needed.

22.10 Instruments/Implants

Standard instrumentation for surgical hip dislocation (see Chap. 7). In addition to the instruments required for the SHD approach, the following special instruments ensure an optimal surgical procedure:

- Pelvic reduction instruments.
  - Jungbluth clamps.
  - Angled Jaw clamps (standard and offset).
  - Weber clamps.
  - Colinear clamps.

  - Farabeuf clamps.
  - Verbrugge forceps.
  - Bone hooks, small and medium.
  - Ball spike pushers.
- Various periosteal elevators.
- Plastic trial acetabular components from Total Hip Arthroplasty (THA) set.
- Plastic femoral head trials from THA set (including large dual mobility trials).
- Schanz pins.

22.11 Access

- Access as for SHD with trochanteric osteotomy (see Chap. 7). In most cases, however, we prefer to follow a curvilinear Kocher-Langenbeck style incision, rather than the traditional straight incision (Fig. 22.2).

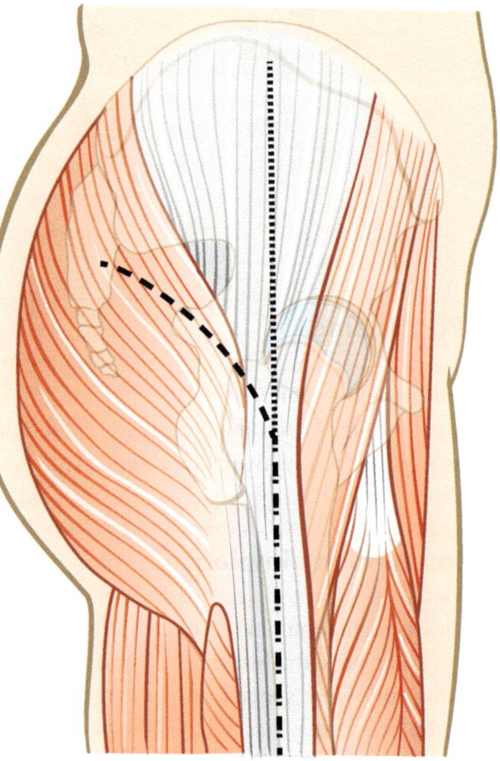

Fig. 22.2 Skin incisions for the Kocher-Langenbeck (dash line) v. the Gibson approach (dotted line)

22.12 Technical Steps of Deep Dissection

- ***Alternative to following the Gibson interval***
  As described in Chap. 7 the Gibson interval is typically used for a SHD in order to protect the fibers of the gluteus maximus muscle. However, a more "traditional" Kocher-Langenbeck approach can be employed by splitting the gluteus maximus muscle, carefully, in line with its fibers. This option is particularly suited to the treatment of fractures where maximal access is needed posteriorly, such as in complex and extensive posterior wall fractures or posterior column fractures.
  The trochanteric osteotomy can be performed as slide or stepped osteotomy, the later increasing the stability of the trochanteric refixation. Predriling screw holes also might be employed to enhance anatomical reduction.
- ***Identification of the sciatic nerve***
  During a traditional SHD, we do not routinely visualize the sciatic nerve. However, in the case of acetabular fractures involving the posterior wall and/or column, we prefer to identify the course of the sciatic nerve as it can occasionally be found entrapped between posterior wall fragments and the posterior column. Identifying the sciatic nerve in this step allows us to release it from any potential entrapment and to monitor the nerve during the surgery.
- ***Exposure of the retroacetabular space***
  In the case of isolated posterior wall fractures, the retroacetabular space will often need to be exposed more fully to ensure adequate reduction and fixation. The interval between the piriformis and the superior gemellus or the interval between the inferior gemellus and obturator externus can both be used to approach the retroacetabular space. You may selectively cut either the piriformis muscle or the conjoint tendon of the obturator internus and gemelli (triceps coxae) to achieve greater exposure.
  In some cases, you may choose to reflect all the short external rotators superior to the obturator externus muscle. At this level, the medial femoral circumflex artery (MFCA) is anterior to the short external rotators, and, if the muscles are detached at least 1.5 cm to 2 cm from their insertion on the greater trochanter, the MFCA should remain well protected. The hip should be in extension and internal rotation, with the knee in approximately 60 degrees of flexion, when releasing the rotators. This puts

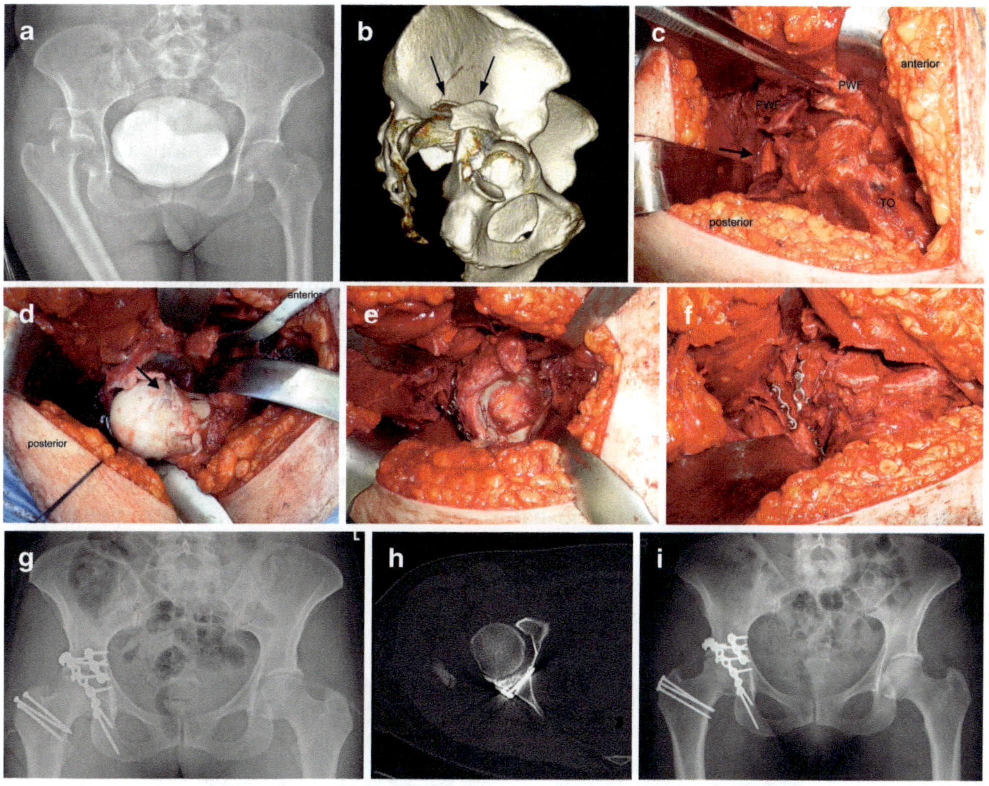

Fig. 22.3 (**a**) Trauma AP pelvis with right traumatic hip dislocation with associated posterior wall fracture (**b**) 3D surface rendered image demonstrating multi fragmentary posterior wall (**c**) Intraoperative photograph depicting trochanteric osteotomy (TO), multiple posterior wall fragments (PWF), and marginal impaction (arrow) (**d**) Surgical dislocation of femoral and demonstrating associated cartilage injury (**e**) Direct visualization of articular reduction following fixation of posterior wall (**f**) Retroacetabular surface with plate and lag screw fixation (**g**) Postoperative AP pelvis with congruent reduction (**h**) Postoperative CT to confirm reduction with confirmation of extra-articular position of the internal fixation (**i**) Radiographic follow-up at union. Congruent joint without heterotopic ossification

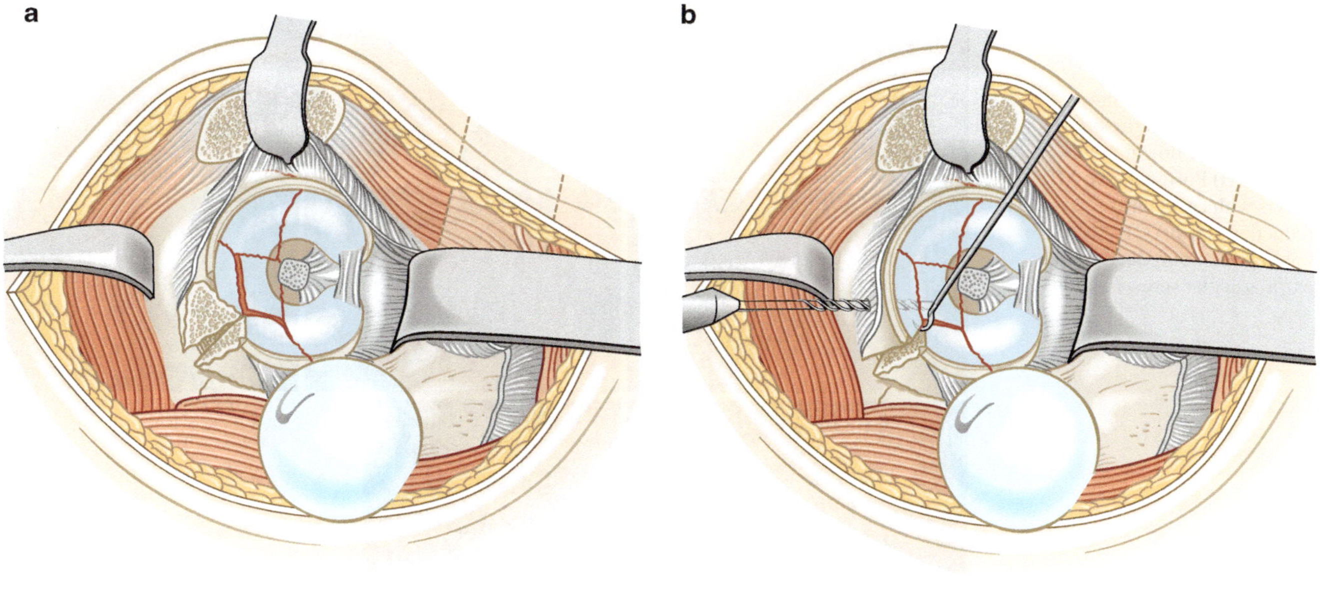

Fig. 22.4 A/B direct visualization of articular surface allowing for reduction and safe placement of internal fixation

the short external rotators under tension but relaxes the sciatic nerve. We never recommend releasing the obturator externus or quadratus femoris muscles. These muscles together protect the course of the MFCA.

- ***Capsulotomy considerations***
  The standard Z-shaped capsulotomy as described in Chap. 7 is routinely used. However, traumatic disruption of the capsule is common in these fractures, and the capsulotomy may be modified to allow for a balance between adequate exposure while preserving vascularity to the acetabular wall fragments.
- ***Evaluation of the fracture pattern following femoral head dislocation***
  With the acetabulum completely exposed, we can analyze the fracture pattern. The extent of displacement, number of free fragments, and degree of impaction can be visualized and the operative plan adjusted accordingly (Fig. 22.3a-i). The acetabular labrum, cartilage, and femoral head cartilage can also be completely assessed for damage. Labral tears may occur with or without traumatic hip dislocations. They are commonly located posteriorly and inferiorly and are predominantly associated with transverse acetabular fractures. Interestingly, acetabular chondral defects are more commonly observed in the superior region.
- ***Treatment options for traumatic injuries***
  The ultimate advantage of SHD is a full 360-degree view of both the acetabular surface and femoral head. This allows the surgeon to perform an anatomic reduction and restoration of the articular surface of the acetabulum under direct visual control, including impacted and intra-articular fragments (Fig. 22.4a, b). This also permits the surgeon to confirm extra-articular screw placement by directly visualizing the joint surface. In addition, other traumatic sequelae such as labral tears and femoral head fractures and cartilage injuries can be addressed simultaneously and under direct visualization.

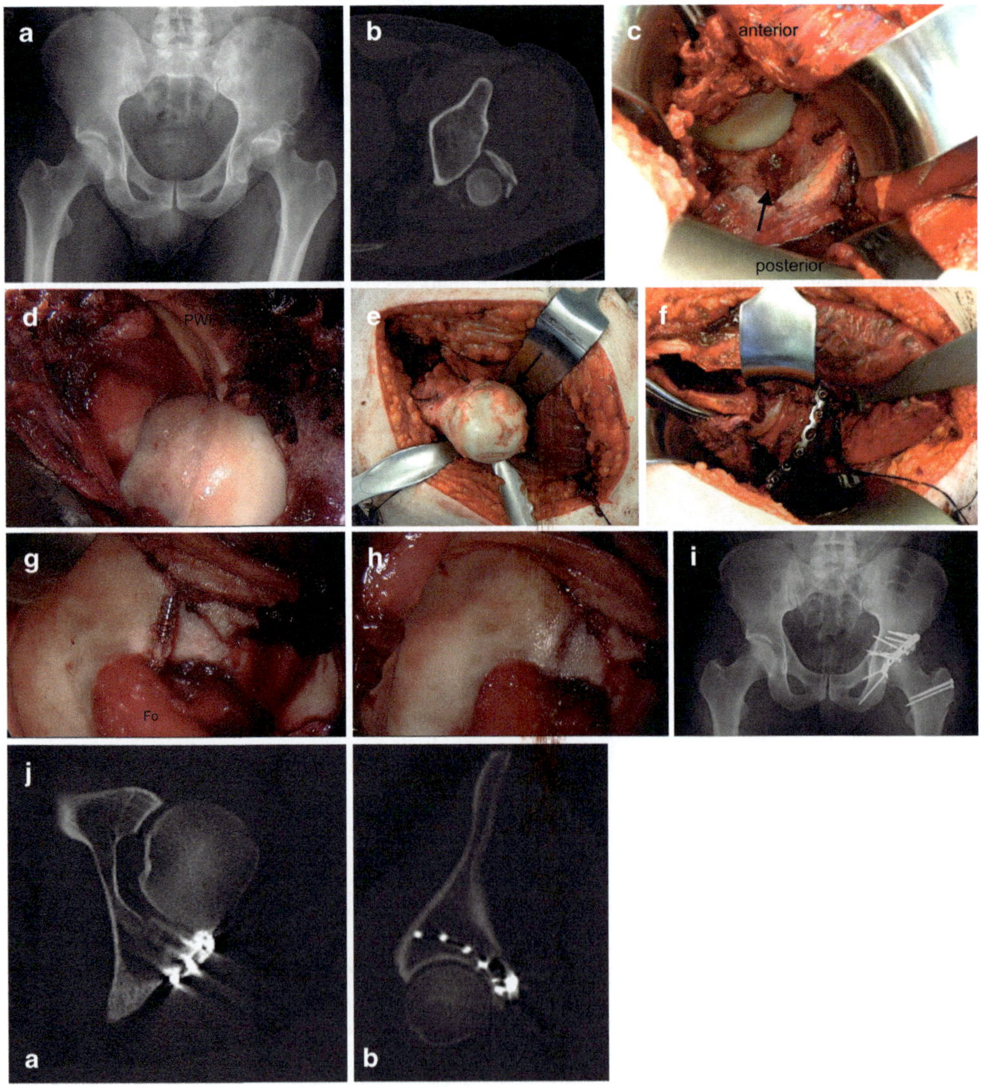

Fig. 22.5 (**a**) AP pelvis with left hip fracture dislocation. Ilioischial and iliopectineal lines are intact. This represents a posterior wall fracture (**b**) CT with head dislocated and surrounding wall fragments (**c**) Impaction of outer ilium (**d**) Dislocated femoral head into wall defect (**e**) Associated femoral head cartilage damage (**f**) Retroacetabular surface following reduction with screw and plate fixation (**g**) Inspection of the joint following fixation confirms intra-articular penetration by a screw (**h**) Following screw removal (**i**) Postoperative AP pelvis with concentric reduction (**ja**, **jb**) CT confirmation of reduction and extra-articular screw fixation

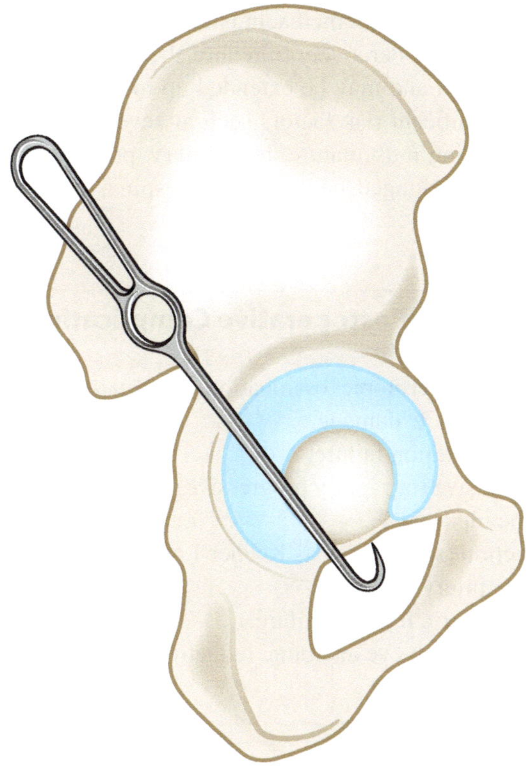

Fig. 22.6 Use of a bone hook to lateralize the ischiopubic or column segment, facilitating reduction of the acetabulum

With the hip in situ, displaced posterior column fractures can be reduced by using reduction forceps, Jungbluth clamps, or Farabeuf clamps. After preliminary fixation, the accuracy of the reduction can be evaluated with the hip dislocated and corrected if needed. Additionally, verification of extra-articular screw placement can be performed with the hip dislocated (Fig. 22.5a-j).

- For transverse and T-shaped fractures, reduction of the anterior column can be achieved with the hip dislocated by placing an elevator or bone hook under the tear drop (Fig. 22.6). Alternatively, applying a reduction clamp superiorly to the supraacetabular region and inferiorly to either the teardrop or the anterior horn of the acetabulum can help with reduction (Fig. 22.7a-c). An anterior column screw may be inserted with the hip dislocated or in situ (Fig. 22.8). This screw typically runs from the posterior aspect of the innominate bone into the anterior column or the superior pubic ramus. In this case direct visual control can again be used to confirm extra-articular screw placement.

Labral tears can be fixed with anchors following standard technique. In case of an extensive rupture, the labrum can be either resected or reconstructed. Certainly, when a labrum is repaired or reconstructed during fracture treatment, the femoral head-neck junction should be dynami-

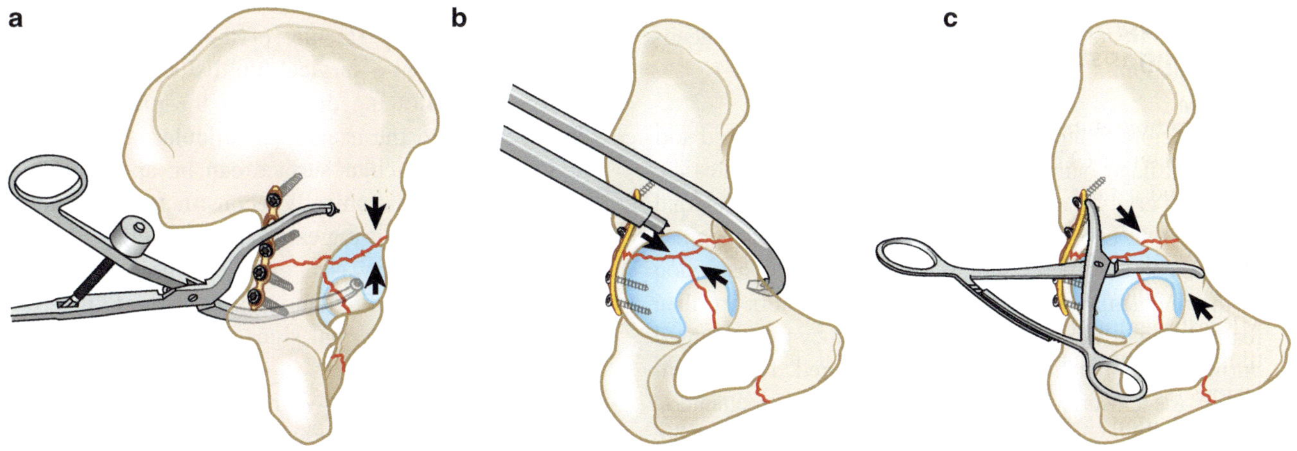

Fig. 22.7 Methods for reducing the anterior column (**a**) Angled jaw reduction forcep placed through the greater sciatic notch (**b**) Colinear clamp placed from the gluteus medius tubercle to the iliopectineal eminence (intrapelvic) (**c**) Pointed reduction forceps (Weber clamp) placed from supraacetabular bone to the superior ramus

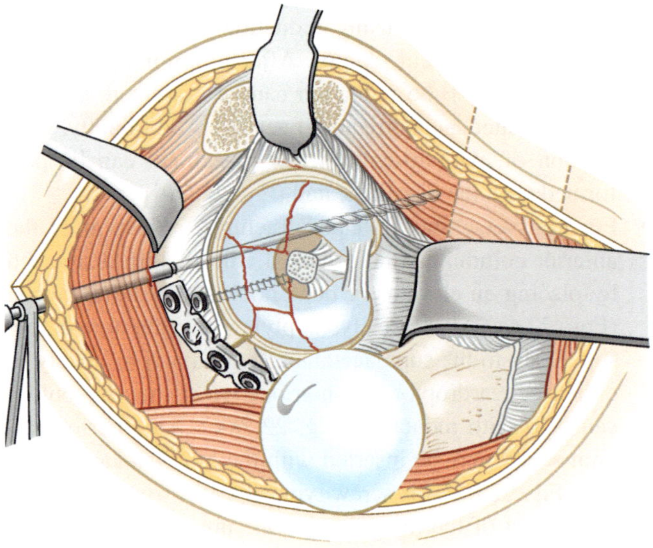

Fig. 22.8 Placement of screw into anterior column may be performed with head dislocated or safe placement of screw confirmed with dislocation

cally assessed to determine the range of motion of the hip joint after fixation. Inadequate femoral offset has been reported in approximately 20% of surgically treated acetabular fractures. A preexisting cam-type deformity can readily be treated with osteoplasty of the femoral head-neck junction.

- ***Closure***
  Once fracture fixation is complete and any associated soft tissue, cartilage, or impingement issues have been addressed, the hip is easily reduced by applying traction and internal rotation to the operative limb. The capsule is loosely approximated with absorbable sutures to prevent any constriction of the retinacular vessels. Short external rotators are then reattached with non-resorbable sutures if they were released during the approach, or traumatically injured. The remainder of the closure, including fixation of the trochanteric fragment, follows the same as for a standard surgical hip dislocation (see Chap. 7). Immediate postoperative imaging includes anteroposterior (AP) and Judet radiographs of the pelvis, as well as a postoperative CT scan.

22.13 Postoperative Follow-Up

- The patient is made 15-kg partial weight bearing for the first 8 weeks with flexion limited to 70°. In addition, continuous passive motion of the hip is used during the hospital stay. Oral indomethacin is administered for the first 2 weeks postoperatively to reduce the risk of heterotopic ossification and may be extended up to 6 weeks in cases with significant risk factors such as severe trauma to the surrounding musculature, head injury, prolonged intubation, or prolonged bed rest due to spinal cord or other injuries.

22.14 Intra-/Postoperative Complications

- Risk of heterotopic ossification, especially in cases of severe muscle damage.
- Risk of fixation failure.
- Progressive (or rapidly progressive) degenerative changes to the hip.
- Infection (similar risk as Kocher-Langenbeck approach).
- Nerve injury.
- Trochanteric fixation failure.
- Failure to achieve anatomic reduction.

22.15 Case Studies

- (Fig. 22.3a-i) A 49-year-old patient sustained an acetabular fracture dislocation following a motor vehicle accident. There was a traumatic posterior hip dislocation with a multifragmentary fracture of the posterior wall. This patient underwent a surgical hip dislocation to treat this injury, and following dislocation the precise extent of damage to both the acetabular articular surface and the femoral head articular surface can be appreciated. The injury could be anatomically reconstructed and stably fixated while also ensuring extra-articular screw placement. Follow-up at 1 year was an excellent clinical result, complete fracture healing, no formation of heterotopic ossification, and minimal signs of posttraumatic degeneration of the joint.
- (Fig. 22.5a-j) Another 49-year-old patient presented with a posterior hip dislocation and posterior wall fracture following a ski injury. Again, a surgical hip dislocation was performed to treat this injury. After exploring the hip joint for associated injuries, fixation of the posterior wall was performed. When assessing the reduction and fixation of the posterior wall, it was noted on dislocation that there was screw penetration into the acetabulum in the peri-fossa area. The location of penetration would have been difficult to assess on intraoperative fluoroscopy but was easily seen with this approach. The position of this screw was then corrected to be extra-articular.

22.16 Controversies

- No significant controversies exist in treating acetabular fractures via SHD separate from any concerns or controversies about the surgical approach itself.

22.17 Expected Outcomes

- The Bern Hip Group began performing SHD for the treatment of acetabular fractures in the mid-1990s. Cumulative 8-year survivorship without joint replacement was 89% in a report on their results with four patients requiring a total hip replacement due to progressive osteoarthritis. Radiologically, the fracture reduction was anatomic in 92.6% of all fractures. No radiological evidence of avascular necrosis of the femoral head was seen. One patient exhibited a stable, asymptomatic nonunion of the trochanteric osteotomy that did not require any surgical revision. Other surgical-related complications were observed including one superior gluteal nerve palsy, one fracture nonunion, and one secondary loss of reduction.

22.18 Outlook

- As our understanding of all the factors that contribute to long-term acceptable outcomes in the treatment of acetabular fractures grows, it becomes clear that perfect restoration of the articular surface is critical for a good outcome. In addition, as we see proportionately greater numbers of elderly patients with operative acetabular fractures, having an approach that seeks to preserve musculature, optimize fracture reduction, and provide the flexibility to pivot to arthroplasty will be a powerful tool to optimize outcomes in our patients.

Further Reading

Gupta S, Singh J, Virk JS. The role of trochanteric flip osteotomy in fixation of certain acetabular fractures. Chin J Traumatol. 2017;20(3):161–5. https://doi.org/10.1016/j.cjtee.2016.11.006.

Keel MJB, Bastian JD, Büchler L, Siebenrock KA. Surgical dislocation of the hip for a locked traumatic posterior dislocation with associated femoral neck and acetabular fractures. J Bone Joint Surg Br. 2010;92(3):442–6. https://doi.org/10.1302/0301-620X.92B3.23016.

Keel MJB, Ecker TM, Siebenrock KA, Bastian JD. Rationales for the Bernese approaches in acetabular surgery. Eur J Trauma Emerg Surg. 2012;38(5):489–98. https://doi.org/10.1007/s00068-012-0229-3.

Masse A, Aprato A, Rollero L, Bersano A, Ganz R. Surgical dislocation technique for the treatment of acetabular fractures. Clin Orthop Relat Res. 2013;471(12):4056–64. https://doi.org/10.1007/s11999-013-3228-8.

Siebenrock KA, Gautier E, Woo AKH, Ganz R. Surgical dislocation of the femoral head for joint debridement and accurate reduction of fractures of the acetabulum. J Orthop Trauma. 2002;16(8):543–52. https://doi.org/10.1097/00005131-200209000-00002.

Siebenrock KA, Keel MJB, Tannast M, Bastian JD. Surgical hip dislocation for exposure of the posterior column. JBJS Essent Surg Tech. 2019;9(1):e2. https://doi.org/10.2106/JBJS.ST.18.00048.

Tannast M, Krüger A, Mack PW, Powell JN, Hosalkar HS, Siebenrock KA. Surgical dislocation of the hip for the fixation of acetabular fractures. J Bone Joint Surg Br. 2010;92(6):842–52. https://doi.org/10.1302/0301-620X.92B6.22994.

Part 6

Tumors

Benign Tumors: In and Around the Hip Joint

23

Ira Zaltz and Hannes A. Rüdiger

23.1 Introduction

Benign intra-articular tumors affecting the hip can be locally aggressive and destructive. They can be difficult to surgically access and to excise completely while maintaining femoral head blood perfusion. Besides this biological aspect, such lesions often create mechanical conflicts within the joint. Failure to achieve complete excision risks recurrence that can affect hip joint health, patient symptoms, and function. While arthroscopic accessibility has improved substantially over the past decade, certain locations and specific types of metaplastic or neoplastic disorders may be more reliably treated using the surgical dislocation as the mode of complete access to the hip joint.

23.2 Background

The surgical hip dislocation (SHD) that was described by Ganz et al. and is an approach that provides complete access to the hip joint while preserving femoral head perfusion. Depending upon the extent of the capsulotomy, literally the entire joint is accessible while preserving the retinacular structure. Considering the treatment of benign intra-articular tumors of synovial, chondrocytic, or osteoblastic origin, not only is safe access to the joint possible, but treatment of associated chondral and labral damage can be undertaken.

I. Zaltz (✉)
Department of Orthopaedic Surgery, C.S. Mott Children's Hospital, University of Michigan, Ann Arbor, MI, USA
e-mail: zaltz@med.umich.edu

H. A. Rüdiger
Hip Service, Department of Orthopedics, Zürich, Switzerland
e-mail: Hannes.Ruediger@kws.ch

23.3 Indications

The indication to utilize SHD to treat intra-articular tumors is dependent upon accurate preoperative diagnosis and precise tumor staging. In general, malignant lesions, whether primary or metastatic are not treated using a SHD due to multicompartment dissection and the risk of iatrogenic cellular contamination and tumor spread. Benign localized or benign aggressive tumors, however, can be safely approached using a surgical dislocation because the extensile approach provides extensive intra-articular and extra-articular access enabling complete tumor excision and treatment of any associated chondral lesions.

23.4 Preoperative/Preinterventional Diagnostics

Benign tumors have characteristic radiographic appearances that generally enable accurate diagnosis and a biopsy is rarely needed (see also Chap. 3). While a complete discussion of the radiographic and MRI appearances of the variety of intra-articular masses is beyond the scope of this chapter, it is essential to emphasize that surgical planning is predicated upon an accurate diagnosis. Failure to accurately diagnose the type of tumor can lead to devastating and potentially life-threatening consequences. Once the diagnosis of a benign intra-articular tumor is established, appropriate management can be planned. Since many benign tumors can lead to advanced cartilage damage and secondary osteoarthritis, it is essential to establish that the articular cartilage is sufficiently preserved or potentially treatable prior to undertaking treatment. Additionally, those tumors that substantially weaken the structural integrity of the femoral head or neck may require mechanical stabilization, and appropriate graft, synthetic or natural, and properly sized implants must be planned preoperatively.

M. Leunig et al. (eds.), *Surgical Hip Dislocation*, https://doi.org/10.1007/978-3-031-70622-6_23

The variety of tumors that may affect the hip include the following:

1. Synovial origin tumors (synovial chondromatosis, pigmented villonodular synovitis, giant cell tumor)
2. Chondrocytic origin (chondroblastoma, osteochondroma/cartilaginous exostosis)
3. Osteocytic origin (osteoblastoma, osteoid osteoma, osteochondroma, dysplasia epiphysealis hemimelica)
4. Vascular origin (simple bone cysts, aneurysmal bone cyst)

The general indication for removal of a benign tumor is dependent upon the type and location. Most patients present primarily with pain or limitation of movement. Suspicion of a tumor is based upon the patient's symptoms and the preoperative plain radiographic assessment of the hip joint. Advanced imaging studies include magnetic resonance imaging and CT scanning that are both essential to diagnosis and staging of the tumor, depending upon the tissue type being evaluated. MRI is usually adequate to the diagnosis and staging of the tumor, as well as to assess the quality of the articular cartilage and labral tissue. CT may be necessary to define anatomically the shape and location of osseous masses or bone cysts as well as to assess their precise size, location, and dimensions. In selected cases an angio-CT may help to better understand the anatomical relation of the lesion with the medial circumflex artery (which may be displaced by the tumor). In addition, CT scanning can help with preoperative diagnosis in specific types of tumors.

23.5 Preoperative Planning/Computer Modeling

Two principles of preoperative planning are necessary when evaluating and planning treatment for patients with nonmalignant intra-articular tumors. First, an accurate diagnosis is essential prior to planning treatment. Since most benign-type tumors have unique MRI and plain radiographic and CT scanning appearance, the diagnosis is usually certain. The precise radiographic findings unique to each tumor are beyond the extent of this chapter; however, it is absolutely mandatory to establish an accurate diagnosis prior to planning a treatment. In rare cases a biopsy is necessary to establish the diagnosis. Planning and execution of the biopsy should be performed under the guidance of specialized orthopedic tumor surgeon. Care has to be taken to keep biopsy track contamination limited in case the lesion turns out malignant. Second, understanding the anatomical location and distribution is needed to plan the surgical approach and excision of the tumor. Some tumors are localized, and access is straightforward, while others can be diffusely spread and localized both inside and outside of the hip joint capsule or in close proximity to the nourishing vessels of the femoral head. Surgical planning, specifically the extent of the capsulotomy and any necessary extra-articular dissection, is dependent upon proper preoperative imaging analysis.

An alternate strategy for classification of benign lesions is based upon anatomic location and helps to determine the surgical strategy:

1. Synovial disorders (e.g., chondromatosis, Pigmented villonodular synovitis (PVNS))
2. Intraosseous lesions (e.g., giant cell tumor of bone or aneurysmal bone cysts)
3. Cortical-based lesions (e.g., exostosis, osteoid osteoma)

23.6 Applied Anatomy

Proper execution of the SHD is dependent upon understanding the skeletal, muscular, neurologic, and vascular anatomy of the proximal femur and hip joint. Specifically, the applied anatomy of the medial femoral circumflex artery (Chap. 6) is essential to performing safe exposure and excision of benign tumors or performing a synovectomy. As certain tissue types, especially synovial origin tumors, can spread diffusely, understanding the location and arborization of the medial femoral circumflex is crucial. In cases of posterior extra-articular spread of the tumor, it is important to understand the anatomy of the sciatic nerve and the extra-articular course of the medial femoral circumflex artery. In cases of anterior extra-articular spread, understanding the location of the femoral nerve and artery will avoid injury, and when the tumor is localized inferior and distal to the hip joint, both the medial femoral circumflex artery and the obturator artery and nerve may be at risk of injury.

23.7 Specific Risks

There are three risks specifically associated with excision of benign intra-articular tumors. First, incomplete tumor excision can lead to recurrence, or persistence of a mechanical conflict (e.g., exostosis). Second, iatrogenic neurovascular injury can lead to osteonecrosis of the femoral head, or paralysis of muscles innervated by the obturator, femoral, or sciatic nerve. Third, when advanced chondral damage is present at the time of tumor excision, pain relief may be inadequate, or the patient can develop significant hip stiffness.

Other risks are generically associated with the SHD and include heterotopic ossification, trochanteric nonunion, and infection.

23.8 Type of Anesthesia

Most SHDs are performed under general anesthesia. Spinal anesthetic and continuous epidural anesthetics can also be utilized depending upon specific medical or anatomic reasons specific to individual patients.

Some centers utilized preoperative regional anesthesia useful for postoperative pain management. These blocks include preoperative fascia iliaca, femoral nerve, sciatic nerve, and intraoperative field blocks.

23.9 Positioning

The patient is positioned in the lateral decubitus position with an axillary role placed beneath the contralateral chest and adequate padding used for the ipsilateral peroneal nerve. The patient should be held in place with a positioner that is familiar to the surgeon. It is crucial that adequate exposure of the hip is not limited by positioning.

23.10 Instruments/Implants

The instruments that are required to perform a SHD are described in detail in Chap. 7 and include an oscillating saw, osteotomes, and screws for fixation of the trochanter. Instruments that are unique to tumor excisions include an assortment of rongeurs, curettes, and burrs. In special circumstances, ablative devices may be required including laser devices or chemicals such as phenol or dehydrated ethanol. In addition, grafting materials such as cancellous allograft or synthetic substances such as calcium sulfate and calcium phosphate may be necessary to fill voids remaining after tumor excision.

23.11 Access

The hip joint is accessed via a transtrochanteric approach (Chap. 7). Due to extra-articular spread of certain tumors, periarticular dissection may be necessary prior to performing an arthrotomy. Regardless of direction of spread, the entire hip joint and surrounding structures are safely accessible using the SHD. Preoperative imaging and accurate anatomic staging are essential for preoperative planning. Extra-articular tumor extension is commonly associated with synovial-based tumors, and complete excision minimizes the risk of recurrence. Therefore, careful radiographic study is needed prior to planning the procedure.

23.12 Technical Steps

The steps for the SHD are described in Chap. 7. Pertinent to benign tumor excision, the periarticular dissection must be performed meticulously based upon the preoperative radiographic staging. Since marginal excision of a benign tumors will enable complete removal, it is important to carefully dissect around the tumor prior to violating the capsule of the mass in order to minimize the risk of tissue contamination. If the tumor is contained within the hip, a standard Z-shaped arthrotomy will permit access to most of the hip joint. In unique circumstances, a circumferential capsulotomy may be necessary so that the posterior femur and posterior capsule can be completely accessed. In cases where a complete capsulotomy is required, the standard Z-shaped capsulotomy is performed, and then the remaining posterior and inferior capsule can be safely divided using an "inside-out" approach such that the posterior and inferior capsule are dissected using a right-angled instrument and then divided using either a scalpel or cautery. To access posterior and posterior-inferior parts of the capsule, excessive adduction should be avoided (a cushion underneath the distal thigh may help).

Management of intraepiphyseal, intraosseous, and periretinacular tumors require special consideration on an individualized basis. Chondroblastoma, the only intraepiphyseal tumor is managed by excision; however, reconstruction is based upon the location within the epiphysis. Those inferior to the fovea can be grafted using either autograft or allograft. Those superior to the fovea, especially when a large part of the articular cartilage may be involved, can be reconstructed using various techniques depending upon the precise size and location of the articular defect. Options include OATS grafting, autografting with (sandwich), Autologous matrix-induced chondrogenesis (AMIC), free osteoarticular allograft, or redirecting femoral osteotomy. Other tumors such as osteoid osteoma or osteoblastoma may be located very close to the vascular retinaculum making the risk of thermal ablation-associated osteonecrosis excessive. It such cases, retinacular damage can be avoided by careful marginal excision or by mobilizing the retinaculum (Chap. 8) in order to safely access the lesion.

Similarly, intraosseous lesions in the neck can be accessed using a SHD. Depending upon the size and location of the lesion, in addition to intralesional grafting, supplemental prophylactic fixation may be necessary to minimize the risk of fracture. The type of fixation is beyond the scope of this text; however, the surgeon must plan the optimal type of fixation. When using a SHD, the entire femur is accessible for application of fixation plates. Prophylactic fixation should only be applied after complete removal of the lesion to avoid spreading of neoplastic tissue.

23.13 Postoperative Follow-Ups

Postoperative radiographic follow-up is required to monitor trochanteric and lesion consolidation in the immediate postoperative period. In certain cases, CT scanning or MRI may be necessary to follow the patient for resolution of the lesion or recurrence of soft tissue growth.

23.14 Intra-/Postoperative Complications

Generally, the SHD is safe and there are few complications. In certain cases of biochemically active tumors (osteoid osteoma), more diffuse bleeding might occur during the approach. There are specific complications that may occur in association with tumor excision including iatrogenic fracture and osteonecrosis. Fracture can occur if an intraosseous femoral neck lesion is large during exposure and mobilization or while treating the lesion. To prevent fractures in large lesions, prophylactic fixation prior to exposure might be required. Osteonecrosis may occur in association with treatment of lesions that are located within the lateral epiphysis or deep to the retinaculum. In theory, retinacular damage can occur during mobilization or lesion removal or following thermal or chemical treatment of lesions in close proximity to the vasculature. Prevention by intimate knowledge of the anatomy and meticulous mobilization of the retinaculum is best. There are certain intraepiphyseal tumors that may pose great risk especially if located immediately adjacent to the entry zone of the retinacular vessels. If larger areas of cancellous bone is exposed, postoperative capsule-osseous adhesions need to be avoided by immediate hip motion postoperatively (Continuous passive motion (CPM)).

23.15 Case Study

Case 1: A 35-year-old female was referred with suspected FAI. Plain X-ray showed ossifications of the acetabular rim and around the fossa (Fig. 23.1a, b). Arthro MRI revealed a borderline pincer-type FAI with a small cam deformity and multiple small free bodies mainly in the fossa, while the cartilage appeared intact (Fig. 23.1c, d). A subsequent CT scan showed multiple chondromas with calcifications in line with a synovial chondromatosis (Fig. 23.1e, f). As an extensive synovectomy was necessary but difficult to perform arthroscopically, a surgical hip dislocation was performed using the technique described in Chap. 7. Multiple free bodies were removed and ossifications around the fossa were trimmed. FAI treatment included trimming of the lateral and anterior acetabular wall, removal of the ossified labrum, and contouring of the head-neck junction (Fig. 23.1g, h). A subtotal synovectomy was performed. Histological analysis revealed a synovial metaplasia in line with a synovial chondromatosis. The trochanteric screws were removed 9 months after surgery (Fig. 23.1j). The patient fully recovered and was pain-free at 1 year after surgery.

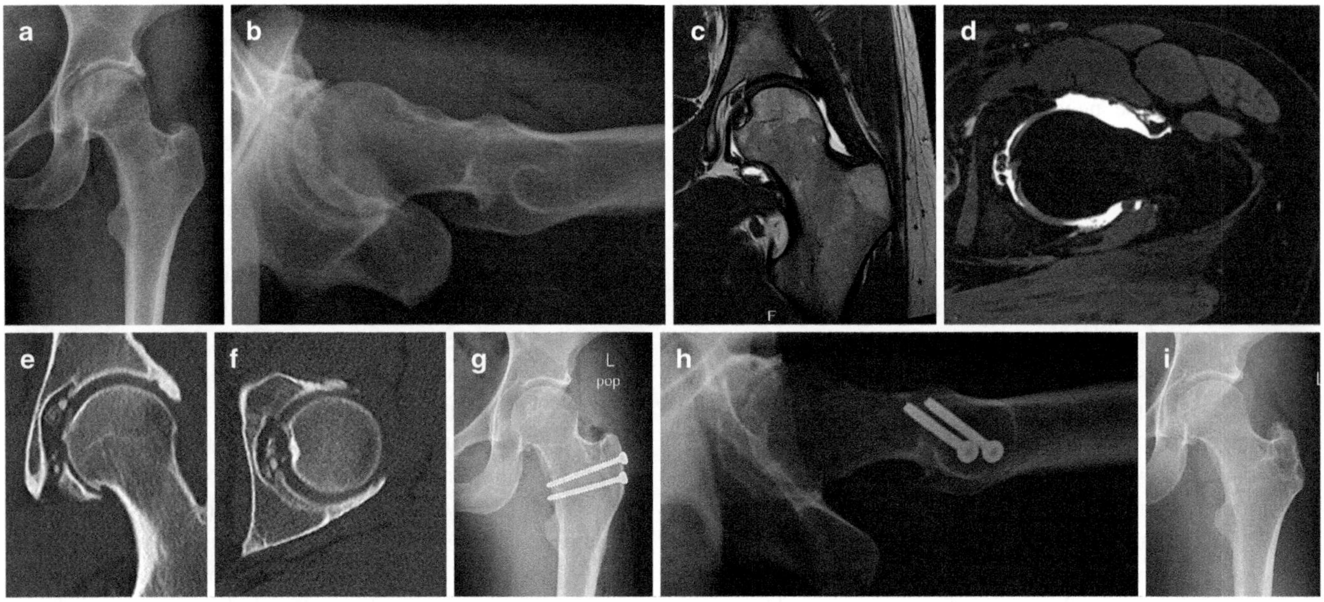

Fig. 23.1 (**a**, **b**) Case 1: Plain AP and cross-table axial views showing ossification of the acetabular rim and around the fossa and s slight cam deformity, (**c**, **d**) Case 1: MR-arthrography reveals free bodies in the fossa and a cam deformity, (**e**, **f**) Case 1: CT scans shows freed bodies with calcifications in line with the diagnosis of a synovial chondromatosis, (**g**, **h**) Case 1: SHD was performed with extensive synovectomy, trimming of the acetabular rim, and resection of the cam deformity, (**i**) Case 1: Nine months after surgery, the trochanteric screws were removed

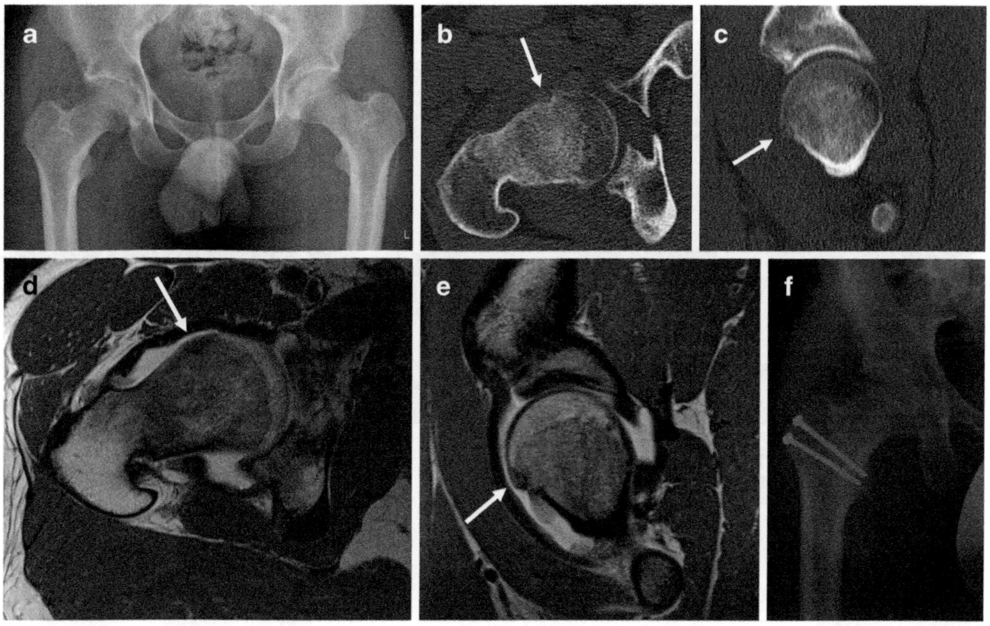

Fig. 23.2 (**a**) Case 2: Plain AP pelvic view without significant impingement configuration, (**b-e**) Case 2: CT and MRI show typical signs of a nidus of an osteoid osteoma with a lytic cortical lesion of less than 1 cm in diameter and a central calcification, (**f**) Case 2: The nidus was removed trough a SHD

Case 2: A 22-year-old male presented with pain in his right hip. Pain increased with activity but was also present at night and was effectively treated with aspirin. Despite some clinical suspicion, there were minimal signs of a femoroacetabular impingement on plane radiographs (Fig. 23.2a). On CT scan there was a nidus with a typical central calcification anterolateral at the head-neck junction (Fig. 23.2b, c). MRI showed significant joint effusion and the presence of a nidus was confirmed. Based on these images, the diagnosis of an osteoid osteoma was established (Fig. 23.2d, e). A surgical hip dislocation was performed as described in Chap. 7 (Fig. 23.2f), the nidus was removed together with reactive synovia, and the femoral offset was improved using a high-speed burr. The patient was pain-free within a few weeks.

Case 3: A 14-year-old boy presented with typical signs of anterior hip impingement. Internal rotation, particularly in flexion, was very limited and painful. Plain radiographs and a CT scan revealed an exostosis just anterior to the lesser trochanter with open femoral and acetabular physis (Fig. 23.3a, b). MRI showed an intact cartilage and only a minimal cartilage cap on the cartilaginous exostosis with a thin pseudobursa covering the lesions. There were no signs of malignancy (Fig. 23.3c). A classic surgical hip dislocation was performed, and the exostosis was resected to correct the mechanical conflict (Fig. 23.3d, e). Due to the large base of the exostosis, involving the anterior part of the calcar and due to the fact that it was a young and active patient, a screw was placed along the calcar for reinforcement to avoid a neck fracture during recovery. All screws were removed 12 months after surgery (Fig. 23.3f, g). The patient did fully recover and was pain-free thereafter.

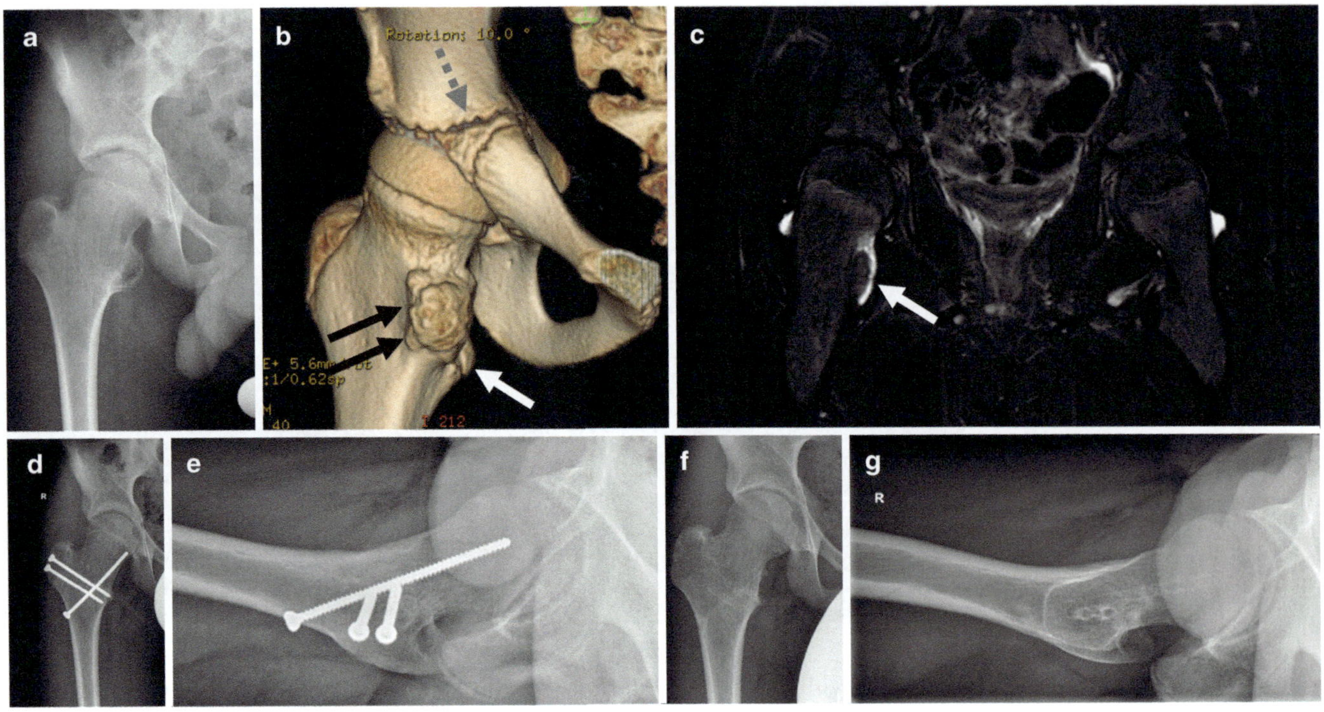

Fig. 23.3 (**a**, **b**) Case 3: Plain AP view and a 3D CT reconstruction showing an exostosis (black double arrows) anterior to the lesser trochanter (white arrow). The acetabular physis are still open (grey dotted arrow), (**c**) Case 3: MRI shows a cartilaginous exostosis with a thin cartilage cap (white arrow), which is covered by a thin pseudobursa. The articular cartilage is intact, (**d**, **e**) Case 3: SHD was performed to resect the exostosis. An additional screw was inserted to reinforce the cortical defect at the femoral neck, (**f**, **g**) Case 3: Twelve months postoperatively, all screws have been removed. The patient was pain free with a normal hip function

23.16 Controversies

There are many approaches to the treatment of benign upper femoral and intra-articular tumors of the hip. This chapter is not meant to be authoritative regarding tumor excision, merely a guide to one surgical approach for treatment. Surgeons who routinely treat such patients have comprehensive training, experience, and judgment. Those surgeons who elect a SHD for access and exposure can utilize this chapter as a guide.

23.17 Expected Outcomes

The ideal outcome following tumor excision is to prevent recurrence and to restore normal hip anatomy and function. The major preoperative determinants of postoperative outcomes are mechanically significant deformities of the hip joint and chondral damage. The outcomes associated with cartilage damage are variable and dependent upon patient age, location, extent, and severity of cartilage damage.

23.18 Future Direction

The benefits of the SHD include complete access the hip joint, periarticular structure, and the entire femur, access to the articular surfaces, and the ability to perform simultaneous tumor excision and reconstructive procedure. There are many other methods used to treat tumors, and future studies will elucidate the benefits of each approach for the management of selected upper femoral tumors.

Further Reading

Ganz R, Gill TJ, Gautier E, Ganz K, Krugel N, Berlemann U. Surgical dislocation of the adult hip a technique with full access to the femoral head and acetabulum without the risk of avascular necrosis. J Bone Joint Surg Br. 2001;83(8):1119–24.

Jellicoe P, Son-Hing J, Hopyan S, Thompson GH. Surgical hip dislocation for removal of intraarticular exostoses: report of two cases. J Pediatr Orthop. 2009;29(4):327–30. https://doi.org/10.1097/BPO.0b013e3181a56b4f.

Mainzer J, Ganz R, Tibor L, Leunig M. Not all hip pain is impingement: femoral neck osteoid Osteoma in a patient with a coexisting cam deformity: a case report. JBJS Case Connect. 2012;2(3):e31. https://doi.org/10.2106/JBJS.CC.K.00101.

Nisar A, Gulhane S, Mahendra A, Meek RM, Patil S. Surgical dislocation of the hip for excision of benign tumours. J Orthop. 2014;11(1):28–36.

Ralf Schoeniger, Douglas D R Naudie, Klaus A Siebenrock, Robert T Trousdale, Reinhold Ganz. Modified complete synovectomy prevents recurrence in synovial chondromatosis of the hip. Clin Orthop Relat Res 2006451:195–200. doi: https://doi.org/10.1097/01.blo.0000229280.53109.d5.

Rego P, Mascarenhas V, Collado D, Coelho A, Barbosa L, Ganz R. Arterial topographic anatomy near the femoral head-neck perforation with surgical relevance. J Bone Joint Surg Am. 2017;99(14):1213–21. https://doi.org/10.2106/JBJS.16.01386.

Rüdiger HAPK, Becce F, Cherix ST. Trans-Foveal approach for curettage and bone grafting of a Giant cell tumour in the femoral head. Hip Int. 2016;26(6):612–4.

Part 7

Total Hip Replacement

24 Transtrochanteric Approach for Primary Total Hip Replacement

Paul E. Beaulé and Hannes A. Rüdiger

24.1 Introduction

With less invasive surgical approaches being used in the majority of primary total hip replacement (THR) today, the trochanteric osteotomy remains a very useful technique in selected and often complex cases. The currently most widely used technique follows largely that of the surgical hip dislocation (SHD) (Chap. 7), which is mostly used in joint preservation surgery. The initial tenet of the trochanteric osteotomy was leaving the attachments of the gluteus medius and minimus to the trochanter. English later modified it by leaving the vastus lateralis attached to the osteotomized fragment while staying extracapsular. As the abductors are retracted anteriorly, this approach allows for an excellent exposure of both the acetabular and the femoral side even in presence of very contract soft tissues or in cases with extremely narrow pelvic-trochanteric clearance. As perfusion of the femoral head and neck is preserved, it may prevent early femoral bone resorption in hip resurfacings or if neck-preserving stems are used.

While the technique allows for advancement of the greater trochanter (e.g., distalization), solid fixation of the trochanteric fragment is pivotal to avoid secondary dislocation of the fragment or pseudarthrosis. Such complications are often cumbersome to treat.

P. E. Beaulé (✉)
University of Ottawa, Ottawa, Canada

Division of Orthopedic Surgery, Hawkesbury and District General Hospital, Hawkesbury, Canada
e-mail: pbeaule@toh.ca

H. A. Rüdiger
Hip Service, Department of Orthopedics, Zürich, Switzerland
e-mail: Hannes.Ruediger@kws.ch

24.2 Background

The classic trochanteric osteotomy was first described by Ollier in 1891 [1] and used by Charnley for THR [2]. In this classic technique, the gluteus medius and minimus muscle remain with the trochanteric fragment. As this osteotomy does exit the trochanter proximal to the vastus ridge, the vastus lateralis remains untouched and attached to the femoral shaft. In 1975, English [3] provided a review of the current techniques of trochanteric osteotomies where he described the preservation of the vastus lateralis attachment to the trochanteric fragment so that the upward pull of the gluteal muscles would be balanced thus minimizing the risk of nonunion. Later, Courpied et al. [4] refined the technique emphasizing the need to preserve the attachment of the short external rotators to the shaft of the femur, while the piriformis tendon is left attached to the trochanteric fragment. Ganz et al. [5] recognized the merits of this approach both from a soft tissue and vascular standpoint and modified it by leaving the piriformis attached to the femoral shaft and limiting the distal extension of the osteotomy to the vastus lateralis ridge. This approach is now known as the surgical hip dislocation (SHD).

24.3 Indications

The transtrochanteric technique, which follows largely the technique for SHD (Chap. 7) provides a wide exposure to the proximal femur and acetabulum while minimizing the risk of damage to neurovascular structures and thus preserves the vascularity to the femoral head.

24.3.1 Indications

- In young adults, with advanced cartilage damage with uncertainty regarding the potential for joint preservation. The decision to either go for joint preservation or arthroplasty can be made intraoperatively.

M. Leunig et al. (eds.), *Surgical Hip Dislocation*, https://doi.org/10.1007/978-3-031-70622-6_24

- A high-riding trochanter with equal leg length with potential pelvi-trochanteric impingement after THR (e.g., Perthes deformities).

24.3.2 Relative Indications

- Severe acetabular protrusion with significant soft tissue contractures and minimal pelvic-trochanteric clearance
- Takedown of a hip fusion
- Hip resurfacing to provide sufficient femoral head and neck vascularity
- Cases of severe heterotopic ossification (Brooker IV) both anterior and posterior to the joint

24.3.3 Contraindications

- Poor bone quality (osteoporosis)
- Severe tendon rupture with advanced fatty degeneration of the abductor muscles

24.4 Preoperative/Pre-interventional Diagnostics

History of previous hip surgery is critical. If a transgluteal (Hardinge type) approach has been used previously, the vitality of the trochanter and/or the abductor apparatus may be impaired. Previous proximal femoral osteotomies may have impaired the bony integrity of the trochanter.

On physical exam, determining abductor function as well as range of motion and previous incisions is important.

On radiographs, one must look at retained internal fixation, bone stock on the acetabular side, deformity of the femur, and finally quality of the bone. Computer tomography can also be helpful to examine if retained fixation blocks the femoral canal as well as determining hip center of rotation. MRI may help to assess soft tissue quality of the abductors. Both computer tomography and MRI allow quantification of femoral torsion, which is often abnormal in these complex cases.

24.5 Preoperative Templating/Computer Modeling

Preoperative templating is essential. Femoral and acetabular centers of rotation are templated as well as approximate implant sizes. In most cases standard primary implants should be considered. In case the femoral torsion needs to be substantially corrected, a cylindric or conic stem as well as a cemented stem can be used. If bone stock is poor, a primary cemented stem may be indicated. It is however important to avoid that cement is pushed between the trochanteric fragment and the femur as this will greatly reduce the chances for bony consolidation. Finally, hip stability can be an issue so that dual mobility options should be available.

24.6 Applied Anatomy

For basic anatomy, see Chaps. 6 and 7. In cases of previous surgery around the trochanter, local soft tissue anatomy might however be significantly altered. In such cases, proximal or distal extension of the approach might aid in identifying anatomical structures.

24.7 Special Risks

Size, thickness, and bony quality of trochanteric fragment which could affect fixation and union of the osteotomy need to be considered when planning a transtrochanteric technique. Insufficient fixation of the fragment (wires or cables are not tightened, screws are not bicortical) and the risk of creating a stress riser by putting screws too close to one another are common pitfalls. Osteopenic or even osteoporotic bone particularly in women, long-standing osteoarthritis (OA), and large abductor tendon ruptures with fatty degeneration are risks for nonunion. Similarly, sclerotic bone after previous surgeries can impact the healing process. In addition, especially when performing hip resurfacing, one can damage the major branch of the medial femoral circumflex artery by exiting the osteotomy intracapsularly proximally. This occurs either by performing the osteotomy too angled toward the femoral neck or creating too thick of a trochanteric fragment. If the osteotomy runs anterior to the piriformis tendon footprint, leaving the tendon attached to the femur, the risk of damaging the perfusion of the femoral head/neck is minimal.

24.8 Type of Anesthesia

While spinal anesthesia is possible, we do prefer general anesthesia. First, it is important to attain full muscle paralysis. Second, the procedure is performed in lateral decubitus position and usually takes more than 90 minutes. Third, these patients are typically children and adolescents.

24.9 Positioning

Although transtrochanteric technique using SHD for THR was initially described in the supine position, most patients would be placed in the lateral decubitus position using a supporting pillow (Chap. 7). As the dislocated hip is placed in external rotation and flexion, the lower leg is placed in a bag attached to the side of the operating table to keep the foot sterile.

24.10 Instruments/Implants

Standard instrumentation for SHD is used (see Chap. 7). In addition to the instruments required for the SHD, wires or cables or screws have to be available. We prefer 4.5 mm over 3.5 mm screws for better stability and smaller risk of screws breakage. In very small bones however, 3.5 mm screws may be preferred.

Depending on the type of THR, specific reamer and broaches are required. A high-speed burr might be advisable to contour the trochanteric fragment against the shoulder of the prosthetic stem.

24.11 Access

As mentioned above the incision is mostly longitudinal and centered over the greater trochanter splitting the iliotibial band distally and tensor fascia proximally between maximus and tensor muscle. This is followed by identifying the vastus tubercle as well as the anterior and posterior aspects of the greater trochanter. At this point one can elect to do a trochanteric slide leaving the vastus lateralis attachment to the trochanter intact as described by English or do a trans-trochanteric osteotomy as described by Ollier, which we do not really perform anymore.

24.12 Technical Steps

The technique follows largely the standard technique of SHD (Chap. 7) originally described by Ganz et al [5].

The posterior aspect of the vastus lateralis muscle is identified and elevated subperiosteally off the femur, close to its attachment on the greater trochanter. A narrow Hohman is placed anteriorly on the femur underneath the vastus lateralis. Next, the piriformis tendon is identified (i.e., the interval between the piriformis tendon and the posterior border of the gluteus minimus muscle). It is important not to dissect soft tissues distal to the piriformis tendon to avoid damage to the medial circumflex artery or its anastomosis from the superior gluteal artery which could affect femoral head perfusion. Using a thin oscillating saw blade, the trochanteric fragment is freed and mobilized in posterior to anterior direction where the leg should be placed in slight internal rotation to ensure an even thickness cut. Leaving a small cuff of gluteus medius tendon attached to the stable part of the posterior trochanter ensures that the attachment of the piriformis tendon remains intact. A step cut may help to later reduce the trochanteric fragment anatomically, which required that no trochanteric advancement is performed (Chap. 12). Likewise, the anterior cortex might be divided by a controlled fracture rather than by saw to increase stability of the trochanteric refixation at the end. The osteotomized fragment is mobilized anteriorly with the gluteus medius and minimus tendons and the vastus lateralis attached to it while bringing the leg in flexion and external rotation, allowing exposure of the anterior hip capsule. Anterior capsulotomy is then performed in a Z or H shape, depending on the expected complexity on the acetabular side. The hip is then dislocated and the femoral neck is cut according to the templating. Meanwhile, the leg is placed in a sterile bag attached to the side of the table. THR components are then implanted.

Solid reattachment of the fragment in the correct position is pivotal. Depending on the case, a repositioning of the fragment may be necessary (e.g., more distal). We generally prefer fixation of the trochanteric fragment with two 4.5 mm steel screws. Usually both screws pass posteriorly of the femoral stem and are aimed toward the lesser trochanter. It is important to have good bicortical purchase of both screws.

Alternatively, wires or cables may be used for trochanteric fixation in complex cases with trochanteric advancement. The downside of this technique is that the medial and lateral circumflex arteries are usually strangled, which may be a problem if a resurfacing prosthesis or a neck-preserving stem is used. While various fixation techniques have been described, we generally use a "belt and suspenders" technique. Simple "Figure of Eight" wire fixation lacks rotational stability and should be avoided. Claw plates are rarely necessary in the primary setting.

24.13 Postoperative Follow-up

An immediate postoperative X-ray (and/or pre-discharge after ambulation) is indispensable. Postoperative partial weight-bearing and a flexion limit of 70° depending on fixation of the trochanteric osteotomy is advised.

Sufficient consolidation of the trochanter can be expected earliest after 6 weeks, in women or patients with long-standing OA after 8+ weeks; strengthening of the abductor muscles should not begin before that time. An X-ray is taken 6 to 8 weeks postop to assess for trochanteric union. Removal of the trochanteric screws may be performed not earlier than 6 to 12 months postoperatively, if necessary.

24.14 Intra-/Postoperative Complications

Although quite popular in the early era of hip replacement surgery, the trochanteric osteotomy is no longer used in standard primary hip arthroplasty and reserved for selected and mostly complex cases. This is due to the delayed rehab process, nonunions of the trochanteric osteotomy, and need for removal of painful internal fixation, this combined with poor rate of healing.

Intraoperative complications include wrong sizing of the trochanteric fragment, fracture of the trochanteric fragment, mal-reduction, and suboptimal/insufficient hardware placement. Postoperatively, irritation due to fixation hardware, nonunion, and secondary migration of the trochanteric fragment may occur. To minimize this risk, we cannot emphasize enough the importance of the thickness of the trochanteric fragment to ensure that fixation purchase is reliable.

24.15 Case Studies

24.15.1 Case 1 (Fig. 24.1)

A 44-year-old former competitive hammer thrower presented with a short acetabular roof (LCE 20°) and painful osteoarthritis of his right hip. Due to incapacitating pain and the advanced cartilage damage, a hip resurfacing was performed with a trochanteric osteotomy at that time using the Birmingham prosthesis (Smith & Nephew). At 12 years the patient is still pain-free with normal metal ion level, and there are no signs of loosening or femoral neck resorption. This indicates that bone perfusion at the medial femoral neck is still intact.

24.15.2 Case 2 (Fig. 24.2)

This 34-year-old female underwent multiple joint-preserving procedures for femoral dysplasia and torsional malalignment including two initial hip arthroscopies followed by a periacetabular osteotomy and a subtrochanteric grafting and stabilization of a fibrous dysplasia in the subtrochanteric region. Despite all these interventions, she continued to suffer from pain requiring crutches. Despite the joint space narrowing of the left hip, MRI showed only mild cartilage damage but a considerable joint effusion. Another joint-preserving surgery (treatment of residual impingement and cartilage lesions) was balanced against THR. A SHD was performed to allow for both options, depending on the intraoperative

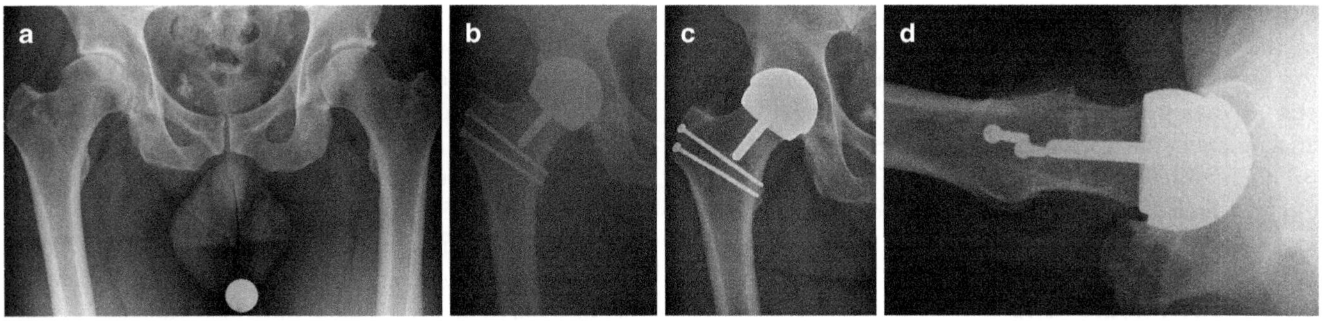

Fig. 24.1 (**a**) Preoperative osteoarthritis of the right hip of a 44-year-old male, (**b**) Postoperative (Day 0) X-ray. To conserve blood supply to the femoral head/neck, a SHD was performed to implant a hip resurfacing prosthesis, (**c**, **d**) 10 years postoperatively no loosening or bone resorption is noted an plain AP and cross-table axial views. (Courtesy of Michael Leunig)

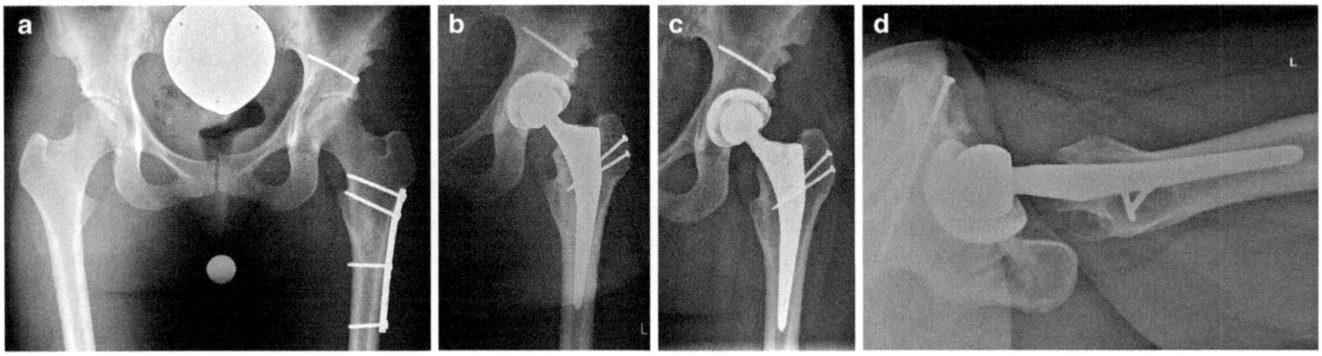

Fig. 24.2 (**a**) Pelvic AP view of a 34-year-old female after periacetabular osteotomy and curettage, bone grafting and plating of fibrous dysplasia in the subtrochanteric region, (**b**) Due to only mild cartilage damage on the MRI, a SHD was performed and the joint intraoperatively evaluated. On intraoperative visual evaluation, degenerative changes were more extensive than expected, and it was opted to perform a THR rather than joint-preserving procedures (Day 0), (**c**, **d**) At 1-year postop, the prosthesis was fully integrated, the trochanteric osteotomy consolidated, and the patient subjectively significantly improved. (Courtesy of Michael Leunig)

findings. Joint inspections revealed advanced cartilage damage on the femoral side and superficial alterations on the acetabular cartilage. It was decided at this point to implant a total hip prosthesis.

24.16 Controversies

Due to the technical complexity and the specific set of complications due to the trochanteric osteotomy of SHD, its use in primary THR has to be carefully balanced against other (more standard) approaches.

24.17 Expected Outcomes

In a more contemporary series of the use of a transtrochanteric technique for primary THR, Bal et al. reported a nonunion rate of 8% with a reoperation rate of 28%. Similarly, Beaulé et al. reported on the SHD technique for hip resurfacing with a 8.7% nonunion rate with 18% requiring screw removal. Treatment of trochanteric nonunions is difficult: Hamadouche et al. reported only a 71% union rate in treatment of trochanteric osteotomy nonunion after THR. Similarly, Stewart et al. reported on a third generation of cable grip system for fixation of trochanteric fragment with a union rate of only 62%.

24.18 Future Direction

SHD will keep its place as surgical approach for THR in very selected and mostly complex cases. With improving the quality of preoperative imaging of cartilage lesions, the indication of explorative SHD to allow for intraoperative decision-making to perform either a joint-preserving procedure or THR will probably decrease in the future.

References

1. Ollier L. Traité des résections et des opérations conservatrices: qu'on peut pratiquer sur le système osseux. Paris: Masson et Cie; 1891.
2. Charnley J. Low friction arthroplasty of the hip: theory and practice. New York: Springer-Verlag; 1979.
3. English TA. The trochanteric approach to the hip for prosthetic replacement. J Bone Joint Surg. 1975;57A:1128–32.
4. Courpied JP, Desportes G, Postel M. Une nouvelle trochanterotomie pour l'abord postero-externe de la hanche. RevChirOrthop. 1991;77:506–12.
5. Ganz R, Gill TJ, Gautier E, Ganz K, Krugel N, Berlemann U. Surgical dislocation of the adult hip. A new technique with full access to the femoral head and acetabulum without the risk of avascular necrosis. J Bone Joint Surg. 2001;83B:1119–24.

Further Reading

Bal BS, Kazmier P, Burd T, Aleto T. Anterior trochanteric slide osteotomy for primary total hip arthroplasty. Review of nonunion and complications. J Arthroplast. 2006;21(1):59–63.

Beaulé PE, Shim P, Banga K. Clinical experience of Ganz surgical dislocation approach for metal-on-metal hip resurfacing. J Arthroplast. 2009;24(6 Suppl):127–31.

Dall DM, Miles AW. Re-attachment of the greater trochanter. The use of the trochanter cable-grip system. J Bone Joint Surg Br. 1983;65(1):55–9.

Hamadouche M, Zniber B, Dumaine V, Kerboull M, Courpied JP. Reattachment of the ununited greater trochanter following total hip arthroplasty. The use of a trochanteric claw plate. J Bone Joint Surg Am. 2003;85(7):1330–7.

Stewart AD, Abdelbary H, Beaulé PE. Trochanteric fixation with a third-generation cable-plate system: an independent experience. J Arthroplast. 2017;32(9):2864–8.

25 Extended Trochanteric Osteotomy (ETO) in Revision THR

Hannes A. Rüdiger and Paul E. Beaulé

25.1 Introduction

Various surgical approaches have been described for revision hip arthroplasty. Approaches using extended trochanteric osteotomies (sometimes referred to as *transfemoral* approaches) offer some specific advantages. These include an excellent exposure to the acetabulum and even more of the femoral medullary canal. Extended trochanteric osteotomies (ETOs) can be performed by following the intermuscular and internervous plane between the superior gluteal nerve (gluteus medius and minimus) and direct nerve branches of the sacral plexus L5-S2 (piriformis and short external rotator muscles). It eases the removal of the cement mantel or well-ingrown stems in the revision setting and allows for preservation of posterior structures and short external rotators and maintains posterior joint stability. It offers the option to change the position of the greater trochanter (e.g., distalization). However, it requires refixation of the osteotomized fragment bearing risks of secondary displacement and non-union during the rehab period.

25.2 Background

Transfemoral approaches have been popularized by Wagner [1], who described in 1987 an extended trochanteric osteotomy with a split of the gluteus medius muscle. The posterior branch of the osteotomy follows from distal to proximal the linea aspera (Fig. 25.1). At the level of the vastus ridge, the osteotomy continues toward the middle of the greater trochanter anterior to the main tendon of the gluteus medius muscle. The fibers of the latter are split longitudinally.

In 1995, Paprosky and his group [2] modified Wagner's technique with a more posterior-based trochanteric fragment. The proximal part of the posterior branch of the ETO is located posterior to the gluteus medius muscle insertion, leaving the abductor tendon and muscles intact. They describe this technique in combination with a posterior approach: "the short external rotators are incised [...] and complete posterior, superior, and inferior capsulotomy is performed." The prosthesis is dislocated posteriorly prior to performing osteotomy.

In 2010, Gross and his group [3] described a further modification, in which the posterior structures are preserved. The osteotomy starts proximal between the piriformis and the gluteus medius tendon. After the trochanteric fragment is elevated and an anterior capsulotomy is performed, the joint is dislocated anteriorly. This technique is hence similar to the surgical hip dislocation, which was described for joint preservation surgery by Ganz et al. (Chap. 7).

The focus of this chapter is on a combination between Gross' and Ganz' techniques.

25.3 Indications

Extended trochanteric osteotomies offer the best exposure to the femoral medullary canal. The trochanteric fragment is retracted anteriorly providing an excellent exposure to the acetabulum without damaging the abductor muscles.

25.3.1 Indications

- Well-ingrown fully hydroxyapatite-coated stems, which are usually laborious to remove by other approaches.
- Cemented stems with well-fixed cement mantels particularly in the distal part of the stem or with long and well-fixed cement plugs distal to the tip of the stem.

H. A. Rüdiger (✉)
Hip Service, Department of Orthopedics, Zürich, Switzerland
e-mail: Hannes.Ruediger@kws.ch

P. E. Beaulé
University of Ottawa, Ottawa, Canada

Division of Orthopedic Surgery, Hawkesbury and District General Hospital, Hawkesbury, Canada
e-mail: pbeaule@toh.ca

M. Leunig et al. (eds.), *Surgical Hip Dislocation*, https://doi.org/10.1007/978-3-031-70622-6_25

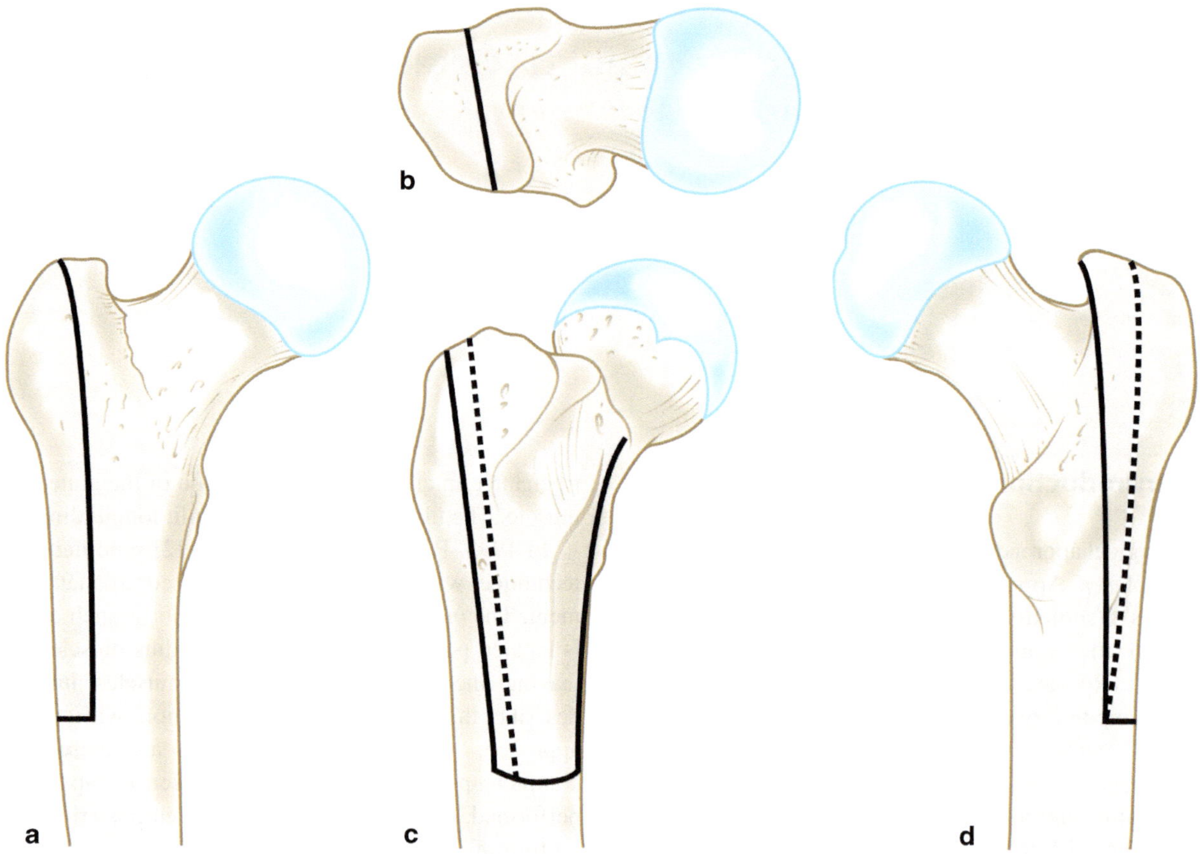

Fig. 25.1 Differences between different types of ETO techniques. The principal difference among the techniques is the posterior branch of the osteotomy. In the variations of Ganz, Gross, or Paprowski, the posterior branch of the osteotomy runs mostly posterior to the gluteus medius main tendon, and its muscle belly is not divided (solid lines). In contrast, in the original Wagner technique, the posterior branch of the osteotomy (dotted line) starts at the tip of the greater trochanter ventral to the main tendon of the gluteus medius (C/D). In order to retract the ETO fragment ventrally, the gluteus muscle is split in line of its fibers

- As ETOs offer also a good exposure of the medial femoral cortex, it may be used for primary total hip replacement (THR) in complex proximal femoral deformities such as severe varus deformities as the deformity may be corrected by a counter osteotomy of the medial femoral cortex, which is then reduced to a distally fixed long revision stem.

25.3.2 Relative Indications

- Large cavitary defects of the acetabulum may be very well addressed using an ETO.

25.3.3 Contraindications

- Large segmental defects of the anterior wall or column are better addressed through other approaches such as the direct anterior or iliofemoral approaches.
- Major tendon avulsions and fatty degeneration of the gluteal muscles. In these cases the vitality of the ETO fragment might be compromised and consolidation of the osteotomy impaired.

25.4 Preoperative/Preinterventional Diagnostics

Patient's history, physical exam, and plain X-rays remain the mainstay of preoperative diagnostics of painful THR. Most cases are further investigated with CT or MRI. With increasing quality of the latter due metal artifacts reducing sequences, it has replaced CT scans in most cases. MRI allows for detection of osteolysis, bone edema, joint effusion, and soft tissue damages. It may also indicate signs of periprosthetic joint infection. Joint aspiration should be indicated generously to exclude periprosthetic joint infection.

25.5 Preoperative Templating/Computer Modeling

Preoperative templating is essential in all cases. Particularly in cases with massive bone loss at the calcar region or the lesser trochanter, reconstruction of the correct leg length can be challenging. It is essential to identify landmarks on the X-ray which are consistently found in situ. Such landmarks may not only include anatomical structures (e.g., calcar osteotomy, lesser trochanter, tip to the greater trochanter) but also metalware from previous surgeries such as wires or screws.

It is highly recommended that the length of the ETO is templated. The position of the distal branch of the osteotomy depends on the need for intramedullary exposure in the given case. The vastus ridge (also called "innominatum") is a reliable landmark from which to measure the distance to the distal end of the ETO. For most uncemented stems, a relatively short ETO may be sufficient. The advantage of a shorter ETO is that the distance of intact diaphyseal bone to the isthmus is large and primary stability of the revision stem is more reliable. On the other hand, fixation of short ETO fragments is more difficult. In general, a minimal distance from the vastus ridge to the distal end of the ETO should be at least 60 mm. This usually allows for one cerclage proximal and at least one cerclage distal to the lesser trochanter.

It is advantageous to decide preoperatively if an ETO is performed, as the posterior soft tissue structures (i.e., posterior capsule and short external rotators) may be preserved if the ETO is performed similar to a surgical hip dislocation (i.e., anterior joint dislocation).

25.6 Applied Anatomy

A profound understanding of the muscle insertions at the level of the proximal femur is essential. The muscle insertions on the ETO fragment include the gluteus medius and minimus muscles as well as the vastus lateralis muscles. The two former muscles have a tendinous insertion at the posterior and anterior facet of the greater trochanter. The vastus lateralis inserts at the vastus ridge and on the periosteum of the lateral femoral cortex.

Preservation of blood supply to the ETO fragment is essential to achieve bony consolidation of the osteotomy. The greater trochanter receives its blood supply through the insertions of the gluteus medius and minimus and vastus lateralis muscles. These muscle insertions must be preserved as much as possible not only for blood supply but also because they give stability to the fragment after fixation with wires and screws. The periosteum underneath the vastus lateralis should likewise be preserved, and stripping should be minimized as much as possible. The superficial fascia of the vastus lateralis inserts along the linea aspera, and its posterolateral femoral insertion runs over the insertion of the gluteus maximus, which is very solid and easy to identify.

Posterior to the greater trochanter are the insertions of the quadratus femoris, the short external rotators (i.e., inferior gemellus, internal obturator, and superior gemellus), and the piriformis muscle located in a line adjacent to the insertion of the posterior capsule. The piriformis muscle is usually easy to identify as it runs directly underneath the most posterior fibers of the gluteus medius and is characterized by a long round tendon, while all the other short rotators do insert with very short and flat tendons. Deep to this muscle layer runs the external obturator muscle from the external face of the obturator membrane to the piriformis fossa at the greater trochanter. As the ETO runs lateral to these insertions, all posterior structures can be preserved in most cases. Lateral and proximal to the piriformis muscle insertion at the tip of the greater trochanter is the footprint of the main tendon of the gluteus medius, which remains attached to the ETO fragment.

The transfemoral approach is an intermuscular and internervous approach: the gluteus maximus muscle is innervated by the inferior gluteal nerve. The gluteus medius and minimus muscles are innervated by the superior gluteal nerve. The piriformis muscle and the short external rotators are innervated by direct branches of the sacral plexus. The vastus lateralis muscle is innervated by branches of the femoral nerve.

The lateral and posterior aspect of the proximal femur is covered by the trochanteric bursa. If possible, we try to preserve the bursa also in revision cases to allow for a sliding surface and to avoid adhesions to the fascia lata.

25.7 Special Risks

A few specific risks are associated with ETO:

- Fracture of the trochanteric fragment. While fractures may occur at every location at the time of surgery, the area distal to the vastus ridge is particularly prone as the cortical bone is thin in this area. It is important to be aware of periprosthetic osteolysis and overall bone quality. The anteroposterior extension of the trochanteric fragment has to be wider in case of poor bone quality. We have observed some fatigue fractures through the trochanter several months after surgery. They are probably the result of impaired vitality of the bone combined with cyclic mechanical loading of the proximal trochanter.

- Endomedullary malalignment of the trochanteric fragment with the new implant can be avoided by using a high-speed burr to remove bone substance blocking reduction of the trochanter to the stable femur.
- Fractures distal to the ETO during stem extraction or reimplantation are prevented by placing a cerclage about 10 to 20 mm distal to the ETO prior to stem extraction.
- Proximal migration of the trochanteric fragment (escape) may occur during the first few weeks after surgery if the fixation of the trochanteric fragment is insufficient. Due to the conical shape of the proximal femur, cerclages may become loose if the trochanteric fragment slides proximally, which in turn may lead to fragment instability and pseudarthrosis of the ETO. Two cerclages in combination with either two trochanteric 3.5 mm screws or a small two-hole ("eight"-) plate in the distal part of the fragment are usually sufficient to prevent proximal sliding.

25.8 Type of Anesthesia

While we do prefer general anesthesia, the procedure may also be performed using spinal anesthesia.

25.9 Positioning

- Surgery is performed in a lateral decubitus position. Radiolucent anterior and posterior supports facilitate the use of an intraoperative fluoroscopy. A tunnel cushion keeps the leg in neutral abduction, which helps to reduce the trochanteric fragment.

25.10 Instruments/Implants

- To perform the osteotomy a short and narrow saw blade, flexible osteotomes (10 mm width, single- and double-edged blades) and wide Lambotte osteotomes (20 to 40 mm width) are useful. A high-speed burr is helpful to clean the medullary canal and to shape the ETO fragment to fit the revision stem.
- Fixation of the osteotomy is performed using large-diameter steel wire cerclages or cable systems. Additional fixation may be achieved with 3.5 mm small fragment steel screws or a two-hole plate distally with monocortical screws (Figs. 25.3 and 25.4).

25.11 Access

A straight incision is centered over the greater trochanter and the fascia lata is exposed. Opening of the fascia lata along the Gibson interval between the gluteus maximus and medius muscles and the tensor fascia latae. The trochanteric bursa is divided over the greater trochanter, and the posterior portion is peeled off the trochanter. If possible, the bursa is preserved and closed at the end after fixation of the trochanteric fragment.

25.12 Technical Steps

- Proximally, the most posterior fibers of the gluteus medius muscle are identified and slightly retracted anteriorly, exposing the piriformis tendon. Between the latter and the gluteus minimus muscle, the joint capsule is exposed. The gluteus minimus is elevated from the lateral capsule. In the revision setting, this interval is often scared. The proximal and posterior branch of the osteotomy is marked using electrocautery between the main tendon of the gluteus medius and the piriformis.
- A subvastus approach is then performed in a distal to proximal direction. The length of the subvastus approach depends on the length of the ETO according to the preoperative templating. The periosteum of the lateral femur is preserved as much as possible to preserve vitality of the ETO fragment. At the templated distance from the vastus ridge to the distal end of the ETO, a Hohmann retractor is placed around the femur anteriorly (Fig. 25.2).
- The distal edges of the ETO are marked with a 3.2 mm drill hole through the cortical bone onto the prosthesis. The holes help prevent unwanted propagation of the osteotomy. The anterior/posterior width of the osteotomy depends on the type of prosthesis to remove and the bone quality. In most cases one third of the diaphyseal circumference is sufficient (Fig. 25.2).
- With a small saw blade, the posterior osteotomy is performed under water cooling to avoid thermal damage. Proximally, the osteotomy runs directly anterior to the insertion of the short external rotators. The distal branch of the ETO is then performed followed by the distal part of the anterior osteotomy (Fig. 25.2).
- To avoid extensive stripping of the vastus lateralis from the lateral femur, the anterior osteotomy is then extended from distal to proximal underneath the vastus lateralis muscle. The osteotomy may be guided anteriorly or posteriorly by single- and double-edged narrow flexible osteotomes. The most proximal portion of the anterior osteotomy is covered by the vastus intermedius muscle (Fig. 25.2).
- Using a blunt clamp, its fibers are split longitudinally, and this part of the osteotomy is performed using a wide Lambotte chisel. This leaves a bony bridge between the ETO fragment and the anterior femoral cortex (Fig. 25.2).
- From posterior two wide Lambotte osteotomes are inserted into the posterior osteotomy, and the trochanteric fragment is carefully elevated. The anterior branch of the

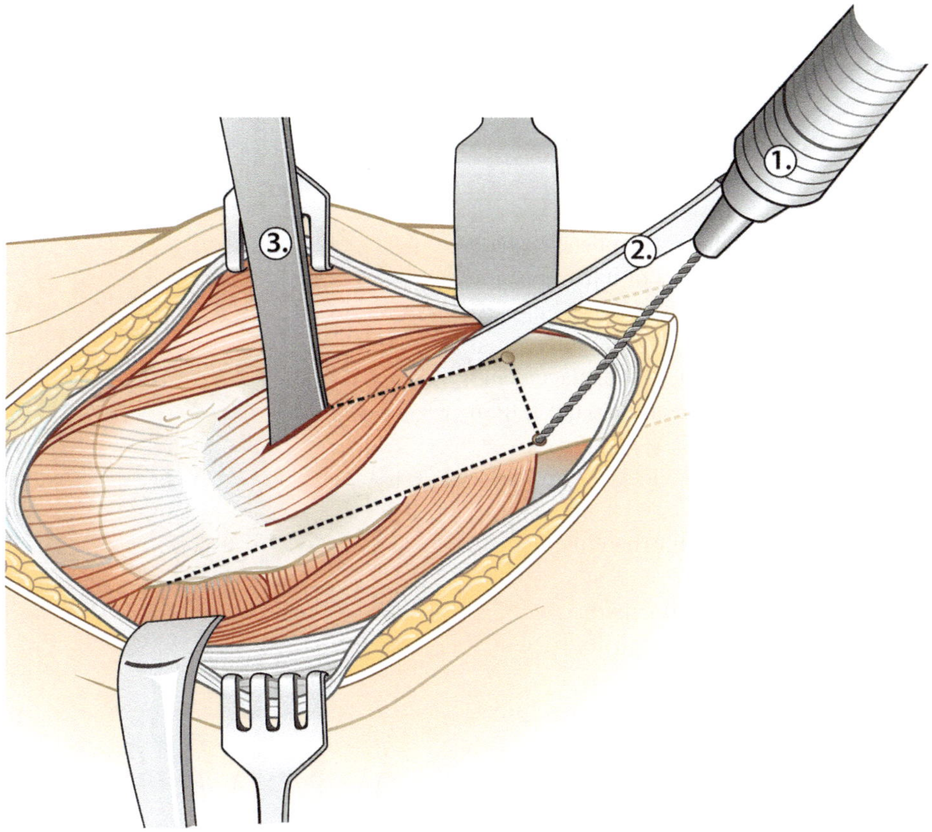

Fig. 25.2 The first osteotomy runs ventral to the linea aspera and ventral of the femoral insertions of the short external rotators from distal to proximal. The two corners distally of the ETO fragment are marked with a 3.2 drill hole. The proximal part of the ventral branch of the osteotomy is performed with a wide Lambotte chisel

ETO is thereby completed by a controlled fracture. This step must be done carefully as transverse fractures of the trochanteric fragment have to be avoided. At the tip of the trochanter, capsular adhesions are divided.

- By gently retracting the trochanteric fragment anteriorly, the lateral and anterior capsule is then exposed including the anterior and lateral acetabular wall. Slight flexion and external rotation allows exposure of the medial capsule. The capsule is then opened from the inferior iliac spine to the lateral femoral neck. The extent of the capsulotomy depends on the specific requirements of the case.
- If an acetabular revision is necessary, a large H-shaped capsulotomy is usually necessary. As the capsule is often thickened and scarred making exposure difficult, thinning of the capsule or even anterior capsular resection may be performed.
- The hip is then dislocated anteriorly with external rotation and flexion. The lower leg is placed in a sterile bag attached to the side of the table.
- After implantation of the prosthesis, the trochanteric fragment is contoured with a high-speed burr (e.g., 9 mm ultra-power) to optimize the contact of the trochanter with the stem. We allow a small gap (1 to 2 mm) of the posterior osteotomy as this assures contact between the trochanteric fragment and the stem.
- The fragment is then fixed with at least two large-diameter cerclage wires (or cables). Here it is key that the cerclages or cables are well tensioned to avoid trochanteric migration. After bending the tensioned wires, they have to be retensioned, as bending frequently reduces the tension (Fig. 25.3).
- To avoid proximal migration of the trochanteric fragment additional fixation such as two trochanteric screws, a two-hole plate distally with monocortical screws or monocortical staples may be applied.
- The trochanteric bursa, if preservable, is closed with 2–0 Vicryl sutures.

25.13 Postoperative Follow-Up

Partial weight-bearing and a flexion limited to 70° for 6 to 8 weeks allows the ETO to heal. Bone quality has to be considered for determining the duration of partial weight-bearing. The distal osteotomy of the ETO is often visible on X-rays for several months.

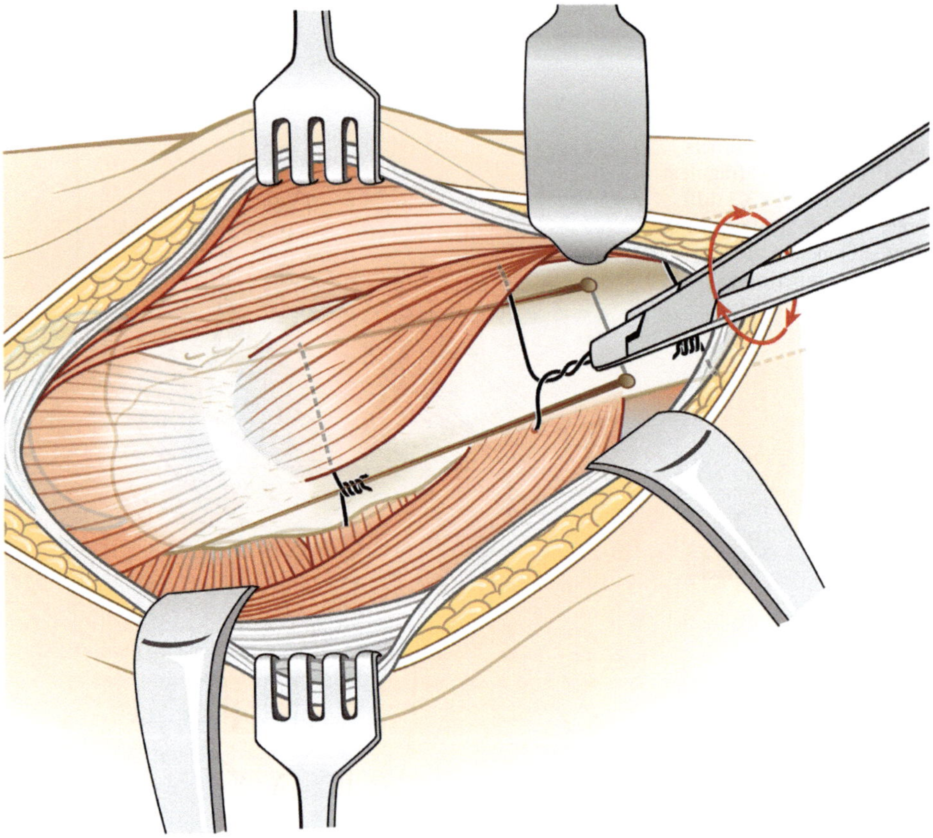

Fig. 25.3 After reduction of the ETO, the fragment is fixed with cerclage wires

25.14 Intra-/Postoperative Complications

- The ETO fragment must be elevated very carefully to prevent a transverse fracture, which may occur in osteolytic zones or in the zone just below the vastus ridge where the cortical bone is thinned out. Completion of the anterior osteotomy as complete as possible with cuts from distal and from proximal (through a split in the vastus intermedius) and the use of very wide Lambotte chisels to elevate the fragment from posteriorly reduces that risk.
- During preparation of the medullary canal and the insertion of the stem, there is a risk of a split fracture distal of the ETO. A prophylactic cerclage about 1 to 2 cm distal to the ETO before the preparation of the canal does usually prevent such fractures.
- Postoperative proximal sliding of the ETO fragment must be prevented by adequate fixation. Usually two wire cerclages and additional screws through the greater trochanter or a small two-hole plate with monocortical screws distally are sufficient. If trochanteric escape occurs, clinical manifestations include pain, limp, reduced abductor strength, and THR instability.
- Migration of the ETO fragment can lead to nonunion and may be associated with development of a Trendelenburg gait pattern. Conservative treatment for 6 to 12 weeks with limited weight-bearing and no active abduction exercises until the fracture has united may be successful.
- Migration >20 mm leads to significant abductor weakness. Treatment with open reduction and internal fixation if adequate fixation is likely to be achieved.

25.15 Case Studies

25.15.1 Case 1 (Fig. 25.4a-d)

A 58-year-old patient presented with constant nagging pain 1 year after primary THR elsewhere. While there were no signs of implant loosening on plain X-ray (A), the MRI showed typical signs of a periprosthetic joint infection including joint effusion, soft tissue, and bone edema and periosteal reaction (B). Joint aspiration revealed an infection with *Staphylococcus capitis*. A one-stage revision as described here including an ETO was performed with

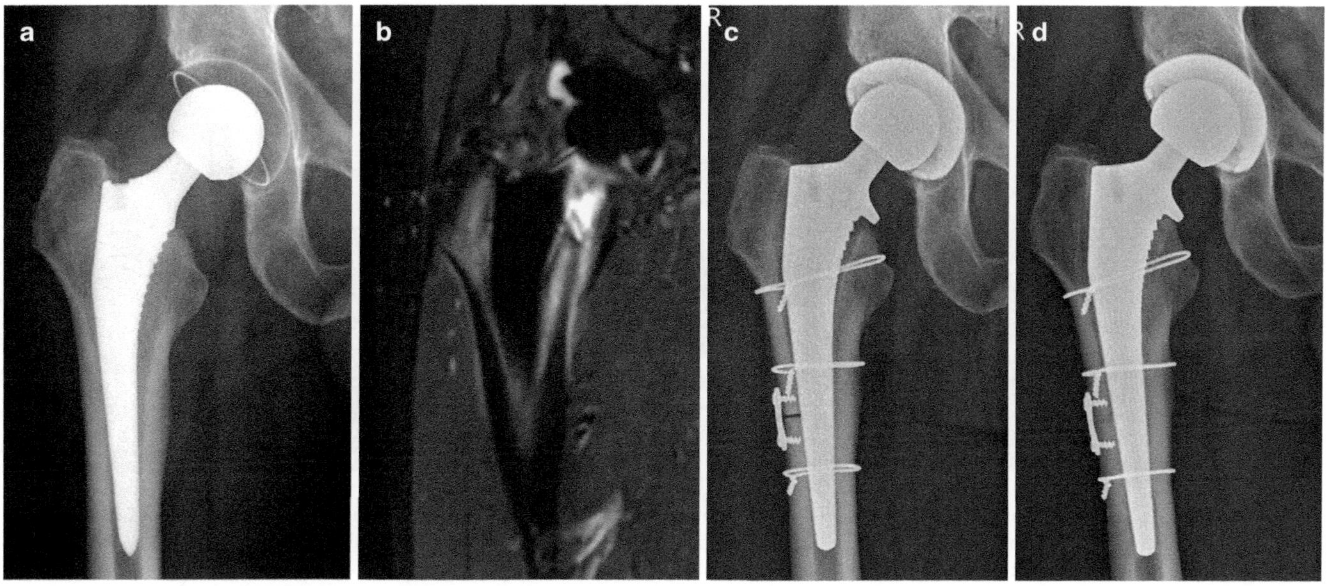

Fig. 25.4 Case 1: Periprosthetic total hip joint infection on plain X-ray (**a**). The MARS MRI shows joint effusion, periprosthetic bone, and soft tissue edema as well as a periosteal reaction at the calcar (**b**). A one-stage revision was performed with an ETO (**c**: day 1). There was no sign of infection and the ETO was fully consolidated at 1 year post-op (**d**)

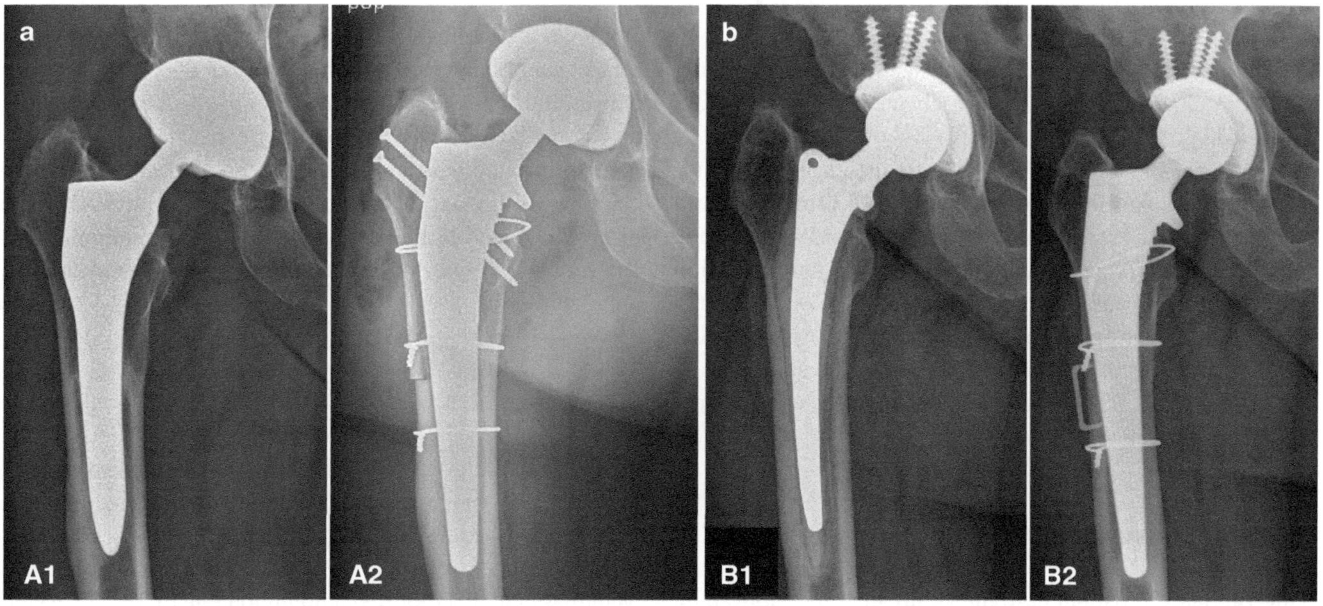

Fig. 25.5 Case 2 (**a**) and Case 3 (**b**): Different types of fixation of the ETO fragment with steel cerclage wires and trochanteric screws (A1, A2 at post-op day 1)) or with a staple (B1, B2 at 1 year post-op)

fixation of the ETO fragment with two cerclage wires and a distal two-hole plate with monocortical screws to avoid proximal sliding. Without any signs of secondary migration of the ETO fragment at 6 weeks post-op (C), the patient was allowed for full weight-bearing. At 1-year post-op, the ETO was consolidated and the implants were fully osteointegrated. In most cases implantation of a primary straight stem is possible, particularly if the medial cortex is intact. In these cases, we prefer to use a collar for additional stability.

25.15.2 Case 2/3 (Fig. 25.5a, b)

We have used various alternatives for trochanteric refixation after ETO including short. Alternatives for fixation of the trochanteric fragments in addition to cerclages wires (or cables) include trochanteric screws (A) or staples (B). A1/2: A 71-year-old female patient presented with increasing mechanical pain 16 years after primary THR. While the stem appeared well integrated in Gruen zones III–V, there was

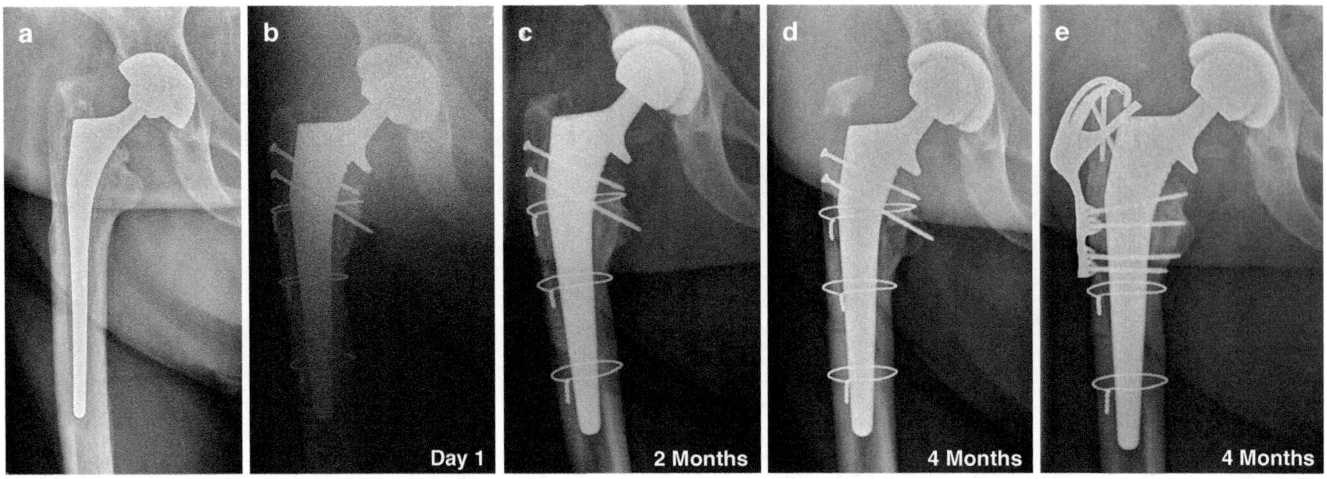

Fig. 25.6 Case 4: Fatigue fracture after total hip revision through an ETO. Periprosthetic joint infection with a cemented stem (**a**). The fragment was fixed with wires and screws (**b**, day 1). At 2 months the position of the fragment remained unchanged, without signs of fractures (**c**). A fatigue fracture then occurred at 4 months (**d**), which was fixed with a claw plate and screws (**e**)

significant stress shielding in zones I, II, VI, and VII. A revision of a total hip through a ETO was performed for aseptic loosening. The trochanteric fragment was stabilized with two wire cerclages and two 3.5 mm steel screws through the greater trochanter into the lesser trochanter. These screws are positioned posteriorly to the stem (A2: post-op day 1). B1/2: (A) a 60-year-old female presented with increasing mechanical pain on weight-bearing 3 years after a primary hybrid cemented THR. Plane X-ray showed for loosening of the cemented stem (B1). There were no signs of joint infection neither on MRI nor on joint aspiration. Refixation of the ETO fragment was performed using two cerclage wires and a monocortical bone staple. The holes for the staples were pre-drilled. The ETO fragment consolidated without any secondary migration at 1 year post-op (B2).

25.15.3 Case 4 (Fig. 25.6)

This 79-year-old patient presented with an aseptic loosening of a cemented stem after previous revision surgery. A total hip revision through a trans-trochanteric approach was performed. The patient recovered well and was allowed full weight-bearing at the clinical and radiological review after 2 months. However, a fatigue fracture of the tip of the greater trochanter occurred after 4 months, which was reduced and fixed with a claw plate.

25.16 Controversies

While an ETO offers excellent exposure to the femoral medullary canal and the acetabulum, the approach is time-consuming, and fractures migration of the trochanteric fragment or nonunion of the osteotomy may occur. Moreover, hardware-related discomfort can occur. These complications can have an impact on the outcome. The unique advantages of an ETO need to be balanced against these specific risks. It is important that the surgeon is familiar with alternative approaches.

25.17 Results

A high rate of union of the ETO has been reported by several authors [3, 4]. In the larges series published to date, the union rate in 612 cases was 98% [4]. Intra- and postoperative fractures have been reported. In a meta-analysis of 19 studies, Malahias et al. [5] reported a nonunion rate of 7% and a stem subsidence of >5 mm in 7%. Abdel MP et al. [4] reported a 10-year implant survivalship free of revision for aseptic loosening of 97% in their series of 612 cases ETO a with femoral revisions. Implant survivorship at 10 years free of revision for any reason and free of any reoperation was 91% and 82%, respectively.

25.18 Future Directions

If proximal femoral bone stock is sufficient and the medial femoral cortex up to the neck osteotomy is solid, we use in most cases a primary stem (with a collar if possible), even if an ETO is performed. While it is essential to achieve a solid primary implant stability, it is not mandatory to use a revision stem longer than the previous stem in every case. We also advise to avoid modular implant systems whenever possible. This trend toward using shorter and non-modular (primary) stems in the revision setting has been called "de-escalation" by Miletic et al. [6].

References

1. Wagner H. Revision prosthesis for the hip joint in severe bone loss. Orthopade. 1987;16(4):295–300.
2. Younger TI, Bradford MS, Magnus RE, Paprosky WG. Extended proximal femoral osteotomy. A new technique for femoral revision arthroplasty. J Arthroplast. 1995;10(3):329–38.
3. Lakstein D, Kosashvili Y, Backstein D, Safir O, Gross AE. Modified extended trochanteric osteotomy with preservation of posterior structures. Hip Int. 2010;20(1):102–8.
4. Abdel MP, Wyles CC, Viste A, Perry KI, Trousdale RT, Berry DJ. Extended trochanteric osteotomy in revision Total hip arthroplasty: contemporary outcomes of 612 hips. J Bone Joint Surg Am. 2021;103(2):162–73.
5. Malahias MA, Gkiatas I, Selemon NA, De Filippis R, Gu A, Greenberg A, Sculco PK. Outcomes and risk factors of extended trochanteric osteotomy in aseptic revision Total hip arthroplasty: a systematic review. J Arthroplast. 2020;35(11):3410–6.
6. Miletic B, May O, Krantz M, Girard J, Pasquier G, Migaud H. De-escalation exchange of loosened locked revision stems to a primary stem design: complications, stem fixation and bone reconstruction in 15 cases. Orthop Traumatol Surg Res. 2012;98(2):138–43.

Further Reading

Levine BR, Della Valle CJ, Hamming M, Sporer SM, Berger RA, Paprosky WG. Use of the extended trochanteric osteotomy in treating prosthetic hip infection. J Arthroplast. 2009;24(1):49–55.

Wronka KS, Cnudde PHJ. Union rates and midterm results after extended trochanteric osteotomy in revision hip arthroplasty. Useful and safe technique. Acta Orthop Belg. 2017;83(1):53–6.

Wronka KS, Gerard-Wilson M, Peel E, Rolfson O, Cnudde PHJ. Extended trochanteric osteotomy: improving the access and reducing the risk in revision THA. EFORT Open Rev. 2020;5(2):104–12.

GPSR Compliance

The European Union's (EU) General Product Safety Regulation (GPSR) is a set of rules that requires consumer products to be safe and our obligations to ensure this.

If you have any concerns about our products, you can contact us on ProductSafety@springernature.com

In case Publisher is established outside the EU, the EU authorized representative is:

Springer Nature Customer Service Center GmbH
Europaplatz 3
69115 Heidelberg, Germany

Batch number: 10776259

Printed by Printforce, the Netherlands